Basal Ganglia: At the Base of Brain and Mind

Basal Ganglia: At the Base of Brain and Mind

Editor: Alvina Evans

AMERICAN
MEDICAL PUBLISHERS
www.americanmedicalpublishers.com

AMERICAN
MEDICAL PUBLISHERS
www.americanmedicalpublishers.com

Cataloging-in-Publication Data

Basal ganglia : at the base of brain and mind / edited by Alvina Evans.
p. cm.
Includes bibliographical references and index.
ISBN 978-1-63927-915-9
1. Basal ganglia. 2. Basal ganglia--Diseases. 3. Cognitive neuroscience.
4. Neuropsychology. I. Evans, Alvina.
QP383.3 .B37 2023
612.825--dc23

American Medical Publishers,
41 Flatbush Avenue,
1st Floor, New York,
NY 11217, USA

ISBN 978-1-63927-915-9 (Hardback)

Contents

Preface

The collection of subcortical nuclei which handle motor control, motor learning, executive behaviors and functions, and emotions is known as the basal ganglia. It is situated at the base of the forebrain and above the midbrain. The striatum, which includes the dorsal striatum and ventral striatum, the globus pallidus, the ventral pallidum, the substantia nigra, and the subthalamic nucleus are its principal functional components. Each of these components has a complicated internal anatomical and neurochemical organization. The striatum gets input from various brain areas beyond the basal ganglia but only provides output to other components of the basal ganglia. The globus pallidus receives input from the striatum and gives inhibitory output to variety motor-related areas. This book explores all the important aspects of the basal ganglia. It elucidates the concepts and innovative models around prospective developments with respect to the latest studies on this topic. This book will prove to be immensely beneficial to students and researchers in this field.

This book is a comprehensive compilation of works of different researchers from varied parts of the world. It includes valuable experiences of the researchers with the sole objective of providing the readers (learners) with a proper knowledge of the concerned field. This book will be beneficial in evoking inspiration and enhancing the knowledge of the interested readers.

In the end, I would like to extend my heartiest thanks to the authors who worked with great determination on their chapters. I also appreciate the publisher's support in the course of the book. I would also like to deeply acknowledge my family who stood by me as a source of inspiration during the project.

Editor

1

High and Low Frequency Stimulation of the Subthalamic Nucleus Induce Prolonged Changes in Subthalamic and Globus Pallidus Neurons

Hagar Lavian[1,2], Hana Ben-Porat[1] and Alon Korngreen[1,2]*

[1] The Leslie and Susan Gonda Interdisciplinary Brain Research Center, Bar-Ilan University, Ramat Gan, Israel
[2] The Mina and Everard Goodman Faculty of Life Sciences, Bar-Ilan University, Ramat Gan, Israel

Correspondence:
Alon Korngreen, The Leslie and Susan Gonda Interdisciplinary Brain Research Center and The Mina and Everard Goodman Faculty of Life Sciences, Bar-Ilan University, Ramat Gan 52900, Israel
e-mail: alon.korngreen@biu.ac.il

High frequency stimulation (HFS) of the subthalamic nucleus (STN) is widely used to treat the symptoms of Parkinson's disease (PD) but the mechanism of this therapy is unclear. Using a rat brain slice preparation maintaining the connectivity between the STN and one of its target nuclei, the globus pallidus (GP), we investigated the effects of high and low frequency stimulation (LFS) (HFS 100 Hz, LFS 10 Hz) on activity of single neurons in the STN and GP. Both HFS and LFS caused changes in firing frequency and pattern of subthalamic and pallidal neurons. These changes were of synaptic origin, as they were abolished by glutamate and GABA antagonists. Both HFS and LFS also induced a long-lasting reduction in firing frequency in STN neurons possibly contending a direct causal link between HFS and the outcome DBS. In the GP both HFS and LFS induced either a long-lasting depression, or less frequently, a long-lasting excitation. Thus, in addition to the intrinsic activation of the stimulated neurons, long-lasting stimulation of the STN may trigger prolonged biochemical processes.

Keywords: subthalamic nucleus, globus pallidus, high frequency stimulation, low frequency stimulation, basal ganglia

INTRODUCTION

High frequency stimulation (HFS) of the subthalamic nucleus (STN) is widely used to treat various basal ganglia disorders, particularly Parkinson's disease (PD; Limousin et al., 1995; Starr et al., 1998). Because both STN lesions and HFS lead to similar amelioration of PD symptoms (Bergman et al., 1990; Benazzouz et al., 1993), it is commonly thought that the alleviating effect of HFS stems from partial or complete inhibition of the STN neurons. Supporting this hypothesis, some *in vivo* studies have shown that HFS in the STN suppressed the firing rate of STN neurons (Tai et al., 2003; Filali et al., 2004). Similarly, HFS of the STN in brain slice preparations inhibited subthalamic neurons (Beurrier et al., 2001; Magarinos-Ascone et al., 2002), supporting the view of inhibition of the STN as the underlying cause for alleviation of PD symptoms. Note, however, that such inhibitory effects have not yet been demonstrated to be specific to stimulation at therapeutic parameters. Furthermore, other *in vivo* studies found that HFS in the STN led to increased glutamate concentration (Windels et al., 2000) or elevated firing rate in STN target nuclei, indicating increased subthalamic activity (Hashimoto et al., 2003). Finally, using optogenetics to selectively inhibit subthalamic neurons did not affect motor symptoms in hemi-parkinsonian rats (Gradinaru et al., 2009). Thus, the effects of HFS in the STN on the firing frequency of its neurons and other basal ganglia neurons are unresolved.

HFS may alleviate PD by changing the firing pattern of STN neurons rather than their firing rate, as HFS in an irregular pattern is not effective in treating PD, as oppose to regular stimulation (Dorval et al., 2010). Indeed, *in vivo* HFS of the STN causes changes in the timing of the firing of STN neurons (Meissner et al., 2005) and of neurons in the external and internal globus pallidus (GP; Hashimoto et al., 2003; Moran et al., 2011).

In contrast with the alleviating effect of HFS, low frequency stimulation (LFS) may worsen PD symptoms (Timmermann et al., 2004). Can this be correlated to cellular changes in STN neurons as observed for HFS? Therefore, to investigate the effects of STN stimulation, we compared the effects of HFS and LFS on the STN and on one of its target nuclei, the GP. Pallidal neurons not only receive glutamatergic input from the STN (Smith and Parent, 1988), but also innervate STN neurons via GABAergic synapses (Shink et al., 1996). We use these two reciprocally connected nuclei as a system for understanding the dynamic changes occurring during repetitive stimulation. Whole-cell recordings were made simultaneously from pallidal and subthalamic neurons in a rat brain slice preparation preserving the connectivity between these two nuclei. Both HFS and LFS led to similar prolonged depression of subthalamic firing. A similar long-term depression was also seen in pallidal neurons but also, less frequently, a long–term excitation.

MATERIALS AND METHODS

IN VITRO SLICE PREPARATION

Brain slices were obtained from 17–22 days old Wistar rats as previously described (Stuart et al., 1993; Bugaysen et al., 2010). Rats were killed by rapid decapitation according to the guidelines of the Bar-Ilan University animal welfare committee. This procedure was approved by the national committee for experiments on laboratory animals at the Israeli Ministry of Health. The brain was quickly removed and placed in ice-cold artificial cerebrospinal fluid (ACSF) containing (in mM): 125 NaCl, 4 KCl, 25 $NaHCO_3$, 1.25 Na_2HPO_4, 2 $CaCl_2$, 2 $MgCl_2$, 25 glucose, and 0.5 Na-ascorbate (pH 7.4 with 95% O_2/5% CO_2). Thick sagittal slices (370 μm) were cut on an HR2 Slicer (Sigman Electronic, Germany) and transferred to a submersion-type chamber, where they were maintained for the remainder of the day in ACSF at room temperature. Experiments were carried out at 37°C, the recording chamber was constantly perfused with oxygenated ACSF.

IN VITRO ELECTROPHYSIOLOGY

Individual GP and STN neurons were visualized using infrared differential interference contrast (IR-DIC) microscopy. Whole-cell recordings were obtained from the soma of GP and STN neurons using patch pipettes (4–8 MΩ) pulled from thick-walled borosilicate glass capillaries (2.0 mm outer diameter, 0.5 mm wall thickness, Hilgenberg, Malsfeld, Germany). The standard pipette solution contained (in mM): 140 K-gluconate, 10 NaCl, 10 HEPES, 4 MgATP, 0.05 SPERMIN, 5 l-glutathione, 0.2 EGTA, and 0.4 GTP (Sigma, pH 7.2 with KOH). The reference electrode was an Ag–AgCl pellet placed in the bath. Voltage signals were amplified by an Axopatch-200B amplifier (Axon Instruments), filtered at 10 kHz and sampled at 20 kHz. The 10-mV liquid junction potential measured under the ionic conditions reported here was not corrected for.

Electrical stimulation was applied via a monopolar 2–3 KΩ Narylene-coated stainless steel microelectrode positioned on the rostrodorsal part of the STN. The anode was an Ag–AgCl pellet placed in the bath. Stimulation pulses consisted of 100–300 μA biphasic currents (200 μs cathodal followed by 200 μs anodal phase). The interval between consecutive pulses was 100 and 10 ms, over 30/20 s leading to stimulation frequencies of 10 (300 stimuli) and 100 Hz (2000 stimuli), respectively. In several experiments the following drugs were added to the ACSF: bicuculline (BCC) methiodide to block GABAa receptors (final concentration 50 μM), D(-)-2-amino-5-phosphonopentanoic acid (APV) (50 μM) and 6-cyano-7-nitroquinoxaline-2,3-dione (CNQX) (15 μM) to block NMDA and AMPA receptors, respectively.

DATA ANALYSIS

All off-line analyses were carried out using Matlab R2007b (Mathworks) and IgorPro 6.0 (WaveMetrics) on a personal computer. Data for each experiment were obtained from at least five rats. All results for each experiment were pooled and displayed as mean ± SD. The pre-stimulus average firing rate was calculated from spikes extracted from 30 s of continuous recording. Firing rate was defined as the time-dependent average firing rate aligned to the stimulation onset. Changes in firing pattern were determined through raster plots and peri-stimulus time histograms (PSTH) from each recording. A t-test gave the significance of changes before and after application of the drugs during stimulation ($^*p < 0.05$ and $^{**}p < 0.01$).

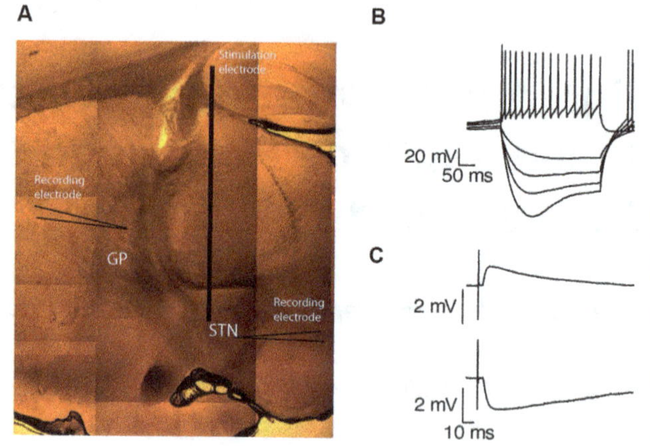

FIGURE 1 | Preservation of functional connectivity between the GP and the STN. (A) A sagittal brain slice containing the STN and the GP. **(B)** Voltage responses of a subthalamic neuron to injection of positive and negative current steps. **(C)** EPSP recorded in the GP in response to STN stimulation (upper trace). IPSP recorded in the STN in response to GP stimulation (lower trace).

RESULTS

The STN was identified as a small oval nucleus above the internal capsule (**Figure 1A**). Neurons in this region were spontaneously active and were characterized by sag current induced by hyperpolarization (**Figure 1B**) and burst firing (n = 39), as previously reported (Nakanishi et al., 1987; Beurrier et al., 1999). The GP was identified rostral to the internal capsule and caudal to the striatum (**Figure 1A**). To assess the connectivity between both nuclei in the slices, subthalamic and pallidal neurons were labeled with biocytin, allowing us to track stained axons. Axons in both directions were best preserved when the sagittal slices were cut at an angle of 17° to the midline. To confirm the functional connectivity in each slice, we placed the stimulating electrode at the center of each nucleus and obtained whole-cell recordings from neurons in the other nucleus. As both subthalamic and pallidal neurons are spontaneously active, recorded neurons were hyperpolarized to identify synaptic activity. Single pulse stimulation of the STN evoked excitatory postsynaptic potentials (EPSPs) in the recorded GP neurons (**Figure 1C**). These EPSPs were abolished after application of APV and CNQX indicating a glutamatergic origin (data not shown). Single pulse stimulation of the GP evoked inhibitory postsynaptic potentials (IPSPs) in the subthalamic neurons, indicating the preservation of GABAergic axons from the GP to the STN (**Figure 1C**).

Whole-cell recordings were obtained from 47 subthalamic and 48 pallidal neurons during repetitive stimulation of the STN at different frequencies. All recorded neurons were labeled with biocytin showing that they lay within the boundaries of the appropriate nucleus. **Figure 2A** shows an example of such simultaneous recording of a subthalamic (i) and a pallidal neuron (ii)

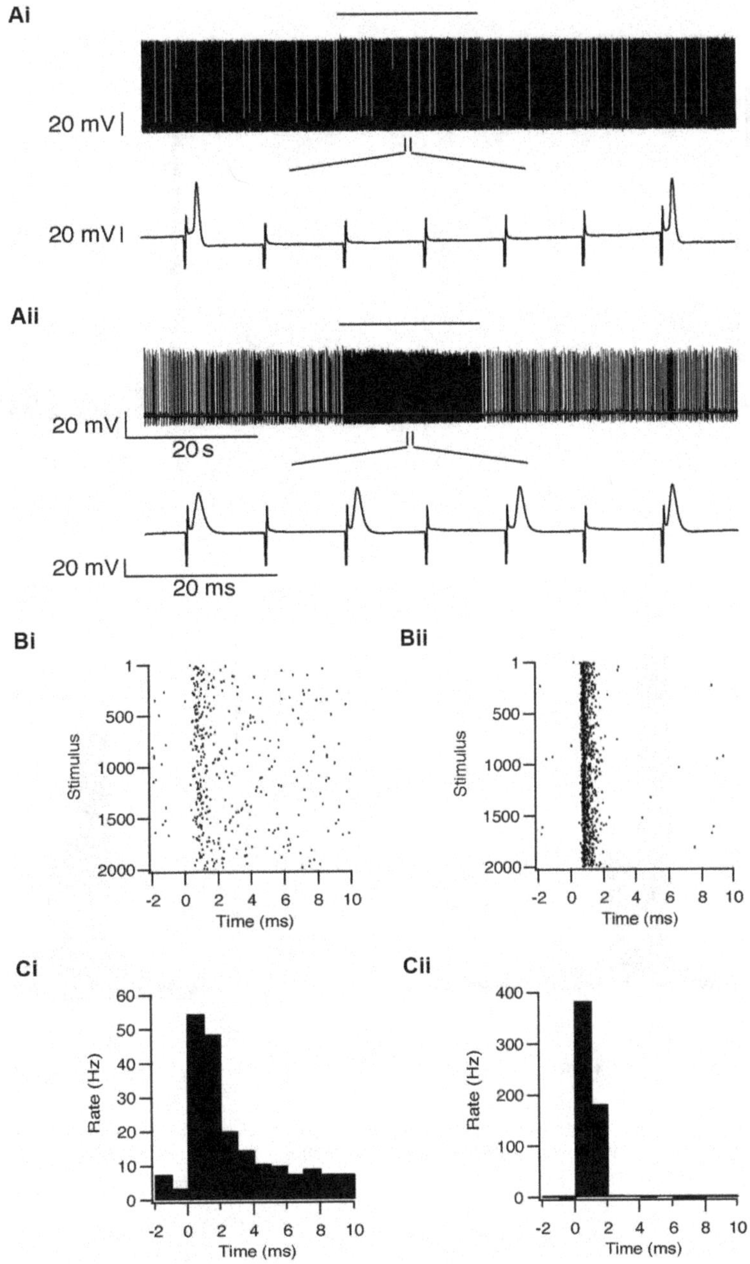

FIGURE 2 | Simultaneous recording from a subthalamic neuron (i) and a pallidal neuron (ii) during repetitive stimulation of the STN. **(A)** Typical responses of a subthalamic and a pallidal neuron to 100 Hz stimulation of the STN. The stimulation artifact was removed to improve visualization of the neuronal activity. Horizontal lines indicate the stimulation period. **(B)** Raster plots of responses to each pulse constructed from all repetitions (n = 2000). **(C)** Peristimulus time histogram (PSTH).

during 100 Hz stimulation of the STN. To investigate the effects of HFS, on the pallidal and subthalamic neurons we recorded simultaneously from both nuclei during 100 Hz stimulation. In order to identify changes in firing pattern, we calculated raster plots and PSTH from each recording (**Figures 2B, C**). HFS evoked significant changes in the firing pattern of most subthalamic (n = 44/47) and pallidal neurons (45/48) (**Figure 3**) as found *in vivo* (Hashimoto et al., 2003; Moran et al., 2011). During the stimulation the firing of neurons from both nuclei became partially locked to the stimulus pulses; population PSTHs showed that the STN and GP firing rate transiently increased at an average latency of 2.6 ± 1 ms and 2.5 ± 0.9 ms, respectively (**Figure 3A**). These latencies are consistent with *in vivo* findings (Kita and Kitai, 1991; Hashimoto et al., 2003; Moran et al., 2011). The effect of LFS was examined using stimulation at 10 Hz. Similar to the responses observed during HFS, most of the subthalamic (28/37) and pallidal (34/44) neurons showed a transient increase in firing rate at an average latency of 2.3 ± 0.8 ms and 2.5 ± 0.6 ms (**Figure 3B**).

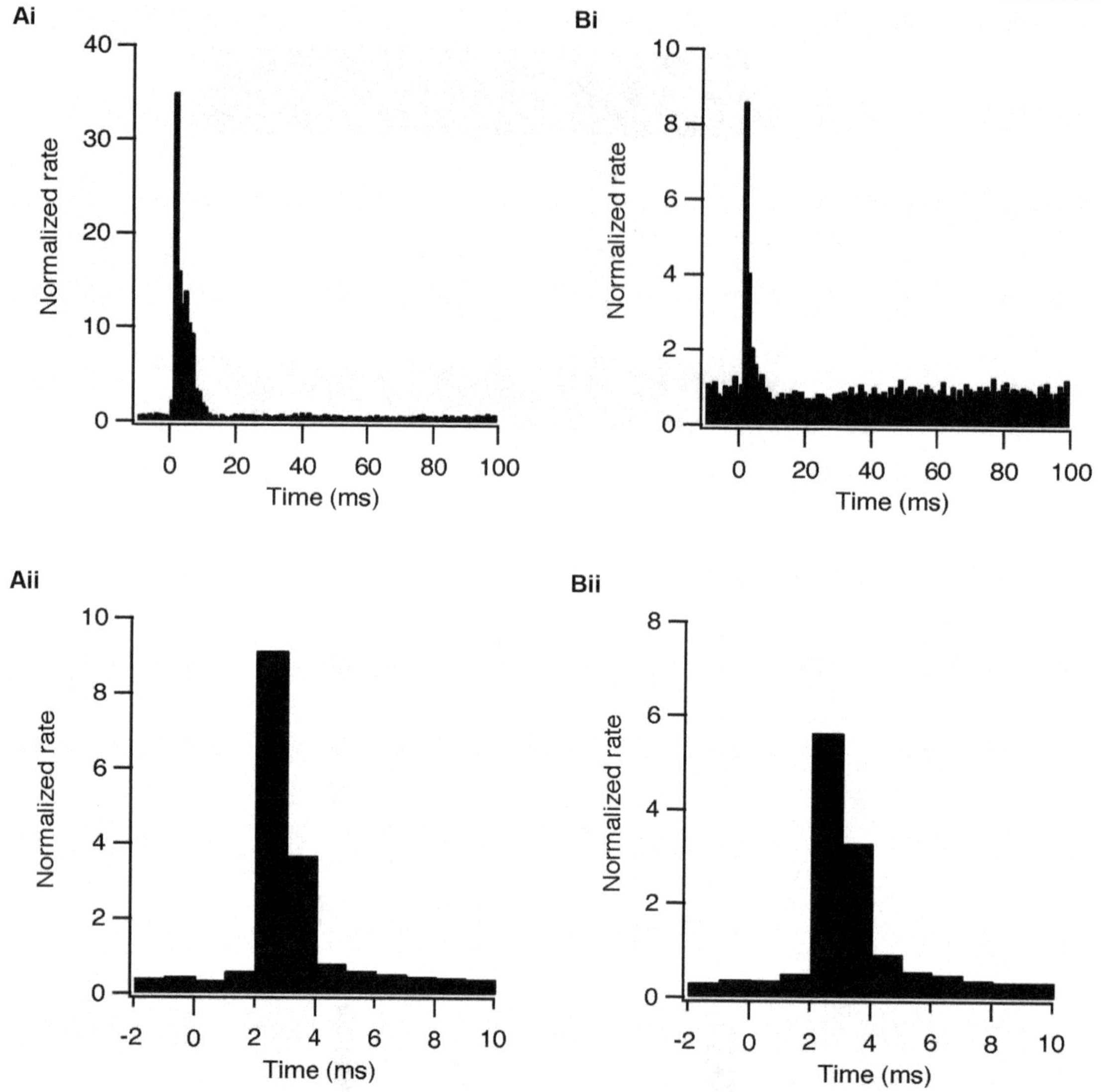

FIGURE 3 | Synaptically locked response during repetitive stimulation of the STN. (A) Population PSTH of subthalamic neurons during 10 (i, $n = 28$) and 100 Hz (ii, $n = 44$) stimulation. **(B)** Population PSTH of pallidal neurons during 10 (i, $n = 34$) and 100 Hz (ii, $n = 45$) stimulation.

The early excitation in the STN evoked by the stimulation protocols could result from intrinsic activation of the subthalamic neurons or from the activation of afferent cortical and thalamic glutamatergic fibers. The early GP excitation could result from antidromic activation of pallidal axons or from the activation of subthalamic fibers. To determine the origin of this excitatory phase APV and CNQX were applied to the slices. These glutamatergic blockers completely abolished this excitatory response in both subthalamic and pallidal neurons (**Figure 4**). That is, rather than activating the neurons intrinsically, the stimulation results in activation of neurons in both nuclei via glutamatergic synapses.

In some cases a transient inhibition followed the initial excitation evoked by each pulse. During HFS, the firing rate of 7/47 subthalamic (15%) and 9/48 pallidal neurons (19%) decreased to a minimum at an average latency of 3.7 ± 0.9 ms and 3.6 ± 0.5 ms, respectively (**Figure 5A**). Single pulses in LFS resulted in inhibition in 9 subthalamic (24%) and 19 pallidal (43%) neurons. This inhibitory phase was abolished by applying BCC (**Figure 5B**) and thus results from the delayed activation of GABAergic synapses. The lower prevalence of inhibition after HFS, compared with LFS, may be due to partial depression of GABAergic synapses due to the high frequency of stimulation.

We next characterized the effect of repetitive STN stimulation on the firing frequency of the subthalamic and pallidal neurons. The population firing rate of the subthalamic neurons increased slightly during both HFS and LFS. In most subthalamic neurons, cessation of stimulation was followed by a prolonged decrease in firing rate. An example of such a prolonged decrease in the firing rate after LFS at 10 Hz is shown in **Figure 6A**. Following 10 Hz stimulation the firing rate of 22/37 subthalamic neurons

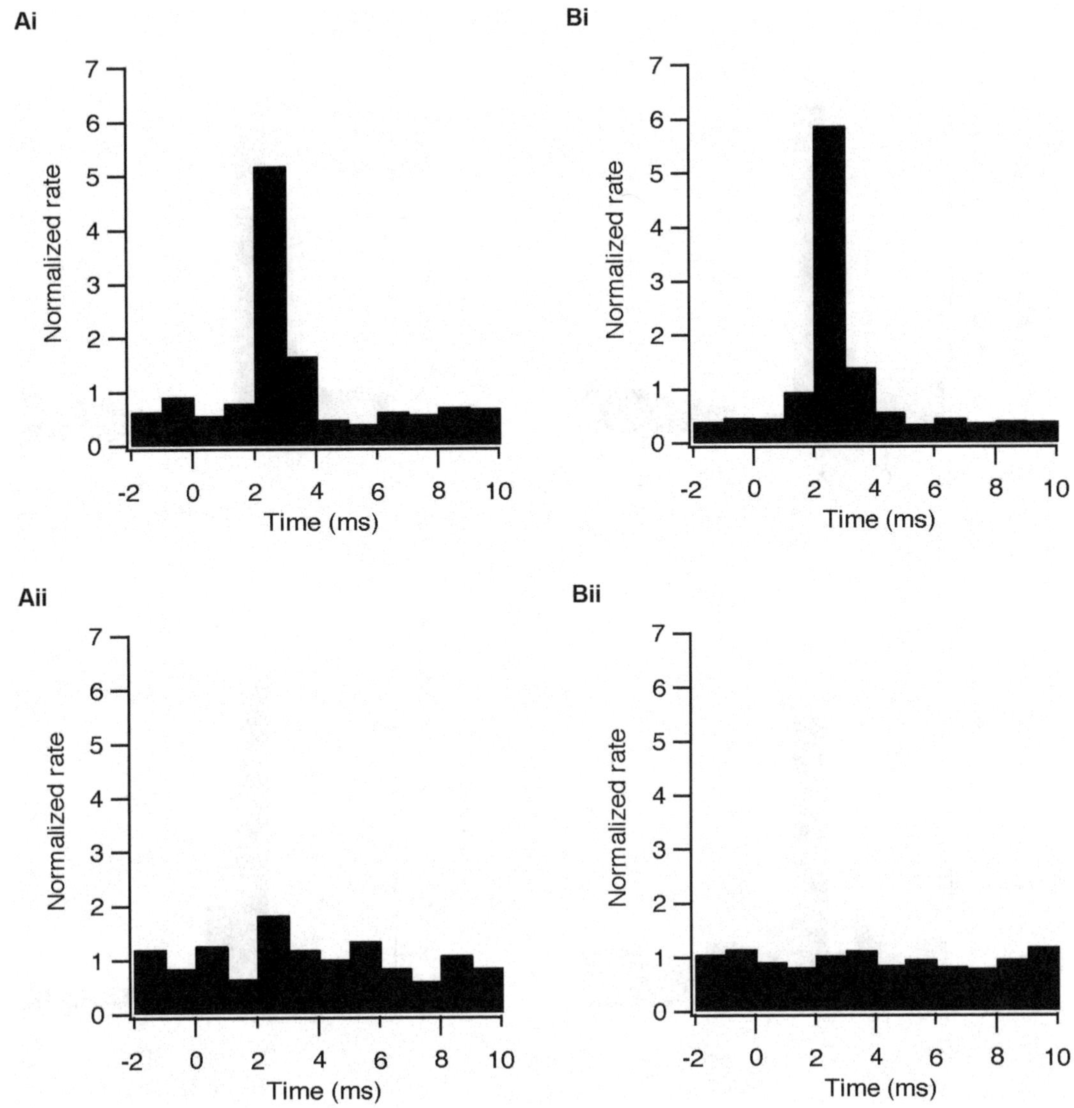

FIGURE 4 | Changes in firing pattern are of synaptic origin. (A) Population PSTH of the response to each pulse of subthalamic (i, $n = 6$) and pallidal (ii, $n = 6$) neurons under control conditions. **(B)** Population PSTH of the same neurons following bath application of 50 μM APV and 15 μM CNQX, showing the absence of transient excitation in the STN ($p < 0.05$) and in the GP ($p < 0.01$) when glutamatergic conductance was blocked (i) sub thalamic and (ii) pallidal.

was reduced by 31 ± 23% ($p < 0.01$); after 100 Hz stimulation the firing rate of 28/47 subthalamic neurons was reduced by 41 ± 26% ($p < 0.01$, **Figures 6B, C**). This prolonged inhibition was evident in cells from different areas within the STN and did not vary with the distance from the stimulation electrode.

Long-term effects were also observed in pallidal neurons. Similar to the responses recorded in the STN, the firing rate of 20/40 pallidal neurons was reduced by 22 ± 20% ($p < 0.01$) after 10 Hz stimulation and after 100 Hz stimulation the firing rate of 25/48 pallidal neurons was reduced by 21 ± 13% ($p < 0.01$) (**Figure 7**). As in the STN, there was no relation between the long-term response and the location of the pallidal neurons. However, in contrast to the STN, approximately a quarter of the pallidal neurons showed the opposite effect, a prolonged increase of firing rate which could be induced by both protocols (**Figure 8**). Following 10 Hz stimulation the firing rate of 9/40 pallidal neurons increased by 17 ± 11% ($p < 0.01$). Following 100 Hz stimulation the firing rate of 11/48 pallidal neurons increased by 24 ± 21% ($p < 0.01$).

DISCUSSION

This study characterized changes in firing of subthalamic and GP neurons during HFS and LFS of the STN. Both HFS and LFS led to significant short-term modulation of firing pattern in both nuclei (**Figures 2, 3**) through the activation of glutamatergic and GABAergic synapses (**Figures 4, 5**). LFS and HFS also induced

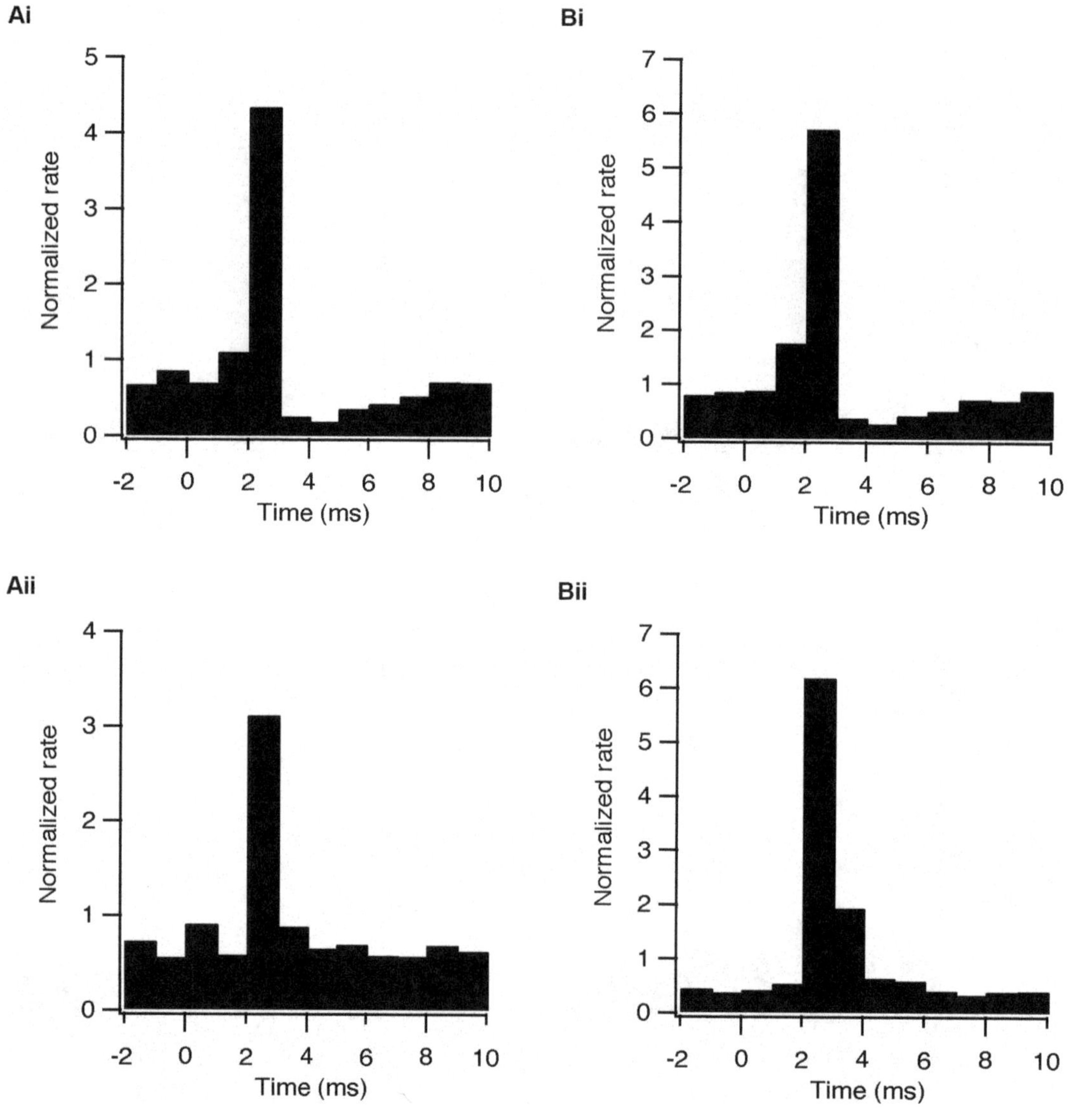

FIGURE 5 | Activation of GABAergic synapses during STN stimulation at 10 and 100 Hz. (A) Population PSTH of the response to each pulse of subthalamic (i, $n = 5$) and pallidal (ii, $n = 7$) neurons under control conditions. **(B)** Population PSTH of the same neurons following bath application of 50 μM BCC, showing the absence of transient inhibition when GABAa receptors were blocked ($p < 0.01$), (i) sub thalamic and (ii) pallidal.

similar long-term effects. In STN, both protocols induced long lasting suppression of firing rate in many neurons (**Figure 6**), while in the GP the same protocols could induce either long-lasting suppression or, less frequently, excitation (**Figures 7, 8**).

Both HFS and LFS activated glutamatergic and GABAergic synapses, thus reshaping the firing pattern of the subthalamic neurons (**Figures 4, 5**). None of the recorded cells was intrinsically activated by the stimulus pulses. These findings fit the changes in firing pattern found *in vivo* HFS studies (Hashimoto et al., 2003). It has also been shown *in vivo* that HFS of the STN raised the glutamate concentration in the GP. This suggests that HFS activates subthalamic neurons, which consequently excite pallidal neurons (Windels et al., 2000). We showed here that the excitation of both subthalamic and pallidal neurons was of glutamatergic origin. Previous findings showed that cortical afferents to the STN are activated antidromically during STN-HFS (Li et al., 2012). Our findings suggest that the activation of these glutamatergic fibers during STN-HFS or LFS consequently excite the subthalamic neurons.

During repetitive stimulation of the STN, the glutamatergic excitation after each pulse was followed by a GABAergic inhibition. Blocking the glutamatergic conduction blocked both excitatory and inhibitory phases (data not shown), indicating the dependence of the inhibitory GABAergic effect on activation of glutamategric fibers. It is possible that, due to differences in the basal activity of the glutamatergic and GABAergic afferents, the stimulus pulses directly activated only glutamatergic synapses, with the delayed GABAergic effect stemming from the increased activity of pallidal neurons. This may be due to differences in the basal activity of the glutamatergic and GABAergic afferents. The

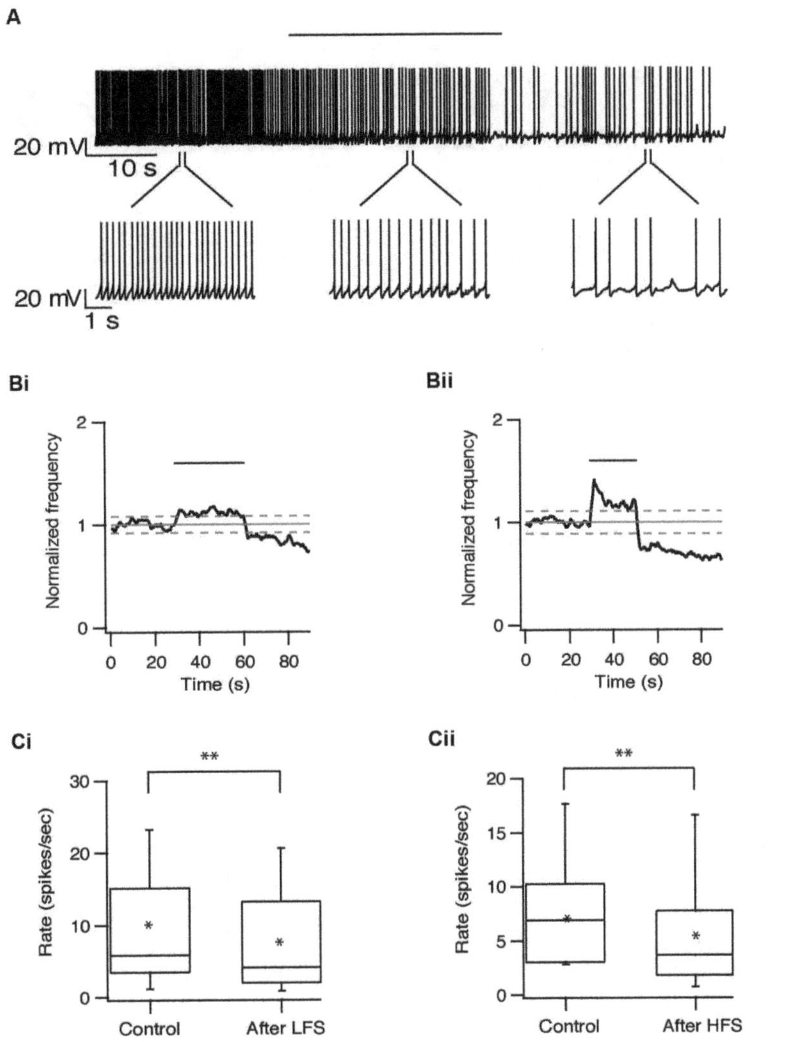

FIGURE 6 | Long-term depression of the STN induced by repetitive stimulation. (A) Representative recording from a subthalamic neuron during 10 Hz stimulation of the STN. Stimulation artifact was removed to improve visualization of the neuronal activity. Horizontal line above indicates the stimulation period. **(B)** Changes in normalized population firing rate of subthalamic neurons in response to each pulse of 10 Hz (i, $n = 22$) and 100 Hz (ii, $n = 28$) stimulation of the STN. Thick and dashed red lines indicate the average ±2 SD of pre-stimulus frequency, respectively. **(C)** Box plots showing the differences in firing rate before and after 10 Hz (i) or 100 Hz (ii) stimulation ($^*p < 0.05$ and $^{**}p < 0.01$).

STN receives glutamatergic inputs from the cortex and thalamus and GABAergic inputs from the GP. Unlike the thalamic and cortical afferents, pallidal neurons fire spontaneously at relatively high rates and thus the GABAergic synapses are partially depressed (Atherton et al., 2013; Bugaysen et al., 2013). As a result, the stimulus pulses may only modulate the activity of the glutamatergic synapses, while the GABAergic synapses remain unaffected. This suggestion is supported by our finding that GABAergic inhibition was present in 24% of subthalamic neurons during 10 Hz stimulation, yet only in 15% neurons during 100 Hz stimulation.

We found no clear dynamic change in the neuronal activity during repetitive stimulation, however there was a significant depression of firing rate following either 100 or 10 Hz stimulation in most subthalamic and pallidal neurons (**Figures 6, 7**). In addition, both HFS and LFS induced prolonged increase of the firing rate in about a quarter of GP neurons but not in STN neurons (**Figure 8**). These results fit the different dynamic and static changes in firing rate induced by similar stimulation protocols applied to the GP (Erez et al., 2009; Bugaysen et al., 2011).

The differences in long-term responses between STN and GP (**Figures 6–8**) may arise from differences between the nuclei. Unlike the homogeneous neuronal population of the STN, the neurons in the GP can be classified into different populations by their electrophysiological and molecular characteristics (Cooper and Stanford, 2000; Bugaysen et al., 2010). These differences may account for the opposing long-term effects observed in the pallidal neurons. On the other hand, the differences in response may be explained by the inner connectivity of the

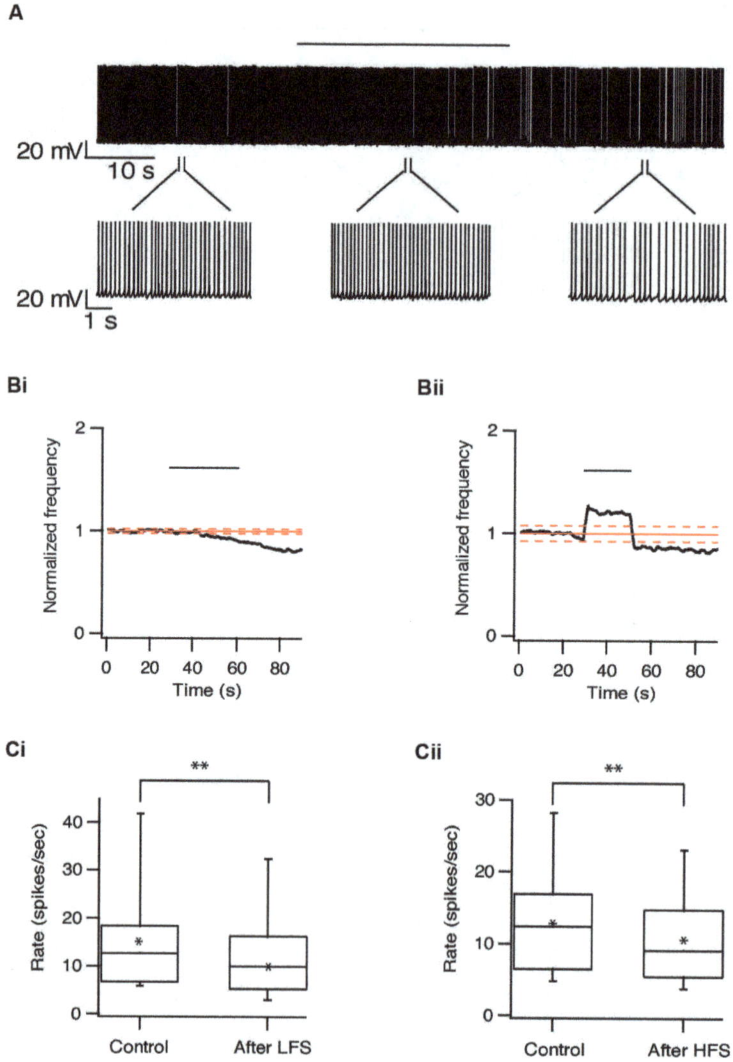

FIGURE 7 | Long-term depression in the GP induced by repetitive stimulation. (A) Representative recording from a pallidal neuron during 10 Hz stimulation of the STN. Stimulation artifact was removed to improve visualization of the neuronal activity. Horizontal line above indicates period of stimulation. **(B)** Changes in normalized population firing rate of pallidal neurons in response to each pulse of 10 Hz (i, $n = 20$) and 100 Hz (ii, $n = 25$) stimulation of the STN. Thick and dashed red lines indicate the average ±2 SD of pre-stimulus frequency, respectively. **(C)** Box plots showing the differences in firing rate before and after 10 Hz (i) or 100 Hz (ii) stimulation ($*p < 0.05$ and $**p < 0.01$).

GP. Pallidal neurons send collaterals to form inhibitory synapses within the GP (Sato et al., 2000; Sadek et al., 2007). We recently showed that a single pallidal neuron can modulate the postsynaptic firing rate of other neurons in the GP (Bugaysen et al., 2013). It is thus possible that the different long-term responses were recorded from neurons receiving different synaptic inputs. One may expect that pallidal neurons receiving direct input from the STN exhibit a prolonged depression similar to that in the subthalamic cells. As the activity of these neurons decreases, other pallidal neurons may increase their firing rate due to disinhibition. This hypothesis remains to be investigated.

As the long-lasting effects observed here after repetitive stimulation were independent of frequency, they may be due to biochemical processes rather than inactivation of the stimulated neurons. Shen et al. (2003) reported that that HFS of the STN *in vitro* induced either long-term depression or long-term potentiation in the subthalamic synapses, implicating synaptic plasticity mechanisms. Here we found no excitatory effect in the STN. It should be pointed out that the experiments reported here were performed in slices obtained from normal rats, and may not represent the effects of STN-HFS and LFS in dopamine depleted preparations. As long-term plasticity mechanisms may be dopamine dependent (Yamawaki et al., 2012; Dupuis et al., 2013), similar measurements from dopamine-depleted slices are further required.

HFS is commonly thought to alleviate PD symptoms through inhibiting STN neurons. *In vitro* studies have shown that HFS of the STN caused complete cessation of firing during or following stimulation (Beurrier et al., 2001). An *in vivo* study showed

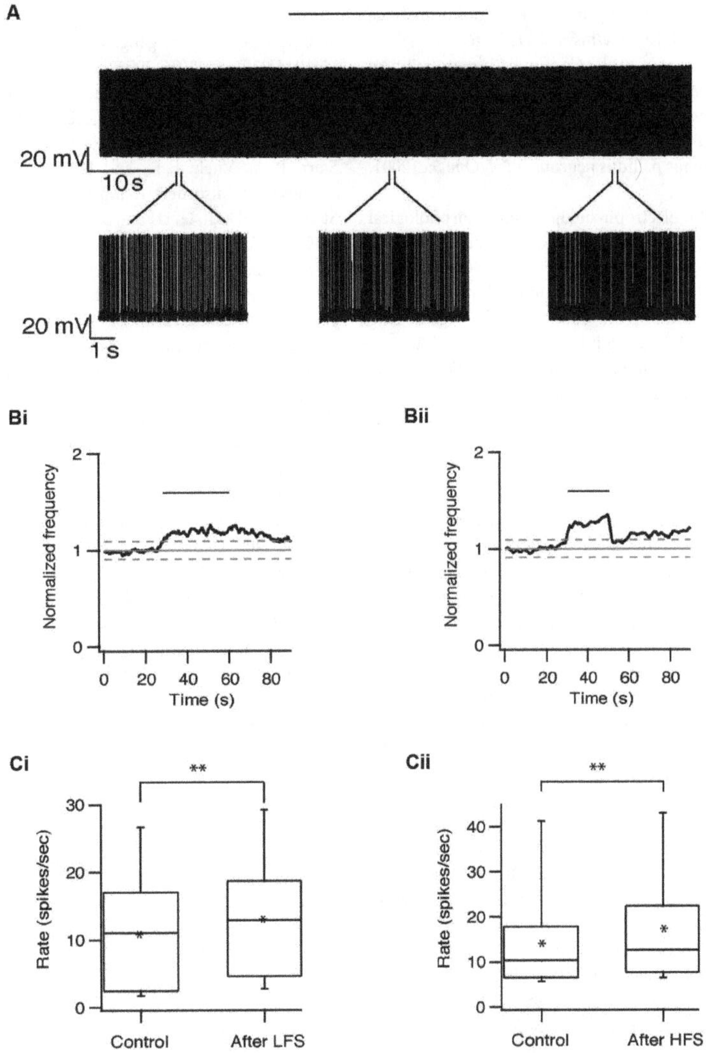

FIGURE 8 | Long-term excitation in the GP induced by repetitive stimulation. (A) Representative recording from a pallidal neuron during 10 Hz stimulation of the STN. Stimulation artifact was removed to improve visualization of the neuronal activity. Horizontal line above indicates period of stimulation. **(B)** Changes in normalized population firing rate of pallidal neurons in response to each pulse of 10 Hz (i, $n = 9$) and 100 Hz (ii, $n = 11$) stimulation of the STN. Thick and dashed red lines indicate the average ±2 SD of pre-stimulus frequency, respectively. **(C)** Box plots showing the differences in firing rate before and after 10 Hz (i) or 100 Hz (ii) stimulation ($*p < 0.05$ and $**p < 0.01$).

decreased firing rate of subthalamic neurons during, but not after, HFS of the STN in 6-hydroxy dopamine (6-OHDA) lesioned rats (Filali et al., 2004). These studies indicate HFS has an inhibitory effect on the STN and suggested that this may plays a role in alleviating PD symptoms. This hypothesis is contended by our results, which, as far we know, are the first demonstrating similar inhibitory effects induced by LFS of the STN. LFS shows no therapeutic effect in PD and may even worsen the symptoms. Therefore the mechanisms underlying the therapeutic effect of HFS in the STN remain to be resolved.

ACKNOWLEDGMENTS

This work was supported by the Legacy Heritage Bio-Medical Program of the Israeli Science Foundation (#981/10) to Alon Korngreen.

REFERENCES

Atherton, J. F., Menard, A., Urbain, N., and Bevan, M. D. (2013). Short-term depression of external globus pallidus-subthalamic nucleus synaptic transmission and implications for patterning subthalamic activity. *J. Neurosci.* 33, 7130–7144. doi: 10.1523/jneurosci.3576-12.2013

Benazzouz, A., Gross, C., Feger, J., Boraud, T., and Bioulac, B. (1993). Reversal of rigidity and improvement in motor performance by subthalamic high-frequency stimulation in MPTP-treated monkeys. *Eur. J. Neurosci.* 5, 382–389. doi: 10.1111/j.1460-9568.1993.tb00505.x

Bergman, H., Wichmann, T., and Delong, M. R. (1990). Reversal of experimental parkinsonism by lesions of the subthalamic nucleus. *Science* 249, 1436–1438. doi: 10.1126/science.2402638

Beurrier, C., Bioulac, B., Audin, J., and Hammond, C. (2001). High-frequency stimulation produces a transient blockade of voltage-gated currents in subthalamic neurons. *J. Neurophysiol.* 85, 1351–1356.

Beurrier, C., Congar, P., Bioulac, B., and Hammond, C. (1999). Subthalamic nucleus neurons switch from single-spike activity to burst-firing mode. *J. Neurosci.* 19, 599–609.

Bugaysen, J., Bar-Gad, I., and Korngreen, A. (2011). The impact of stimulation induced short-term synaptic plasticity on firing patterns in the globus pallidus of the rat. *Front. Syst. Neurosci.* 5:16. doi: 10.3389/fnsys.2011.00016

Bugaysen, J., Bar-Gad, I., and Korngreen, A. (2013). Continuous modulation of action potential firing by a unitary GABAergic connection in the globus pallidus in vitro. *J. Neurosci.* 33, 12805–12809. doi: 10.1523/jneurosci.1970-13.2013

Bugaysen, J., Bronfeld, M., Tischler, H., Bar-Gad, I., and Korngreen, A. (2010). Electrophysiological characteristics of globus pallidus neurons. *PLoS One* 5:e12001. doi: 10.1371/journal.pone.0012001

Cooper, A. J., and Stanford, I. M. (2000). Electrophysiological and morphological characteristics of three subtypes of rat globus pallidus neurone in vitro. *J. Physiol.* 527(Pt. 2), 291–304. doi: 10.1111/j.1469-7793.2000.t01-1-00291.x

Dorval, A. D., Kuncel, A. M., Birdno, M. J., Turner, D. A., and Grill, W. M. (2010). Deep brain stimulation alleviates parkinsonian bradykinesia by regularizing pallidal activity. *J. Neurophysiol.* 104, 911–921. doi: 10.1152/jn.00103.2010

Dupuis, J. P., Feyder, M., Miguelez, C., Garcia, L., Morin, S., Choquet, D., et al. (2013). Dopamine-dependent long-term depression at subthalamo-nigral synapses is lost in experimental parkinsonism. *J. Neurosci.* 33, 14331–14341. doi: 10.1523/jneurosci.1681-13.2013

Erez, Y., Czitron, H., Mccairn, K., Belelovsky, K., and Bar-Gad, I. (2009). Short-term depression of synaptic transmission during stimulation in the globus pallidus of 1-methyl-4-phenyl-1,2,3,6-tetrahydropyridine-treated primates. *J. Neurosci.* 29, 7797–7802. doi: 10.1523/jneurosci.0401-09.2009

Filali, M., Hutchison, W. D., Palter, V. N., Lozano, A. M., and Dostrovsky, J. O. (2004). Stimulation-induced inhibition of neuronal firing in human subthalamic nucleus. *Exp. Brain Res.* 156, 274–281. doi: 10.1007/s00221-003-1784-y

Gradinaru, V., Mogri, M., Thompson, K. R., Henderson, J. M., and Deisseroth, K. (2009). Optical deconstruction of parkinsonian neural circuitry. *Science* 324, 354–359. doi: 10.1016/s0513-5117(09)79065-9

Hashimoto, T., Elder, C. M., Okun, M. S., Patrick, S. K., and Vitek, J. L. (2003). Stimulation of the subthalamic nucleus changes the firing pattern of pallidal neurons. *J. Neurosci.* 23, 1916–1923.

Kita, H., and Kitai, S. T. (1991). Intracellular study of rat globus pallidus neurons: membrane properties and responses to neostriatal, subthalamic and nigral stimulation. *Brain Res.* 564, 296–305. doi: 10.1016/0006-8993(91)91466-e

Li, Q., Ke, Y., Chan, D. C., Qian, Z. M., Yung, K. K., Ko, H., et al. (2012). Therapeutic deep brain stimulation in Parkinsonian rats directly influences motor cortex. *Neuron* 76, 1030–1041. doi: 10.1016/j.neuron.2012.09.032

Limousin, P., Pollak, P., Benazzouz, A., Hoffmann, D., Broussolle, E., Perret, J. E., et al. (1995). Bilateral subthalamic nucleus stimulation for severe Parkinson's disease. *Mov. Disord.* 10, 672–674. doi: 10.1002/mds.870100523

Magarinos-Ascone, C., Pazo, J. H., Macadar, O., and Buno, W. (2002). High-frequency stimulation of the subthalamic nucleus silences subthalamic neurons: a possible cellular mechanism in Parkinson's disease. *Neuroscience* 115, 1109–1117. doi: 10.1016/s0306-4522(02)00538-9

Meissner, W., Leblois, A., Hansel, D., Bioulac, B., Gross, C. E., Benazzouz, A., et al. (2005). Subthalamic high frequency stimulation resets subthalamic firing and reduces abnormal oscillations. *Brain* 128, 2372–2382. doi: 10.1093/brain/awh616

Moran, A., Stein, E., Tischler, H., Belelovsky, K., and Bar-Gad, I. (2011). Dynamic stereotypic responses of Basal Ganglia neurons to subthalamic nucleus high-frequency stimulation in the parkinsonian primate. *Front. Syst. Neurosci.* 5:21. doi: 10.3389/fnsys.2011.00021

Nakanishi, H., Kita, H., and Kitai, S. T. (1987). Electrical membrane properties of rat subthalamic neurons in an in vitro slice preparation. *Brain Res.* 437, 35–44. doi: 10.1016/0006-8993(87)91524-1

Sadek, A. R., Magill, P. J., and Bolam, J. P. (2007). A single-cell analysis of intrinsic connectivity in the rat globus pallidus. *J. Neurosci.* 27, 6352–6362. doi: 10.1523/jneurosci.0953-07.2007

Sato, F., Lavallee, P., Levesque, M., and Parent, A. (2000). Single-axon tracing study of neurons of the external segment of the globus pallidus in primate. *J. Comp. Neurol.* 417, 17–31. doi: 10.1002/(SICI)1096-9861(20000131)417:1<17::AID-CNE2>3.0.CO;2-I

Shen, K. Z., Zhu, Z. T., Munhall, A., and Johnson, S. W. (2003). Synaptic plasticity in rat subthalamic nucleus induced by high-frequency stimulation. *Synapse* 50, 314–319. doi: 10.1002/syn.10274

Shink, E., Bevan, M. D., Bolam, J. P., and Smith, Y. (1996). The subthalamic nucleus and the external pallidum: two tightly interconnected structures that control the output of the basal ganglia in the monkey. *Neuroscience* 73, 335–357. doi: 10.1016/0306-4522(96)00022-x

Smith, Y., and Parent, A. (1988). Neurons of the subthalamic nucleus in primates display glutamate but not GABA immunoreactivity. *Brain Res.* 453, 353–356. doi: 10.1016/0006-8993(88)90177-1

Starr, P. A., Vitek, J. L., and Bakay, R. A. (1998). Deep brain stimulation for movement disorders. *Neurosurg. Clin. N. Am.* 9, 381–402.

Stuart, G. J., Dodt, H. U., and Sakmann, B. (1993). Patch-clamp recordings from the soma and dendrites of neurons in brain slices using infrared video microscopy. *Pflugers Arch.* 423, 511–518. doi: 10.1007/bf00374949

Tai, C. H., Boraud, T., Bezard, E., Bioulac, B., Gross, C., and Benazzouz, A. (2003). Electrophysiological and metabolic evidence that high-frequency stimulation of the subthalamic nucleus bridles neuronal activity in the subthalamic nucleus and the substantia nigra reticulata. *FASEB J.* 17, 1820–1830. doi: 10.1096/fj.03-0163com

Timmermann, L., Wojtecki, L., Gross, J., Lehrke, R., Voges, J., Maarouf, M., et al. (2004). Ten-Hertz stimulation of subthalamic nucleus deteriorates motor symptoms in Parkinson's disease. *Mov. Disord.* 19, 1328–1333. doi: 10.1002/mds.20198

Windels, F., Bruet, N., Poupard, A., Urbain, N., Chouvet, G., Feuerstein, C., et al. (2000). Effects of high frequency stimulation of subthalamic nucleus on extracellular glutamate and GABA in substantia nigra and globus pallidus in the normal rat. *Eur. J. Neurosci.* 12, 4141–4146. doi: 10.1046/j.1460-9568.2000.00296.x

Yamawaki, N., Magill, P. J., Woodhall, G. L., Hall, S. D., and Stanford, I. M. (2012). Frequency selectivity and dopamine-dependence of plasticity at glutamatergic synapses in the subthalamic nucleus. *Neuroscience* 203, 1–11. doi: 10.1016/j.neuroscience.2011.12.027

2

Subthalamic Nucleus Long-Range Synchronization—An Independent Hallmark of Human Parkinson's Disease

***Shay Moshel*[1,2,3,4*†], *Reuben R. Shamir*[1,3†], *Aeyal Raz*[5], *Fernando R. de Noriega*[6], *Renana Eitan*[7], *Hagai Bergman*[1,2,3] and *Zvi Israel*[6]**

[1] *Department of Medical Neurobiology, IMRIC, The Hebrew University-Hadassah Medical School, Jerusalem, Israel*
[2] *The Interdisciplinary Center for Neural Computation, The Hebrew University, Jerusalem, Israel*
[3] *The Edmond and Lily Safra Center for Brain Sciences, The Hebrew University, Jerusalem, Israel*
[4] *The Research Laboratory of Brain Imaging and Stimulation, The Jerusalem Mental Health Center, Kfar-Shaul Etanim, Hebrew University-Hadassah Medical School, Jerusalem, Israel*
[5] *Department of Anesthesiology, University of Wisconsin School of Medicine and Public Health, Madison, WI, USA*
[6] *Department of Neurosurgery, Center for Functional and Restorative Neurosurgery, Hadassah University Hospital, Jerusalem, Israel*
[7] *Department of Psychiatry, Hadassah University Hospital, Jerusalem, Israel*

Correspondence:
Shay Moshel, The Interdisciplinary Center for Neural Computation and the Edmond and Lily Safra Center for Brain Sciences and the Department of Medical Neurobiology, The Hebrew University - Hadassah Medical School, Building 3, PO Box 12272, Jerusalem 91120, Israel
e-mail: shaymoshel@gmail.com
† These authors have contributed equally to this work.

Beta-band synchronous oscillations in the dorsolateral region of the subthalamic nucleus (STN) of human patients with Parkinson's disease (PD) have been frequently reported. However, the correlation between STN oscillations and synchronization has not been thoroughly explored. The simultaneous recordings of 2390 multi-unit pairs recorded by two parallel microelectrodes (separated by fixed distance of 2 mm, $n = 72$ trajectories with two electrode tracks >4 mm STN span) in 57 PD patients undergoing STN deep brain stimulation surgery were analyzed. Automatic procedures were utilized to divide the STN into dorsolateral oscillatory and ventromedial non-oscillatory regions, and to quantify the intensity of STN oscillations and synchronicity. Finally, the synchronicity of simultaneously vs. non-simultaneously recorded pairs were compared using a shuffling procedure. Synchronization was observed predominately in the beta range and only between multi-unit pairs in the dorsolateral oscillatory region ($n = 615$). In paired recordings between sites in the dorsolateral and ventromedial ($n = 548$) and ventromedial-ventromedial region pairs ($n = 1227$), no synchronization was observed. Oscillation and synchronicity intensity decline along the STN dorsolateral-ventromedial axis suggesting a fuzzy border between the STN regions. Synchronization strength was significantly correlated to the oscillation power, but synchronization was no longer observed following shuffling. We conclude that STN long-range beta oscillatory synchronization is due to increased neuronal coupling in the Parkinsonian brain and does not merely reflect the outcome of oscillations at similar frequency. The neural synchronization in the dorsolateral (probably the motor domain) STN probably augments the pathological changes in firing rate and patterns of subthalamic neurons in PD patients.

Keywords: Parkinson's disease, subthalamic nucleus, deep brain stimulation, oscillations, synchronization

INTRODUCTION

The subthalamic nucleus (STN) plays a critical role in the control of basal ganglia activity (Kitai and Kita, 1987; Nambu et al., 2002). In Parkinson's disease (PD), midbrain dopaminergic neurons degenerate, leading to a cascade of physiological changes that strongly affect the STN (Bergman et al., 1994; Hamani et al., 2004). Inactivation (Bergman et al., 1990; Aziz et al., 1991; Alvarez et al., 2009) and deep brain stimulation (DBS, Benazzouz et al., 1993; Pollak et al., 1993; Benabid et al., 1994; Weaver et al., 2009; Follett et al., 2010; Moro et al., 2010; Williams et al., 2010; Bronstein et al., 2011; Lhommée et al., 2012; Odekerken et al., 2013; Schuepbach et al., 2013) of the STN are highly effective in the management of advanced PD.

Neuronal oscillations, at the level of action-potential (spike) discharge (Rodriguez-Oroz et al., 2001; Kuhn et al., 2005; Moran et al., 2008; Zaidel et al., 2010; Guo et al., 2012; Lourens et al., 2013) and local field potential (Kuhn et al., 2009; Chen et al., 2010; Giannicola et al., 2010; Rosa et al., 2011) have been observed in physiological studies of the STN of PD patients undergoing DBS surgery. LFPs span the frequency range of 1–70 Hz [or 1–400 Hz, if one include the high gamma peaks reported at 65–90 Hz and 250–350 Hz (Danish et al., 2007), but see (Yuval-Greenberg et al., 2008) for possible confounding factors in the high frequency regime of LFP], whereas spikes have their maximal power around 1000 Hz. Thus, although LFP oscillations have been thought to imply spike synchronization (Brown and Williams, 2005; Hammond et al., 2007; de-Solages et al., 2011), they more likely represent sub-threshold phenomena such as synaptic activity (Belitski et al., 2010; Buzsaki et al., 2012) which is probably correlated with spike activity.

Conclusive evidence of the correlation (and causality) between neuronal oscillations and synchronization in the PD STN has remained elusive. Physiological studies of neuronal synchronization in the STN of the MPTP primate model are not yet reported. Robust oscillatory synchronization patterns of STN spiking activity have been reported in the 6-hydroxydopamine rodent model of Parkinsonism (Machado et al., 2006; Mallet et al., 2008a,b; Lintas et al., 2012). In human PD patients, oscillatory synchronization of spiking activity has been reported in several studies (Levy et al., 2000, 2002a,b; Amirnovin et al., 2004; Weinberger et al., 2006; Hanson et al., 2012; Alavi et al., 2013; Lourens et al., 2013) but there have been no detailed descriptions of the dependence of the neuronal synchronization on the oscillatory activity or the spatial properties of the neuronal pairs (e.g., simultaneous recording of neurons from the oscillatory and non-oscillatory regions of the STN, see below).

Previous studies have shown that the STN of PD patients can be divided into a dorso-lateral oscillatory region (DLOR) and ventro-medial non-oscillatory region (VMNR) (Moran et al., 2008; Zaidel et al., 2010; Seifried et al., 2012; Guo et al., 2013). The first aim of this study was to explore the properties of neuronal (spike) synchronization of the STN of human PD patients, principally within and between the different STN domains. The second goal was to further explore the relationship between oscillations and synchronization phenomena in the neural activity of the STN.

To overcome the inherent technical difficulties of spike isolation (Joshua et al., 2007; Hill et al., 2011) and spike sorting (Lewicki, 1998) in the electrically noisy environment of the human operating room, and to increase the sensitivity of correlation analysis (Bedenbaugh and Gerstein, 1997; Gerstein, 2000) this study used the unresolved collective (multi-unit) spiking activity recorded by two different microelectrodes exploring the boundaries and the domains of the STN during DBS procedures. This enabled the exploration of the properties of long-range correlation in the STN, in contrast to correlation studies of the activity recorded by a single electrode (e.g., Moran et al., 2008) which can only reveal short range correlations.

MATERIALS AND METHODS

PATIENTS AND SURGERY

Simultaneous microelectrode recordings from two electrodes in patients with Parkinson's disease (PD) undergoing surgery for subthalamic nucleus (STN) deep brain stimulation (DBS) were analyzed in this study. All patients met accepted criteria for STN DBS and signed informed consent for surgery. Microelectrode recording is performed to accurately localize STN borders and domains, in order to optimize the placement of the DBS electrode and thus enhance the therapeutic effects of the DBS procedure. The data collection was therefore done as part of our routine procedures and not part of a clinical trial. This study was authorized and approved by the Institutional Review Board of Hadassah University Hospital in accordance with the Helsinki Declaration (reference codes: 0545-08-HMO and HMO: 10-18.01.08).

Surgery was performed using a CRW stereotactic frame (Radionics, Burlington, MA, USA). STN target coordinates were chosen as a composite of the indirect anterior commissure-posterior commissure (AC-PC) atlas- based location and direct (1.5 or 3 Tesla) T2 magnetic resonance imaging (MRI), using Framelink 4 or 5 software (Medtronic, Minneapolis, USA). The recordings used in this study were made while the patients were awake without sedation. The patient's level of awareness was continuously assessed clinically and, if drowsy, the patient was stimulated and awoken through conversation by a member of the surgical team. Data were obtained while the patients were off dopaminergic medication, which was stopped 12 h prior to surgery.

MICROELECTRODE RECORDINGS

Data were acquired with the MicroGuide system (Alpha-Omega Engineering, Nazareth, Israel). Neurophysiological activity was recorded using polyamide coated tungsten microelectrodes (Alpha Omega) with impedance mean $\pm$ standard deviation (*SD*) of 0.60 ± 0.11 MΩ (measured at 1 kHz at the beginning of each trajectory). The signal was amplified by 10,000, band-passed filtered from 250 to 6000 Hz using four-pole Butterworth filter hardware, and sampled at 48 kHz by a 12-bit A/D converter (using ± 5 V input range). Local field potentials were not recorded due to constraints of electrical noise in the operating room.

Microelectrode recording was performed using two parallel microelectrodes starting 10 mm above the estimated center of the dorsolateral STN target, based on the pre-operative T2 MRI image. The two electrodes were simultaneously advanced, and therefore the distance between the two electrodes was fixed (2 mm) during all recordings. Trajectories followed a double-oblique approach (approximately 60° from the axial AC-PC plane and 15° from the mid-sagittal plane) toward the STN target. The angles of the trajectory were slightly modified to avoid the cortical sulci, the ventricles and major blood vessels as revealed by gadolinium-enhanced T1 MRI (Machado et al., 2006). The "central" electrode was directed at the center of the STN target, and an "anterior" (ventral) electrode was located 2 mm anterior to the central electrode. Typically, the electrodes were advanced in steps of $\sim 100 \mu m$ between successive recordings sites within the STN. Only trajectories where both electrodes had passed through the STN for at least 4 mm were used in this study (yielding 72 trajectories of 2 electrodes from 57 PD patients undergoing bilateral STN deep brain stimulation surgery). After identification of the STN ventral border by the electro-physiologist, the STN and its sub- regions were automatically detected using the Hidden Markov model (HMM) method (Zaidel et al., 2009).

DATABASE

We studied 72 STN trajectories (each of 2 electrodes) from 57 PD patients, 40 males and 17 females, aged 58.9 ± 10.3 years (mean $\pm$ standard deviation, *SD*) and with disease duration of 10.3 ± 4.7 years (mean $\pm$ *SD*). The UPDRS motor part score, UPDRS III, was 49.2 ± 17.8 (mean $\pm$ *SD*) when assessed off dopamine replacement therapy before surgery. Patient details and clinical effects of the surgery are given at **Table 1**.

The minimal recording time duration of a STN pair to be included in this study was 5 s (analysis of the subset of recording with minimal recording duration of 10 s reveal similar results, data not shown). A total of 2390 multi-unit pair sites, in which both electrodes were judged to be inside the STN for the minimal

Table 1 | Summary of clinical data, before and after the DBS surgery, include medical treatment [total daily levodopa equivalent dose (LED)] and the motor part of patients rate scale for Parkinson; The Unified Parkinson's Disease Rating Scale, part 3 (UPDRS III; maximum value is equal to 108).

Patient number	Age (years)	Disease duration (years)	Gender	UPDRS III							Medications (LED) daily doses		
				Before DBS (Med: On\Off)		After DBS: (Stim\Med: On\Off)							
				On	Off	On, On	On, Off	Off, On	Off, Off	Months since DBS	Before STN DBS	After STN DBS	Months Since DBS
1	62	8	M	10	39.5	21	23	34	34	12	400	1100	8
2	73	10	M	23	58.5	NA	NA	NA	NA	NA	675	200	NA
3	51	14	F	17	99	2	16	9	46	13	1700	875	NA
4	68	9	M	NA	NA	NA	NA	NA	NA	NA	1662.5	1246.9	6
5	31	13	F	19	62	14	11		53	12	NA	0	NA
6	58	22	M	22.5	54	5	14	61	64	8	2575	900	8
7	73	6	M	22	55	5	18	NA	NA	4	1700	700	NA
8	75	8	F	17	51	17	21	24	37	8	1400.1	897.75	7
9	61	5	F	38	73	1	10		47	8	1250	125	5
10	56	8	M	29	70	NA	NA	NA	NA	NA	875	250	NA
11	63	12	F	19	49	5	16			3	890	459	NA
12	49	10	M	NA	NA	NA	NA	NA	NA	NA	900	NA	NA
13	64	11	F	3	21	2	4	7	21	5	1505	437.5	4
14	61	6	M	32	60	10	14	51	61	3	700	200	2
15	39	10	F	16	47	5	18	27	57	5	512.5	307.5	3
16	61	11	M	10	44	NA	NA	NA	NA	NA	500	510	NA
17	73	20	M	16	60	NA	NA	NA	NA	NA	1496	NA	NA
18	56	13	F	NA	NA	NA	NA	NA	NA	NA	NA	NA	NA
19	62	17	M	22	72	NA	NA	NA	NA	NA	1550	250	NA
20	70	13	F	13	41	NA	NA	NA	NA	NA	400	NA	NA
21	53	9	M	10	41	NA	NA	NA	NA	NA	375	NA	NA
22	72	8	M	4	17	NA	NA	NA	NA	NA	1125	NA	NA
23	50	8	F	NA	NA	NA	NA	NA	NA	NA	550	NA	NA
24	62	5	M	NA	NA	NA	NA	NA	NA	NA	NA	NA	NA
25	58	7	M	14	42	NA	NA	NA	NA	NA	300	NA	NA
26	63	12	M	19	55	NA	NA	NA	NA	NA	1105	NA	NA
27	52	5	M	3	26	NA	NA	NA	NA	NA	650	NA	NA
28	53	10	F	9	42	NA	NA	NA	NA	NA	770	NA	NA
29	74	9	F	42	73	NA	NA	NA	NA	NA	1250	NA	NA
30	57	7	M	37	78	NA	NA	NA	NA	NA	1370	NA	NA

(Continued)

Table 1 | Continued

Patient number	Age (years)	Disease duration (years)	Gender	UPDRS III							Medications (LED) daily doses		
				Before DBS (Med: On\Off)		After DBS: (Stim\Med: On\Off)							
				On	Off	On, On	On, Off	Off, On	Off, Off	Months since DBS	Before STN DBS	After STN DBS	Months Since DBS
31	67	9	M	14	34	NA	NA	NA	NA	NA	1000	NA	NA
32	59	10	M	13	47	NA	NA	NA	NA	NA	NA	NA	NA
33	55	8	M	22	69	NA	NA	NA	NA	NA	1480	NA	NA
34	53	8	M	32	49	NA	NA	NA	NA	NA	750	NA	NA
35	51	NA	M	29	43	NA	NA	NA	NA	NA	562.5	NA	NA
36	61	5	M	0	0	NA	NA	NA	NA	NA	NA	NA	NA
37	53	3	M	6	49	NA	NA	NA	NA	NA	200	NA	NA
38	NA	4	M	34	56	NA	NA	NA	NA	NA	850	NA	NA
39	74	15	M	31	57	NA	NA	NA	NA	NA	750	NA	NA
40	71	22	M	35	51	NA	NA	NA	NA	NA	2000	NA	NA
41	66	3.5	F	16	46	NA	NA	NA	NA	NA	750	NA	NA
42	66	10	M	11	63	NA	NA	NA	NA	NA	600	NA	NA
43	71	NA	F	6.5	28.5	15	23	56	59	28	1525	100	NA
44	51	12	M	NA	NA	4	3	48	31	23	1025	731.5	10
45	46	NA	M	1	25.5	NA	NA	NA	NA	NA	900	NA	NA
46	60	11	M	10.5	42.5	NA	NA	NA	NA	NA	1064	399	24
47	59	6	M	15.5	40.5	23	29	40	38	20	500	250	NA
48	56	10	M	6.5	37.5	12	20	23	31	26	900	675	NA
49	72	16	M	NA	NA	NA	NA	NA	NA	NA	1500	200	23
50	54	5	F	11	43.5	10	14	NA	60	22	850	600	NA
51	55	NA	M	7.5	36.5	NA	NA	NA	NA	NA	1150	450	NA
52	47	8	M	7.5	51	NA	NA	NA	NA	NA	1200	722.12	NA
53	42	9	F	4.5	43	NA	NA	NA	NA	NA	187	250	NA
54	29	9	M	NA	NA	NA	NA	NA	NA	NA	1200	612.5	NA
55	69	12	M	7.5	28.5	12	13	27	21	14	1609.5	768.13	NA
56	53	20	M	39.5	83	NA	NA	NA	NA	NA	2200	537.5	NA
57	61	22	F	15.5	56.5	NA	NA	NA	NA	NA	1000	500	18
Mean	58.9	10.3	M40/F17	17.2	49.2	9.58	15.7	34	44	12.588	1037.3	508.48	9.83
STD	10.3	4.7		11.1	17.8	6.75	6.65	18	15	8.3221	516.56	309.06	7.6

Mean and STD are respectively for the mean and standard deviation of each column values.

duration, were studied. The same data base was used for the single site (oscillation) analysis, yielding 4780 single STN sites. Recording (and analysis) time duration of the STN pairs equaled 23.7 ± 25.3 s (mean ± *SD*).

ANALYSIS OF SYNCHRONIZATION AND OSCILLATIONS

All data analysis utilized custom-made MATLAB 7.10b (R2010.b) routines. The local field potential frequency domain was filtered out by the recording apparatus. Burst frequencies below the range of the operating room band-pass filter (250–6000 Hz) could be detected using the rectified signal, which follows the envelope of multi-unit activity (Moran et al., 2008; Halliday and Farmer, 2010; Moran and Bar-Gad, 2010; Zaidel et al., 2010). The raw 250–6000 Hz analog signal was therefore rectified by the "absolute" operator and the global mean was subtracted. Thus, the resulting analysis represents only spike activity.

The average power spectrum density (PSD) at each site was calculated using Welch's method with a 1.5 s Hamming window (50% overlap), after removing the local window mean, and with a 131,072 FFT points (nfft), yielding spectral resolution of 1/3 Hz [nfft = 2^round(log2(Fs/f_res)), where *Fs* = sampling frequency and f_res is the spectral resolution]. PSD amplitude is affected by the amplitude of the recorded neural activity, which is impacted by non-physiological factors such as the impedance of the electrode (Zaidel et al., 2010). To create homogenous PSD results for all recorded sites, the "relative" (normalized) power spectral density was calculated by dividing it by the total power of the signal between 0 and 3000 Hz. This relative, or normalized, power spectral density therefore estimates the spectral peak in relation to the other peaks in the spectrogram.

To compute coherence, the magnitude squared (MS-) coherence method (Kay, 1988; Miller and Sigvardt, 1998) was used. Welch's method was utilized, with a 1.5 s Hamming window (50% overlap), after removing the local window mean and with a spectral resolution of 1/3 Hz (same conventions as for PSD). Coherence values are limited (by definition) between 0 and 1. All coherence averages were therefore calculated in Fisher's transform domain (Miranda de Sa et al., 2009) and then reversed.

By definition, the removal of each window mean in the spectrum and the coherence analysis eliminate any power at 0 Hz (DC). We therefore start all the spectrum and coherence plot of this manuscript at 1 Hz.

A constant baseline level emerged in our coherence results (e.g., **Figures 4A,B**). This baseline probably resulted from the finite sampling of two "random noise" sources. To verify this, pairs of Gaussian random noise sources were simulated. The simulated data were subjected to the same filters and absolute operator as the real neuronal data and the same analysis tools. The magnitude of the coherence baseline dropped exponentially as time duration increased. Therefore, the baseline level seen in the STN coherence is most likely due to the finite (and relatively) short duration (mean = 23.7 s) of the recordings in human patients. The coherence functions were normalized by the subtraction of the average coherence of the randomly shuffled (10,000 times) pairs from the same STN domain. Note that the normalized coherence functions can therefore display negative coherence values.

SYNCHRONIZATION AND OSCILLATION STRENGTH (*SYNC* AND *OSCIL SCORES*)

Rosenberg and Halliday (Halliday et al., 1995, 2000; Farmer et al., 1997; Farmer, 1998) proposed a very useful method to estimate coherence significance. However, this method employs a threshold confidence level, and does not offer a quantitative measure of synchronization strength. Therefore, a *Z*-score like method (effective *Z*-score: Z^*) was devised to determine the synchronization and oscillation strength. The *Z*-score of a given parameter is defined as the number of standard deviations above (or below) the mean. In this case the parameter was the maximum value (peak value) of the smoothed PSD or coherence (see below). However, instead of using the standard deviation of the entire frequency range, a *tail* standard deviation (σ_{tail}) was defined in the frequency range of 35 to 70 Hz. In this range, no coherence or power spectrum phenomena were observed in our dataset (**Figures 1D, 2A–C, 3A,B, 4B**). To smooth the coherence, a simple moving average (SMA) was calculated, with a window size of 23 samples (7.67 Hz), and a delta of one sample (i.e., the frequency resolution of 1/3 Hz). The synchronization strength or score was defined as $Z^* = (\mathrm{MAX}(\mathrm{SMA}(C\ (f))) - \mu/\sigma_{tail})$. MAX(SMA (C (f))) is the maximum value of the coherence after smoothing with the moving average, and μ is the coherence mean. To find the frequency in which the spectrum or the coherence achieved maximal value, the arg-max(SMA($C(f)$)) was calculated. The coherence ($C(f)$) maximal peaks were defined in the smoothed coherence function with minimal distances of 5 Hz between them. The search for the coherence peak was started at the lower frequency, and progressed to the largest value of the smoothed coherence function. All calculations (max, mean and arg-max) were performed in the frequency range between 1 and 70 Hz. Negative scores were found in a few cases, due to residual high power at the low (1–2 Hz) frequency range, and these were ignored.

To determine the oscillation strength, the same effective *Z*-score as for the synchronization was used and defined as the *oscil score*. The maximum value of the smoothed PSD (by a simple moving average, with window size of 23 samples, and delta of one sample, i.e., 1/3 Hz), and the *tail* standard deviation (σ_{tail}) in the frequency range of 35–70 Hz were calculated. The *oscil score* was defined as $Z^* = (\mathrm{MAX}(\mathrm{SMA}(\mathrm{PSD}\ (f))) - \mu/\sigma_{tail})$. MAX(SMA(PSD (f))) is the maximum value of the PSD after smoothing with the moving average; μ is the PSD mean.

To explore the relationship between oscillation and synchronization a statistical measure of the oscillation strength of the two oscillatory sites was used. The average PSD* = (PSD1 + PSD2)/2 was calculated, where PSD1 and PSD2 were the power spectrum densities of each site in the neuronal pair, and the *oscil score* of PSD* was calculated. Additionally, other estimates of *oscil scores* of the two sites were calculated as: $min(oscil_1, oscil_2)$; $max(oscil_1, oscil_2)$; and as the geometric mean of the two scores where $oscil_1$, $oscil_2$ were the *oscil scores* of each PSD site. The geometric mean was calculated as: oscil = sign($oscil1 * oscil2$) * GeoMean($|oscil1|$, $|oscil2|$), where *sign* was the sign operator of $oscil_1$ and $oscil_2$ product, in the case of negative values.

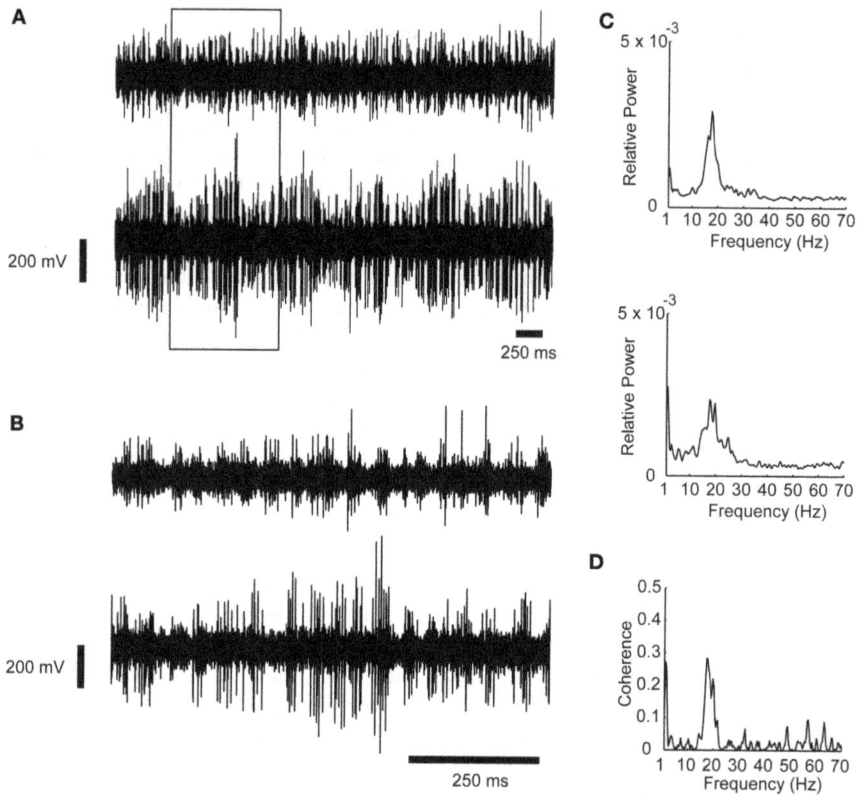

FIGURE 1 | An example of synchronous oscillations between two recording sites in the STN. (A) Raw analog data. Data is recorded by two microelectrodes separated horizontally by a distance of 2 mm, hardware band pass filtered between 250 and 6000 Hz, and digitally sampled at 48 KHz. The 1 s data in the rectangle is expanded in **(B)**. **(C)** Power spectrum of the recording shown in **(A)**. **(D)** Coherence function of the two STN sites. Oscillations scores = 31.57 and 17.13 respectively; Synchronization score = 4.89.

Synchronization or oscillations were defined to be significant when the scores reached the $Z^* \geq 2$ (i.e., the coherence or the PSD peak value was higher than 2 *SD* of the mean values of these functions).

COHERENCE CONFIDENCE LEVEL

To assess the validation of *sync score* the confidence level (CL) of the coherence analysis (Halliday et al., 1995) was used. We divided the microelectrode records of duration R into L non-overlapped disjoint segments of duration S (R = L*S). The total spectrum was calculated using the average of the magnitude-squared (MS) of the discrete Fourier transform (periodogram), after removing the local mean in each segment S. Each segment contained S = 2^16 samples with a frequency resolution of 0.7336 Hz. Only complete segments were analyzed; data points at the end of the record that did not make a complete segment were not included in the analysis. The procedures were implemented using Neurospec free MATLAB toolbox: http://www.neurospec.org. To obtain the approximate confidence interval for 95% and 99% from the data points, the level thresholds: $CL_{95} = 1 - 0.05^{1/(L-1)}$ and $CL_{99} = 1 - 0.01^{1/(L-1)}$, respectively, were used. **Figure 4B** depicts examples of the relations between MS-coherence estimates (*Z*-scores) we used in the manuscript with coherence confidence levels of 95% and 99% respectively.

ASSESSING THE CAUSAL RELATIONS BETWEEN OSCILLATIONS AND SYNCHRONY

Spurious synchronization can arise from non-coupled oscillatory sites that oscillate in the same frequency bands (i.e., two atomic clocks might be synchronized due to their exact frequency although there is no physical coupling between them (Strogatz, 2003). To rule out this spurious oscillation-synchronization, the mean coherence of randomly shuffled pairs (10,000 times) was calculated for each category (all pairs, DLOR-DLOR, VMNR-VMNR, and DLOR-VMNR) of the STN. The shuffling was performed using the Mersenne Twister algorithm (Matsumoto and Nishimura, 1998) with a different seed number in each iteration.

RESULTS

SYNCHRONIZATION OCCURS ONLY BETWEEN DLOR PAIRS

Figure 1 show an example of synchronous oscillatory activity as recorded by two electrodes inserted into the STN of a PD patient during DBS procedures. The raw analog data is shown in two time scales in **Figures 1A,B**. The power spectrums and the coherence function of this recording are shown in **Figures 1C,D**, respectively. One can easily observe the synchronous oscillations in the beta range (~20 Hz) in this example.

To explore the properties of STN neuronal synchronization, STN spiking activity simultaneously recorded from two electrodes was analyzed (**Figure 2**). In total, 2390 multi-unit pairs along 72 STN trajectories (with >4 mm STN span in both electrodes) from 57 PD patients undergoing DBS surgery were included in the analysis.

Previous physiological studies of the basal ganglia in the rodent (Mallet et al., 2008a,b) and primate (Bergman et al., 1994; Nini et al., 1995; Raz et al., 1996, 2000, 2001; Goldberg et al., 2002) models of PD have indicated abnormal synchronicity of basal ganglia neurons as one of the major changes occurring in the network following dopamine depletion. Nevertheless, when the neuronal synchronization of simultaneously recorded STN sites (over the entire STN 2390 pairs) was measured, no distinguishable synchronization was found.

The STN can be spatially differentiated into sub-regions according to neural activity (Zaidel et al., 2010). Two areas could be robustly discriminated in our recording: the dorsolateral oscillatory region (DLOR, $n = 1778$ sites, **Figure 3A**) and the ventromedial non-oscillatory region (VMNR, $n = 3002$ sites, **Figure 3B**). **Figures 3C,D** show the distribution of the *oscil scores* in the DLOR and VMNR, respectively. As expected, significantly

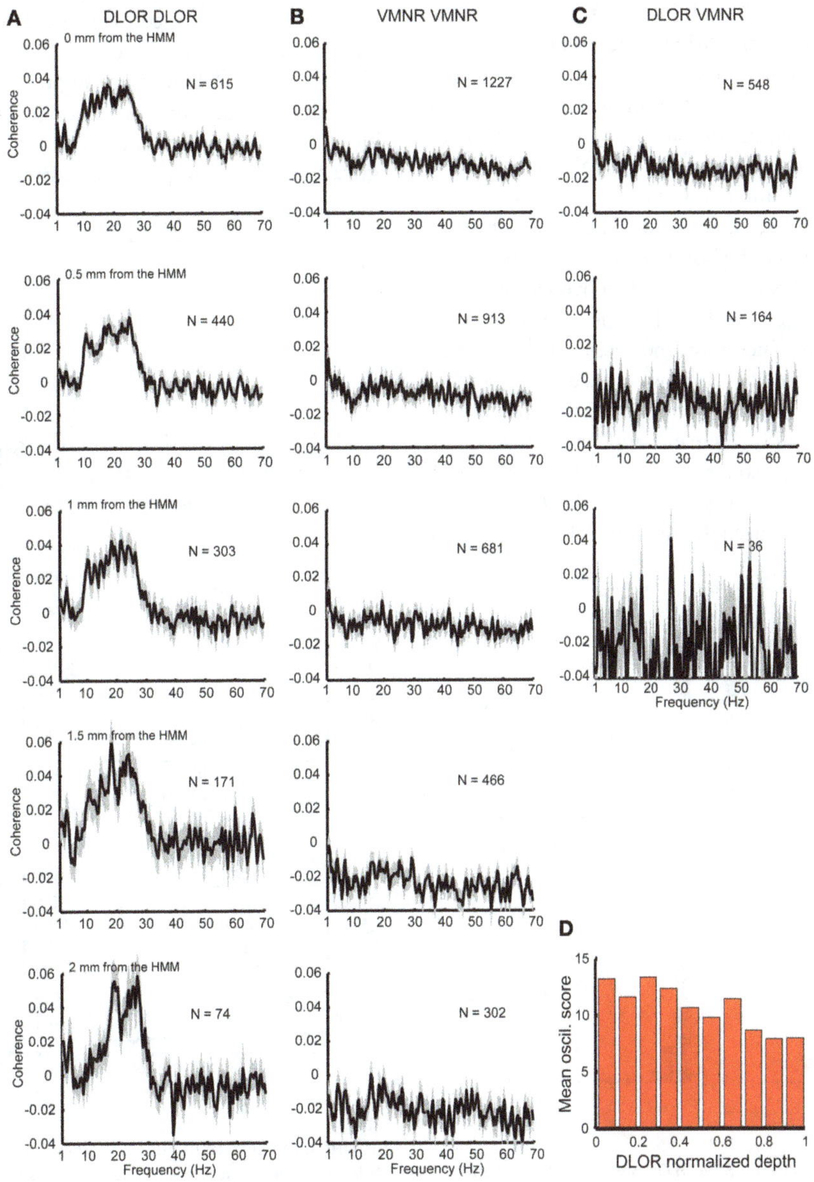

FIGURE 2 | Synchronization found only between sites in the DLOR. (A) Substantial coherence at beta frequency range exists between sites within the DLOR (from the STN entrance to the DLOR\VMNR border). However, the relative coherence is around zero in the beta range for pairs recording from the VMNR **(B)**, or between sites of the DLOR and VMNR **(C)**. HMM was used to automatically define the DLOR-VMNR border. The first row is calculated using the HMM defined border, and lower rows calculated with a progressively increasing gap from the HMM border. *N* is the number of pairs, and the shaded areas represent the standard error of the mean (SEM) of the relative coherence function for each population. **(D)** Distribution of oscillations scores along the normalized DLOR depth. For each trajectory the DLOR length was normalized for 0-entry, 1-end of DLOR.

higher *oscil score* values were observed in the DLOR than in the VMNR.

The division of the STN into the DLOR and VMNR domains enabled testing of the synchronization of STN pairs from the same and different regions. Significant synchronization, mainly in the frequency band of 8–30 Hz was found, but only between pairs in the DLOR itself (DLOR-DLOR, $n = 615$ pairs, **Figure 2A**, upper subplot). This synchronization was not observed in pairs of electrodes at DLOR and VMNR ($n = 548$ pairs, **Figure 2B**, upper subplot) or in the VMNR ($n = 1227$ pairs, **Figure 2C**, upper subplot). This finding is consistent with previous multiple electrode studies of the human Parkinsonian STN (Levy et al., 2000, 2002a,b; Amirnovin et al., 2004; Weinberger et al., 2006, 2009; Alavi et al., 2013; Lourens et al., 2013) which reported coherence between STN oscillations in a small fraction of STN pairs. However, our findings indicated that the topographical location of the STN electrodes affected the probability of finding a correlation between STN sites, and coherence was only and robustly found between DLOR-DLOR multi-unit pairs.

Recent imaging studies (Lambert et al., 2012; Haynes and Haber, 2013) have clarified that the boundaries between the functional subdomains of the STN are fuzzy, and an overlap of motor and non-motor projections can be found in the transition areas between the STN domains. Therefore, the average coherence at the dorsolateral and ventromedial STN was tested with increasing gaps (0.5–2 mm) from the HMM borders. These results are shown in the lower five rows of **Figure 2**, and reveal a sharpening and increase of the average coherence peak in the STN DLOR when the gap is increased. Similarly, when the *oscillation scores* are calculated along the normalized depth of the DLOR, a gradual decrease in the oscillatory scores is observed as the DLOR lower border is approached (**Figure 2D**).

The above results were obtained by averaging over pairs recorded for different durations. The average coherence results (**Figure 2**) was further compared to the average coherence results of the same pairs with homogenous intervals (only the first 10 s of each recording was included, and recordings with durations shorter than 10s were excluded). Similar results (data not shown) were obtained.

SYNCHRONIZATION vs. OSCILLATIONS IN THE DLOR AREA

Next, correlation between the oscillations and synchronization in the STN was analyzed. The oscillation and synchronization strengths were calculated using the *oscil* and *sync scores* for each pair in the DLOR area. **Figures 4A,B** depict three examples of power spectrum and coherence function of STN activity with their relative *oscil* and *sync scores*, respectively. See also **Figure 1** for an example of a simultaneous recording of two

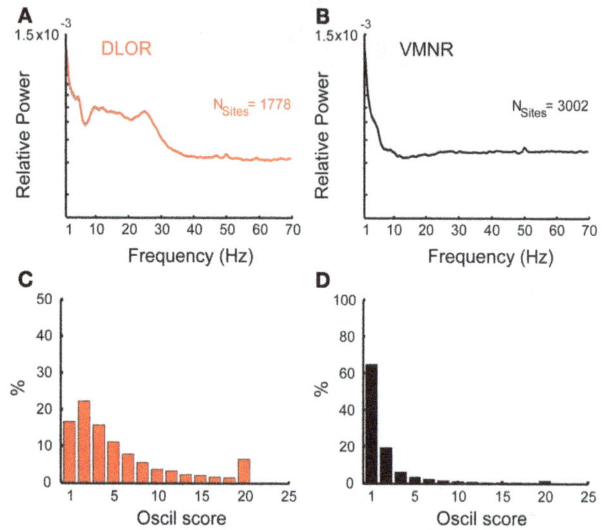

FIGURE 3 | Oscillatory activity in the STN DLOR and VMNR. Average power spectra of STN activity of DLOR **(A)** and VMNR **(B)** recordings. The shaded areas represent the standard error of the mean (SEM) of the spectrum function for each population. N_{sites} is the number of sites averaged. **(C,D)** Distribution of the *oscil scores* in the DLOR and the VMNR recordings. Note the different scales of the *Y*-axes. *Oscil scores* below zero and above 20 ($n = 68$ and 153 out 4780) are appended to the first and last bin respectively to enhance visualization of the results.

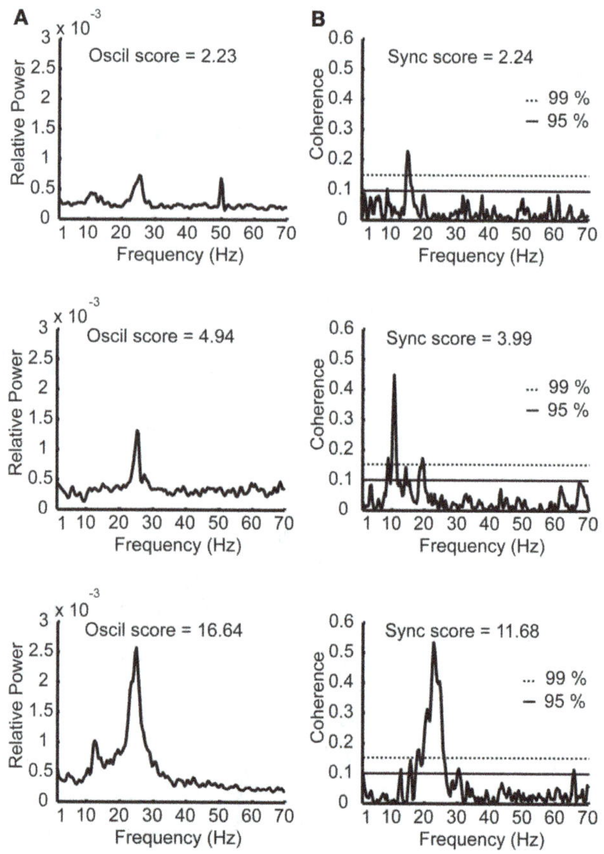

FIGURE 4 | Examples of power spectra and coherence functions with different oscillation and synchronization scores. (A) Three examples of power spectra with low, medium, and high oscillation (*oscil*) scores. **(B)** Three examples of STN coherence functions with low, medium, and high synchronization (*sync*) scores. The dashed horizontal and continuous lines denote the confidence interval of 99 and 95% respectively. Sampling duration equals 33.4, 14.5, and 35.1 s for the power spectra examples and 40.2, 41.5, and 40.6 s for the coherence examples (yielding similar confidence intervals for the coherence functions).

sites in the STN, and their corresponding values of *oscil* and *sync scores*.

Figure 5B depicts the scatter plot of the *oscil* and *sync scores* for all DLOR pairs. Different indicators for the oscillation strength of pairs of STN sites were used: the minimal and maximal *oscil score*, the arithmetic average of the PSDs, and the geometric mean of *oscil scores*. In all cases, the scatter plot of the *sync score* vs. the *oscil score* of the pairs within the DLOR area ($n = 615$) indicated a significant correlation ($r > 0.24$, $p < 0.001$) between the synchronization and the oscillations. Here (**Figure 5B**) we show only the data for the arithmetic mean of the *oscil. scores*.

The correlation between the oscillation and synchronization strength could imply that the synchronization pattern was dependent on the homogeneity of the neuronal oscillations within the DLOR. If the neural oscillations in different sites of the STN of a single patient have a very stable and equal frequency, the existence of synchronization may not be the result of physical coupling between the STN neurons. Therefore, the DLOR pairs of each trajectory were randomly shuffled and the synchronization between the shuffled (non-simultaneously recorded) pairs was re-quantified in each trajectory. After shuffling, the oscillations remained in the same frequency band, but the synchronization was no longer apparent. **Figures 5A,C** show the average coherence functions before and after shuffling of the DLOR-DLOR pairs ($n = 615$), respectively. **Figures 6A,B** depict the average *sync* and *oscil scores* before and after shuffling in the STN DLOR and the VMNR. As expected, shuffling had no significant effect on the *oscil score* in either area (oscillation is a property of a single element and therefore should not be affected by the shuffling procedure). However, the average *sync score* of the DLOR pairs, but not the VMNR pairs declined significantly after the shuffling procedure (**Figure 6A**). Finally, **Figure 5D** depicts the scatter plot of the *sync* and *oscil scores* of the shuffled pairs within the DLOR. The Spearman correlation between the *sync score* and *oscill score* dropped dramatically from $r1 = 0.34$ to $r2 = 0.05$ ($p < 0.001$ for the null assumption that r1=r2). The mean PSD estimate for the average *oscil score* (as in **Figure 5B**) was used for this analysis. Similar results were obtained for the other indicators of oscillation strength of the STN pairs.

COHERENCE IS MAINLY IN THE BETA FREQUENCY RANGE

Next, the frequency value where each spectrum (**Figure 7A**) and coherence (**Figure 7C**) reached its maximal value was calculated. In both cases, a bi-modal distribution was observed, with a dominance of tremor frequency (3–7 Hz) and beta (12–30 Hz) oscillations, for the auto-spectrums and the coherence functions, respectively. **Figures 7B,D** show the scatterplot of the maximal *oscil* and *sync scores*, respectively, as a function of their frequency. While the *oscil scores* had similar values in the beta and the tremor range, the values of the maximal *sync scores* were much higher in the beta than in the tremor range. These results are in line with our previous primate studies (Raz et al., 2000) that revealed

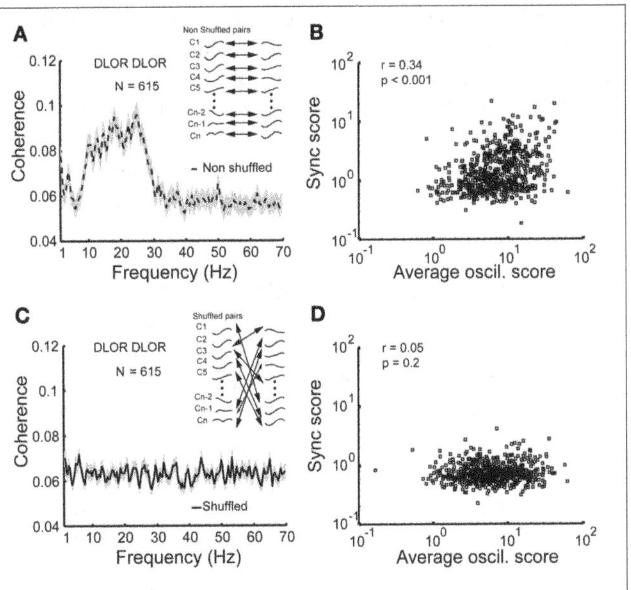

FIGURE 5 | Synchronization is no longer apparent between non-simultaneously recorded (shuffled) STN DLOR pairs. (A) A significant average coherence between non-shuffled pairs within the STN DLOR. $N = 615$ represents the number of DLOR-DLOR pairs. **(B)** Scatter plot of synchronization *(sync)* and oscillation *(oscil)* scores in the STN DLOR reveals that the two measures are correlated. Each square represents the synchronization (*Y*-axis) vs. average (arithmetic mean) of the two oscillation scores of one of the 615 pairs within the DLOR. *r* is the Spearman correlation coefficient and *p* is the probability that $r = 0$ (no correlation between the scores). **(C)** Synchronization is no longer seen between non-simultaneously recorded (shuffled) STN DLOR-DLOR pairs. Inset: Schematic illustration of the shuffling procedure. The shuffling procedure was repeated 10,000 times for each pair. **(D)** Scatter plot of shuffled oscil-sync score values. Same conventions as in **(B)**.

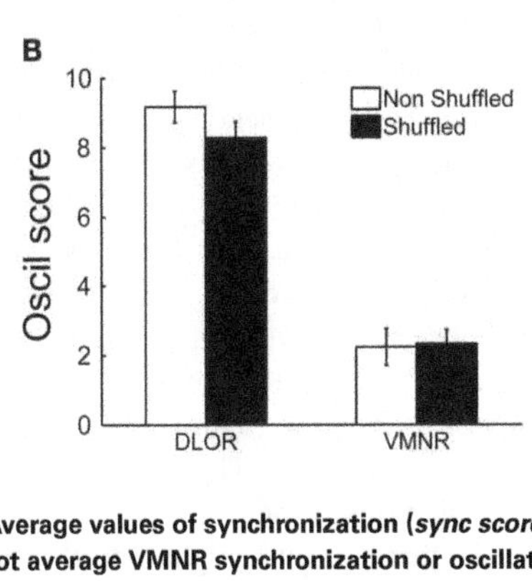

FIGURE 6 | Average values of synchronization (*sync score*) in the DLOR, but not average VMNR synchronization or oscillations scores in both STN domains, are affected by the shuffling procedures. (A) Synchronization (*Sync*) scores before (white) and after (black) shuffling, lines indicate standard error of the mean (SEM). **(B)** Oscillation (*Oscil*) scores before and after shuffling. Same conventions as in **(A)**.

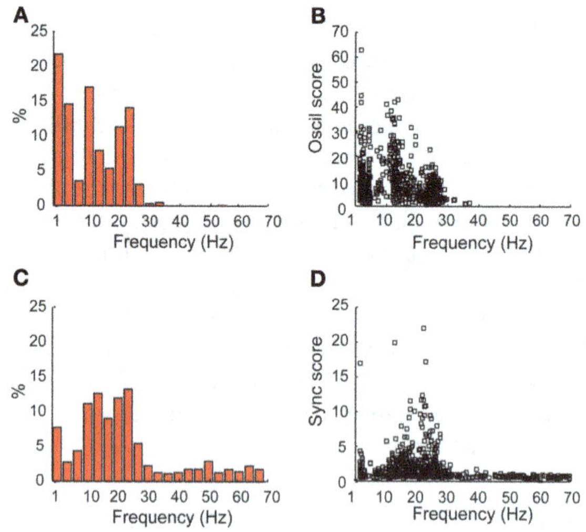

FIGURE 7 | Dominance of coherence at the beta frequency range vs. tremor frequency and beta oscillations in the power spectrums in the STN DLOR. (A) Frequency distribution of the frequencies with maximal power in the power spectrums of STN DLOR recording sites. **(B)** Scatter plot of oscillations (*oscil*) scores vs. the frequency with maximal power. **(C,D)** show the frequency distribution and scatter plot, respectively, for the coherence, same conventions as in **(A,B)**. $N = 1230$ single DLOR sites and 615 DLOR-DLOR pairs.

mainly 5 Hz peaks in the auto-correlations vs. higher frequencies (10 Hz) in the cross-correlations functions of pallidal units and pairs recorded in the globus pallidus after MPTP treatment. However, we cannot rule out the possibility that the 10 Hz activity in this study is not tremor related and a harmonic feature (or n:m locking) of the tremor or of the neuronal oscillations at the tremor frequency.

LACK OF POSITIVE CORRELATION BETWEEN THE STN *OSCIL* AND *SYNC SCORES* vs. PD SYMPTOMS

Previous studies have suggested that STN oscillations and synchronization are correlated with tremor in PD patients (Levy et al., 2002a). This would indicate that the STN synchronized oscillations are driven by the tremor (which may be generated by an independent neuronal loop). The above findings of robust synchronization in the beta rather than in the tremor frequency range (**Figure 7D**) are not in line with this hypothesis. Nevertheless, we looked for correlations between the *oscil* and *sync scores* of our patients and their pre-operative (OFF medication) UPDRS scores. We did not find significant positive correlation between the average *oscil score* and *sync scores* of STN activity and the UPDRS scores of the tremor in the contra-lateral upper limb(s), all tremor (including axial) scores, and all UPDRS III motor scores. There is a trend for STN synchronized beta oscillations to be more robust in patients with less tremor. While these results might point to a correlation between STN beta oscillations and akinetic/rigid Parkinsonian symptoms (an issue that requires clarification in future studies with bigger sample of patients and with intra-operative clinical assessment), they definitely indicate that the STN beta synchronized oscillations are not a by-product of the PD tremor.

DISCUSSION

In this manuscript, synchronization within the human Parkinsonian subthalamic nucleus was investigated. No significant synchronization was found over the STN as a whole. After dividing the STN into two electro-physiologically distinct regions, the dorsolateral oscillatory region (DLOR) and the ventromedial non-oscillatory region (VMNR), significant synchronization in the beta range was observed, however, only within the DLOR. The strength of the DLOR synchronization was correlated with the strength of the oscillations of the multi-unit pairs. Nevertheless, shuffling between DLOR pairs abolished synchronization, suggesting that STN synchronization is an independent phenomenon and not a mere reflection of neuronal oscillations at similar frequencies.

Previous studies have shown significant spatial overlap between the DLOR and the STN sensorimotor area (Rodriguez-Oroz et al., 2001; Zaidel et al., 2010). The finding that the STN VMNR (considered to be part of the limbic and associative basal ganglia network) remains unsynchronized is consistent with the predominantly motor nature of PD. However, the (normal) lack of synchronization in the STN VMNR may be due to a selection bias of our DBS patients. Since conventional inclusion criteria were used to select candidates for DBS, patients were usually severely motor-impaired and had few of the non-motor features of the disease. Furthermore, the DLOR may reflect the pathological area of the STN which progressively invades the limbic domains of the STN as the disease advances. Finally, our results are in line with a fuzzy rather than a sharp boundary between the STN sub-domains (Lambert et al., 2012; Haynes and Haber, 2013).

THE STN SPIKING POPULATION ACTIVITY IS SYNCHRONIZED

In this study population spiking (multi-unit) activity was used as a measure of the spiking activity of the STN rather than the more classical parameter of single unit activity (Perkel et al., 1967; Abeles, 1982; Lemon, 1984; Eggermont, 1990). This was primarily for practical reasons. The goal of physiological recording in the operating room (OR) is to enable better identification of the borders of the subthalamic nucleus and its sub-regions. The electrode is therefore advanced in 100 μm steps rather than 2–5 μm steps as is customary in the research laboratory setup. The sampling duration at each step is also limited (Shamir et al., 2012) and the OR conditions often do not allow stable recordings (as compared to 30–90 min stable recordings in a research setting). On the other hand, the cross-correlation of composite spike trains derived from several un-discriminated cells recorded on a single electrode (multi-unit activity) enhances the sensitivity of correlation methods. First, the higher discharge rate of multi vs. single unit recording reduces the asymmetric sensitivity of correlation methods to excitation vs. inhibition (Aertsen and Gerstein, 1985). Second, multi-unit cross-correlation can be a more sensitive detector of a neuronal relationship than single-unit cross-correlation (Bedenbaugh and Gerstein, 1997). Thus, use of a multi-unit signal is warranted for both practical and theoretical reasons. Furthermore, the use of signals recorded by two different electrodes in this study reveal the long range (2 mm) synchronization of STN DLOR. It is hoped that future studies of STN units using objective metrics for quantification of the quality of the unit isolation (Joshua et al., 2007; Hill et al., 2011) will shed more light on synchronization in the STN and other basal ganglia structures of human patients.

SYNCHRONIZATION ONLY OCCURS BETWEEN DLOR PAIRS IN THE STN

Early studies described neuronal synchronization in the STN as an epiphenomenon found mainly in patients presenting with tremor (Levy et al., 2000, 2002a). More recent studies (Hanson et al., 2012; Alavi et al., 2013; Lourens et al., 2013) have reported that synchronization can be found between some but not all STN pairs. On the other hand, beta-band LFP and spike oscillations have been described as a consistent feature of human PD in the dopamine depleted state (Brown and Williams, 2005; Foffani et al., 2005; Little et al., 2012). Moreover, many studies have documented the consistency of beta-band oscillations in both the spatial and temporal domains (Bronte-Stewart et al., 2009; de-Solages et al., 2010; Zaidel et al., 2010; Abosch et al., 2012; Little et al., 2012). In this study, synchronization within the Parkinsonian STN DLOR was indeed found to correlate with oscillations. However, the shuffling procedure revealed that STN synchronization was not due to independent oscillators with a similar oscillation frequency (Strogatz, 2003). If this had been the case, a significant synchronization should also have been observed between the shuffled (non-simultaneously recorded pairs of the same patient) DLOR-DLOR pairs. Thus, the synchronization of the simultaneously recorded STN pairs probably reflects the increased coupling between these neurons in the dopamine depleted state of Parkinson's disease. This increased coupling is probably due to the increased efficacy of the common inputs to the STN cells, either from the cortex (Nambu, 2004; Kita and Kita, 2012) or from the external segment of the globus pallidus (Plenz and Kitai, 1999; Tachibana et al., 2011). However, at this stage the possibility of increased coupling by lateral connectivity within the STN cannot be ruled out (Parent et al., 2000; Parent and Parent, 2007).

The finding that most of the energy of the STN synchronous oscillations is in the beta range suggest that these oscillations are not generated by feedback of the peripheral tremor. It is interesting to note that synchronous oscillations in the basal ganglia of MPTP treated primates are mainly found in the 10 Hz domain, where human oscillations span the full beta range (12–30 Hz). Future studies should reveal if this is due to species difference, or due to differences between the MPTP model and human idiopathic Parkinson's disease.

CONCLUDING NOTES

In this study we show that the STN domain most affected by PD dopamine depletion (the DLOR, probably the STN motor domain) exhibited both oscillations and synchronization. This suggests that synchronization reflects an additional property of the Parkinsonian STN. Previous studies in the basal ganglia of MPTP treated primates have demonstrated that synchronization can be completely independent of oscillatory activity (Heimer et al., 2002). The previous and the current findings can serve to recast the relationship between oscillations and synchronization in the Parkinsonian basal ganglia (Raz et al., 2000; Amirnovin et al., 2004; Moran et al., 2008). In addition to changes in discharge rate and pattern, synchronization within the STN may be another pathophysiological marker of Parkinson's disease. The potential consequences of synchronization (as opposed to other attributes like rate and pattern change) are probably mainly due to reduced information capacity of the basal ganglia neurons. However, the different pathological changes in the parkinsonian basal ganglia are probably not mutually exclusive. Synchronized oscillations have stronger effects than less synchronized oscillations and completely unsynchronized oscillations might have no effect on target neurons. Furthermore, future studies toward adaptive DBS (Rosin et al., 2011) should investigate which of the pathophysiological changes in the STN activity might be used as the optimal trigger for closed loop DBS.

ACKNOWLEDGMENTS

This work was supported partially by the Vorst Family Foundation for Parkinson Research, by the Simone and Bernard Guttman chair of Brain Research, and the generous support of the Rosetrees and Dekker foundations (to Hagai Bergman) as well as by the ELSC post-doctorate fellowships to Shay Moshel and Reuben R. Shamir and the PATH and Bloom foundations of London to Zvi Israel. We would like to thank Prof. Y. Ritov for statistical advice and Dr. S. Freeman and E. Singer for help in scientific editing.

AUTHOR CONTRIBUTIONS

Shay Moshel and Reuben R. Shamir claim for equal contribution. Shay Moshel did the data analysis, and wrote the manuscript together with Hagai Bergman and Zvi Israel. Reuben R. Shamir handled the database and collected part of the data. AR initiated the study and helped in the collection of data. Hagai Bergman, Renana Eitan, Fernando R. de Noriega, and Zvi Israel collected the data. All authors discussed the results, reviewed the manuscript, and made their comments.

REFERENCES

Abeles, M. (1982). *Local Cortical Circuits*. Berlin; Heidelberg; New York: Springer-Verlag. doi: 10.1007/978-3-642-81708-3

Abosch, A., Lanctin, D., Onaran, I., Eberly, L., Spaniol, M., and Ince, N. F. (2012). Long-term recordings of local field potentials from implanted deep brain stimulation electrodes. *Neurosurgery* 71, 804–814. doi: 10.1227/NEU.0b013e3182676b91

Aertsen, A. M., and Gerstein, G. L. (1985). Evaluation of neuronal connectivity: sensitivity of cross-correlation. *Brain Res.* 340, 341–354. doi: 10.1016/0006-8993(85)90931-X

Alavi, M., Dostrovsky, J. O., Hodaie, M., Lozano, A. M., and Hutchison, W. D. (2013). Spatial extent of beta oscillatory activity in and between the subthalamic nucleus and substantia nigra pars reticulata of Parkinson's disease patients. *Exp. Neurol.* 245, 60–71. doi: 10.1016/j.expneurol.2012.09.021

Alvarez, L., Macias, R., Pavon, N., Lopez, G., Rodriguez-Oroz, M. C., Rodriguez, R., et al. (2009). Therapeutic efficacy of unilateral subthalamotomy in Parkinson's disease: results in 89 patients followed for up to 36 months. *J. Neurol. Neurosurg. Psychiatry* 80, 979–985. doi: 10.1136/jnnp.2008.154948

Amirnovin, R., Williams, Z. M., Cosgrove, G. R., and Eskandar, E. N. (2004). Visually guided movements suppress subthalamic oscillations in Parkinson's disease patients. *J. Neurosci.* 24, 11302–11306. doi: 10.1523/JNEUROSCI.3242-04.2004

Aziz, T. Z., Peggs, D., Sambrook, M. A., and Crossman, A. R. (1991). Lesion of the subthalamic nucleus for the alleviation of 1-methyl-4-phenyl-1,2,3,6-tetrahydropyridine (MPTP)-induced parkinsonism in the primate. *Mov. Disord.* 6, 288–292. doi: 10.1002/mds.870060404

Bedenbaugh, P., and Gerstein, G. L. (1997). Multiunit normalized cross correlation differs from the average single-unit normalized correlation. *Neural comput.* 9, 1265–1275. doi: 10.1162/neco.1997.9.6.1265

Belitski, A., Panzeri, S., Magri, C., Logothetis, N. K., and Kayser, C. (2010). Sensory information in local field potentials and spikes from visual and auditory cortices: time scales and frequency bands. *J. Comput. Neurosci.* 29, 533–545. doi: 10.1007/s10827-010-0230-y

Benabid, A. L., Pollak, P., Gross, C., Hoffmann, D., Benazzouz, A., Gao, D. M., et al. (1994). Acute and long-term effects of subthalamic nucleus stimulation in Parkinson's disease. *Stereotact. Funct. Neurosurg.* 62, 76–84. doi: 10.1159/000098600

Benazzouz, A., Gross, C., Feger, J., Boraud, T., and Bioulac, B. (1993). Reversal of rigidity and improvement in motor performance by subthalamic high-frequency stimulation in MPTP-treated monkeys. *Eur. J. Neurosci.* 5, 382–389. doi: 10.1111/j.1460-9568.1993.tb00505.x

Bergman, H., Wichmann, T., and DeLong, M. R. (1990). Reversal of experimental parkinsonism by lesions of the subthalamic nucleus. *Science* 249, 1436–1438. doi: 10.1126/science.2402638

Bergman, H., Wichmann, T., Karmon, B., and DeLong, M. R. (1994). The primate subthalamic nucleus. II. Neuronal activity in the MPTP model of parkinsonism. *J. Neurophysiol.* 72, 507–520.

Bronstein, J. M., Tagliati, M., Alterman, R. L., Lozano, A. M., Volkmann, J., Stefani, A., et al. (2011). Deep brain stimulation for Parkinson disease: an expert consensus and review of key issues. *Arch. Neurol.* 68, 165. doi: 10.1001/archneurol.2010.260

Bronte-Stewart, H., Barberini, C., Koop, M. M., Hill, B. C., Henderson, J. M., and Wingeier, B. (2009). The STN beta-band profile in Parkinson's disease is stationary and shows prolonged attenuation after deep brain stimulation. *Exp. Neurol.* 215, 20–28. doi: 10.1016/j.expneurol.2008.09.008

Brown, P., and Williams, D. (2005). Basal ganglia local field potential activity: Character and functional significance in the human. *Clin. Neurophysiol* 116, 2510–2519. doi: 10.1016/j.clinph.2005.05.009

Buzsaki, G., Anastassiou, C. A., and Koch, C. (2012). The origin of extracellular fields and currents - EEG, ECoG, LFP and spikes. *Nat. Rev. Neurosci.* 13, 407–420. doi: 10.1038/nrn3241

Chen, C. C., Hsu, Y. T., Chan, H. L., Chiou, S. M., Tu, P. H., Lee, S. T., et al. (2010). Complexity of subthalamic 13–35 Hz oscillatory activity directly correlates with clinical impairment in patients with Parkinson's disease. *Exp. Neurol.* 224, 234–240. doi: 10.1016/j.expneurol.2010.03.015

Danish, S. F., Moyer, J. T., Finkel, L. H., Baltuch, G. H., Jaggi, J. L., Priori, A., et al. (2007). High-frequency oscillations (>200 Hz) in the human non-parkinsonian subthalamic nucleus. *Brain Res. Bull.* 74, 84–90. doi: 10.1016/j.brainresbull.2007.05.006

de-Solages, C., Hill, B. C., Koop, M. M., Henderson, J. M., and Bronte-Stewart, H. (2010). Bilateral symmetry and coherence of subthalamic nuclei beta band activity in Parkinson's disease. *Exp. Neurol.* 221, 260–266. doi: 10.1016/j.expneurol.2009.11.012

de-Solages, C., Hill, B. C., Yu, H., Henderson, J. M., and Bronte-Stewart, H. (2011). Maximal subthalamic beta hypersynchrony of the local field potential in Parkinson's disease is located in the central region of the nucleus. *J. Neurol. Neurosurg. Psychiatry* 82, 1387–1389. doi: 10.1136/jnnp.2010.223107

Eggermont, J. J. (1990). *The Correlative Brain. Theory and Experiment in Neuronal Interaction.* Berlin: Springer-Verlag. doi: 10.1007/978-3-642-51033-5

Farmer, S. F. (1998). Rhythmicity, synchronization and binding in human and primate motor systems. *J. Physiol. Lond.* 509, 3–14. doi: 10.1111/j.1469-7793.1998.003bo.x

Farmer, S. F., Halliday, D. M., Conway, B. A., Stephens, J. A., and Rosenberg, J. R. (1997). A review of recent applications of cross-correlation methodologies to human motor unit recording. *J. Neurosci. Methods* 74, 175–187. doi: 10.1016/S0165-0270(97)02248-6

Foffani, G., Bianchi, A. M., Baselli, G., and Priori, A. (2005). Movement-related frequency modulation of beta oscillatory activity in the human subthalamic nucleus. *J. Physiol.* 568, 699–711. doi: 10.1113/jphysiol.2005.089722

Follett, K. A., Weaver, F. M., Stern, M., Hur, K., Harris, C. L., Luo, P., et al. (2010). Pallidal versus subthalamic deep-brain stimulation for Parkinson's disease. *N. Engl. J. Med.* 362, 2077–2091. doi: 10.1056/NEJMoa0907083

Gerstein, G. L. (2000). Cross-correlation measures of unresolved multi-neuron recordings. *J. Neurosci. Methods* 100, 41–51. doi: 10.1016/S0165-0270(00)00226-0

Giannicola, G., Marceglia, S., Rossi, L., Mrakic-Sposta, S., Rampini, P., Tamma, F., et al. (2010). The effects of levodopa and ongoing deep brain stimulation on subthalamic beta oscillations in Parkinson's disease. *Exp. Neurol.* 226, 120–127. doi: 10.1016/j.expneurol.2010.08.011

Goldberg, J. A., Maraton, S., Boraud, T., Haber, S. N., Vaadia, E., and Bergman, H. (2002). Enhanced synchrony among primary motor cortex neurons in the MPTP primate model of Parkinson's disease. *J. Neurosci.* 22, 4639–4653.

Guo, S., Zhuang, P., Hallett, M., Zheng, Z., Zhang, Y., Li, J., et al. (2013). Subthalamic deep brain stimulation for Parkinson's disease: correlation between locations of oscillatory activity and optimal site of stimulation. *Parkinsonism Relat. Disord.* 19, 109–114. doi: 10.1016/j.parkreldis.2012.08.005

Guo, S., Zhuang, P., Zheng, Z., Zhang, Y., Li, J., and Li, Y. (2012). Neuronal firing patterns in the subthalamic nucleus in patients with akinetic-rigid-type Parkinson's disease. *J. Clin. Neurosci.* 19, 1404–1407. doi: 10.1016/j.jocn.2011.11.038

Halliday, D. M., Conway, B. A., Farmer, S. F., Shahani, U., Russell, A. J., and Rosenberg, J. R. (2000). Coherence between low-frequency activation of the motor cortex and tremor in patients with essential tremor. *Lancet* 355, 1149–1153. doi: 10.1016/S0140-6736(00)02064-X

Halliday, D. M., and Farmer, S. F. (2010). On the need for rectification of surface EMG. *J. Neurophysiol.*103, 3547–3549. doi: 10.1152/jn.00222.2010

Halliday, D. M., Rosenberg, J. R., Amjad, A. M., Breeze, P., Conway, B. A., and Farmer, S. F. (1995). A framework for the analysis of mixed time series/point process data–theory and application to the study of physiological tremor, single motor unit discharges and electromyograms. *Prog. Biophys. Mol. Biol.* 64, 237–278. doi: 10.1016/S0079-6107(96)00009-0

Hamani, C., Saint-Cyr, J. A., Fraser, J., Kaplitt, M., and Lozano, A. M. (2004). The subthalamic nucleus in the context of movement disorders. *Brain* 127, 4–20. doi: 10.1093/brain/awh029

Hammond, C., Bergman, H., and Brown, P. (2007). Pathological synchronization in Parkinson's disease: networks, models and treatments. *Trends Neurosci.* 30, 357–364. doi: 10.1016/j.tins.2007.05.004

Hanson, T. L., Fuller, A. M., Lebedev, M. A., Turner, D. A., and Nicolelis, M. A. (2012). Subcortical neuronal ensembles: an analysis of motor task association, tremor, oscillations, and synchrony in human patients. *J. Neurosci.* 32, 8620–8632. doi: 10.1523/JNEUROSCI.0750-12.2012

Haynes, W. I., and Haber, S. N. (2013). The organization of prefrontal-subthalamic inputs in primates provides an anatomical substrate for both functional specificity and integration: implications for Basal Ganglia models and deep brain stimulation. *J. Neurosci.* 33, 4804–4814. doi: 10.1523/JNEUROSCI.4674-12.2013

Heimer, G., Bar-Gad, I., Goldberg, J. A., and Bergman, H. (2002). Dopamine replacement therapy reverses abnormal synchronization of pallidal neurons in the 1-methyl-4-phenyl-1,2,3,6-tetrahydropyridine primate model of parkinsonism. *J. Neurosci.* 22, 7850–7855.

Hill, D. N., Mehta, S. B., and Kleinfeld, D. (2011). Quality metrics to accompany spike sorting of extracellular signals. *J. Neurosci.* 31, 8699–8705. doi: 10.1523/JNEUROSCI.0971-11.2011

Joshua, M., Elias, S., Levine, O., and Bergman, H. (2007). Quantifying the isolation quality of extracellularly recorded action potentials. *J. Neurosci. Methods* 163, 267–282. doi: 10.1016/j.jneumeth.2007.03.012

Kay, S. M. (1988). *Modern Spectral Estimation: Theory and Application.* Englewood Cliffs, NJ: Prentice Hall.

Kita, T., and Kita, H. (2012). The subthalamic nucleus is one of multiple innervation sites for long-range corticofugal axons: a single-axon tracing study in the rat. *J. Neurosci.* 32, 5990–5999. doi: 10.1523/JNEUROSCI.5717-11.2012

Kitai, S. T., and Kita, H. (1987). "Anatomy and physiology of the subthalamic nucleus: a driving force of the basal ganglia," in *The Basal Ganglia. II. Structure and Function: Current Concepts* eds M. B. Carpenter and A. Jayaraman (New York, NY: Plenum), 357–373. doi: 10.1007/978-1-4684-5347-8_25

Kuhn, A. A., Trottenberg, T., Kivi, A., Kupsch, A., Schneider, G. H., and Brown, P. (2005). The relationship between local field potential and neuronal discharge in the subthalamic nucleus of patients with Parkinson's disease. *Exp. Neurol.* 194, 212–220. doi: 10.1016/j.expneurol.2005.02.010

Kuhn, A. A., Tsui, A., Aziz, T., Ray, N., Brucke, C., Kupsch, A., et al. (2009). Pathological synchronisation in the subthalamic nucleus of patients with Parkinson's disease relates to both bradykinesia and rigidity. *Exp. Neurol.* 215, 380–387. doi: 10.1016/j.expneurol.2008.11.008

Lambert, C., Zrinzo, L., Nagy, Z., Lutti, A., Hariz, M., Foltynie, T., et al. (2012). Confirmation of functional zones within the human subthalamic nucleus: patterns of connectivity and sub-parcellation using diffusion weighted imaging. Neuroimage 60, 83–94. doi: 10.1016/j.neuroimage.2011.11.082

Lemon, R. (1984). *Methods for Neuronal Recording in Conscious Animals.* New York, NY: John Wiley & Sons.

Levy, R., Hutchison, W. D., Lozano, A. M., and Dostrovsky, J. O. (2002a). Synchronized neuronal discharge in the basal ganglia of parkinsonian patients is limited to oscillatory activity. *J. Neurosci.* 22, 2855–2861.

Levy, R., Ashby, P., Hutchison, W. D., Lang, A. E., Lozano, A. M., and Dostrovsky, J. O. (2002b). Dependence of subthalamic nucleus oscillations on movement and dopamine in Parkinson's disease. *Brain* 125, 1196–1209. doi: 10.1093/brain/awf128

Levy, R., Hutchison, W. D., Lozano, A. M., and Dostrovsky, J. O. (2000). High-frequency synchronization of neuronal activity in the subthalamic nucleus of parkinsonian patients with limb tremor. *J. Neurosci.* 20, 7766–7775.

Lewicki, M. S. (1998). A review of methods for spike sorting: the detection and classification of neural action potentials. *Network* 9, R53–R78. doi: 10.1088/0954-898X/9/4/001

Lhommée, E., Klinger, H., Thobois, S., Schmitt, E., Ardouin, C., Bichon, A., et al. (2012). Subthalamic stimulation in Parkinson's disease: restoring the balance of motivated behaviours. *Brain* 135, 1463–1477. doi: 10.1093/brain/aws078

Lintas, A., Silkis, I. G., Alberi, L., and Villa, A. E. (2012). Dopamine deficiency increases synchronized activity in the rat subthalamic nucleus. *Brain Res.* 1434, 142–151. doi: 10.1016/j.brainres.2011.09.005

Little, S., Pogosyan, A., Kuhn, A. A., and Brown, P. (2012). Beta band stability over time correlates with Parkinsonian rigidity and bradykinesia. *Exp. Neurol.* 236, 383–388. doi: 10.1016/j.expneurol.2012.04.024

Lourens, M. A., Meijer, H. G., Contarino, M. F., van den Munckhof, P., Schuurman, P. R., van Gils, S. A., et al. (2013). Functional neuronal activity and connectivity within the subthalamic nucleus in Parkinson's disease. *Clin. Neurophysiol.* 124, 967–981. doi: 10.1016/j.clinph.2012.10.018

Machado, A., Rezai, A. R., Kopell, B. H., Gross, R. E., Sharan, A. D., and Benabid, A. L. (2006). Deep brain stimulation for Parkinson's disease: Surgical technique and perioperative management. *Mov. Disord.* 21, S247–S258. doi: 10.1002/mds.20959

Mallet, N., Pogosyan, A., Marton, L. F., Bolam, J. P., Brown, P., and Magill, P. J. (2008a). Parkinsonian beta oscillations in the external globus pallidus and their relationship with subthalamic nucleus activity. *J. Neurosci.* 28, 14245–14258. doi: 10.1523/JNEUROSCI.4199-08.2008

Mallet, N., Pogosyan, A., Sharott, A., Csicsvari, J., Bolam, J. P., Brown, P., et al. (2008b). Disrupted dopamine transmission and the emergence of exaggerated beta oscillations in subthalamic nucleus and cerebral cortex. *J. Neurosci.* 28, 4795–4806. doi: 10.1523/JNEUROSCI.0123-08.2008

Matsumoto, M., and Nishimura, T. (1998). Mersenne twister: a 623-dimensionally equidistributed uniform pseudo-random number generator. *ACM Trans. Model. Comput. Simulat.* 8, 3–30. doi: 10.1145/272991.272995

Miller, W. L., and Sigvardt, K. A. (1998). Spectral analysis of oscillatory neural circuits. *J. Neurosci. Methods* 80, 113–128. doi: 10.1016/S0165-0270(97)00185-4

Miranda de Sa, A. M., Ferreira, D. D., Dias, E. W., Mendes, E. M., and Felix, L. B. (2009). Coherence estimate between a random and a periodic signal: Bias, variance, analytical critical values, and normalizing transforms. *J. Franklin Inst. Eng.Appl. Math.* 346, 841–853. doi: 10.1016/j.jfranklin.2009.07.009

Moran, A., and Bar-Gad, I. (2010). Revealing neuronal functional organization through the relation between multi-scale oscillatory extracellular signals. *J. Neurosci. Methods* 186, 116–129. doi: 10.1016/j.jneumeth.2009.10.024

Moran, A., Bergman, H., Israel, Z., and Bar-Gad, I. (2008). Subthalamic nucleus functional organization revealed by parkinsonian neuronal oscillations and synchrony. *Brain* 131, 3395–3409. doi: 10.1093/brain/awn270

Moro, E., Lozano, A. M., Pollak, P., Agid, Y., Rehncrona, S., Volkmann, J., et al. (2010). Long-term results of a multicenter study on subthalamic and pallidal stimulation in Parkinson's disease. *Mov. Disord.* 25, 578–586. doi: 10.1002/mds.22735

Nambu, A. (2004). A new dynamic model of the cortico-basal ganglia loop. *Prog. Brain Res.* 143, 461–466. doi: 10.1016/S0079-6123(03)43043-4

Nambu, A., Tokuno, H., and Takada, M. (2002). Functional significance of the cortico-subthalamo-pallidal 'hyperdirect' pathway. *Neurosci. Res.* 43, 111–117. doi: 10.1016/S0168-0102(02)00027-5

Nini, A., Feingold, A., Slovin, H., and Bergman, H. (1995). Neurons in the globus pallidus do not show correlated activity in the normal monkey, but phase-locked oscillations appear in the MPTP model of parkinsonism. *J. Neurophysiol.* 74, 1800–1805.

Odekerken, V. J., van, L. T., Staal, M. J., Mosch, A., Hoffmann, C. F., Nijssen, P. C., et al. (2013). Subthalamic nucleus versus globus pallidus bilateral deep brain stimulation for advanced Parkinson's disease (NSTAPS study): a randomised controlled trial. *Lancet Neurol.* 12, 37–44. doi: 10.1016/S1474-4422(12)70264-8

Parent, A., Sato, F., Wu, Y., Gauthier, J., Levesque, M., and Parent, M. (2000). Organization of the basal ganglia: the importance of axonal collateralization. *Trends Neurosci.* 23, S20–S27. doi: 10.1016/S1471-1931(00)00022-7

Parent, M., and Parent, A. (2007). The microcircuitry of primate subthalamic nucleus. *Parkinsonism Relat. Disord.* 13(Suppl. 3), S292–S295. doi: 10.1016/S1353-8020(08)70018-X

Perkel, D. H., Gerstein, G. L., and Moore, G. P. (1967). Neuronal spike trains and stochastic point processes. II. Simultaneous spike trains. *Biophys. J.* 7, 419–440. doi: 10.1016/S0006-3495(67)86597-4

Plenz, D., and Kitai, S. T. (1999). A basal ganglia pacemaker formed by the subthalamic nucleus and external globus pallidus. *Nature* 400, 677–682. doi: 10.1038/23281

Pollak, P., Benabid, A. L., Gross, C., Gao, D. M., Laurent, A., Benazzouz, A., et al. (1993). Effects of the stimulation of the subthalamic nucleus in Parkinson disease. *Rev. Neurol. Paris* 149, 175–176.

Raz, A., Feingold, A., Zelanskaya, V., Vaadia, E., and Bergman, H. (1996). Neuronal synchronization of tonically active neurons in the striatum of normal and parkinsonian primates. *J. Neurophysiol.* 76, 2083–2088.

Raz, A., Frechter-Mazar, V., Feingold, A., Abeles, M., Vaadia, E., and Bergman, H. (2001). Activity of pallidal and striatal tonically active neurons is correlated in mptp-treated monkeys but not in normal monkeys. *J. Neurosci.* 21:RC128.

Raz, A., Vaadia, E., and Bergman, H. (2000). Firing patterns and correlations of spontaneous discharge of pallidal neurons in the normal and the tremulous 1-methyl-4-phenyl-1,2,3,6-tetrahydropyridine vervet model of parkinsonism. *J. Neurosci.* 20, 8559–8571.

Rodriguez-Oroz, M. C., Rodriguez, M., Guridi, J., Mewes, K., Chockkman, V., Vitek, J., et al. (2001). The subthalamic nucleus in Parkinson's disease: somatotopic organization and physiological characteristics. *Brain* 124, 1777–1790. doi: 10.1093/brain/124.9.1777

Rosa, M., Giannicola, G., Servello, D., Marceglia, S., Pacchetti, C., Porta, M., et al. (2011). Subthalamic local field beta oscillations during ongoing deep brain stimulation in Parkinson's disease in hyperacute and chronic phases. *Neurosignals* 19, 151–162. doi: 10.1159/000328508

Rosin, B., Slovik, M., Mitelman, R., Rivlin-Etzion, M., Haber, S. N., Israel, Z., et al. (2011). Closed-loop deep brain stimulation is superior in ameliorating parkinsonism. *Neuron* 72, 370–384. doi: 10.1016/j.neuron.2011.08.023

Schuepbach, W. M., Rau, J., Knudsen, K., Volkmann, J., Krack, P., Timmermann, L., et al. (2013). Neurostimulation for Parkinson's disease with early motor complications. *N. Engl. J. Med.* 368, 610–622. doi: 10.1056/NEJMoa1205158

Seifried, C., Weise, L., Hartmann, R., Gasser, T., Baudrexel, S., Szelenyi, A., et al. (2012). Intraoperative microelectrode recording for the delineation of subthalamic nucleus topography in Parkinson's disease. *Brain Stimul.* 5, 378–387. doi: 10.1016/j.brs.2011.06.002

Shamir, R. R., Zaidel, A., Joskowicz, L., Bergman, H., and Israel, Z. (2012). Microelectrode recording duration and spatial density determine the detection accuracy of the subthalamic nucleus. *Stereotact. Funct. Neurosurg.* 90, 325–334. doi: 10.1159/000338252

Strogatz, S. (2003). *Sync - The Emerging Science of Spontaneous Order.* London: Penguin books.

Tachibana, Y., Iwamuro, H., Kita, H., Takada, M., and Nambu, A. (2011). Subthalamo-pallidal interactions underlying parkinsonian neuronal oscillations in the primate basal ganglia. *Eur. J. Neurosci.* 34, 1470–1484. doi: 10.1111/j.1460-9568.2011.07865.x

Weaver, F. M., Follett, K., Stern, M., Hur, K., Harris, C., Marks, W. J., Jr. et al. (2009). Bilateral deep brain stimulation vs best medical therapy for patients with advanced Parkinson disease: a randomized controlled trial. *JAMA* 301, 63–73. doi: 10.1001/jama.2008.929

Weinberger, M., Hutchison, W. D., Lozano, A. M., Hodaie, M., and Dostrovsky, J. O. (2009). Increased gamma oscillatory activity in the subthalamic nucleus during tremor in Parkinson's disease patients. *J. Neurophysiol.* 101, 789–802. doi: 10.1152/jn.90837.2008

Weinberger, M., Mahant, N., Hutchison, W. D., Lozano, A. M., Moro, E., Hodaie, M., et al. (2006). Beta oscillatory activity in the subthalamic nucleus and its relation to dopaminergic response in Parkinson's disease. *J. Neurophysiol.* 96, 3248–3256. doi: 10.1152/jn.00697.2006

Williams, A., Gill, S., Varma, T., Jenkinson, C., Quinn, N., Mitchell, R., et al. (2010). Deep brain stimulation plus best medical therapy versus best medical therapy alone for advanced Parkinson's disease (PD SURG trial): a randomised, open-label trial. *Lancet Neurol.* 9, 581–591. doi: 10.1016/S1474-4422(10)70093-4

Yuval-Greenberg, S., Tomer, O., Keren, A. S., Nelken, I., and Deouell, L. Y. (2008). Transient induced gamma-band response in EEG as a manifestation of miniature saccades. *Neuron* 58, 429–441. doi: 10.1016/j.neuron.2008.03.027

Zaidel, A., Spivak, A., Grieb, B., Bergman, H., and Israel, Z. (2010). Subthalamic span of beta oscillations predicts deep brain stimulation efficacy for patients with Parkinson's disease. *Brain* 133, 2007–2021. doi: 10.1093/brain/awq144

Zaidel, A., Spivak, A., Shpigelman, L., Bergman, H., and Israel, Z. (2009). Delimiting subterritories of the human subthalamic nucleus by means of microelectrode recordings and a Hidden Markov Model. *Mov. Disord.* 24, 1785–1793. doi: 10.1002/mds.22674

3

Exploring the Cognitive and Motor Functions of the Basal Ganglia: An Integrative Review of Computational Cognitive Neuroscience Models

Sebastien Helie[1]*, Srinivasa Chakravarthy[2] and Ahmed A. Moustafa[3]

[1] Department of Psychological Sciences, Purdue University, West Lafayette, IN, USA
[2] Department of Biotechnology, Indian Institute of Technology, Madras, India
[3] Marcs Institute for Brain and Behaviour and School of Social Sciences and Psychology, University of Western Sydney, Sydney, NSW, Australia

***Correspondence:**
Sebastien Helie, Department of Psychological Sciences, Purdue University, 703 Third Street, West Lafayette, IN 47907, USA
e-mail: shelie@purdue.edu

Many computational models of the basal ganglia (BG) have been proposed over the past twenty-five years. While computational neuroscience models have focused on closely matching the neurobiology of the BG, *computational cognitive neuroscience* (CCN) models have focused on how the BG can be used to implement cognitive and motor functions. This review article focuses on CCN models of the BG and how they use the neuroanatomy of the BG to account for cognitive and motor functions such as categorization, instrumental conditioning, probabilistic learning, working memory, sequence learning, automaticity, reaching, handwriting, and eye saccades. A total of 19 BG models accounting for one or more of these functions are reviewed and compared. The review concludes with a discussion of the limitations of existing CCN models of the BG and prescriptions for future modeling, including the need for computational models of the BG that can simultaneously account for cognitive and motor functions, and the need for a more complete specification of the role of the BG in behavioral functions.

Keywords: basal ganglia, computational cognitive neuroscience, cognitive function, motor function, Parkinson's disease

INTRODUCTION

The basal ganglia (BG) are a group of nuclei at the base of the forebrain that are strongly connected to the cortex. While the role of the BG had historically been restricted to motor function, a substantive amount of recent research suggests that the BG are also involved in a variety of cognitive functions (Steiner and Tseng, 2010). Behavioral and neural experiments with human and non-human animals have informed our understanding of the BG function for over a century, and the past two decades have seen an increased use of computational models to simulate the anatomy and functionality of the BG. The most anatomically detailed computational neuroscience models seldom go as far as simulating complex animal behavior (because of complexity issues), but simpler (less anatomically detailed) models can be used to simultaneously account for some anatomical details and complex animal behavior. The strength of these later *computational cognitive neuroscience* (CCN) models lies in that they can simultaneously account for both neuroscience data and behavioral data (Ashby and Helie, 2011).

This review article focuses on CCN models of the BG and classifies existing models according to cognitive and motor function. The remainder of this article is organized as follows. First, the anatomy that is usually included in CCN models of the BG is reviewed. This anatomy section is incomplete by design, as only details that are simulated to account for specific cognitive or motor function are included. Next, we review CCN models used to simulate six different cognitive functions, namely categorization, instrumental conditioning, probabilistic learning, working memory, sequence learning, and automaticity. This presentation is followed by CCN models of motor function. Computational cognitive neuroscience models of motor functions are separated into models of reaching, handwriting, and eye saccades. The review concludes with a discussion of the limitations of existing CCN models of the BG and prescriptions for future modeling. Future directions emphasize the need for CCN models of the BG that can simultaneously account for cognitive and motor functions, and the need for a more complete specification of the role of the BG in the reviewed functions.

NEUROANATOMY OF THE BASAL GANGLIA

The BG include the striatum (caudate, putamen, nucleus accumbens), the globus pallidus (GP), the subthalamic nucleus (STN), the substantia nigra (SN), the ventral tegmental area, and the olfactory tubercle (see **Figure 1**). The striatum receives the majority of afferent connections whereas the internal segment of the GP Globus pallidus (internal) (GPi) and SN pars reticulate (SNr) are the sources of the majority of efferent connections that target cortical regions via the thalamus. Based on both structural and functional evidence, the striatum is often divided into a ventral and a dorsal part. The ventral striatum includes the nucleus accumbens, ventromedial portions of the caudate and putamen, and the olfactory tubercle. The dorsal striatum, which is usually

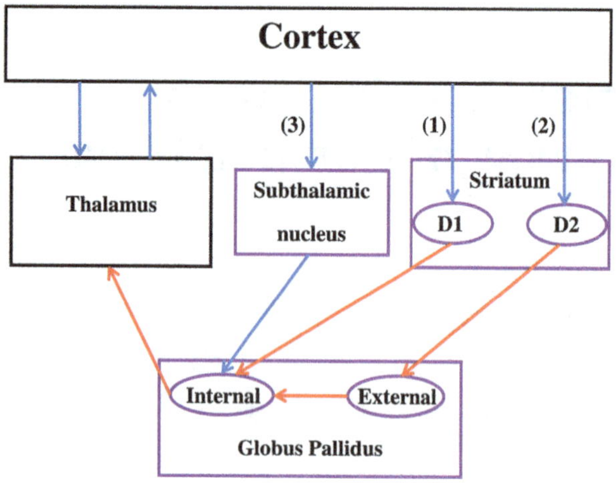

FIGURE 1 | Functional anatomy of the basal ganglia. Note that only subdivisions included in most of the reviewed CCN models are represented. Purple boxes correspond to areas of the BG while black boxes are not included in the BG. Blue arrows represent excitatory (glutamatergic) connections while red arrows represent inhibitory (GABA) connections. The direct pathway **(1)** passes through the D1 receptors in the striatum, the indirect pathway **(2)** passes through the D2 receptors in the striatum, and the hyperdirect pathway **(3)** passes through the STN. If the thalamic projections target the same cortical region that initially targeted the striatum, the circuit is called a closed loop. Otherwise, the circuit is an opened loop.

the main focus of CCN models of the BG, includes the remainder of the caudate and putamen.

Virtually all of the neocortex sends excitatory (glutamatergic) projections to the striatum (Reiner, 2010). Corticostriatal input is massively convergent with estimates ranging from 5,000 to 10,000 cortical neurons converging on a single striatal medium spiny neuron (MSN; the main striatal projection neurons) (Kincaid et al., 1998). Classically, corticostriatal organization is thought to follow a fairly strict spatial topography (Kemp and Powell, 1970). Along the rostral-to-caudal extent of the BG, the cortical afferents tend be more prevalent from rostral-to-caudal cortical regions. For instance, ventral striatum receives input predominantly from orbitofrontal cortex, ventromedial prefrontal cortex, and anterior cingulate cortex (ACC). As one moves caudally within the striatum, inputs from areas 9, 46, and 8 become more prevalent (Haber et al., 2006; Calzavara et al., 2007), followed by inputs from premotor regions (area 6) with the most caudal motor and somatosensory cortical regions projecting preferentially to the caudal putamen (Flaherty and Graybiel, 1994). Spatial topography holds as you continue rostrally and ventrally through parietal and temporal cortices as well as other extrastriate visual areas (Kemp and Powell, 1970; Yeterian and Pandya, 1993, 1995, 1998).

The thalamus provides another major source of input to the BG (Wilson, 2004), with the majority of thalamostriatal projections originating from the parafascicular-centromedian (CMPf) complex (Smith et al., 2010). Thalamic input to the striatum synapses on both MSNs and cholinergic tonically active neurons (TANs; a class of large-body interneurons) (Smith et al., 2004), with the latter likely playing an important role in modulating cortico-striatal synaptic plasticity (Ashby and Crossley, 2011). Finally, thalamic input to the striatum is in a position to modulate BG function by virtue of cortico-thalamo-striatal connections and striatal-thalamo-striatal feedback (Smith et al., 2010).

The BG also receives dopaminergic input that plays a critical role in modulating striatal activity. Dopamine is projected from the ventral tegmental area and SN pars compacta to the BG and prefrontal cortex, among other brain regions. Dopamine firing patterns fluctuate between two different modes: phasic and tonic. While the phasic mode is fast-acting and spans milliseconds, the tonic mode is long-acting and can span minutes or hours. The dissociable function of both phasic and tonic dopamine is debatable (Dreher and Burnod, 2002; Assadi et al., 2009; Moustafa et al., 2013). However, various studies suggest that phasic dopamine plays a key role in synaptic plasticity and reinforcement learning (Wickens et al., 1996; Reynolds et al., 2001), while tonic dopamine is important for speeding-up reaction times (Niv et al., 2007; Moustafa et al., 2008) and controlling the signal-to-noise ratio (Durstewitz and Seamans, 2008).

Information flow through the BG follows two distinct pathways (see **Figure 1**). Striatal MSNs in the direct pathway project directly to the output nuclei (e.g., GPi) and selectively express D1-like receptors (i.e., D1 and D5; Gerfen et al., 1990). The striatal MSNs in the indirect pathway project to the external segment of the GP Globus pallidus (external) (GPe) prior to reaching the output nuclei of the BG (e.g., GPi), and selectively express D2-like receptors (i.e., D2, D3, and D4; Gerfen and Young, 1988). In addition to the direct and indirect pathways, the STN is another major input structure of the BG receiving extensive cortical and thalamic input. This so-called hyperdirect pathway provides a means by which frontal cortical regions can monosynapically influence STN function (Nambu et al., 2002).

With abundant dopamine receptors in the BG affecting the dynamics of the different pathways, most CCN models of the BG include a role for dopamine. One important way of testing whether the hypothesized role for dopamine in the model is adequate is to simulate the model under dopamine-depleted conditions. Specifically, reducing the amount of dopamine available in the model should produce Parkinsonian symptoms. Parkinson's disease (PD) is caused by the accelerated death of dopamine producing neurons. The pattern of cell loss is opposite to that of, and more severe than in, normal aging. Within the SN pars compacta, cell loss is predominately found in the ventral tier with less (but still extensive) damage in the dorsal tier (Fearnley and Lees, 1991; Gibb and Lees, 1991). In contrast, normal aging yields substantially less cell loss and in a dorsal-to-ventral pattern. Parkinsonian motor symptoms appear after a loss of 60–70% of SN pars compacta cells and 70–80% of dopamine levels in striatal nuclei (Bernheimer et al., 1973; Gibb and Lees, 1991). Motor symptoms include tremor, rigidity, bradykinesia, and akinesia. In addition to motor deficits, non-demented PD patients present cognitive symptoms that resemble those observed in patients with frontal damage. Numerous studies documenting cognitive deficits of PD patients have revealed impairment in a variety of tasks related to memory, learning, visuospatial skills, and attention (e.g., Gotham et al., 1988; Price et al., 2009).

COGNITIVE FUNCTION

While many cognitive functions have been attributed to the BG (for a review, see Steiner and Tseng, 2010), relatively few have been modeled and numerically simulated using CCN models, i.e., models that can simultaneously account for both neurobiological and behavioral data. Hence, this review does not constitute an attempt at reviewing all the cognitive and motor functions attributed to the BG: the focus is on CCN models of the BG. Note that the model descriptions included are conceptual, in that implementation details and mathematical formulations are not discussed. The reader is referred to the cited original papers for model details and equations. **Table 1** summarizes the reviewed models along with their respective components.

CATEGORIZATION

Categorization is the ubiquitous process by which individual items are grouped to form categories. The massive convergence of cortico-striatal connectivity makes the BG an ideal site for categorization, and much research supports the role of the BG in category learning (for a review, see Seger, 2008).

Models

One of the earliest and most prominent neurobiological models of categorization is called COVIS (Ashby et al., 1998). COVIS is a multiple-system theory that was originally developed to account for the many behavioral dissociations between verbal and non-verbal categorization (as described by the general recognition theory; Ashby and Gott, 1988). COVIS includes an hypothesis-testing system and a procedural learning system. The hypothesis-testing system can quickly learn a small set of (e.g., verbal) categories (those that can be found by hypothesis-testing and often be verbally described) while the procedural learning system can learn any type of arbitrary categories in a slow trial-and-error manner (e.g., non-verbal). Each categorization system relies on a separate brain circuit but, interestingly, they both include the BG. In the hypothesis-testing system, the BG is used to support working memory maintenance and for rule switching. In the procedural system, the BG is used to learn stimulus—response associations. The COVIS model of categorization has been used to simulate a large number of category learning experiments and made several behavioral predictions, many of which have been later confirmed by empirical experiments (for a review, Maddox and Ashby, 2004). For example, COVIS predicts that delaying the feedback in verbal categorization should not affect performance (because the hypothesis-testing system relies on working memory) whereas delaying feedback in non-verbal categorization should impair learning (because the procedural learning system relies on dopamine-mediated reinforcement learning in the BG). This prediction was confirmed in Ashby et al. (2003). In addition, reducing dopamine levels in COVIS can account for many cognitive symptoms in PD patients such as perseveration, reduced sensitivity to negative feedback, and others (see Helie et al., 2012a,b). Likewise, dopamine elevation can account for the effect of positive affect on verbal category learning (Helie et al., 2012b). While most COVIS simulations have used a rate version of the model, a spiking version of the procedural-learning system has been used to account for some categorization results and extended to account for instrumental conditioning (Ashby and Crossley, 2011) and automaticity (Ashby et al., 2007).

As an alternative, Moustafa and Gluck (2011a,b) proposed a computational model of the striatum and prefrontal cortex that focuses on the dopamine projections to these areas as well as their interactions during multi-cue category learning. In this task, participants learn to select and pay attention to a single cue among a multi-cue pattern, and then make a categorization response. Participants learn this task via corrective feedback. In the model, the prefrontal cortex is essential for attentional selection while

Table 1 | Summary of the basal ganglia components included in the reviewed models.

	DP (1)	IP (2)	HP (3)	Str	GPi	GPe	STN
Cognitive							
Ashby et al. (1998)	X			X	X		
Moustafa and Gluck (2011a)	X			X			
Ashby and Crossley (2011)	X			X	X		
Frank (2005)	X	X		X	X	X	
Guthrie et al. (2013)	X		X	X	X		X
Monchi et al. (2000)	X			X	X		
Ashby et al. (2005)	X			X	X		
Frank et al. (2001)	X			X	X		
Moustafa and Maida (2007)	X			X			
Schroll et al. (2012)	X		X	X	X	X	X
Nakahara et al. (2001)	X		X	X			
Ashby et al. (2007)	X			X	X		
Chersi et al. (2013)	X	X	X	X	*	X	X
Motor							
Bischoff (1998)	X	X		X	X	X	X
Magdoom et al. (2011)	X	X		X			
Gangadhar et al. (2008)		X				X	X
Contreras-Vidal and Stelmach (1995)	X	X	X	X	X	X	X
Dominey and Arbib (1992)	X			X	*		
Krishnan et al. (2011)	X	X		X	*	X	X

*Note. DP = Direct pathway [(1) in **Figure 1**]; IP = Indirect pathway [(2) in **Figure 1**]; HP = Hyperdirect pathway [(3) in **Figure 1**]; Str = Striatum; GPi = Globus pallidus (internal); GPe = Globus pallidus (external); STN = Subthalamic nucleus. * These models used the substantia nigra pars reticulate (SNr) as their output node of the basal ganglia. In this context, the SNr is functionally equivalent to the GPi.*

the striatum is used for motor response selection. Similar to COVIS, the Moustafa and Gluck (2011a,b) model can account for categorization deficits in PD patients by reducing dopamine levels in both the BG and prefrontal cortex, which is in agreement with empirical results (Kaasinen et al., 2001; Silberstein et al., 2005). Additionally, the Moustafa and Gluck (2011a,b) model can account for some effects of dopaminergic and anticholinergic medication. The Moustafa and Gluck (2011a,b) model assumes that the administration of anticholinergic medications in PD interferes with hippocampal function, which is also in agreement with empirical studies (Meco et al., 1984; Pondal et al., 1996; Ehrt et al., 2010; Herzallah et al., 2010). In contrast, the current version of COVIS has not been used to simulate medication effects in PD.

Synthesis

The reviewed models of categorization both agree that the BG, and its interaction with the prefrontal cortex, are essential for category learning. Furthermore, they agree that dopamine levels in both the BG and prefrontal cortex are important. While COVIS (Ashby et al., 1998) has been used to simulate a wider range of categorization tasks, the Moustafa and Gluck (2011a,b) model has been used to simulate more details in a smaller subset. For example, one limitation of the Moustafa and Gluck (2011a,b) model is that it does not simulate complex multi-cue learning tasks that involve paying attention to more than one stimulus (which can be done using COVIS). However, the Moustafa and Gluck (2011a,b) model can simulate the effect of dopaminergic medication, whereas COVIS has not been used to simulate medication effects. One important difference between the COVIS and Moustafa and Gluck (2011a,b) model is that COVIS assigns a different role for BG and cortical dopamine, namely error signal and signal gain (respectively). In contrast, Moustafa and Gluck (2011a,b) assign both of these roles to dopamine in both the BG and the prefrontal cortex. In addition, an important limitation of both models is that they oversimplify the anatomy of the BG by not including the indirect and hyperdirect pathways. Future work aimed at increasing the biological accuracy of COVIS and the Moustafa and Gluck (2011a,b) models may highlight some additional key differences between the modeling approaches and allow for selecting the most appropriate BG model of categorization.

INSTRUMENTAL CONDITIONING

Instrumental conditioning (also called "operant" conditioning) is a process by which animals learn to behave in a way that will maximize reward and minimize punishment. In a typical instrumental conditioning experiment, a neutral environment is altered and begins generating rewards (acquisition phase). Next, the reward is removed from the environment and the environment reverts to its neutral state (extinction phase). Extinction is usually followed by a reacquisition phase, where the reward is introduced again in the same neutral environment. Typically, a new behavior is learned during the acquisition phase, and progressively disappears during the extinction phase. The behavior reappears during the reacquisition phase, usually at a much faster rate than during the initial acquisition phase. This phenomenon is called *fast reacquisition.* Much evidence implicates the BG in instrumental conditioning (e.g., O'Doherty et al., 2004; Yin et al., 2005), but the neurobiology underlying extinction and fast reacquisition is poorly understood.

Models

Ashby and Crossley (2011) proposed a spiking model of the direct pathway of the BG (see **Figure 1**) inspired by the COVIS procedural learning system (Ashby et al., 1998) to account for instrumental conditioning. The Ashby and Crossley (2011) model focuses on the TANs, a population of cholinergic interneurons in the striatum that is rarely included in CCN models of the BG. Pakhotin and Bracci (2007) have shown that TANs play an important role in inhibiting cortical activation of the MSNs (i.e., the projection neurons generally modeled in the direct and indirect pathways). As suggested by their name, TANs have a high baseline firing rate, but they learn to pause in rewarding contexts (Apicella, 2007). Ashby and Crossley (2011) suggest that one possible role for the TANs is to protect striatal learning from catastrophic interference and allow for fast reacquisition. In addition to the direct pathway, the Ashby and Crossley (2011) model includes a sensory association area, the supplementary motor area (SMA), and the CMPf complex.

The Ashby and Crossley (2011) model is an opened loop through the BG (from sensory association cortex to the SMA). The stimulus activates the sensory association cortex, which in turn activates the striatum and the direct pathway of the BG. At the same time, the context activates the CMPf complex, which transmits activation to the TANs (this pathway is not included in **Figure 1**). At the beginning of an experiment, the simulated subject does not know that the context is rewarding. Hence, the TANs do not pause, and the MSNs in the direct pathway cannot be activated by the sensory association cortex. This prevents stimulus—response association learning. During the acquisition phase, the TANs quickly learn that the context is rewarding and pause. The MSNs are thus released from inhibition and the model learns to produce the rewarding behavior using reinforcement learning. Next, during the extinction phase, the TANs learn that the context is no longer rewarding and stop pausing. This change inhibits the MSNs and interrupts cortico-striatal learning. Hence, the associations that were learned during the acquisition phase are protected. Finally, during the reacquisition phase, the context becomes rewarding again, and the TANs learn to pause. The MSNs are released from inhibition, and the learned associations are in the same state as in the acquisition phase, which produces fast reacquisition. Using this process, the model has been used to reproduce the acquisition, extinction, and fast reacquisition phases typical of instrumental conditioning and single-cell recording data from TANs showing that the cells learn to pause in rewarding contexts (Ashby and Crossley, 2011).

Synthesis

The Ashby and Crossley (2011) model is the only CCN model of instrumental conditioning that can simultaneously account for behavioral (e.g., fast reacquisition) and single-cell data (from the TANs). This model constitutes an important step in that it provides an implementation and numerical simulation of the theory that TANs learn to pause in rewarding contexts, and how this can affect reinforcement learning in the BG. However, the neuroanatomy of the BG was simplified in that only the direct pathway through one of the cortico-BG loops was included. It is unclear at this time how the TANs' dynamics would affect the indirect pathway, or how the model would behave if more than one loops was included. Future work is needed to verify how the theory implemented in Ashby and Crossley (2011) behaves in a more detailed model of the BG.

PROBABILISTIC LEARNING

Probabilistic learning typically refers to tasks where the association between the response and the reward is uncertain. Unlike most categorization experiments, the same response to the same stimulus can result in different outcomes on different trials. While probabilistic learning has been shown to rely on the BG since the mid-1990s (Knowlton et al., 1996), it took a decade before CCN models of the BG were used to attempt to account for probabilistic learning.

Models

The Frank (2005) model was originally proposed to account for cognitive deficits in parkinsonism. The model includes both the direct and indirect pathways through the BG (see **Figure 1**), the premotor cortex, and an unspecified input area (probably located in posterior cortex) (so the model is an opened loop). In the Frank (2005) model, the input activates both the premotor cortex and the striatum. However, cortical activation is insufficient to produce a response, so BG processing is required to gate the correct response. The focus of the model is on: (1) the role of the indirect pathway in probabilistic learning and (2) the role of dopamine in probabilistic learning. In the Frank (2005) model, the direct pathway is in charge of selecting the appropriate action (Go) whereas the indirect pathway is in charge of inhibiting inappropriate actions (NoGo). The direct and indirect pathways converge in the GPi and compete to control GPi activation, and eventually the response. Simulation results show that removing the indirect pathway in the model reduces performance, suggesting that both the direct and indirect pathways are essential in probabilistic learning. In addition, the effect of the indirect pathway needs to be specific to each action (so that the indirect pathway can individually inhibit each action).

As described in the neuroanatomy section above, the competition between the direct and indirect pathways is modulated by dopamine (the second focus of the Frank (2005) model). Specifically, higher dopamine levels increase activation in the direct pathway (e.g., through D1 receptors) and reduces activation in the indirect pathway (e.g., through D2 receptors). Hence, dopamine release following unexpected rewards results in long-term potentiation (LTP) in the direct pathway and long-term depression (LTD) in the indirect pathway. In contrast, dopamine dips following the unexpected absence of a reward reduces activation and produces LTD in the direct pathway but increases activation and produces LTP in the indirect pathway. The simulation results suggest that the dynamic range of the dopamine signal is crucial in probabilistic learning and reversal learning (e.g., when the response—reward associations are changed during learning). Reducing (to simulate PD) or increasing (to simulate medication overdose) dopamine levels can result in simulated Parkinsonian symptoms (Frank, 2005).

Another interesting model of probabilistic learning was recently proposed by Guthrie et al. (2013). The Guthrie et al. (2013) model is based on an earlier computational neuroscience model of the BG that focuses on the interaction between the direct and hyperdirect pathways (Leblois et al., 2006). The Guthrie et al. (2013) model includes two cortico-BG closed-loop that interact in the striatum. The first loop is called the "cognitive" loop and is used to identify the visual symbols used in the probabilistic learning task. The second loop is called the "motor" loop and is used to select a response based on the observed symbols. Some of the corticostriatal projections affect both loops, but the rest of the circuit is segregated. In both loops, the direct pathway is in charge of selecting the correct channel (i.e., identifying the symbols or the response) while the hyperdirect pathway sends non-specific inhibition to the GPi to produce a center-surround decision process. All corticostriatal synapses are plastic (using dopamine-mediated reinforcement learning) and the cognitive loop gradually learns to bias the motor loop, thus producing faster reaction times. The model successfully reproduces both neural firing rates and behavioral data in the double-arm bandit task.

The categorization models reviewed earlier have also been applied to probabilistic learning. The Moustafa and Gluck (2011a) model focused on the role of dopamine in probabilistic learning. In addition to simulating probabilistic learning with normal dopamine levels, Moustafa and Gluck (2011a) have simulated the effect of decreased dopamine (as in PD) and the effect of dopaminergic medication in both the BG and prefrontal cortex. The COVIS model has also been used to simulate probabilistic learning (Helie et al., 2012a). While COVIS was not used to simulate medication effects, the model could account for probabilistic learning with normal and reduced (as in PD) dopamine levels (with a dosage effect such that lowest levels of dopamine produced worst performance; see Knowlton et al., 1996).

Synthesis

The reviewed models of probabilistic learning tend to be more biologically detailed than the reviewed models of categorization. Specifically, the Frank (2005) model includes the direct and indirect pathways, whereas the Guthrie et al. (2013) model includes the direct and hyperdirect pathways. In contrast, COVIS (Ashby et al., 1998) and the Moustafa and Gluck (2011a,b) models only included the direct pathway. Interestingly, however, the Frank (2005) model does not include the same details as the Guthrie et al. (2013) model. Both models include the direct pathway for action selection, and use dopamine-mediated reinforcement learning to learn corticostriatal synapses. However, the Frank (2005) model uses the indirect pathway as a channel-specific excitatory process to cancel inappropriate actions whereas Guthrie et al. (2013) use the hyperdirect pathway as a non-specific excitatory process to cancel inappropriate actions. Neither model includes both the indirect and hyperdirect pathways. While there is agreement on the need for an excitatory process to enhance the contrast between the selected and non-selected actions, the exact process is still to be determined.

While the categorization models only included the direct pathway of the BG, one of their strengths is that, in addition to their generality, they also include other brain areas. For instance, Unlike the Frank (2005) model, the Moustafa and Gluck (2011a,b) model simulates the role of prefrontal cortex and its dopamine projections, which is in agreement with empirical studies (Mulder et al., 2003; Histed et al., 2009). Also, analysis of the parameter space in the COVIS simulations challenges the role of the BG for procedural learning in probabilistic learning, and suggests instead that the BG are used for hypothesis-testing in this task (Gluck et al., 2002). So, both categorization models agree on an important role for the prefrontal cortex in probabilistic learning, and this role is missing from both the Frank (2005) and the Guthrie et al. (2013) models. The most productive future approach might be to add a prefrontal cortex to the existing probabilistic learning models and see how this addition affects the dynamic of the different BG pathways.

WORKING MEMORY

Working memory is a cognitive function used to maintain and manipulate information in real-time for a short duration (seconds). While working memory has traditionally been associated with the prefrontal cortex (Fuster, 2008), Monchi et al. (2000) proposed that the BG may be required to maintain information in prefrontal cortex.

Models

The Monchi et al. (2000) model was originally proposed to account for working memory deficits in PD and schizophrenia. The model includes three BG-thalamocortical closed loops: two with the prefrontal cortex (one for spatial information and the other for object information), and one through the ACC (for strategy selection). In all three cases, only the direct pathway through the BG was included (see **Figure 1**). The role of the two prefrontal-BG loops is to maintain working memory information about the stimuli, whereas the ACC maintains the adopted strategy by inhibiting all the prefrontal cortex loops except one (i.e., representing the selected strategy). Visual input to the BG comes from the posterior parietal cortex (spatial) and inferior temporal cortex (object). The model output is located in the premotor cortex, and the nucleus accumbens (not shown in **Figure 1**) is used to provide feedback. In the model, the visual stimulus is input to the prefrontal cortex loops, and the stimulus activity is propagated through the direct pathway of the BG. As a result, the thalamus is released from GPi inhibition, and activation produced by the stimulus in the prefrontal cortex reverberates through closed-loops with the thalamus. When a response is required, the prefrontal cortex transfers its activation to the premotor cortex. If the response is incorrect, the nucleus accumbens sends a feedback signal to the ACC loop, which selects a new strategy by switching its inhibition to different prefrontal cortex loops. The Monchi et al. (2000) model has been used to simulate a delayed response task and the Wisconsin Card Sorting Test. Interestingly, reducing the connection strengths within the BG-thalamocortical loops produces Parkinsonian symptoms, whereas reducing nucleus accumbens activity produces deficits similar to those observed in schizophrenia (Monchi et al., 2000).

Five years later, Ashby et al. (2005) proposed the FROST model to account for intact spatial working memory maintenance. Similar to the Monchi et al. (2000) model, FROST includes the direct pathway of the BG (see **Figure 1**), and working memory maintenance relies on reverberating activation between the prefrontal cortex and the thalamus. However, unlike in the Monchi et al. (2000) model, only one prefrontal cortex loop is included, and thalamic activation is not sufficient to maintain prefrontal activity: a second set of closed-loops between the prefrontal cortex and posterior cortex needs to be simultaneously activated to maintain working memory information. In Ashby et al. (2005), the focus is on simulating spatial working memory tasks, and the area of posterior cortex required for working memory maintenance is the posterior parietal cortex. However, it is likely the case that the specific location in posterior cortex depends on what information is being maintained. For instance, if the items being maintained in working memory were objects, then it is likely that the posterior cortex area involved would be inferior temporal cortex. Another difference between FROST and the Monchi et al. (2000) model is that the striatum in FROST is activated by a different population of prefrontal neurons (separate from the working memory maintenance prefrontal population) whereas the same prefrontal neurons are used to activate the striatum and maintain information in Monchi et al. (2000). As a result, the striatum becomes activated only after the stimulus has disappeared in FROST, whereas the striatum becomes activated as soon as the stimulus appears in Monchi et al. (2000). These differences between FROST and Monchi et al. (2000) were motivated by recent single-cell recording results reviewed in Ashby et al. (2005). FROST has been used to reproduce single-cell recordings from many experiments in several brain regions, in addition to accounting for working memory capacity limitation and the relation between memory span and the ability to ignore distracting information (Ashby et al., 2005).

One common theme of the two previous models is that working memory activity is maintained by closed-loops between the thalamus and prefrontal cortex, and the main role of the BG is to release the thalamus from inhibition and allow for the reverberating activation to take place. However, this view was challenged by Frank et al. (2001) who proposed a model of BG-prefrontal cortex interaction in working memory. Specifically, Frank et al. (2001) argued that in order for the thalamus to contribute to working memory maintenance in the way described by the previous models, it would need to have a dedicated number of cells comparable to the number of cells dedicated to working memory in prefrontal cortex (which is unlikely). Instead, the Frank et al. (2001) model proposes that working memory maintenance is accomplished by reverberating loops between two cell populations within the prefrontal cortex. Similar to Monchi et al. (2000) and FROST (Ashby et al., 2005), the Frank et al. (2001) model includes the direct pathway through the BG (see **Figure 1**), but the role of the direct pathway is to "turn on the switch" on the prefrontal cortex cells and allow for reverberating activation. The "switch" can only be turned on if the prefrontal cortex cells from one population simultaneously receive activation from the BG and the other prefrontal cortex cell population. Once the switch is "on", the BG is no longer required for working memory maintenance. The Frank et al. (2001) model has been used to simulate the 1-2-AX task, a working memory task that requires maintenance but also switching and selecting new items (Frank et al., 2001). Specifically, the 1-2-AX task requires the subject to maintain two cues in working memory in order to correctly select a response to a target sequence. The identity of the target sequence depends on the previous cue, which is used to trigger selection and switching.

One topic that was not addressed by any of the previous models of working memory is learning. How can the brain learn what is important, and what needs to be maintained in working memory? Moustafa and Maida (2007) proposed a computational model of prefrontal cortex and BG interactions that is similar to the Frank et al. (2001) model except that Moustafa and Maida (2007) also simulate: (a) temporal difference learning based on phasic dopamine signaling and (b) more than one corticostriatal loops that are responsible for both motor and cognitive processes. Specifically, the model includes a cortico-striatal motor loop and a cortico-striatal cognitive loop whose functions are action selection (choosing motor responses) and cognitive selection (choosing the perceptual information to be maintained in working memory), respectively. The model can account for the separate roles of the motor and cognitive loops in working memory maintenance, including delayed-response tasks.

Schroll et al. (2012) recently proposed a CCN model of working memory to address the problem of learning complex working memory tasks. The Schroll et al. (2012) model includes two separate BG-thalamocortical closed loops, one through the prefrontal cortex for maintenance and another through motor cortex to produce a response. Only the direct pathways were used for maintenance and response selection, but the hyperdirect pathway was also included in the prefrontal loop as a reset mechanism (see **Figure 1**). Specifically, visual information enters the model through the inferior temporal cortex, which then activates the lateral prefrontal cortex. This activation is transferred through the direct pathway of the BG and releases the thalamus from inhibition, which in turn activates the lateral prefrontal cortex. In the Schroll et al. (2012) model, working memory activation in the prefrontal cortex is maintained by a reverberating activation loop through the direct pathway, so the BG does not only act as a gating mechanism but is part of the maintenance loop (unlike Monchi et al., 2000; Frank et al., 2001; Ashby et al., 2005). At any moment, the prefrontal cortex can activate the STN, which increases activation in the GPi and interrupt working memory maintenance (i.e., the reset mechanism). More importantly, the connectivity between the prefrontal cortex and the striatum and the connections between the prefrontal cortex and the STN are learned using dopamine-mediated reinforcement learning. Hence, the model can automatically adapt and only maintain information that is rewarded in working memory. The model has been used to simulate a delayed response task, a delayed alternation task, and the 1-2-AX task (Schroll et al., 2012).

Synthesis

Working memory is one of the most active areas for CCN modeling of the BG. Five different models were reviewed, each having both commonalities and differences. First, all five models focused on the interaction between the BG and the prefrontal cortex, but only included the direct pathway of the BG for working memory maintenance and response selection. Hence, the neuroanatomy of the BG was not very detailed. Also, all models except Schroll et al. (2012) used the BG as a gating mechanism that turns working memory maintenance "on" or "off". The main difference is that Monchi et al. (2000) and Ashby et al. (2005) used the BG to gate closed loops between the prefrontal cortex and the thalamus, whereas Frank et al. (2001) and Moustafa and Maida (2007) used the BG to gate closed loop between two populations of prefrontal cortex units. This differs from Schroll et al. (2012) where the BG was not used for gating, but instead was part of the working memory maintenance mechanism itself (i.e., the closed loop went through the BG). In all cases, however, working memory maintenance was achieved by closed loop through the prefrontal cortex.

Another important difference between the models is that the Ashby et al. (2005) and the Moustafa and Maida (2007) models focused on simple maintenance tasks. In contrast, the Monchi et al. (2000), Frank et al. (2001), and Schroll et al. (2012) models were able to simulate more complex tasks involving hierarchical structures and switching. Only the Moustafa and Maida (2007) and the Schroll et al. (2012) models include learning mechanisms that allowed for selecting the relevant information that needs to be maintained in working memory. The other models assumed a pre-filtering of the information.

Interestingly, there seems to be a progression and a building up of knowledge related to CCN models of working memory. The Schroll et al. (2012) model is the most recent, and also the most detailed. It is the only model that can learn and simulate complex tasks. However, this model departs from all the others in that the BG is not used as a gating mechanism but is part of the maintenance mechanism. This departure from previous modeling is not extensively discussed in Schroll et al. (2012), and it is unclear at this point what motivated this departure. More work is needed to determine which of these two roles the BG play in working memory, but the overlap in the models, and the progression in functionality, suggest a steady progress in CCN modeling of working memory.

SEQUENCE LEARNING

Almost all our everyday behaviors and cognitive activities can be interpreted as a sequence of steps that bring us closer to achieving a goal. One key question is how can we learn to chain these sequences of substeps? Miyachi et al. (1997, 2002) have gathered much data suggesting that the BG is important in learning such sequences.

Models

Nakahara et al. (2001) formalized Miyachi et al. (1997, 2002) findings into a CCN model. According to Nakahara et al. (2001), sequences are learned in both visual and motor coordinates. The visual sequences are learned by a BG-thalamocortical closed-loop linking the anterior striatum with the dorsolateral prefrontal cortex while motor sequences are learned by a BG-thalamocortical closed-loop linking the posterior striatum with the SMA. Only the direct pathway through the BG is included in each loop (see **Figure 1**), and both the visual and motor loops learn every sequence in parallel using reinforcement learning. The visual loop learns faster than the motor loop, and response coordination between the loops is controlled by the pre-SMA. According to Nakahara et al. (2001), the visual loop relies on working memory and is important for rapid acquisition of sequences. However, the motor loop is more reliable and produces movement more rapidly after training. As a result, control is gradually transferred from the visual loop to the motor loop in the Nakahara et al. (2001) model. The Nakahara et al. (2001) model has been used to account for: (1) the time course of learning (including single-cell recordings and lesion studies); (2) the effect of opposite hand use; (3) the effect of sequence reversal; and (4) the change in brain locus from early to late sequence production (Nakahara et al., 2001).

Synthesis

The Nakahara et al. (2001) model is interesting for several reasons. First, it successfully accounts for lesion data, single-cell recordings, and behavioral phenomena. In addition, the transition from a visual loop to a motor loop represents an early attempt at bridging the gap between cognitive and motor functions of the BG. However, a recent study by Desmurget and Turner (2010) challenges the generality of the Nakahara et al. (2001) model. Specifically, Desmurget and Turner (2010) had monkeys perform a sequence of visually-cued joystick movements aimed at moving a cursor into a pre-determined part of a computer screen. After some training, muscimol was injected into the motor segment of the GPi to functionally disconnect the BG from the frontal cortex. The results show that the kinematics of the movements were impaired, but not sequence knowledge. Desmurget and Turner (2010) interpreted these results as suggesting that the BG contributes to motor execution in automatic sequence production, but not to the motor sequencing or the storage of the overlearned sequence. This result is problematic for the Nakahara et al. (2001) model.

AUTOMATICITY

Automaticity results from overtraining in a task until performance requires little attentional resources and becomes highly rigid (Helie et al., 2010; Helie and Cousineau, 2011). Many computational models of automaticity development have assigned a role for the BG.

Models

First, in the Nakahara et al. (2001) model of sequence learning (above), automaticity in sequence production is characterized by a gradual transfer from the visual loop (which learns sequences in visual coordinates) to the motor loop (which learns sequences in motor coordinates). This corresponds well with the results of Miyachi et al. (1997, 2002), who showed using single-cell recordings that task-sensitive cells in early learning are mostly located in the anterior striatum whereas selective cells in late sequence production are mostly located in the posterior striatum (Miyachi et al., 2002). This specialization of the striatum is further supported by inactivation studies where muscimol (a GABA agonist) was injected in different parts of the striatum in early and late sequence production. Well-learned sequence production was selectively disrupted by muscimol injection in the middle-posterior putamen while early sequence production was selectively disrupted by muscimol injection in the anterior caudate and putamen (Miyachi et al., 1997).

However, a recent study by Desmurget and Turner (2010) challenges the generality of the Nakahara et al. (2001) model. Specifically, injecting muscimol into the motor segment of the GPi to functionally disconnect the BG from the frontal cortex affects the kinematics of the movements but not sequence knowledge. These results suggest that the BG contributes to motor execution in automatic sequence production, but not to the motor sequencing or the storage of the overlearned sequence. Interestingly, the results of Desmurget and Turner (2010) are consistent with a neurobiological model of automaticity in perceptual categorization (SPEED) (Ashby et al., 2007). SPEED uses the procedural system of COVIS (Ashby et al., 1998) (i.e., the direct pathway of an opened loop between posterior cortex and premotor areas) but also includes a Hebbian learning mechanism between posterior cortex and premotor areas. The role of the BG in SPEED is to learn to produce the correct categorization responses early in training to ensure that the correct motor plan in the premotor areas is consistently activated shortly after the visual representation in associative cortex (using dopamine-mediated reinforcement learning). This consistent association between associative and premotor cortical activity triggers Hebbian learning between associative cortex (stimulus) and the premotor areas (response), and the direct cortico-cortical connections eventually become strong enough so that the BG is no longer required to produce a response. When responding becomes purely cortical, the skill is said to be "automatic" [note that this is different from Nakahara et al. (2001), in which the posterior striatum is still required for automatic sequence production]. SPEED has been used to simulate single-cell recordings data in many categorization experiments, as well as human reaction times and accuracies in categorization (Ashby et al., 2007; Helie and Ashby, 2009).

While the Hikosaka et al. (2000) and SPEED models can account for how behavior becomes automatic, they cannot account for how automatic responses are overridden by goal-directed behavior when needed (e.g., when the stimulus—response associations change). Chersi et al. (2013) proposed a computational model of automaticity in instrumental conditioning that can account for the change back to goal-directed behavior when needed. The Chersi et al. (2013) model includes the prefrontal cortex (for goal representation), the motor cortex (for action representation), the sensory cortex (for stimulus representation), the BG (for action selection), and the thalamus (to relay information between the BG and the motor cortex). Two sets of connections are plastic: (1) connections from the prefrontal cortex to the motor cortex (to learn goal—response associations) and (2) connections from the sensory cortex to the striatum (to learn stimulus—response associations). According to this model, the stimulus activates the sensory cortex, which in turn activates a goal in prefrontal cortex and action representations in the striatum. For automatic behavior, the striatal activation propagates through both the direct and indirect pathways (see **Figure 1**) of the BG and an action is selected by inhibiting all but one action at the output level (SNr, but it is functionally equivalent to the GPi shown in **Figure 1**). The action that is not inhibited activates the appropriate response in motor cortex (through the thalamus). For goal-directed behaviors, the prefrontal activation propagates to the appropriate action in motor cortex. When an automatic action needs to be overwritten by a goal-directed behavior, the prefrontal cortex sends activation to the STN, which hyperpolarizes the SNr and prevents the BG from controlling the motor response (Chersi et al., 2013). The model has been successfully used to account for the development of automaticity in an instrumental conditioning task and the reversal of stimulus—response associations after automaticity had developed (Chersi et al., 2013).

Synthesis

The Nakahara et al. (2001) and the Chersi et al. (2013) models both assign the role of producing automatic behavior to the BG. However, this "classic" role of the BG in automaticity is difficult to reconcile with the Desmurget and Turner (2010) data. As an alternative, SPEED (Ashby et al., 2007) also assigns an important role to the BG in automaticity, but this role is restricted to training automatic cortico-cortical projections that can account for automaticity. Simply put, the BG is required to learn automatic behaviors, but the BG is no longer required to produce automatic behaviors once the cortico-cortical connectivity is sufficiently strong. The SPEED model can account for the Desmurget and Turner (2010) data, but it includes only the direct pathway of one loop through the BG. In contrast, the Nakahara et al. (2001) model includes two loops through the BG (only the direct pathways) and the Chersi et al. (2013) model includes both the direct and indirect pathways, but only one loop through the BG (similar to SPEED). In addition to being the most biologically detailed, the Chersi et al. (2013) model is the only reviewed model that can override automatic behavior using goal-directed behavior. This is an important function that was not accounted for by the previous models. However, like the Nakahara et al. (2001) model, the Chersi et al. (2013) model cannot account for the Desmurget and Turner (2010) data. To summarize, each one of these models was designed to account for a different aspect of automatic behavior, and successfully accounts for the aspect of automaticity for which it was designed. The next step is to explore how each one of these candidate models can account for the missing function/data that was the focus of the other candidate models.

MOTOR FUNCTION

This section describes motor functions that have been attributed to the BG and that have been simulated using CCN models. Hence, computational models that focus only on modeling biological data or motor function (e.g., kinematics) were not included. Similar to the section reviewing cognitive functions above, the model descriptions are conceptual, in that implementation details and formalities are not discussed. The reader is referred to the cited original papers for details and equations. **Table 1** summarizes the reviewed models along with their respective components.

REACHING

The BG has been implicated in reaching movements for many years (for a review, see Bischoff, 1998). Not surprisingly, PD patients show unmistakable changes in reaching movements, which can be used for diagnostic purposes (Brown and Jahanshahi, 1996). Simple reaching movements in PD patients show longer reaction times and movement times than normal controls. This reduced movement speed seen in PD reaching is called bradykinesia. From a physiological perspective, a typical reaching movement under normal conditions consists of a sequence of agonist-antagonist bursts. In contrast, a PD reaching movement is generally multi-staged and involves multiple agonist bursts. Furthermore, PD reaching movements have greater variability of hand position for larger movements (Sheridan and Flowers, 1990). PD patients also show impairment in sequential movements (Weiss et al., 1997). For example, during movements aimed at reaching a glass of water, PD patients exhibit an inordinately long pause between the reaching and retrieval of the glass.

Models

Several computational models relating dopamine deficiencies to impaired reaching movements have been proposed. One of the first models of PD reaching movements is the model of Bischoff (1998). Bischoff (1998) model includes the prefrontal cortex (for working memory/learning), the SMA (for sequence generation), the pre-SMA (for sequence preparation), motor cortex (for movement parameters), the thalamus (to filter information from the BG to cortex), and the BG. The BG model assigns complementary roles to the direct and indirect pathways (see **Figure 1**). According to Bischoff (1998), the role of the direct pathway is to inform the motor cortex of the movement's next sensory state, while the role of the indirect pathway is to inhibit competing movements. The function of dopamine is to keep the balance between the two pathways, which is impaired in PD. The Bischoff (1998) model was used to simulate the reciprocal aiming task, a task where subjects are asked to alternatively tap a stylus between two targets as quickly as possible. Reducing the dopamine levels in the simulation reproduced bradykinesia and the exaggerated pauses in sequential movements observed in PD.

Magdoom et al. (2011) also proposed a model of the role of the BG in PD reaching movements. The model is cast in the framework of reinforcement learning and focuses on interactions between the motor cortex and the BG. The Magdoom et al. (2011) model uses the classical interpretations of BG pathways according to which the direct pathway facilitates movement, (i.e., the "Go" pathway), while the indirect pathway inhibits movements (i.e., the "NoGo" pathway). Switching between the two pathways is thought to be driven by striatal dopamine levels. However, Magdoom et al. (2011) also deviate from the classical "Go"/"NoGo" model of the BG by adding an intermediate regime called the *explore* regime. The explore regime is used to control the stochasticity of action selection when the gradient is absent or too weak to allow for reinforcement learning. The indirect pathway is proposed to be the substrate supporting the explore regime. Simulations show that under dopamine-deficient conditions of PD, the model spends less time in the "Go" regime while spending more time in the remaining two regimes. These regime changes were used to account for a variety of features of impaired reaching movements in PD including movement undershoot (Van Gemmert et al., 2003), bradykinesia, and increased path variability (Sheridan and Flowers, 1990).

Synthesis

Two models that highlight the role of the BG in reaching were reviewed. The Bischoff (1998) model includes, in addition to the BG, cortical areas such as prefrontal areas, the SMA and the pre-SMA. The model captures bradykinesia and abnormal pauses in sequential movements under Parkinsonian conditions. The reaching model of Magdoom et al. (2011) also incorporates the BG and the motor cortex. However, the Magdoom et al. (2011) model is cast in the framework of reinforcement learning, whereas there is no learning in the Bischoff (1998) model. Focus on learning makes the Magdoom et al. (2011) model consistent with the proposed role of BG in error correction (Lawrence, 2000). As a result, the Magdoom et al. (2011) model is more general and is consistent with the view that a wide range of BG functions can be explained within the framework of reinforcement learning (Chakravarthy et al., 2010). The compatibility of the Magdoom et al. (2011) model with other CCN models of BG function may facilitate integration to achieve a more complete model of BG function.

HANDWRITING

Handwriting is a fine motor skill. PD patients often exhibit an impaired form of handwriting, known as micrographia, characterized by reduced letter size, a "kinky" handwriting contour, and abnormal fluctuations in velocity and acceleration (Teulings and Stelmach, 1991; Van Gemmert et al., 1999; Gangadhar et al., 2009). As a result, handwriting features like stroke size, peak acceleration, and stroke duration have been attributed to the BG and used for diagnosis of PD (Phillips et al., 1991; Van Gemmert et al., 2003).

Models

Although models of PD handwriting are scanty, extensive work has been done on modeling handwriting generation. One of the earliest insights into modeling handwriting consisted of performing a Fourier-like resolution of handwriting into oscillatory components (Hollerbach, 1981). This notion has led to the development of oscillatory or spiking neural network models of handwriting generation that can be trained to produce single characters (Schomaker, 1991; Kalveram, 1998). However, the models of Schomaker (1991) and Kalveram (1998) suffered from the absence of a plausible procedure for initializing the phases of neural oscillators, a difficulty that was solved in an oscillatory neural network model of handwriting generation proposed by Gangadhar et al. (2007).

While the above-described models did not explicitly include the BG, Gangadhar et al. (2008) combined the Gangadhar et al. (2007) handwriting generation model with a model of the BG. Similar to handwriting patterns observed in PD patients, the Gangadhar et al. (2008) model exhibits micrographia under conditions of reduced dopamine. Another significant feature of the model is the role of the dynamics of the STN and the GPe, which are connected as a loop to produce complex oscillations. Under pathological conditions, the oscillations of the STN and the GPe in the model are highly correlated, resembling the correlated neural firing from STN and GPe neurons under dopamine-deficient conditions observed in real electrophysiology experiments (Bergman et al., 1994; Brown et al., 2001). Under the influence of correlated oscillations of STN and GPe, the Gangadhar et al. (2008) model produces handwriting with large fluctuations in velocity in addition to diminutive letter size.

As another example, Contreras-Vidal and Stelmach (1995) attached a BG model to the VITE-WRITE model (Bullock et al., 1993) to simulate PD handwriting. The Contreras-Vidal and Stelmach (1995) model includes the direct, indirect, and hyperdirect pathways of the BG (see **Figure 1**), the SMA, and other motor and premotor areas. The role of the SMA is to read-in the next motor subprogram from the movement plan, while the role of the other motor and premotor areas is to produce the movement selected by the SMA. The role of the BG is to modulate the dynamics of the formation of movement trajectories (produced by VITE-WRITE). Reducing dopamine in the model to simulate PD results in reduced letter size, as observed in PD patients.

Synthesis

Two models of PD handwriting were reviewed above. The model of Contreras-Vidal and Stelmach (1995) combines the VITE-WRITE model (Bullock et al., 1993) with a BG model. The essence of the model consists of showing that dopamine reduction in PD causes an imbalance in the outputs of the direct and indirect pathways. Although constructed out of considerably different modeling components, the model of Gangadhar et al. (2008) also shows an imbalance in the activations of the direct and indirect pathways under simulated PD conditions, which causes a reduction in letter size. In addition, Gangadhar et al. (2008) also account for the oscillations in STN-GPe interaction. Loss of complexity in these oscillations under PD conditions were linked to higher velocity fluctuations and distorted handwriting contour in PD handwriting. To summarize, the indirect pathway appears to be critical in accounting for handwriting.

EYE SACCADES

Eye saccades are rapid, darting eye movements that shift the fovea to points of interest in the visual scene. There is an extensive cortical and subcortical network that is responsible for saccade generation, and the BG play a key role among the subcortical substrates for saccade generation (Hikosaka et al., 2000). The influence of BG on saccades is propagated via the superior colliculus, a midbrain nucleus with a central role in saccade generation (not shown in **Figure 1**). Studies on Parkinsonian monkeys prepared by MPTP (a neurotoxin used to destroy dopaminergic neurons) infusion have observed prolonged saccades, longer reaction times, smaller peak velocities, and smaller amplitudes (Kato et al., 1995). Smaller peak velocities and smaller amplitudes in PD saccades may be comparable to bradykinesia and hypometria found in

PD reaching movements. Similarly, analogous to PD tremor in extremities, some PD patients exhibit square-wave jerks in visually guided saccades (Rascol et al., 1991).

Models

Computational modeling literature that specifically focuses on the role of BG in saccade generation is rather limited. Dominey and Arbib (1992) proposed a model of the role of the BG in sequential saccade generation. Their model includes a number of relevant neural substrates such as the superior colliculus, thalamus, frontal eye fields, and the BG. In the Dominey and Arbib (1992) model, the BG is used as an indirect link between the frontal eye field and the superior colliculus, and its main function is to prevent saccades while a target stimulus is foveated. As such, only the direct pathway through the BG is modeled. The Dominey and Arbib (1992) model has been used to simulate simple saccade data, memory saccade data, double saccade data, compensatory saccade data, and lesion data.

Two decades later, Krishnan et al. (2011) proposed a model of the role of the BG in saccade generation using the principle of reinforcement learning. Similar to their model of PD reaching movement (Magdoom et al., 2011), the indirect pathway serves as an explorer that drives the saccades toward more rewarding targets. The model was able to successfully simulate two forms of visual search, namely feature search and conjunction search, a sequential saccade task, and a directional saccade task. When PD-related changes were incorporated in the model by reducing BG output, the model exhibited increased search times (Krishnan et al., 2011).

Synthesis

Two models of the role of BG in saccade generation were reviewed above (Dominey and Arbib, 1992; Krishnan et al., 2011). Both models can account for a range of saccade data in normal and lesioned/pathological conditions. The anatomical components incorporated by the two models are also quite similar. However, there are two main distinguishing features between the two models. One of these features is anatomical: the Dominey and Arbib (1992) model does not include the indirect pathway in the BG, whereas the indirect pathway plays a key role in the Krishnan et al. (2011) model. The second feature is functional: the Dominey and Arbib (1992) model does not involve learning, while that of Krishnan et al. (2011) model is based on reinforcement learning. These key differences make the Krishnan et al. (2011) model more biologically and functionally detailed.

GENERAL DISCUSSION

This article presented a review of CCN models of cognitive and motor functions. The 19 reviewed models were organized to highlight BG functionality and classified according to six cognitive functions (i.e., categorization, instrumental conditioning, probabilistic learning, working memory, sequence learning, and automaticity) and three motor functions (i.e., reaching, handwriting, and visual saccades). On the one hand, some of the reviewed models are standalone models of specific functions of BG, e.g., the reaching model of Bischoff (1998). On the other hand, there are models that are specific instances of a more general learning framework applied to BG function. COVIS (Ashby et al., 1998, 2007; Ashby and Crossley, 2011), and the models of Chakravarthy and colleagues (Krishnan et al., 2011; Magdoom et al., 2011) belong to the second category. For example, both the models of Krishnan et al. (2011) and Magdoom et al. (2011) used a nearly identical reinforcement learning-based approach to account for the specific motor functions of reaching and saccade generation. A review article by Chakravarthy et al. (2010) proposes that an expanded framework based on reinforcement learning, adapted to BG anatomy and physiology, can be used to explain a wide variety of BG functions. Such a proposal needs a more extensive modeling and experimental investigation for further confirmation. However, interestingly, CCN models accounting for more than one function were accounting for more than one cognitive function or more than one motor function. None of the reviewed CCN models could account for at least one motor and one cognitive function simultaneously. This may be a serious limitation as behavioral experiments are beginning to reveal important interactions between motor and cognitive processes. Below, we discuss how cognitive processes might impact motor function, and point to novel directions for computational modeling studies.

INTERACTION OF MOTOR AND COGNITIVE PROCESSES

While none of the models included simultaneously accounted cognitive and motor functions, they all had a cognitive and motor component. For example, the Ashby and Crossley (2011) model made a cognitive decision, but it also included premotor areas associated with the response. It just did not include a detailed model of the motor response (e.g., how is the left button pressed). Likewise, the Gangadhar et al. (2007) has to include a cognitive component specifying what character is to be drawn. However, the focus is on how the movement is produced. Perhaps the model that comes closest to integrating motor and cognitive functions is the model of Guthrie et al. (2013). In this model, both a cognitive and a motor decision are taken, and the interaction between these decisions is accounted for. However, this model does not include a detailed simulation of how the movement is produced. Therefore, it was only discussed in the context of cognitive function.

One way to explore how cognitive and motor functions interact is to explore disease states. For example, akinesia and bradykinesia in PD are arguably associated with BG (and corticostriatal circuits) dysfunction, while tremor is perhaps associated with cerebellar, thalamic, and STN abnormalities (Kassubek et al., 2002; Probst-Cousin et al., 2003; Weinberger et al., 2009; Zaidel et al., 2009; Mure et al., 2011). For example, Schillaci et al. (2011) found that PD patients with akinesia and rigidity as the predominant symptoms have significantly more widespread dopamine loss in the striatum than PD patients with tremor as the predominant symptom. Because these different brain areas (e.g., striatum, cerebellum) are also involved in different cognitive functions, it is reasonable to hypothesize that different PD motor symptoms may be associated with different cognitive impairments. Accordingly, Jankovic et al. (1990) found that PD patients with predominant tremor are less cognitively impaired than patients with bradykinesia. Below we explore some specific PD motor symptoms and their relation to cognition.

Akinesia

Experimental studies have shown that PD patients with severe akinesia are generally more cognitively impaired than PD patients with predominant tremor (Vakil and Herishanu-Naaman, 1998; Poletti et al., 2011, 2012; Poletti and Bonuccelli, 2013). For instance, PD patients with severe akinesia and rigidity symptoms are more impaired than PD patients with severe resting tremor at working memory tasks (Moustafa et al., 2013). Likewise, studies have shown that PD patients with tremor are usually less cognitively impaired than PD patients with akinesia or gait dysfunction (Burn et al., 2006; Lyros et al., 2008; Oh et al., 2009; Domellof et al., 2011). For example, Vakil and Herishanu-Naaman (1998) found that tremor-dominant PD patients are less impaired at procedural learning than akinesia-dominant PD patients.

Most motor models of the BG and corticostriatal circuit function have been able to explain the occurrence of akinesia and bradykinesia, but not tremor (Obeso et al., 2008). We suggest that motor performance may rely on cognitive processes in two different ways: (a) maintenance of motor plans in working memory while performing a sequence of movements, such as hand/leg movement, grasping, or reaching (Hayhoe et al., 2002; Ohbayashi et al., 2003; Piek et al., 2004; Issen and Knill, 2012); or (b) maintenance of goals in working memory while performing a motor act, such as maintaining the goal of grasping the cup in working memory while moving the hands (Batuev, 1989; McIntyre et al., 1998; Matsumoto et al., 2003). This relationship between cognitive and motor processes could explain why some cognitive training programs are effective at treating motor dysfunction in PD patients (Disbrow et al., 2012). Although this is speculative, computational models are needed to explicitly study the complex relationship between motor and cognitive processes in healthy subjects and PD patients.

Freezing of gait

Freezing of gait—paroxysmal cessation of motor output—is a common symptom in advanced PD (Hoehn and Yahr stage 2+) (Giladi et al., 1992). Freezing of gait is debilitating since it often leads to falls and, importantly, is not manageable by common psychopharmacological medications (Giladi et al., 1992; Matar et al., 2013).

Research shows that perceptual and cognitive factors play a role in successful locomotion and the occurrence of freezing of gait episodes in PD patients (Lewis and Barker, 2009; Naismith et al., 2010; Matar et al., 2013). For example, providing auditory or visual cues or instructions can often reduce the occurrence of freezing behavior in PD patients (Lewis and Barker, 2009). Other studies found that walking dysfunction in PD is related to difficulty in resolving response interference produced by distractors (Plotnik et al., 2011; Vandenbossche et al., 2011). Locomotive dysfunction in PD is associated with brain volume changes (Kostic et al., 2012; Tessitore et al., 2012) and aberrant neural activity within the prefrontal cortex (Matsui et al., 2005; Shine et al., 2013), suggesting a role for cognitive processes in locomotion.

There are currently no computational models that simulate the role of cognitive processes in the occurrence of freezing of gait in PD patients. Prior computational models of BG-cortex interactions have focused on the simulation of cognitive processes (O'Reilly and Frank, 2006), learning, or simple action selection in static environments (Gurney et al., 2001) without considering how cognitive factors might affect motor actions such as locomotion. Future models should simulate how the cortex represents multiple inputs (including perceptual and cognitive) that feed into the BG, which is important for action selection (e.g., move right, left, forward, etc.). Future models should also be more dynamical in that they should continuously receive and update perceptual input from the environment and produce motor output (step right, left, . . .), which then takes the model to a new perceptual input, and so forth.

WHAT IS THE ROLE OF THE BASAL GANGLIA IN COGNITIVE AND MOTOR FUNCTION?

In addition to the current unavailability of CCN models of the BG that can simultaneously account for cognitive and motor function, another limitation of the current state of BG modeling is the absence of consensus on the specific function of the BG in a given task. For example, many CCN models of working memory assign a role for the BG, but some models use the BG as a gating mechanism allowing for thalamo-cortical loops (e.g., Monchi et al., 2000; Ashby et al., 2005), while others use the BG as a gating mechanism for cortico-cortical loops (e.g., Frank et al., 2001) or as the actual maintenance mechanism (Schroll et al., 2012). As with many other cognitive and motor functions, CCN models are critical in pinpointing the specific function of the BG in the cognitive task (e.g., working memory). Computational models can be simulated to identify the consequences of different design choices, and these predictions need to be tested empirically. While models tend to do very well at simulating the function that motivated the model, it is unclear at this point how the model can handle other (different) functions. One way to select useful BG CCN models is to consider generalization capabilities. Towards this end, general integrative frameworks are most useful. For example, the reinforcement learning approach of Chakravarthy and colleagues (Krishnan et al., 2011; Magdoom et al., 2011) or the COVIS-based approach of Ashby and colleagues (Ashby et al., 1998; Apicella, 2007; Ashby and Crossley, 2011) are useful because they have been used to account for functions that were outside of the original scope of the model. Other models of cognitive and motor functions need to be generalized to account for data for which they were not originally designed to build biological "cognitive architectures". Frameworks that are already general should attempt to bridge the gap between CCN models of cognitive function and CCN models of motor function. This could be achieved by integrating existing models. For example, a detailed CCN model of motor function could be added to the COVIS framework. Likewise, a detailed CCN model of cognitive function could be added to the reinforcement-learning-based approach of Chakravarthy and colleagues. While more data will help in eliminating some of the candidate CCN BG models, generalization and integration will be required to avoid overfitting the model to the available data.

REFERENCES

Apicella, P. (2007). Leading tonically active neurons of the striatum from reward detection to context recognition. *Trends Neurosci.* 30, 299–306. doi: 10.1016/j.tins.2007.03.011

Ashby, F. G., Alfonso-Reese, L. A., Turken, A. U., and Waldron, E. M. (1998). A neuropsychological theory of multiple systems in category learning. *Psychol. Rev.* 105, 442–481. doi: 10.1037//0033-295x.105.3.442

Ashby, F. G., and Crossley, M. J. (2011). A computational model of how cholinergic interneurons protect striatal-dependent learning. *J. Cogn. Neurosci.* 23, 1549–1566. doi: 10.1162/jocn.2010.21523

Ashby, F. G., Ell, S. W., Valentin, V. V., and Casale, M. B. (2005). FROST: a distributed neurocomputational model of working memory maintenance. *J. Cogn. Neurosci.* 17, 1728–1743. doi: 10.1162/089892905774589271

Ashby, F. G., Ell, S. W., and Waldron, E. M. (2003). Procedural learning in perceptual categorization. *Mem. Cognit.* 31, 1114–1125. doi: 10.3758/bf03196132

Ashby, F. G., Ennis, J. M., and Spiering, B. J. (2007). A neurobiological theory of automaticity in perceptual categorization. *Psychol. Rev.* 114, 632–656. doi: 10.1037/0033-295x.114.3.632

Ashby, F. G., and Gott, R. E. (1988). Decision rules in the perception and categorization of multidimensional stimuli. *J. Exp. Psychol. Learn. Mem. Cogn.* 14, 33–53. doi: 10.1037/0278-7393.14.1.33

Ashby, F. G., and Helie, S. (2011). A tutorial on computational cognitive neuroscience: modeling the neurodynamics of cognition. *J. Math. Psychol.* 55, 273–289. doi: 10.1016/j.jmp.2011.04.003

Assadi, S. M., Yucel, M., and Pantelis, C. (2009). Dopamine modulates neural networks involved in effort-based decision-making. *Neurosci. Biobehav. Rev.* 33, 383–393. doi: 10.1016/j.neubiorev.2008.10.010

Batuev, A. S. (1989). Neuronal mechanisms of goal-directed behaviour in monkeys. *Int. J. Neurosci.* 44, 59–66. doi: 10.3109/00207458908986183

Bergman, H., Whichman, T., Karmon, B., and DeLong, M. R. (1994). The primate subthalamic nucleus. II. neural activity in MPTP model of Parkinsonism. *J. Neurophysiol.* 72, 507–520.

Bernheimer, H., Birkmayer, W., Hornykiewicz, O., Jellinger, K., and Seitelberger, F. (1973). Brain dopamine and the syndromes of Parkinson and huntington clinical, morphological and neurochemical correlations. *J. Neurol. Sci.* 20, 415–455. doi: 10.1016/0022-510x(73)90175-5

Bischoff, A. (1998). *Modeling the Basal Ganglia in the Control of Arm Movements.* Doctoral Dissertation, University of Southern California.

Brown, P., Olivero, A., Mazzone, P., Insola, A., Tonali, P., and Lazzaro, V. D. (2001). Dopamine dependency of oscillations in between subthalamic neucleus and pallidum in Parkinson's disease. *J. Neurosci.* 21, 1033–1038.

Brown, R. G., and Jahanshahi, M. (1996). Cognitive-motor function in Parkinson's disease. *Eur. Neurol.* 36, 24–31. doi: 10.1159/000118880

Bullock, D., Grossberg, S., and Mannes, C. (1993). A neural network model for cursive script production. *Biol. Cybern.* 70, 15–28. doi: 10.1007/bf00202562

Burn, D. J., Rowan, E. N., Allan, L. M., Molloy, S., O'Brien, J. T., and McKeith, I. G. (2006). Motor subtype and cognitive decline in Parkinson's disease, Parkinson's disease with dementia and dementia with Lewy bodies. *J. Neurol. Neurosurg. Psychiatry* 77, 585–589. doi: 10.1136/jnnp.2005.081711

Calzavara, R., Mailly, P., and Haber, S. N. (2007). Relationship between the corticostriatal terminals from areas 9 and 46 and those from area 8A, dorsal and rostral premotor cortex and area 24c: an anatomical substrate for cognition to action. *Eur. J. Neurosci.* 26, 2005–2024. doi: 10.1111/j.1460-9568.2007.05825.x

Chakravarthy, V., Joseph, D., and Bapi, R. S. (2010). What do the basal ganglia do? A modeling perspective. *Biol. Cybern.* 103, 237–253. doi: 10.1007/s00422-010-0401-y

Chersi, F., Mirolli, M., Pezzulo, G., and Baldassarre, G. (2013). A spiking model of the cortico-basal ganglia circuits for goal-directed and habitual action learning. *Neural Netw.* 41, 212–224. doi: 10.1016/j.neunet.2012.11.009

Contreras-Vidal, J., and Stelmach, G. (1995). A neural model of basal ganglia-thalamocortical relations in normal and Parkinsonian movement. *Biol. Cybern.* 73, 467–476. doi: 10.1007/bf00201481

Desmurget, M., and Turner, R. S. (2010). Motor sequences and the basal ganglia: kinematics, not habits. *J. Neurosci.* 30, 7685–7690. doi: 10.1523/jneurosci.0163-10.2010

Disbrow, E. A., Russo, K. A., Higginson, C. I., Yund, E. W., Ventura, M. I., Zhang, L., et al. (2012). Efficacy of tailored computer-based neurorehabilitation for improvement of movement initiation in Parkinson's disease. *Brain Res.* 1452, 151–164. doi: 10.1016/j.brainres.2012.02.073

Domellof, M. E., Elgh, E., and Forsgren, L. (2011). The relation between cognition and motor dysfunction in drug-naive newly diagnosed patients with Parkinson's disease. *Mov. Disord.* 26, 2183–2189. doi: 10.1002/mds.23814

Dominey, P. F., and Arbib, M. A. (1992). A cortico-subcortical model for generation of spatially accurate sequential saccades. *Cereb. Cortex* 2, 153–175. doi: 10.1093/cercor/2.2.153

Dreher, J. C., and Burnod, Y. (2002). An integrative theory of the phasic and tonic modes of dopamine modulation in the prefrontal cortex. *Neural Netw.* 15, 583–602. doi: 10.1016/s0893-6080(02)00051-5

Durstewitz, D., and Seamans, J. K. (2008). The dual-state theory of prefrontal cortex dopamine function with relevance to catechol-o-methyltransferase genotypes and schizophrenia. *Biol. Psychiatry* 64, 739–749. doi: 10.1016/j.biopsych.2008.05.015

Ehrt, U., Broich, K., Larsen, J. P., Ballard, C., and Aarsland, D. (2010). Use of drugs with anticholinergic effect and impact on cognition in Parkinson's disease: a cohort study. *J. Neurol. Neurosurg. Psychiatry* 81, 160–165. doi: 10.1136/jnnp.2009.186239

Fearnley, J. M., and Lees, A. J. (1991). Ageing and Parkinson's disease: substantia nigra regional selectivity. *Brain* 114, 2283–2301. doi: 10.1093/brain/114.5.2283

Flaherty, A. W., and Graybiel, A. M. (1994). Input-output organization of the sensorimotor striatum in the squirrel monkey. *J. Neurosci.* 14, 599–610.

Frank, M. J. (2005). Dynamic dopamine modulation in the basal ganglia: a neurocomputational account of cognitive deficits in medicated and nonmedicated Parkinsonism. *J. Cogn. Neurosci.* 17, 51–72. doi: 10.1162/0898929052880093

Frank, M. J., Loughry, B., and O'Reilly, R. C. (2001). Interactions between frontal cortex and basal ganglia in working memory: a computational model. *Cogn. Affect. Behav. Neurosci.* 1, 137–160. doi: 10.3758/cabn.1.2.137

Fuster, J. M. (2008). *The Prefrontal Cortex.* 4th Edn. Singapore: Academic Press.

Gangadhar, G., Joseph, D., and Chakravarthy, V. S. (2007). An oscillatory neuromotor model of handwriting generation. *Int. J. Document Anal. Recognition* 10, 69–84. doi: 10.1007/s10032-007-0046-0

Gangadhar, G., Joseph, D., and Chakravarthy, V. S. (2008). Understanding Parkinsonian handwriting using a computational model of basal ganglia. *Neural Comput.* 20, 2491–2525. doi: 10.1162/neco.2008.03-07-498

Gangadhar, G., Joseph, D., Srinivasan, A. V., Subramanian, D., Keshavan, S., and Chakravarthy, V. S. (2009). A computational model of Parkinsonian handwriting that high lights the role of the indirect pathway in the basal ganglia. *Hum. Mov. Sci.* 28, 602–618. doi: 10.1016/j.humov.2009.07.008

Gerfen, C. R., Engber, T. M., Mahan, L. C., Susel, Z., Chase, T. N., Monsma, F. J., et al. (1990). D1 and D2 dopamine receptor-regulated gene expression of striatonigral and striatopallidal neurons. *Science* 250, 1429–1432. doi: 10.1126/science.2147780

Gerfen, C. R., and Young, W. S. (1988). Distribution of striatonigral and striatopallidal peptidergic neurons in both patch and matrix compartments: an in situ hybridization histochemistry and fluorescent retrograde tracing study. *Brain Res.* 460, 161–167. doi: 10.1016/0006-8993(88)91217-6

Gibb, W. R., and Lees, A. J. (1991). Anatomy, pigmentation, ventral and dorsal subpopulations of the substantia nigra and differential cell death in Parkinson's disease. *J. Neurol. Neurosurg. Psychiatry* 54, 388–396. doi: 10.1136/jnnp.54.5.388

Giladi, N., McMahon, D., Przedborski, S., Flaster, E., Guillory, S., Kostic, V., et al. (1992). Motor blocks in Parkinson's disease. *Neurology* 42, 333–339. doi: 10.1212/WNL.42.2.333

Gluck, M. A., Shohamy, D., and Myers, C. (2002). How do people solve the "Weather Prediction" Task?: individual variability in strategies for probabilistic category learning. *Learn. Mem.* 9, 408–418. doi: 10.1101/lm.45202

Gotham, A. M., Brown, R. G., and Marsden, C. D. (1988). "Frontal" cognitive function in patients with Parkinson's disease "on"and "off" levodopa. *Brain* 111, 299–321. doi: 10.1093/brain/111.2.299

Gurney, K., Prescott, T. J., and Redgrave, P. (2001). A computational model of action selection in the basal ganglia. II. Analysis and simulation of behaviour. *Biol. Cybern.* 84, 411–423. doi: 10.1007/pl00007985

Guthrie, M., Leblois, A., Garenne, A., and Boraud, T. (2013). Interaction between cognitive and motor cortico-basal ganglia loops during decision making: a computational study. *J. Neurophysiol.* 109, 3025–3040. doi: 10.1152/jn.00026.2013

Haber, S. N., Kim, K. S., Mailly, P., and Calzavara, R. (2006). Reward-related cortical inputs define a large striatal region in primates that interface with associative cortical connections, providing a substrate for incentive-based learning. *J. Neurosci.* 26, 8368–8376. doi: 10.1523/jneurosci.0271-06.2006

Hayhoe, M., Aivar, P., Shrivastavah, A., and Mruczek, R. (2002). Visual short-term memory and motor planning. *Prog. Brain Res.* 140, 349–363. doi: 10.1016/s0079-6123(02)40062-3

Helie, S., and Ashby, G. F. (2009). "A neurocomputational model of automaticity and maintenance of abstract rules," in *Proceedings of the International Joint Conference on Neural Networks (IEEE Press)*, 1192–1198.

Helie, S., and Cousineau, D. (2011). The cognitive neuroscience of automaticity: behavioral and brain signatures. *Cogn. Sci.* 6, 25–43.

Helie, S., Paul, E. J., and Ashby, F. G. (2012a). A neurocomputational account of cognitive deficits in Parkinson's disease. *Neuropsychologia* 50, 2290–2302. doi: 10.1016/j.neuropsychologia.2012.05.033

Helie, S., Paul, E. J., and Ashby, F. G. (2012b). Simulating the effect of dopamine imbalance on cognition: from positive affect to Parkinson's disease. *Neural. Netw.* 32, 74–85. doi: 10.1016/j.neunet.2012.02.033

Helie, S., Waldschmidt, J. G., and Ashby, F. G. (2010). Automaticity in rule-based and information-integration categorization. *Atten. Percept. Psychophys.* 72, 1013–1031. doi: 10.3758/app.72.4.1013

Herzallah, M. M., Moustafa, A. A., Misk, A. J., Al-Dweib, L. H., Abdelrazeq, S. A., Myers, C. E., et al. (2010). Depression impairs learning whereas anticholinergics impair transfer generalization in Parkinson patients tested on dopaminergic medications. *Cogn. Behav. Neurol.* 23, 98–105. doi: 10.1097/wnn.0b013e3181df3048

Hikosaka, O., Takikawa, Y., and Kawagoe, R. (2000). Role of the basal ganglia in the control of purposive saccadic eye movements. *Physiol. Rev.* 80, 953–978.

Histed, M. H., Pasupathy, A., and Miller, E. K. (2009). Learning substrates in the primate prefrontal cortex and striatum: sustained activity related to successful actions. *Neuron* 63, 244–253. doi: 10.1016/j.neuron.2009.06.019

Hollerbach, J. M. (1981). An oscillation theory of handwriting. *Biol. Cybern.* 39, 139–156. doi: 10.1007/bf00336740

Issen, L. A., and Knill, D. C. (2012). Decoupling eye and hand movement control: visual short-term memory influences reach planning more than saccade planning. *J. Vis.* 12, 1–13. doi: 10.1167/12.1.3

Jankovic, J., McDermott, M., Carter, J., Gauthier, S., Goetz, C., Golbe, L., et al. (1990). Variable expression of Parkinson's disease: a base-line analysis of the DATATOP cohort. *Neurology* 40, 1529–1534. doi: 10.1212/wnl.40.10.1529

Kaasinen, V., Nurmi, E., Bergman, J., Eskola, O., Solin, O., Sonninen, P., et al. (2001). Personality traits and brain dopaminergic function in Parkinson's disease. *Proc. Natl. Acad. Sci. U S A* 98, 13272–13277. doi: 10.1073/pnas.231313198

Kalveram, K. T. (1998). "A neural oscillator model learning given trajectories, or how an allo-imitation algorithm can be implemented into a motor controller," in *Motor Behavior and Human Skill: A Multi-Disciplinary Approach*, ed J. Piek (Champaign, IL, USA: Human Kinetics Publishers), 127–140.

Kassubek, J., Juengling, F. D., Hellwig, B., Spreer, J., and Lucking, C. H. (2002). Thalamic gray matter changes in unilateral Parkinsonian resting tremor: a voxel-based morphometric analysis of 3-dimensional magnetic resonance imaging. *Neurosci. Lett.* 323, 29–32. doi: 10.1016/s0304-3940(02)00111-8

Kato, M., Miyashita, N., Hikosaka, O., Matsumura, M., Usui, S., and Kori, A. (1995). Eye movements in monkeys with local dopamine depletion in caudate nucleus.I. Deficits in spontaneous saccades. *J. Neurosci.* 15, 912–927.

Kemp, J. M., and Powell, T. P. S. (1970). The cortico-striate projections in the monkey. *Brain* 93, 525–546. doi: 10.1093/brain/93.3.525

Kincaid, A. E., Zheng, T., and Wilson, C. J. (1998). Connectivity and convergence of single corticostriatal axons. *J. Neurosci.* 18, 4722–4731.

Knowlton, B. J., Mangels, J. A., and Squire, L. R. (1996). A neostriatal habit learning system in humans. *Science* 273, 1399–1402. doi: 10.1126/science.273.5280.1399

Kostic, V. S., Agosta, F., Pievani, M., Stefanova, E., Jecmenica-Lukic, M., Scarale, A., et al. (2012). Pattern of brain tissue loss associated with freezing of gait in Parkinson disease. *Neurology* 78, 409–416. doi: 10.1212/wnl.0b013e318245d23c

Krishnan, R., Ratnadurai, S., Subramanian, D., Chakravarthy, V. S., and Rengaswamy, M. (2011). Modeling the role of basal ganglia in saccade generation: is the indirect pathway the explorer? *Neural Netw.* 24, 801–813. doi: 10.1016/j.neunet.2011.06.002

Lawrence, A. D. (2000). Error correction and the basal ganglia: similar computations for action, cognition and emotion? *Trends Cogn. Sci.* 4, 365–367. doi: 10.1016/s1364-6613(00)01535-7

Leblois, A., Boraud, T., Meissner, W., Bergman, H., and Hansel, D. (2006). Competition between feedback loops underlies normal and pathological dynamics in the basal ganglia. *J. Neurosci.* 26, 3567–3583. doi: 10.1523/jneurosci.5050-05.2006

Lewis, S. J., and Barker, R. A. (2009). A pathophysiological model of freezing of gait in Parkinson's disease. *Parkinsonism Relat. Disord.* 15, 333–338. doi: 10.1016/j.parkreldis.2008.08.006

Lyros, E., Messinis, L., and Papathanasopoulos, P. (2008). Does motor subtype influence neurocognitive performance in Parkinson's disease without dementia? *Eur. J. Neurol.* 15, 262–267. doi: 10.1111/j.1468-1331.2007.02046.x

Maddox, W. T., and Ashby, F. G. (2004). Dissociating explicit and procedural-learning based systems of perceptual category learning. *Behav. Processes* 66, 309–332. doi: 10.1016/j.beproc.2004.03.011

Magdoom, M., Subramanian, D., Chakravarthy, V. S., Ravindran, B., Amari, S., and Meenakshisundaram, N. (2011). Modeling basal ganglia for understanding Parkinsonian reaching movements. *Neural Comput.* 23, 477–516. doi: 10.1162/neco_a_00073

Matar, E., Shine, J. M., Naismith, S. L., and Lewis, S. J. (2013). Using virtual reality to explore the role of conflict resolution and environmental salience in freezing of gait in Parkinson's disease. *Parkinsonism Relat. Disord.* 19, 937–942. doi: 10.1016/j.parkreldis.2013.06.002

Matsui, H., Udaka, F., Miyoshi, T., Hara, N., Tamaura, A., Oda, M., et al. (2005). Three-dimensional stereotactic surface projection study of freezing of gait and brain perfusion image in Parkinson's disease. *Mov. Disord.* 20, 1272–1277. doi: 10.1002/mds.20520

Matsumoto, K., Suzuki, W., and Tanaka, K. (2003). Neuronal correlates of goal-based motor selection in the prefrontal cortex. *Science* 301, 229–232. doi: 10.1126/science.1084204

McIntyre, J., Stratta, F., and Lacquaniti, F. (1998). Short-term memory for reaching to visual targets: psychophysical evidence for body-centered reference frames. *J. Neurosci.* 18, 8423–8435.

Meco, G., Casacchia, M., Lazzari, R., Franzese, A., Castellana, F., Carta, A., et al. (1984). Mental impairment in Parkinson's disease. The role of anticholinergic drugs. *Acta Psychiatr. Belg.* 84, 325–335.

Miyachi, S., Hikosaka, O., and Lu, X. (2002). Differential activation of monkey striatal neurons in the early and late stages of procedural learning. *Exp. Brain Res.* 146, 122–126. doi: 10.1007/s00221-002-1213-7

Miyachi, S., Hikosaka, O., Miyashita, K., Kárádi, Z., and Rand, M. K. (1997). Differential roles of monkey striatum in learning of sequential hand movement. *Exp. Brain Res.* 115, 1–5. doi: 10.1007/pl00005669

Monchi, O., Taylor, J. G., and Dagher, A. (2000). A neural model of working memory processes in normal subjects, Parkinson's disease and schizophrenia for fMRI design and predictions. *Neural Netw.* 13, 953–973. doi: 10.1016/s0893-6080(00)00058-7

Moustafa, A. A., Bell, P., Eissa, A. M., and Hewedi, D. H. (2013). The effects of clinical motor variables and medication dosage on working memory in Parkinson's disease. *Brain Cogn.* 82, 137–145. doi: 10.1016/j.bandc.2013.04.001

Moustafa, A. A., Cohen, M. X., Sherman, S. J., and Frank, M. J. (2008). A role for dopamine in temporal decision making and reward maximization in Parkinsonism. *J. Neurosci.* 28, 12294–12304. doi: 10.1523/jneurosci.3116-08.2008

Moustafa, A. A., and Gluck, M. A. (2011a). A neurocomputational model of dopamine and prefrontal-striatal interactions during multi-cue category learning by Parkinson's patients. *J. Cogn. Neurosci.* 23, 151–167. doi: 10.1162/jocn.2010.21420

Moustafa, A. A., and Gluck, M. A. (2011b). Computational cognitive models of prefrontal-striatal-hippocampal interactions in Parkinson's disease and schizophrenia. *Neural Netw.* 24, 575–591. doi: 10.1016/j.neunet.2011.02.006

Moustafa, Herzallah, M. M., and Gluck, M. A. (2013). Dissociating the cognitive effects of levodopa versus dopamine agonists in a neurocomputational model of learning in Parkinson's disease. *Neurodegener. Dis.* 11, 102–111. doi: 10.1159/000341999

Moustafa, A. A., and Maida, A. S. (2007). Using TD learning to simulate working memory performance in a model of the prefrontal cortex and basal ganglia. *Cogn. Syst. Res.* 8, 262–281. doi: 10.1016/j.cogsys.2007.02.001

Mulder, A. B., Nordquist, R. E., Orgut, O., and Pennartz, C. M. (2003). Learning-related changes in response patterns of prefrontal neurons during instrumental conditioning. *Behav. Brain Res.* 146, 77–88. doi: 10.1016/j.bbr.2003.09.016

Mure, H., Hirano, S., Tang, C. C., Isaias, I. U., Antonini, A., Ma, Y., et al. (2011). Parkinson's disease tremor-related metabolic network: characterization, progression and treatment effects. *Neuroimage* 54, 1244–1253. doi: 10.1016/j.neuroimage.2010.09.028

Naismith, S. L., Shine, J. M., and Lewis, S. J. (2010). The specific contributions of set-shifting to freezing of gait in Parkinson's disease. *Mov. Disord.* 25, 1000–1004. doi: 10.1002/mds.23005

Nakahara, H., Doya, K., and Hikosaka, O. (2001). Parallel cortico-basal ganglia mechanisms for acquisition and execution of visuomotor sequences-a computational approach. *J. Cogn. Neurosci.* 13, 626–647. doi: 10.1162/089892901750363208

Nambu, A., Tokuno, H., and Takada, M. (2002). Functional significance of the cortico-subthalamo-pallidal 'hyperdirect' pathway. *Neurosci. Res.* 43, 111–117. doi: 10.1016/s0168-0102(02)00027-5

Niv, Y., Daw, N. D., Joel, D., and Dayan, P. (2007). Tonic dopamine: opportunity costs and the control of response vigor. *Psychopharmacology (Berl)* 191, 507–520. doi: 10.1007/s00213-006-0502-4

Obeso, J. A., Marin, C., Rodriguez-Oroz, C., Blesa, J., Benitez-Temino, B., Mena-Segovia, J., et al. (2008). The basal ganglia in Parkinson's disease: current concepts and unexplained observations. *Ann. Neurol.* 64, S30–S46. doi: 10.1002/ana.21481

O'Doherty, J., Dayan, P., Schultz, J., Deichmann, R., Friston, K., and Dolan, R. J. (2004). Dissociable roles of ventral and dorsal striatum in instrumental conditioning. *Science* 304, 452–454. doi: 10.1126/science.1094285

Oh, J. Y., Kim, Y. S., Choi, B. H., Sohn, E. H., and Lee, A. Y. (2009). Relationship between clinical phenotypes and cognitive impairment in Parkinson's disease (PD). *Arch. Gerontol. Geriatr.* 49, 351–354. doi: 10.1016/j.archger.2008.11.013

Ohbayashi, M., Ohki, K., and Miyashita, Y. (2003). Conversion of working memory to motor sequence in the monkey premotor cortex. *Science* 301, 233–236. doi: 10.1126/science.1084884

O'Reilly, R. C., and Frank, M. J. (2006). Making working memory work: a computational model of learning in the prefrontal cortex and basal ganglia. *Neural Comput.* 18, 283–328. doi: 10.1162/089976606775093909

Pakhotin, P., and Bracci, E. (2007). Cholinergic interneurons control the excitatory input to the striatum. *J. Neurosci.* 27, 391–400. doi: 10.1523/jneurosci.3709-06.2007

Piek, J. P., Dyck, M. J., Nieman, A., Anderson, M., Hay, D., Smith, L. M., et al. (2004). The relationship between motor coordination, executive functioning and attention in school aged children. *Arch. Clin. Neuropsychol.* 19, 1063–1076. doi: 10.1016/j.acn.2003.12.007

Phillips, J. G., Stelmach, G. E., and Teasdale, N. (1991). What can indices of handwriting quality tell us about Parkinsonian handwriting? *Hum. Mov. Sci.* 10, 301–314. doi: 10.1016/0167-9457(91)90009-m

Plotnik, M., Giladi, N., Dagan, Y., and Hausdorff, J. M. (2011). Postural instability and fall risk in Parkinson's disease: impaired dual tasking, pacing and bilateral coordination of gait during the "ON" medication state. *Exp. Brain Res.* 210, 529–538. doi: 10.1007/s00221-011-2551-0

Poletti, M., and Bonuccelli, U. (2013). Acute and chronic cognitive effects of levodopa and dopamine agonists in patients with Parkinson's disease: a review. *Ther. Adv. Psychopharmacol.* 3, 101–113. doi: 10.1177/2045125312470130

Poletti, M., Emre, M., and Bonuccelli, U. (2011). Mild cognitive impairment and cognitive reserve in Parkinson's disease. *Parkinsonism Relat. Disord.* 17, 579–586. doi: 10.1016/j.parkreldis.2011.03.013

Poletti, M., Frosini, D., Pagni, C., Baldacci, F., Nicoletti, V., Tognoni, G., et al. (2012). Mild cognitive impairment and cognitive-motor relationships in newly diagnosed drug-naive patients with Parkinson's disease. *J. Neurol. Neurosurg. Psychiatry* 83, 601–606. doi: 10.1136/jnnp-2011-301874

Pondal, M., Del Ser, T., and Bermejo, F. (1996). Anticholinergic therapy and dementia in patients with Parkinson's disease. *J. Neurol.* 243, 543–546. doi: 10.1007/bf00886877

Price, A., Filoteo, J. V., and Maddox, W. T. (2009). Rule-based category learning in patients with Parkinson's disease. *Neuropsychologia* 47, 1213–1226. doi: 10.1016/j.neuropsychologia.2009.01.031

Probst-Cousin, S., Druschky, A., and Neundorfer, B. (2003). Disappearance of resting tremor after "stereotaxic" thalamic stroke. *Neurology* 61, 1013–1014. doi: 10.1212/01.wnl.0000086810.14643.fc

Rascol, O., Sabatini, U., Simonetta-Moreau, M., Montastruc, L., Rascol, A., Clanet, M. (1991). Square wave jerks in Parkinsonian syndromes. *J. Neurol. Neurosurg. Psychiatry* 54, 599–602. doi: 10.1136/jnnp.54.7.599

Reiner, A. (2010). "Organization of corticostriatal projection neuron types," in *Handbook of Basal Ganglia Structure and Function*, eds H. Steiner and K. Y. Tseng (New York, NY: Academic Press), 323–340.

Reynolds, J. N. J., Hyland, B. I., and Wickens, J. R. (2001). A cellular mechanism of reward-related learning. *Nature* 413, 67–70. doi: 10.1038/35092560

Schillaci, O., Chiaravalloti, A., Pierantozzi, M., Di Pietro, B., Koch, G., Bruni, C., et al. (2011). Different patterns of nigrostriatal degeneration in tremor type versus the akinetic-rigid and mixed types of Parkinson's disease at the early stages: molecular imaging with 123I-FP-CIT SPECT. *Int. J. Mol. Med.* 28, 881–886. doi: 10.3892/ijmm.2011.764

Schomaker, L. R. B. (1991). *Simulation and Recognition of Handwriting Movements: A Vertical Approach to Modeling Human Motor Behavior.* (Doctoral Dissertation, Nijmegen University).

Schroll, H., Vitay, J., and Hamker, F. H. (2012). Working memory and response selection: a computational account of interactions among cortico-basal ganglio-thalamic loops. *Neural Netw.* 26, 59–74. doi: 10.1016/j.neunet.2011.10.008

Seger, C. A. (2008). How do the basal ganglia contribute to categorization? Their roles in generalization, response selection and learning via feedback. *Neurosci. Biobehav. Rev.* 32, 265–278. doi: 10.1016/j.neubiorev.2007.07.010

Sheridan, M. R., and Flowers, K. A. (1990). Movement variability and bradykinesia in Parkinson's disease. *Brain* 113, 1149–1161. doi: 10.1093/brain/113.4.1149

Shine, J. M., Matar, E., and Lewis, S. J. G. (2013). Differential neural activation patterns in patients with Parkinson's disease and freezing of gait in response to concurrent cognitive and motor load. *PLoS One* 8:e52602. doi: 10.1371/journal.pone.0052602

Silberstein, P., Pogosyan, A., Kuhn, A. A., Hotton, G., Tisch, S., Kupsch, A., et al. (2005). Cortico-cortical coupling in Parkinson's disease and its modulation by therapy. *Brain* 128, 1277–1291. doi: 10.1093/brain/awh480

Smith, Y., Galvan, A., Raju, D., and Wichmann, T. (2010). "Anatomical and functional organization of the thalamostriatal systems," in *Handbook of Basal Ganglia Structure and Function*, eds H. Steiner and K. Y. Tseng (New York, NY: Academic Press), 381–396.

Smith, Y., Raju, D. V., Pare, J. F., and Sidibe, M. (2004). The thalamostriatal system: a highly specific network of the basal ganglia circuitry. *Trends Neurosci.* 27, 520–527. doi: 10.1016/j.tins.2004.07.004

Steiner, H., and Tseng, K. Y. (2010). *Handbook of Basal Ganglia Structure and Function.* New York: Academic Press.

Tessitore, A., Amboni, M., Cirillo, G., Corbo, D., Picillo, M., Russo, A., et al. (2012). Regional gray matter atrophy in patients with Parkinson disease and freezing of gait. *AJNR Am. J. Neuroradiol.* 33, 1804–1809. doi: 10.3174/ajnr.a3066

Teulings, H. L., and Stelmach, G. E. (1991). Control of stroke size, peak acceleration and stroke duration in Parkinsonian handwriting. *Hum. Mov. Sci.* 10, 315–334. doi: 10.1016/0167-9457(91)90010-u

Vakil, E., and Herishanu-Naaman, S. (1998). Declarative and procedural learning in Parkinson's disease patients having tremor or bradykinesia as the predominant symptom. *Cortex* 34, 611–620. doi: 10.1016/s0010-9452(08)70518-5

Vandenbossche, J., Deroost, N., Soetens, E., Spildooren, J., Vercruysse, S., Nieuwboer, A., et al. (2011). Freezing of gait in Parkinson disease is associated with impaired conflict resolution. *Neurorehabil. Neural Repair* 25, 765–773. doi: 10.1177/1545968311403493

Van Gemmert, A. W. A., Adler, C. H., and Stelmach, G. E. (2003). Parkinson's disease patients undershoot target size in handwriting and similar tasks. *J. Neurol. Neurosurg. Psychiatry* 74, 1502–1508. doi: 10.1136/jnnp.74.11.1502

Van Gemmert, A. W. A., Teulings, H. L., Contreras-Vidal, J. L., and Stelmach, G. E. (1999). Parkinson's disease and the control of size and speed in handwriting. *Neuropsychologia* 37, 685–694. doi: 10.1016/s0028-3932(98)00122-5

Weinberger, M., Hutchison, W. D., Lozano, A. M., Hodaie, M., and Dostrovsky, J. O. (2009). Increased gamma oscillatory activity in the subthalamic nucleus during tremor in Parkinson's disease patients. *J. Neurophysiol.* 101, 789–802. doi: 10.1152/jn.90837.2008

Weiss, P., Stelmach, G. E., and Hefter, H. (1997). Programming of a movement sequence in Parkinson's disease. *Brain* 120, 91–102. doi: 10.1093/brain/120.1.91

Wickens, J. R., Begg, A. J., and Arbuthnott, G. W. (1996). Dopamine reverses the depression of rat corticostriatal synapses which normally follows high-frequency stimulation of cortex in vitro. *Neuroscience* 70, 1–5. doi: 10.1016/0306-4522(95)00436-m

Wilson, C. J. (2004). "Basal ganglia," in *The Synaptic Organization of the Brain*, ed G. M. Shepherd (New York: Oxford University Press), 361–414.

Yeterian, E. H., and Pandya, D. N. (1993). Striatal connections of the parietal association cortices in rhesus monkeys. *J. Comp. Neurol.* 332, 175–197. doi: 10.1002/cne.903320204

Yeterian, E. H., and Pandya, D. N. (1995). Corticostriatal connections of extrastriate visual areas in rhesus monkeys. *J. Comp. Neurol.* 352, 436–457. doi: 10.1002/cne.903520309

Yeterian, E. H., and Pandya, D. N. (1998). Corticostriatal connections of the superior temporal region in rhesus monkeys. *J. Comp. Neurol.* 399, 384–402. doi: 10.1002/(sici)1096-9861(19980928)399:3<384::aid-cne7>3.0.co;2-x

Yin, H. H., Ostlund, S. B., Knowlton, B. J., and Balleine, B. W. (2005). The role of the dorsomedial striatum in instrumental conditioning. *Eur. J. Neurosci.* 22, 513–523. doi: 10.1111/j.1460-9568.2005.04218.x

Zaidel, A., Arkadir, D., Israel, Z., and Bergman, H. (2009). Akineto-rigid vs. tremor syndromes in Parkinsonism. *Curr. Opin. Neurol.* 22, 387–393. doi: 10.1097/wco.0b013e32832d9d67

4

Electrophysiological Characterization of Entopeduncular Nucleus Neurons in Anesthetized and Freely Moving Rats

Liora Benhamou and Dana Cohen*

The Leslie and Susan Gonda Multidisciplinary Brain Research Center, Bar-Ilan University, Ramat-Gan, Israel

Correspondence:
Dana Cohen, The Leslie and Susan Gonda Multidisciplinary Brain Research Center, Bar-Ilan University, No. 901, Ramat-Gan 52900, Israel
e-mail: danacoh@gmail.com

The EntoPeduncular nucleus (EP), which is homologous to the internal segment of the Globus Pallidus (GPi) in primates, is one of the two basal ganglia (BG) output nuclei. Despite their importance in cortico-BG information processing, EP neurons have rarely been investigated in rats and there is no available electrophysiological characterization of EP neurons *in vivo*. We recorded and analyzed the activity of EP neurons in freely moving as well as anesthetized rats, and compared their activity patterns. Examination of neuronal firing statistics during wakefulness suggested that similar to neurons recorded in the primate GPi, EP neurons are a single population characterized by Poisson-like firing. Under isoflurane anesthesia the firing rate of EP neurons decreased substantially and their coefficient of variation and relative duration of quiescence periods increased. Investigation of the relationship between firing rate and depth of anesthesia revealed two distinct neuronal groups: one that decreased its firing rate with the increase in anesthesia level, and a second group where the firing rate was independent of anesthesia level. *Post-hoc* examination of the firing properties of the two groups showed that they were statistically distinct. These results may thus help reconcile *in vitro* studies in rats and primates which have reported two distinct neuronal populations, and *in vivo* studies in behaving primates indicating one homogeneous population. Our data support the existence of two distinct neuronal populations in the rat EP that can be distinguished by their characteristic firing response to anesthesia.

Keywords: basal ganglia, electrophysiology, anesthesia, extracellular recording, firing patterns, neuronal population

INTRODUCTION

The Basal Ganglia (BG), a group of subcortical nuclei, process and integrate motor, cognitive, and limbic information arriving from most cortical areas and the thalamus via a network of segregated pathways (Alexander et al., 1986; Alexander and Crutcher, 1990; Deniau et al., 1996; Kitano et al., 1998). The globus pallidus internal segment (GPi), which is one of the two output stations of the BG, projects to the cortex through different thalamic nuclei, and influences information processing in these targets (Kravitz et al., 2010; Kojima et al., 2013). The GPi is thought to participate in motor control especially in movement initiation, sequential organization of movement and action selection (Horak and Anderson, 1984; Mink, 1996; Redgrave et al., 1999). GPi lesions cause motor disturbances such as reduced speed and acceleration, resulting in hypometria (Turner and Anderson, 2005; Turner and Desmurget, 2010). By contrast, ablation of the GPi has been shown to improve the conditions of patients suffering from Parkinson's disease, which suggests that abnormal information processing in the GPi may have a greater influence on motor behavior than its silencing (Obeso et al., 2009). Additionally, it has been shown that GPi neurons process sensory information related to reward consumption (Lidsky, 1975), and that they are also tuned to reward predicting targets (Hong and Hikosaka, 2008), reward probability (Joshua et al., 2009) and that their activity facilitates response variability required for associative learning (Sheth et al., 2011). Moreover, it has been suggested that the GPi neurons may initiate reward related signals through their effect on the lateral habenula (LHb) (Hong and Hikosaka, 2008). Overall, the complexity of BG information processing encourages further examination of information flow through the different BG nuclei.

Primate GPi neurons are anatomically and biochemically comparable to the neurons of the GPe, a central station of the BG. However, extracellular electrophysiological characterizations of the firing properties of GPe neurons suggest there are two distinct neuronal groups of neurons dubbed high frequency pausers and low frequency bursters, whereas a similar analysis of GPi neurons reveals only one neuronal population (DeLong, 1971). GPi neurons display continuous high rate discharges of about 60 spikes/s with rapid firing rate fluctuations ranging from 10 to 107 spikes/s but without displaying pauses or prolonged silences as is the case for GPe neurons (DeLong, 1971). Other studies have reported that GPi neurons display uncorrelated non-synchronous activity (Bar-Gad et al., 2003a) and that they exhibit slow oscillations in the multisecond range (Wichmann et al., 2002). Currently there is no established characterization of neuronal activity in EntoPeduncular (EP) neurons in freely moving rats.

In general, the rodent and primate BG share similar cell types and connectivity. Thus comparative studies may help clarify the nature, role and features of the computation taking place in these structures. We previously compared the rat Globus Pallidus (GP) activity to the GPe, its primate homologue (Benhamou et al., 2012) and showed that like the primate GPe, the rat GP comprised two neuronal populations. Although the neuronal firing rates in the GP were substantially lower than those observed in the GPe, both species displayed similar firing pattern characteristics. Since the EP is homologous to the primate GPi, it was hypothesized that an extracellular electrophysiological characterization of the firing properties of EP would reveal a single population. Contrary to this assumption, however, anatomical tracing studies in primates, cats, and rats have reported that based on their projection target sites, it is likely that the GPi/EP neurons form two neuronal populations (Nauta, 1974; Filion and Harnois, 1978; van der Kooy and Carter, 1981; Tokuno et al., 1988; Parent et al., 2001). These anatomical studies were corroborated by a study in slice preparation of the rat EP that described two distinct neuronal populations based on their intrinsic electrical properties (Nakanishi et al., 1990).

Here, we characterize and compare neuronal activity recorded chronically in the EP of freely moving rats during wakefulness and under different levels of isoflurane anesthesia. Considering the similarity in the electrophysiological properties of GPe neurons between rats and primates (Benhamou et al., 2012) we hypothesized that rat EP neurons would display similar properties to those observed in primate GPi. During wakefulness, the recorded neurons displayed tonic activity with near Poissonian firing. The distributions of neuronal statistics such as firing rate (FR), coefficient of variation (CV), fano factor (FF) and relative duration of quiescence periods (Silence Index) calculated in freely moving animals were spread along a continuum, thus suggesting that this sample was composed of one neuronal population. By contrast, the characterization of neuronal activity measured under different levels of anesthesia revealed two distinct groups: one that decreased firing rate correlatively with anesthesia level and a second whose firing rate was independent of anesthesia. *Post-hoc* examination of the two population statistics revealed that despite being spread over a continuum, the characteristics of the two populations were significantly different. Our data thus suggest the existence of two neuronal populations in the rat EP that can only be distinguished under anesthesia.

MATERIALS AND METHODS

All procedures were carried out in accordance with the National Institutes of Health Guide for the Care and Use of Laboratory Animals and the Bar-Ilan University Guidelines for the Use and Care of Laboratory Animals in Research.

SURGICAL PROCEDURE

The surgical procedure was previously described (Nicolelis et al., 1997; Jacobson et al., 2009). In brief, four adult male Long-Evans rats (Harlan) weighing 450 g on average (range: 430–480 g) were sedated with 5% isoflurane and were then injected i.m. with ketamine HCl and xylazine HCl (100 and 10 mg/kg, respectively). Supplementary injections of xylazine and ketamine were administrated if required. Rats were maintained by a stereotaxic frame (Kopf Instruments, USA). After sterilization, the rat's head was incised and the skull surface revealed. Connective tissue was then removed and the skull surface cleaned. Two bilateral craniotomies slightly larger than the electrode were made above the EP (anteroposterior (AP): 2.4 mm, mediolateral (ML): 3.0 mm, dorsoventral (DV): −7.0 mm). Eight Formvar coated Nichrome wires (coated diameter: 0.0015″, A-M Systems, Inc.) placed in a 27 Gauge cannulae were slowly introduced into the EP through each craniotomy independently. Electrodes (impedance 0.1–0.2 MΩ at 1 kHz) were cemented in place with dental acrylic, leaving the upper part of the connectors exposed.

At the end of experiment, the rats were anesthetized with 5% isoflurane, then ketamine, xylazine and morphine (3 mg/Kg) were injected i.p and electrolytic lesions made before perfusion with 4% formaldehyde. The brain was fixated with 20% sucrose and sectioned with cryostat in 60 μm slices. Electrode positions were confirmed histologically using a microscope (NikonEclipse E400, 1x/400).

DATA COLLECTION

Following about 10 days of recovery from surgery, the activity of EP neurons was recorded in four adult male Long-Evans rats. Within each session the rats were anesthetized with gradually decreasing doses of isoflurane (4% to 1% by steps of 1%) followed by a period of wakefulness during which the rats moved around in the recording chamber rather than remained immobile. Based on our observations of the elapsed time from anesthesia removal until animals started to walk freely in the recording chamber we estimated a recovery time of 5 min for each alteration in isoflurane level thus allowing neuronal activity to physiologically adjust to the different levels. Hence, data collection started after a 5 min intermission following each transition in anesthesia depth. Neural activity was amplified, band-pass filtered at 150–8000 Hz and sampled at 40 kHz using a multichannel acquisition processor system (MAP system; Plexon Inc, Dallas, TX, USA). Offline sorting was performed on all continuously recorded units (OfflineSorter V2.8.8; Plexon, Dallas, TX) and the data were analyzed using custom-written MATLAB software (R2010b, MathWorks Inc., Natick, MA).

DATA ANALYSIS

STATISTICAL ANALYSIS

All the data reported are presented as the mean ± SEM. Unless stated otherwise, statistically significant differences between parameters were assessed by the non-parametric test Kruskal-Wallis with the Tukey-Kramer multiple comparison correction.

In order to identify significant nonlinear correlation between firing rate and isoflurane, we used the a-parametric Kendall-Tau correlation test (Matlab function: corr with type Kendall; $p < 0.05$). The Kendall-tau test provides a coefficient that represents the degree of concordance between two columns of ranked data. It is similar to the non-parametric Spearman's ρ-test but it enables easier interpretation of the correlation value. Specifically, it is the difference between the probability that the observed data are in the same order and the probability that the observed data are not in the same order.

WAVEFORM PARAMETERS

The waveform parameters consisted of the valley to peak ratio, valley to peak duration, valley width, zero-cross, and peak and valley amplitudes. The valley is the minimal amplitude time point and the peak is the first maximum observed after the valley time point. Valley width quantifies the duration of the extracellular waveform at its half amplitude, the valley to peak ratio is the valley amplitude divided by the absolute value of the peak amplitude, and zero-cross is the time elapsed between the two time points around the valley in which the amplitude equals zero (see inset in **Figure 3A**).

FIRING PARAMETERS

The firing parameters included the CV, FF, FR, refractory period and mode Inter-Spike Interval (ISI). The term CV defines the standard deviation of the ISI distribution divided by its mean. The FF is the variance of the spike count distribution calculated in non-overlapping time windows, divided by its mean (window duration equals the median ISI of each neuron). The FR is the total number of spikes divided by the total recording time (spike count rate). The refractory period defines the time in ms elapsed from 0 on the neurons' auto-correlogram to attain its half height at stable state. Mode ISI describes the mode value of the ISI distribution using 5 ms precision bins.

AUTO- AND CROSS-CORRELATIONS

Autocorrelation and crosscorrelation functions were calculated for latencies of 1000 ms and 500 ms respectively (bin size equals 1 ms).

For the cross-correlation functions, upper and lower confidence levels were calculated as follows: the mean and standard deviation of the cross-correlograms at time ±4–5 s were calculated. The probability that the signal crossed a specified limit in 1% of the bins over 1 s in every bin according to the Bonferroni correction for multiple comparisons was calculated in the following manner: $p = \frac{0.01}{Nbins}$. Assuming a normal distribution, we obtained the number of standard deviations (Z-value) required to attain the probability p and drew the lower and upper confidence levels at the ordinates corresponding to the mean $\pm Z$ standard deviations.

SILENCE INDEX

The increase in CV indicated that under anesthesia neuronal firing could not be modeled by a Poisson distribution. Therefore to enable comparison between neuronal relative quiescence periods while taking into account the different firing rates we created the Silence Index which normalized the relative quiescence time of a neuron with that expected from a Poisson neuron having the same firing rate. The proportion of time taken by the longest 5% of the ISIs relative to the whole recording time was calculated for the real neuron and its Poisson model neuron. Then the value of the real neuron was divided by that of its Poisson model. Values substantially higher than 1 indicate that the neuron tended to be more silent than a Poisson neuron with the same firing rate, suggesting that the real neuron compensated its prolonged silent periods by a higher firing rate during non-quiescent periods in order to obtain a similar firing rate.

RESULTS

We recorded the activity of 38 single neurons in the EP of four rats and characterized their waveforms and firing parameters during different levels of isoflurane anesthesia and wakefulness. The electrode placement in the EP was verified histologically by making an electrolytic lesion via the electrodes that displayed neuronal activity during recording sessions (see Section Materials and Methods). An example of the placement of an implanted electrode in the EP is shown in **Figure 1A**. Its corresponding coronal slice taken from a rat atlas (Paxinos, 2007) is shown in **Figure 1B**. In each session neuronal activity was recorded during five states: four levels of isoflurane anesthesia (1%, 2%, 3% and 4%), and wakefulness, during which the animal could move freely in the recording chamber. Neuronal activity was recorded throughout each session with a 5 min intermission following each transition in anesthesia depth, thus allowing neuronal activity to physiologically adjust to the different levels (see Section Materials and Methods). Overall, in each state we analyzed neuronal activity for an average time of 511 ± 24.47 s.

We first analyzed neuronal activity in the awake state to test whether as in primates the properties of the recorded population are uniformly distributed despite the possibility of including two subtypes as suggested by anatomical studies (Nakanishi et al., 1990; Parent et al., 2001). Initial observations indicated that all the recorded neurons displayed similar waveform shapes composed of a sharp narrow valley that was followed by a slightly longer duration peak. Waveform shapes of three EP neuronal exemplars are shown in **Figure 2A**. The waveforms were characterized by the following parameters described in the Materials and Methods section (see also inset in **Figure 2A**): the valley width at half amplitude (142 ± 4.43 μs), the waveform duration measured from the first valley to the following peak (258 ± 11 μs), the valley to peak amplitude ratio (0.67 ± 0.03), and the zero-crossing duration (275 ± 12 μs). Additionally, the neurons had an average refractory period of 6.97 ± 4.61 ms (mean ± std). Examination of the firing patterns displayed by EP neurons showed that these neurons fired tonically at a relatively high rate (26.0 ± 3.1 spikes/s; **Figure 2B**). Their firing was irregular as reflected in the relatively flat autocorrelograms over more than 1 s (see examples in **Figure 2C**). Of the 24 neuronal pairs recorded simultaneously during wakefulness, none showed a peak in the cross-correlogram suggesting that EP neurons did not interact with one another or that their interactions were negligible. Like their waveforms, EP neurons displayed homogenous firing patterns characterized by the following parameters: CV = 1.08 ± 0.08, FF = 1.02 ± 0.09, mode ISI = 19.2 ± 1.5 ms, and a Silence Index = 1.06 ± 0.05. The distributions of these parameters are shown in **Figures 2D–H**. Overall, the relatively narrow distributions with a single peak characteristic of these firing pattern statistics suggest that the recorded population was composed of a single cell type that fired in a Poissonian manner most of the time.

We then examined the effect of isoflurane anesthesia on the properties of the EP neurons. The isoflurane did not influence the waveform shapes of the neurons, and all the measured parameters remained unchanged (valley width: $p = 0.27$, valley to peak duration: $p = 0.94$, zero-cross $p = 0.62$, valley to peak

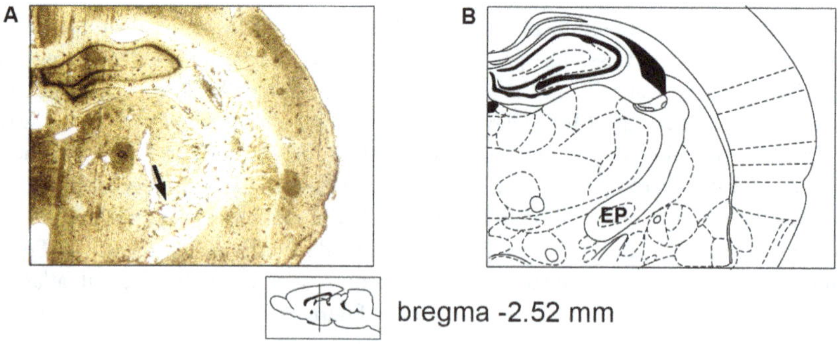

FIGURE 1 | Electrode placement verification. (A) A 60 micron slice showing electrode positioning in the rat EP following electrolytic lesion (marked by an arrow). **(B)** Appropriate coronal section from the rat atlas (Bregma: −2.52 mm; Paxinos, 2007).

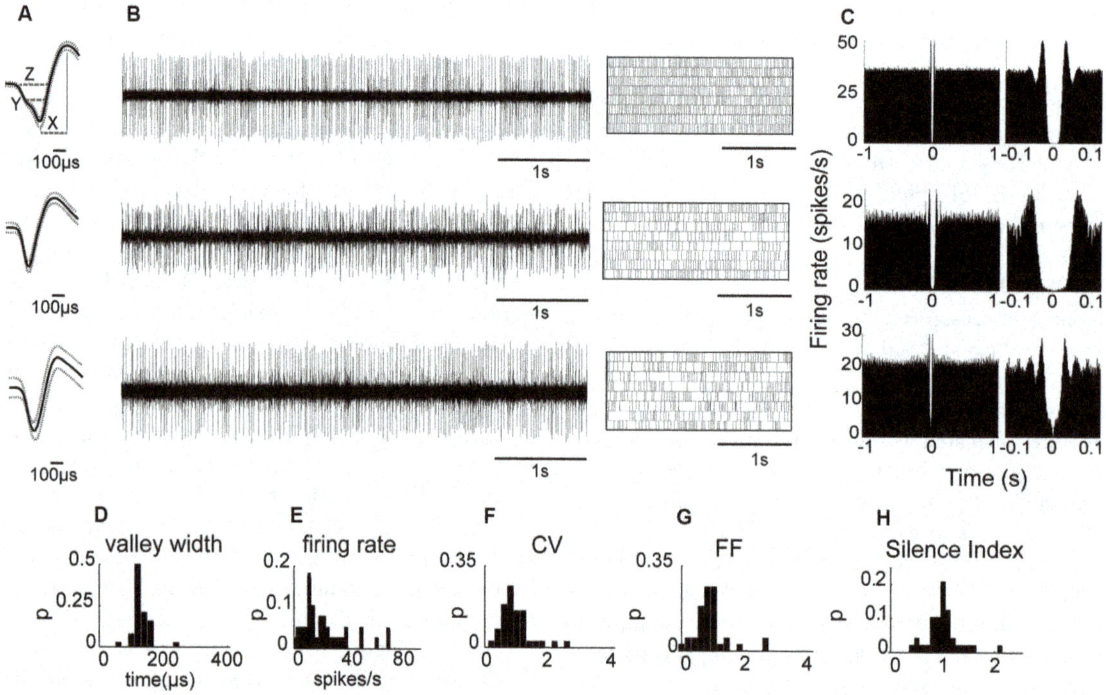

FIGURE 2 | EP neuronal firing characteristics in awake rats. (A) Examples of the firing of three EP neurons. From left to right: Average waveform. Inset (top): *X* represents the valley to peak duration, *Y* the valley width and *Z* the zero-cross parameter. **(B)** Continuous raw signal during 5 s (left) and spike train during 20 s (right). **(C)** Autocorrelation using a time window of ±1 s (left) and autocorrelation with *x*-axis expanded to 0.1 s (right) of the same neuron. **(D–H)** Waveform and firing parameter histograms.

amplitude ratio: $p = 0.97$) indicating that the recordings were stable throughout the sessions. By contrast, firing patterns varied substantially with isoflurane administration (see **Table 1**). The firing rate decreased significantly during anesthesia (14.8 ± 1.5 spikes/s) relative to wakefulness (26.0 ± 3.1 spike/s; Kruskal Wallis; $p = 0.00009$) as shown in **Figure 3A** and in the example shown below of neuronal firing recorded during wakefulness and under anesthesia (**Figure 3E**). Additionally, the CV values were substantially higher during anesthesia (2.40 ± 0.28) relative to wakefulness (1.08 ± 0.08; $p = 0.03$; **Figure 3B**). The increase in the CV values combined with the decrease in FR suggested that EP neurons ceased firing for durations longer than expected from irregular Poisson firing. Indeed, the Silence Index measured during isoflurane administration (1.51 ± 0.09) was substantially higher than during wakefulness (1.06 ± 0.05; **Figure 3D**; $p = 0.048$). An example of the ISI histogram of one EP neuron is shown during anesthesia and wakefulness and illustrates the long tail of ISI observed under anesthesia (**Figure 3F**). The FF values within the population did not change with isoflurane administration (**Figure 3C**; $p = 0.75$), and the neuronal pairwise interactions ($n = 24$) continued to be void.

Table 1 | Firing parameters across conditions (mean ± sem).

Parameter \ Condition	Wakefulness Isoflurane 0%	Isoflurane 1%	Isoflurane 2%	Isoflurane 3%	Isoflurane 4%
Number of neurons	38	34	29	22	15
CV	1.08 ± 0.08	1.78 ± 0.28	2.25 ± 0.59	2.76 ± 0.68	3.59 ± 0.92
FF	1.02 ± 0.09	1.05 ± 0.12	0.98 ± 0.11	0.99 ± 0.11	1.10 ± 0.19
Firing rate (spikes/s)	26.00 ± 3.13	18.14 ± 3.20	14.26 ± 2.70	12.60 ± 2.16	11.40 ± 2.65
Silence Index	1.06 ± 0.05	1.32 ± 0.12	1.56 ± 0.19	1.57 ± 0.19	1.79 ± 0.26

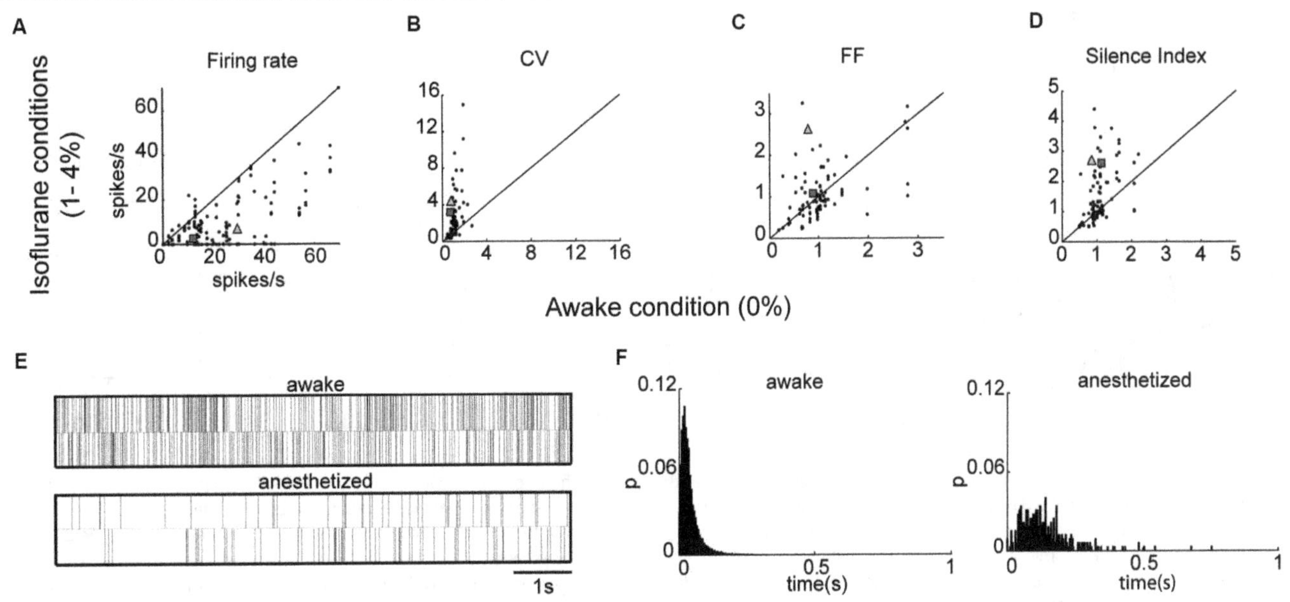

FIGURE 3 | EP neuronal firing characteristics in anesthetized rats. (A) Firing rate under anesthesia vs. firing rate during the awake state. **(B–D)** Same as **A** for CV **(B)**, FF **(C)** and Silence Index **(D)**. **(E)** Representative spike train examples over 20 s of the corresponding neuron marked by a blue triangle in **A–D**. **(F)** ISI histograms of the corresponding neuron marked by a red rectangle in **A–D**.

Examination of the relationship between the neuronal firing rate and the different levels of anesthesia revealed two types of EP neurons: one type (Group I) whose firing rate decreased as the anesthesia level increased, and a second type (Group II) whose firing rate was uncorrelated with anesthesia level. Neuronal spike trains representative of the two groups are shown in **Figure 4A.** The a-parametric Kendall Tau correlation test which identifies significant nonlinear correlations ($p < 0.05$) was used to determine which of the neurons decreased its firing rate with the increase in isoflurane level (see Section Materials and Methods). Observation of the Tau correlation factor showed that none of the neurons increased its firing rate with anesthesia (Tau values < 0); however, only those that substantially and monotonically decreased firing rate (values ~ -1) were identified as significant (red color; **Figure 4B**). Similar results were obtained using the Spearman's ρ rank correlation test. Group I comprised 37% (14/38) of the EP neurons whereas Group II comprised the remaining 63% (24/38) of the recorded population. Statistical examination of the influence of isoflurane administration on the two groups revealed a main effect for both group type and anesthesia level (a two-way ANOVA with Tukey-Kramer correction for multiple comparisons; $p < 0.0001$). *Post-hoc* examination of the firing rate showed that during wakefulness Group I displayed a significantly higher firing rate than Group II. Moreover, the firing rate of Group I gradually decreased and reached significance at isoflurane level of 2% relative to wakefulness whereas the firing rate of Group II decreased abruptly with anesthesia administration and remained constant during all isoflurane levels (**Figure 4C**).

Taking into consideration that neurons with similar firing rates can display different firing patterns and *vice versa* neurons with different firing rates can display similar firing patterns we tested whether the two groups display similar firing pattern characteristics. Specifically, we statistically compared the values of the firing pattern parameters CV, FF and silence index between the two groups which seemed non-separable in the awake state. Although both groups significantly decreased their firing rate in response to anesthesia they were characterized by different firing pattern parameters (**Figures 4D–F**). Group I displayed lower values of CV (1.70 ± 0.34), Silence Index (1.26 ± 0.11), and FF (0.91 ± 0.08) compared to Group II (CV: 2.25 ± 0.27; $p = 0.004$; Silence Index: 1.47 ± 0.08, $p = 0.014$; and FF: 1.09 ± 0.06, $p = 0.008$). These data suggest that the two groups may reflect the

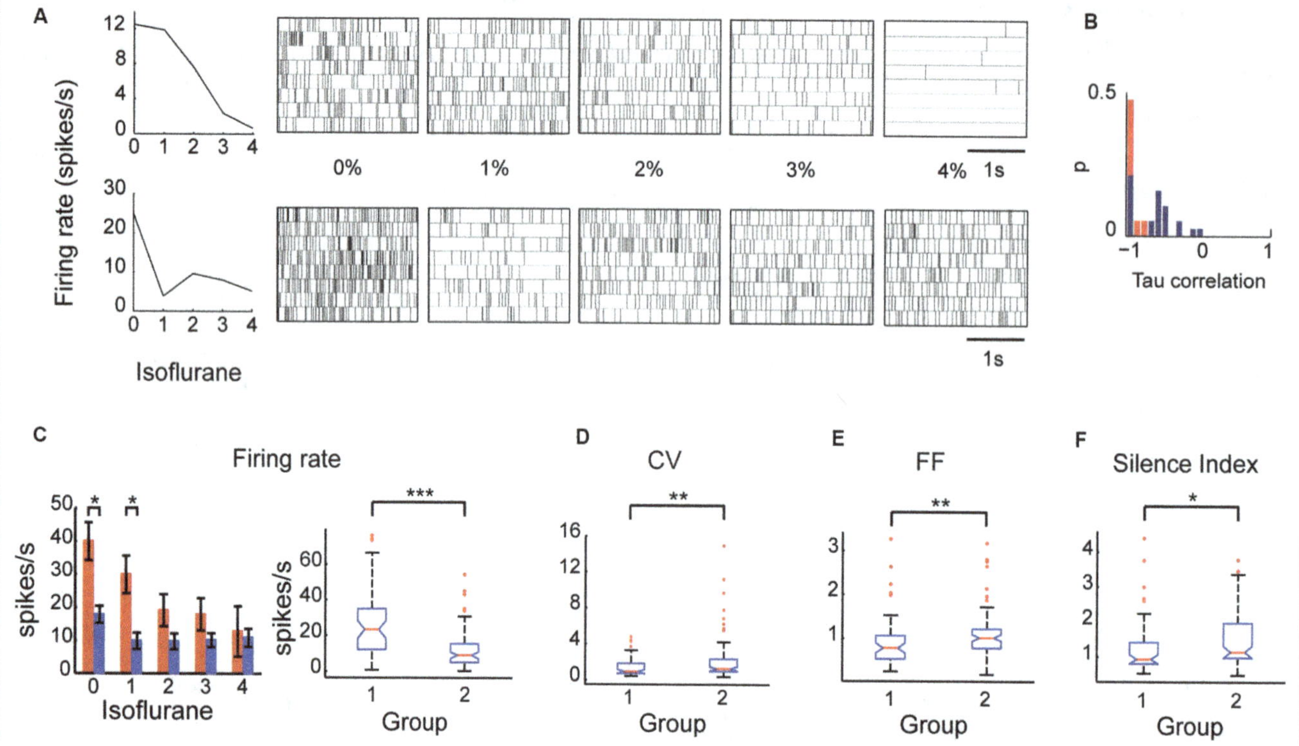

FIGURE 4 | Firing properties of EP neuronal subpopulations: Group I and Group II. (A) An example of two neurons—one that decreased its firing rate correlatively with the increase in isoflurane level (top) and another that decreased its firing rate abruptly with isoflurane administration (bottom)—and their corresponding spike trains over 20 s. **(B)** Tau correlation histogram: red represents the neurons identified as displaying a correlated firing rate to isoflurane levels by the Kendall Tau correlation test. **(C)** (left) Average firing rate of the two groups (Group I is shown in red and Group II is shown in blue) during five states of anesthesia. (right) The boxplots depict the firing rate medians of the two groups under all conditions with the edges at the 25th and 75th percentiles. Vertical lines mark the 5th and the 95th percentiles. Red asterisks mark outliers. **(D–F)** Boxplots of CV **(D)**, FF **(E)**, and Silence Index **(F)** of the two groups under all conditions (* $p < 0.05$; ** $p < 0.01$; *** $p < 0.001$).

existence of two subpopulations of neurons in the EP that could only be distinguished by their characteristic electrophysiological properties during different levels of anesthesia.

DISCUSSION

In this study we characterized neuronal activity in the EP of anesthetized and freely moving rats. Our results show that in freely moving animals, EP neurons displayed a high firing rate of 26 ± 3.1 spikes/s (range: 2.23–76.13 spikes/s, median: 20.30 spikes/s) whereas administration of isoflurane anesthesia induced a significant decrease in the firing rate to an average of 14.8 ± 1.5 spikes/s (range: 0.2–74.4 spikes/s, median: 9.27 spikes/s). This decrease in firing rate occurred either gradually as more anesthesia was delivered, or abruptly with the transition between wakefulness and the first level of anesthesia and then remained relatively stable regardless of the anesthesia level. Based on this distinction in the neurons' responses to anesthesia, we classified the EP neurons into two groups: Group I and Group II. Although examination of the firing properties of EP neurons during wakefulness indicated a homogenous population characterized by near Poissonian tonic firing and a lack of interactions, further examination suggested otherwise; the newly defined groups had significantly different firing pattern properties. Our results provide evidence for the potential existence of two distinct subpopulations within the rat EP that could be distinguished by their electrophysiological characteristics during isoflurane anesthesia.

Analysis of EP neurons recorded during wakefulness without a-priori classifying them into two distinct groups based on their anesthesia response curves revealed a seemingly homogeneous population. Similarly, extracellular recordings in the primate GPi revealed one homogenous neuronal population (DeLong, 1971). The firing pattern characteristics of GPi neurons excluding firing rate described in later studies by DeLong (1971) and others (Joshua et al., 2009; Sheth et al., 2011) are similar in nature to those observed in this study. Additionally, EP neurons were uncorrelated and apparently did not interact with one another as was previously observed in primates (Bar-Gad et al., 2003a), strengthening the view that the BG act as a decorrelating and dimensionality reduction system (Bar-Gad et al., 2003b). Under isoflurane, EP neurons increased their CV and Silence Index and decreased FR indicating that in that condition these neurons displayed a higher firing variability and pauses longer than expected from a Poissonian firing. A similar result was obtained in humans under Propofol anesthesia which inhibited GPi neurons, and in addition to inducing long pauses, increased their burst index (Hutchison et al., 2003).

The main difference between the neuronal activity of EP neurons and that of the GPi neurons is their average firing rate, which was 26.0 ± 3.1 spikes/s in EP and 63 spikes/s in GPi (DeLong, 1971). In a previous study we characterized neuronal activity of GP neurons in freely moving rats and compared the results to those obtained in primate GPe neurons using the same methodology (Benhamou et al., 2012). The outcome of that study showed that similarly to primates, rat GP neurons could be divided into two distinct neuronal populations based on their characteristic firing patterns. Two measures diverged from primates: the first was the average firing rate that appeared to be much lower in rats (20.07 spikes/s) than in primates (55 spikes/s), and the second was that the two subpopulations represented different proportions (rats: 73.5 vs. 26.5%; primates: 85 vs. 15%, for high frequency pausers and low frequency bursters, respectively (DeLong, 1971; Bugaysen et al., 2010; Benhamou et al., 2012). It should be noted that the proportions of these subpopulations resembled the *in vitro* proportions reported in rodents (Kita and Kitai, 1991; Cooper and Stanford, 2000). The current results further support the view that firing patterns rather than firing rates and subpopulation proportions are important to the preservation of BG information processing and especially the GP and EP, and are therefore conserved across species.

Isoflurane administration substantially altered the firing patterns displayed by EP neurons. Isoflurane is minimally metabolized in the body and has a low blood-gas partition coefficient (1.4) so that it has a very low solubility in blood and changes in concentrations are rapid. In the present experiment, we estimated a recovery time of 5 min based on our observations of the time it took animals to walk normally in the recording chamber following the removal of 1% isoflurane anesthesia. Recently, a median recovery time of 330 s has been reported when animals were placed under 1.5% isoflurane for 40 min (Taylor et al., 2013). Therefore, we cannot rule out that some of the anesthesia evoked effects may have had a longer lasting influence on the electrophysiological characteristics of EP neurons. Such a case however would have likely minimized rather than enhanced or caused the observed differences between the two groups because of residual effect averaging.

In vitro studies in rodents, cats and primates have reported the presence of two neuronal populations based either on their biophysical properties (Nakanishi et al., 1990) or on their projections' target sites (Nauta, 1974; Filion and Harnois, 1978; van der Kooy and Carter, 1981; Tokuno et al., 1988; Parent et al., 2001). On one hand, a proportion of 2/3 to 1/3 was found in rats based on the EP projections to the LHb and to the thalamus, respectively (van der Kooy and Carter, 1981). On the other hand, when the identification of two types of neurons was based on their membrane electrical properties a different proportion of division into types was reported; namely, 79.6% of type I neurons and 16.6% of type II neurons (Nakanishi et al., 1990). By taking into account that the intracellular recording method may create a sampling bias and consequently skew the data toward more accessible neurons, it is plausible that despite the difference in proportions the two studies dealt with the same neuronal types (i.e., that EP neurons projecting to different targets may be biophysically distinct). Isoflurane operates by altering neuronal membrane excitability (Franks and Lieb, 1994; Arhem et al., 2003) suggesting that neurons with different membrane properties may display different response curves under anesthesia. Therefore, based on the sensitivity of the membrane excitability to isoflurane and the similarity between the reported proportions of the two identified neuronal populations and the proportions observed in this study (63% in Group II and 37% in Group I) it is possible that the neurons comprising Group I are those projecting to the thalamus and those comprising Group II project to the LHb.

A complementary factor which may accentuate the differences between the firing properties of EP neurons is the different origin of their inputs; pallidohabenular neurons receive afferents from striatofugal neurons in the patch compartment whereas pallidothalamic neurons receive afferents from the matrix compartment (Rajakumar et al., 1993). It remains unknown however whether medium spiny neurons in the patch compartment respond to anesthesia differently than medium spiny neurons in the matrix. Another possible partition of EP neurons into subpopulations is based on their neurotransmitters; pallidothalamic neurons seem to comprise mainly GABAergic projections whereas the majority of the pallidohabenular projections in rats are non-GABAergic (Araki et al., 1984), and are possibly cholinergic (Moriizumi and Hattori, 1992). However, the release of different neurotransmitters is less likely to account for the observed differences in the groups' response curves and would yield a different group ratio (~1:1; GABAergic vs. non-GABAergic neurons) than the observed ratio (2:1; pallidohabenular vs. pallidothalamic). Therefore, a classification of Group I and Group II as GABAergic and possibly cholinergic neurons is less probable.

Primate and cat pallidohabenular neurons, which are far less abundant (10 and 16% of the neurons, respectively) than rat pallidohabenular neurons (2/3 of the neurons), have lower baseline firing rates (33 spikes/s) than presumed motor GPi neurons (77 spikes/s) (Larsen and Mcbride, 1979; Hong and Hikosaka, 2008). In the current study we found that 63% of the neurons (Group II neurons) had significantly lower firing rates than Group I neurons in awake rats (Group II: 17.8 ± 2.5 spikes/s; and Group I: 40.0 ± 5.7 spikes/s). The similarity in the observed firing rate imbalance between the two identified groups in rats and between the habenular projecting GPi neurons and motor neurons in primates lends additional support to the hypothesis that the Group II neurons reported in this study are habenular projecting EP neurons whereas the Group I neurons are thalamus projecting EP neurons. By taking into account the small size of rat EP in the rostro-caudal axis (600–800 μm) it seems that confirmation of this hypothesis could be obtained by optogenetic activation of identified habenular projecting EP neurons or by their antidromic activation via stimulation of the LHb. If confirmed, the simple procedure of isoflurane administration or possibly other kinds of anesthesia would permit selective access to limbic vs. motor information processing in the rat EP and primate GPi.

CONCLUSION

Our results suggest that: (1) firing patterns are preserved in the rat EP compared to primate GPi whereas firing rate and subpopulation ratio are not; and (2) the use of isoflurane anesthesia may provide an easy method to accentuate electrophysiological differences in the EP neurons and consequently enable their classification into two distinct neuronal populations. In so doing our results potentially reconcile *in vitro* studies performed in cat and rodent EP, and primate GPi where two subpopulations of neurons have been identified, and electrophysiological studies in behaving primates where only one homogeneous neuronal population has been reported. Further experiments are required to determine whether these two populations of neurons correspond to pallidohabenular and pallidothalamic neurons, and investigate whether their information processing capacity and contribution to behavior are similar or different in nature.

ACKNOWLEDGMENTS

The study was financed in part by a REALNET (FP7-ICT270434) grant from the European Commission. The authors declare no competing financial interests.

REFERENCES

Alexander, G. E., and Crutcher, M. D. (1990). Functional architecture of basal ganglia circuits: neural substrates of parallel processing. *Trends Neurosci.* 13, 266–271. doi: 10.1016/0166-2236(90)90107-l

Alexander, G. E., Delong, M. R., and Strick, P. L. (1986). Parallel organization of functionally segregated circuits linking basal ganglia and cortex. *Annu. Rev. Neurosci.* 9, 357–381. doi: 10.1146/annurev.neuro.9.1.357

Araki, M., Mcgeer, P. L., and Mcgeer, E. G. (1984). Retrograde HRP tracing combined with a pharmacohistochemical method for GABA transaminase for the identification of presumptive GABAergic projections to the habenula. *Brain Res.* 304, 271–277. doi: 10.1016/0006-8993(84)90330-5

Arhem, P., Klement, G., and Nilsson, J. (2003). Mechanisms of anesthesia: towards integrating network, cellular and molecular level modeling. *Neuropsychopharmacology* 28(Suppl. 1), S40–S47. doi: 10.1038/sj.npp.1300142

Bar-Gad, I., Heimer, G., Ritov, Y., and Bergman, H. (2003a). Functional correlations between neighboring neurons in the primate globus pallidus are weak or nonexistent. *J. Neurosci.* 23, 4012–4016.

Bar-Gad, I., Morris, G., and Bergman, H. (2003b). Information processing, dimensionality reduction and reinforcement learning in the basal ganglia. *Prog. Neurobiol.* 71, 439–473. doi: 10.1016/j.pneurobio.2003.12.001

Benhamou, L., Bronfeld, M., Bar-Gad, I., and Cohen, D. (2012). Globus Pallidus external segment neuron classification in freely moving rats: a comparison to primates. *PLoS One* 7:e45421. doi: 10.1371/journal.pone.0045421

Bugaysen, J., Bronfeld, M., Tischler, H., Bar-Gad, I., and Korngreen, A. (2010). Electrophysiological characteristics of globus pallidus neurons. *PLoS One* 5:e12001. doi: 10.1371/journal.pone.0012001

Cooper, A. J., and Stanford, I. M. (2000). Electrophysiological and morphological characteristics of three subtypes of rat globus pallidus neurone in vitro. *J. Physiol.* 527(Pt. 2), 291–304. doi: 10.1111/j.1469-7793.2000.t01-1-00291.x

DeLong, M. R. (1971). Activity of pallidal neurons during movement. *J. Neurophysiol.* 34, 414–427.

Deniau, J. M., Menetrey, A., and Charpier, S. (1996). The lamellar organization of the rat substantia nigra pars reticulata: segregated patterns of striatal afferents and relationship to the topography of corticostriatal projections. *Neuroscience* 73, 761–781. doi: 10.1016/0306-4522(96)00088-7

Filion, M., and Harnois, C. (1978). A comparison of projections of entopeduncular neurons to the thalamus, the midbrain and the habenula in the cat. *J. Comp. Neurol.* 181, 763–780. doi: 10.1002/cne.901810406

Franks, N. P., and Lieb, W. R. (1994). Molecular and cellular mechanisms of general anaesthesia. *Nature* 367, 607–614. doi: 10.1038/367607a0

Hong, S., and Hikosaka, O. (2008). The globus pallidus sends reward-related signals to the lateral habenula. *Neuron* 60, 720–729. doi: 10.1016/j.neuron.2008.09.035

Horak, F. B., and Anderson, M. E. (1984). Influence of globus pallidus on arm movements in monkeys. I. Effects of kainic acid-induced lesions. *J. Neurophysiol.* 52, 290–304.

Hutchison, W. D., Lang, A. E., Dostrovsky, J. O., and Lozano, A. M. (2003). Pallidal neuronal activity: implications for models of dystonia. *Ann. Neurol.* 53, 480–488. doi: 10.1002/ana.10474

Jacobson, G. A., Lev, I., Yarom, Y., and Cohen, D. (2009). Invariant phase structure of olivo-cerebellar oscillations and its putative role in temporal pattern generation. *Proc. Natl. Acad. Sci. U S A* 106, 3579–3584. doi: 10.1073/pnas.0806661106

Joshua, M., Adler, A., Rosin, B., Vaadia, E., and Bergman, H. (2009). Encoding of probabilistic rewarding and aversive events by pallidal and 'nigral neurons. *J. Neurophysiol.* 101, 758–772. doi: 10.1152/jn.90764.2008

Kita, H., and Kitai, S. T. (1991). Intracellular study of rat globus pallidus neurons: membrane properties and responses to neostriatal, subthalamic and nigral stimulation. *Brain Res.* 564, 296–305. doi: 10.1016/0006-8993(91)91466-e

Kitano, H., Tanibuchi, I., and Jinnai, K. (1998). The distribution of neurons in the substantia nigra pars reticulata with input from the motor, premotor and prefrontal areas of the cerebral cortex in monkeys. *Brain Res.* 784, 228–238. doi: 10.1016/s0006-8993(97)01332-2

Kojima, S., Kao, M. H., and Doupe, A. J. (2013). Task-related "cortical" bursting depends critically on basal ganglia input and is linked to vocal plasticity. *Proc. Natl. Acad. Sci. U S A* 110, 4756–4761. doi: 10.1073/pnas.1216308110

Kravitz, A. V., Freeze, B. S., Parker, P. R., Kay, K., Thwin, M. T., Deisseroth, K., et al. (2010). Regulation of parkinsonian motor behaviours by optogenetic control of basal ganglia circuitry. *Nature* 466, 622–626. doi: 10.1038/nature09159

Larsen, K. D., and Mcbride, R. L. (1979). The organization of feline entopeduncular nucleus projections: anatomical studies. *J. Comp. Neurol.* 184, 293–308. doi: 10.1002/cne.901840206

Lidsky, T. I. (1975). Pallidal and entopeduncular single unit activity in cats during drinking. *Electroencephalogr. Clin. Neurophysiol.* 39, 79–84. doi: 10.1016/0013-4694(75)90129-7

Mink, J. W. (1996). The basal ganglia: focused selection and inhibition of competing motor programs. *Prog. Neurobiol.* 50, 381–425. doi: 10.1016/s0301-0082(96)00042-1

Moriizumi, T., and Hattori, T. (1992). Choline acetyltransferase-immunoreactive neurons in the rat entopeduncular nucleus. *Neuroscience* 46, 721–728. doi: 10.1016/0306-4522(92)90158-x

Nakanishi, H., Kita, H., and Kitai, S. T. (1990). Intracellular study of rat entopeduncular nucleus neurons in an in vitro slice preparation: electrical membrane properties. *Brain Res.* 527, 81–88. doi: 10.1016/0006-8993(90)91063-m

Nauta, H. J. (1974). Evidence of a pallidohabenular pathway in the cat. *J. Comp. Neurol.* 156, 19–27. doi: 10.1002/cne.901560103

Nicolelis, M. A., Ghazanfar, A. A., Faggin, B. M., Votaw, S., and Oliveira, L. M. (1997). Reconstructing the engram: simultaneous, multisite, many single neuron recordings. *Neuron* 18, 529–537. doi: 10.1016/s0896-6273(00)80295-0

Obeso, J. A., Jahanshahi, M., Alvarez, L., Macias, R., Pedroso, I., Wilkinson, L., et al. (2009). What can man do without basal ganglia motor output? The effect of combined unilateral subthalamotomy and pallidotomy in a patient with Parkinson's disease. *Exp. Neurol.* 220, 283–292. doi: 10.1016/j.expneurol.2009.08.030

Parent, M., Levesque, M., and Parent, A. (2001). Two types of projection neurons in the internal pallidum of primates: single-axon tracing and three-dimensional reconstruction. *J. Comp. Neurol.* 439, 162–175. doi: 10.1002/cne.1340

Paxinos, G. A. W. C. (2007). *The Rat Brain in Stereotaxic Coordinates.* 6th Edn. New York: Elsevier.

Rajakumar, N., Elisevich, K., and Flumerfelt, B. A. (1993). Compartmental origin of the striato-entopeduncular projection in the rat. *J. Comp. Neurol.* 331, 286–296. doi: 10.1002/cne.903310210

Redgrave, P., Prescott, T. J., and Gurney, K. (1999). The basal ganglia: a vertebrate solution to the selection problem? *Neuroscience* 89, 1009–1023. doi: 10.1016/s0306-4522(98)00319-4

Sheth, S. A., Abuelem, T., Gale, J. T., and Eskandar, E. N. (2011). Basal ganglia neurons dynamically facilitate exploration during associative learning. *J. Neurosci.* 31, 4878–4885. doi: 10.1523/jneurosci.3658-10.2011

Taylor, N. E., Chemali, J. J., Brown, E. N., and Solt, K. (2013). Activation of D1 dopamine receptors induces emergence from isoflurane general anesthesia. *Anesthesiology* 118, 30–39. doi: 10.1097/aln.0b013e318278c896

Tokuno, H., Moriizumi, T., Kudo, M., Kitao, Y., and Nakamura, Y. (1988). Ultrastructural differences between pallidohabenular terminals and pallidothalamic terminals. *Brain Res.* 474, 390–393. doi: 10.1016/0006-8993(88)90457-x

Turner, R. S., and Anderson, M. E. (2005). Context-dependent modulation of movement-related discharge in the primate globus pallidus. *J. Neurosci.* 25, 2965–2976. doi: 10.1523/jneurosci.4036-04.2005

Turner, R. S., and Desmurget, M. (2010). Basal ganglia contributions to motor control: a vigorous tutor. *Curr. Opin. Neurobiol.* 20, 704–716. doi: 10.1016/j.conb.2010.08.022

van der Kooy, D., and Carter, D. A. (1981). The organization of the efferent projections and striatal afferents of the entopeduncular nucleus and adjacent areas in the rat. *Brain Res.* 211, 15–36. doi: 10.1016/0006-8993(81)90064-0

Wichmann, T., Kliem, M. A., and Soares, J. (2002). Slow oscillatory discharge in the primate basal ganglia. *J. Neurophysiol.* 87, 1145–1148.

5

Fronto-Striatal Gray Matter Contributions to Discrimination Learning in Parkinson's Disease

Claire O'Callaghan*[1,2]*, Ahmed A. Moustafa*[3]*, Sanne de Wit*[4]*, James M. Shine*[5]*, Trevor W. Robbins*[6]*, Simon J. G. Lewis*[5] *and Michael Hornberger*[1,2,7,8]

[1] *Neuroscience Research Australia, Sydney, NSW, Australia*
[2] *Faculty of Medicine, School of Medical Sciences, University of New South Wales, Sydney, NSW, Australia*
[3] *School of Social Sciences and Psychology and the Marcs Institute for Brain and Behaviour, University of Western Sydney, Sydney, NSW, Australia*
[4] *Cognitive Science Center Amsterdam and Department of Clinical Psychology, University of Amsterdam, Amsterdam, Netherlands*
[5] *Parkinson's Disease Clinic, Brain and Mind Research Institute, University of Sydney, Sydney, NSW, Australia*
[6] *Department of Psychology, Behavioural and Clinical Neuroscience Institute, University of Cambridge, Cambridge, UK*
[7] *ARC Centre of Excellence in Cognition and its Disorders, Sydney, NSW, Australia*
[8] *Department of Clinical Neurosciences, University of Cambridge, Cambridge, UK*

***Correspondence:**
Michael Hornberger, Neuroscience Research Australia, Cnr Barker and Easy Street, Randwick, Sydney, NSW 2031, Australia
e-mail: m.hornberger@neura.edu.au

Discrimination learning deficits in Parkinson's disease (PD) have been well-established. Using both behavioral patient studies and computational approaches, these deficits have typically been attributed to dopamine imbalance across the basal ganglia. However, this explanation of impaired learning in PD does not account for the possible contribution of other pathological changes that occur in the disease process, importantly including gray matter loss. To address this gap in the literature, the current study explored the relationship between fronto-striatal gray matter atrophy and learning in PD. We employed a discrimination learning task and computational modeling in order to assess learning rates in non-demented PD patients. Behaviorally, we confirmed that learning rates were reduced in patients relative to controls. Furthermore, voxel-based morphometry imaging analysis demonstrated that this learning impairment was directly related to gray matter loss in discrete fronto-striatal regions (specifically, the ventromedial prefrontal cortex, inferior frontal gyrus and nucleus accumbens). These findings suggest that dopaminergic imbalance may not be the sole determinant of discrimination learning deficits in PD, and highlight the importance of factoring in the broader pathological changes when constructing models of learning in PD.

Keywords: Parkinson's disease, discrimination learning, goal-directed learning, computational modeling, voxel-based morphometry, fronto-striatal

INTRODUCTION

Parkinson's disease (PD) is a neurodegenerative condition characterized by hallmark motor disturbances, with its primary neuropathology in the nigrostriatal pathway. This leads to severe dopamine depletion in the dorsal striatum, while the ventral striatum is relatively preserved in the earlier disease stages (Jellinger, 2001). In PD, both the progressive dopamine depletion in the basal ganglia and the concurrent beneficial and deleterious effects of dopamine replacement medications, have been associated with a range of distinct learning impairments (for reviews, see Price et al., 2009; Foerde and Shohamy, 2011b). These dopamine dependent learning deficits in PD have been informative in the development of theoretical accounts of learning function and have provided important advances and testable predictions for computational explanations of learning (Frank, 2005). In particular, PD has been associated with acquisition deficits in feedback-based discrimination learning (Myers et al., 2003; de Wit et al., 2011), which have also been described via computational approaches (Moustafa et al., 2010).

Feedback-based and trial-and-error learning is presumed to be mediated by relative patterns of tonic vs. phasic dopamine activity occurring in response to environmental reinforcers (Schultz, 2002; Bromberg-Martin et al., 2010). Indeed, current accounts of discrimination learning in PD have been derived through ON- vs. OFF-medication patient studies and through computational models, which have established a role for basal ganglia dopamine imbalance as a crucial factor underpinning the feedback-based learning deficits (Frank et al., 2004; Shohamy et al., 2006). Whilst such explanations of learning deficits based on dopaminergic imbalance do accord with the biological characteristics of PD, these theories have not addressed the potential contributions of other prevalent pathological effects in PD. For example, in addition to the characteristic dopamine depletion PD is also associated with gray matter loss and reduced white matter integrity (Duncan et al., 2013). Significantly, regions of gray matter loss in PD involve systems that are implicated in a range of higher level cognitive functions (including learning), and it is only more recently that direct associations between volumetric reductions and specific cognitive deficits have been confirmed in early stage, non-demented PD (Filoteo et al., 2013; O'Callaghan et al., 2013).

Given the known volumetric brain changes in PD and the possibility that they may directly affect learning processes, exploring this relationship to inform future learning theories and computational approaches that rely on PD as a model is now vital. In the current study, we directly examined this issue by combining voxel-based morphometry analysis with a computational modeling technique in order to determine how fronto-striatal gray matter reductions relate to acquisition efficiency on a discrimination learning task. We hypothesized PD patients would show impaired learning acquisition rates and that these impairments would be associated with volumetric reductions in fronto-striatal regions that are crucial for feedback-based learning and reward processing.

MATERIALS AND METHODS

CASE SELECTION

Seventeen non-demented PD patients were recruited from the Brain and Mind Institute Parkinson's Disease Research Clinic; all satisfied UKPDS Brain Bank criteria for diagnosis of PD (Gibb and Lees, 1988) and were between Hoehn and Yahr stages I and III (Hoehn and Yahr, 1967). Motor score from the Unified Parkinson's Disease Rating Scale (UPDRS-III) (Goetz et al., 2008) is also reported. One patient was untreated; three were on levodopa monotherapy and two were taking levodopa plus an adjuvant; nine patients were on levodopa plus a dopamine agonist, and in this group four were also taking an adjuvant and one was taking a monoamine oxidase inhibitor; one patient was on a dopamine agonist plus a monoamine oxidase inhibitor and one was taking a monoamine oxidase inhibitor only. Treated patients performed behavioral testing in the ON state, having taken their usual medications. L-dopa daily dose equivalents (DDE mg/day) were calculated for treated patients. Patients with overt clinical depression were not included in the study and a measure of affective disturbance was obtained (Beck Depression Inventory-II; BDI-II, Beck et al., 1996). Eleven age- and education-matched healthy controls were selected from a volunteer panel. See **Table 1** for demographic details and clinical characteristics.

The research study was approved by the Human Ethics Committees of the Central and South Eastern Sydney Area Health Services and the Universities of Sydney and New South Wales, and complies with the statement on human experimentation issued by the National Health and Medical Research Council of Australia.

Table 1 | Mean (SD) values for Controls and PD patients on demographics, clinical characteristics and discrimination learning measures.

Demographics, clinical characteristics and executive function	Controls	PD	$F/\chi 2$-values
N	11	17	–
Sex (M:F)	3:8	13:4	–
Age (years)	66.3 (7.2)	66.4 (8.4)	n.s.
Education (years)[a]	14.9 (2.0)	14.1 (3.6)	n.s.
MMSE (max. 30)[a]	29.6 (0.71)	28.6 (1.6)	n.s.
Disease duration (years since diagnosis)	–	5.6 (5.4)	–
Hoehn and Yahr stage	–	2.1 (0.52)	–
UPDRS III	–	29.2 (12.8)	–
Dopamine dose equivalent (mg/day)	–	616.1 (453.1)	–
BDI-II	–	10.6 (6.9)	–
EXECUTIVE FUNCTION			
Digit span forwards	11.4 (1.8)	10.9 (2.3)	n.s.
Digit span backwards	9.1 (2.1)	7.4 (1.8)	*
Letter fluency	49.0 (15.9)	41.2 (13.5)	n.s.
Trail making test B-A	24.5 (19.4)	41.8 (25.0)	n.s.
DISCRIMINATION LEARNING			
Overall accuracy (%)	82.3 (10.6)	71.9 (19.6)	n.s.
Learning rate	0.217 (0.036)	0.163 (0.041)	**
Exploration[a]	0.70 (0.26)	0.85 (0.30)	n.s.

*n.s., non significant, *$p < 0.05$, **$p < 0.001$; F-values indicate significant differences across groups, otherwise due to unequal variance $\chi 2$ indicates differences across groups[a]. MMSE, Mini-Mental State Examination; UPDRS III, Motor score from the Unified Parkinson's Disease Rating Scale; BDI-II, Beck Depression Inventory II.*

NEUROPSYCHOLOGICAL ASSESSMENT

All patients and controls were administered the Mini Mental State Examination (MMSE; Folstein et al., 1975) to determine their overall cognitive functioning. For detailed measurement of executive function, patients and controls underwent a battery of tests including Verbal Fluency [measured by the number of words produced in 60 s, beginning with F, A, and S (Benton et al., 1994)]; the Trail-Making test (time B-A) to assess speeded set-shifting (Reitan and Wolfson, 1985); and a Digit Span task, with digits repeated in their original order (forwards) and in reverse order (backwards) (Wechsler, 1997) to assess attention span and working memory.

DISCRIMINATION LEARNING TASK

We administered a discrimination learning task developed by de Wit and colleagues, which was an abbreviated version of a more extensive instrumental learning measure described by de Wit et al. (2007). The task was computer based and programmed using Visual Basic 6.0, with keyboard response keys *z* and *m* programmed to register a *left* or *right* response.

Discrimination learning tasks involve a discriminative stimulus that signals whether or not a certain response will lead to a particular outcome; stimuli are presumed to have acquired discriminative control over instrumental performance when correct responding occurs in the presence of a given stimulus (i.e., when the stimulus: response-outcome contingency is acquired) (Bouton, 2007). In the current discrimination learning task, for each trial the discriminative stimulus consisted of a colored icon depicting a piece of a fruit on the front of a box. There were six possible fruits that could be pictured on the outside of the box (i.e., strawberry, lemon, grape, kiwi, melon, and orange). Subjects were required to make either a *left* or *right* response in order to "open" the box and obtain the outcome/reward inside (the outcome being a different fruit, i.e., coconut, pear, pineapple, cherry, banana, and apple). Each of the six stimulus fruits were associated with a particular correct response (i.e., *left* or *right*) that would result in obtaining the reward/outcome. These contingencies were kept constant, for example a *left* response to the strawberry stimulus would always result in the box opening to reveal an outcome/reward, whereas if a *right* response was made to the strawberry stimulus, the box would open to reveal nothing inside. Additional feedback was provided as the opened box revealing the reward was paired with a positive sound and points displayed on the screen, whereas the opened box with nothing inside was paired with a negative sound effect. The initial fruit stimulus remained on the screen until subjects made a response and faster correct responses earned more points (in the range from 1 to 5). The outcome fruit was presented for 1 s, and inter-trial intervals were fixed at 1.5 s.

Subjects were instructed at the outset of the task that they would need to determine the correct response for each stimulus fruit via a trial and error process. It was emphasized that these contingencies would not change throughout the trials, so that it would be possible for them to learn these stimulus-response associations. They were also encouraged to memorise the stimulus: response-outcome associations, as they would be questioned on them at the end.

Each subject completed 96 trials, comprising of eight 12-trial blocks during which each of the six possible stimulus-response pairs was presented twice in a randomized order; three of the stimulus fruits were associated with a correct *left* response and the other three were associated with a correct *right* response. Across subjects, the particular fruits that served as the stimulus and those that served as the outcome were counterbalanced. From the discrimination learning task, we derived a binary outcome measure of either 1 or 0 for each trial (1 indicating a correct response for that trial, 0 an incorrect response). Finally, after completing the trials, patients were asked to fill in pencil and paper questionnaires that probed explicit knowledge of the stimulus: response-outcome contingencies. These questionnaires were divided into three parts (each with six items), assessing knowledge of: (1) stimulus-response knowledge; (2) response-outcome; and (3) stimulus-outcome. In part (1), subjects were shown pictures of each stimulus fruit one at a time and they were asked to verbally indicate whether a *left* or *right* response was associated with obtaining a reward for each stimulus. A similar procedure was followed in part (2), as subjects were shown each reward/outcome and asked to indicate whether a *left* or *right* response had been necessary to successfully achieve that reward. In part (3), subjects were shown each stimulus fruit alongside an array of all possible reward fruits and they selected the reward that had been paired with each particular stimulus.

COMPUTATIONAL MODEL

Given the insufficiency of classical statistical methods in extracting learning rates and trial-by-trial responses, we applied the reinforcement Q-learning model to the outcome measures generated from the discrimination learning task, for each subject's pattern of correct and incorrect responses across the 96 trials (Sutton and Barto, 1998). The input of this model is a trial-by-trial sequence of responses for each subject, while the output is the learning rate and exploration parameter values, which cannot be obtained from regular statistical analysis of behavioral data. Previous research has used similar computational models to fit model parameter values for each subject in genetic (Frank et al., 2007) and patient studies (Gold et al., 2012). The rationale for applying the Q-learning model to the behavioral data is to disentangle each subject's performance to different components, and also to determine which model parameters can better account for variations in behavioral performance across different groups. Here, we attempt to understand the observed behavioral results using the computational reinforcement Q-learning model (Watkins and Dayan, 1992; Sutton and Barto, 1998; Frank et al., 2007) and specifically, we have fitted our behavioral data using a Q-learning model (Frank et al., 2007).

By using the reinforcement Q-learning model, we fit individual subject's trial-by-trial data, which culminates in two parameter values that correspond to the subject's learning rate and exploration/exploitation bias. The learning rate parameter modulates the degree to which feedback on the current trial is used to adjust expectations for future trials. The exploration parameter indicates whether the subject is more likely to choose the same or a different response as on previous trials with the same stimulus. A small exploration/exploitation parameter indicates exploitation (i.e., increased likelihood that subjects will choose the same response as previously made, when presented with the same stimulus), and a large value indicates exploration (i.e., increased likelihood they will choose a different response when presented with the same stimulus). In principle, impaired feedback learning can occur because of small learning rate or decreased likelihood to explore alternative responses at the expense of exploiting previously erroneous response strategies.

Specifically, we compute a weight (W) value for selecting each stimulus i during trial t, such that the value of the chosen stimulus is modified by reinforcement feedback:

$$PE(t) = US(t) - W(t)$$

where $PE(t)$ is the prediction error at time t; $US(t)$ is feedback presented at time t, and is equal to 1 for positive and 0 for negative feedback. W-values are computed using the following equation.

$$W_i(t+1) = W_i(t) + \alpha PE(t)$$

where α is learning rate (for more details, see Frank et al., 2007).

We have modeled choice by using a softmax logistic function, with inverse gain (exploration) parameter β, such that the probability of choosing A over B was computed as:

$$P_A(t) = \frac{e^{W_A(t)/\beta}}{e^{W_A(t)/\beta} + e^{W_B(t)/\beta}}$$

Each participant's trial-by-trial choices were fitted with two free parameters, α and β, which were selected to maximize fit to participant's sequence of choices in the task. β is an inverse gain parameter and reflects the participant's tendency to either exploit (i.e., to choose the response with the currently highest W-value) or explore (i.e., to randomly choose a category).

We then fitted the model to each participant's data, by searching through the space of each of these two parameters from 0 to

1 with a step size of 0.01. We then optimized the log likelihood estimate (LLE) at trial t:

$$\text{LLE} = \text{Log}\,(\Pi_t P(t))$$

where t is trial number (for a total of 96 trials). For each participant, the best fitting parameter values are those associated with maximum LLE. Equivalently, maximum LLE is the most predictive of the participant's responses in the task. In this model, the best fitting parameter values to each participant's behavioral data accommodate trial-by-trial adaptations in response to feedback given based on participants' choices. In addition, we predict that these values will explain differences in learning efficiency between patients and controls.

Finally, to validate our model we compared our results with a random responder model. Specifically, we calculated the pseudo-R^2 measure, which is (LLE-r)/r, where r is the log likelihood of the data under a model of purely random choices, in which $p = 0.5$ for all trials (Camerer and Ho, 1999; Daw et al., 2006). The resulting pseudo-R^2 statistic reveals how well the model fits the data compared to a model predicting chance performance and is independent of the number of trials to be fit in each set (see Frank et al., 2007, for discussion).

BEHAVIORAL ANALYSES

Data were analyzed using SPSS19.0 (SPSS Inc., Chicago, Ill., USA). Parametric demographic and neuropsychological data were compared across the groups via One-Way ANOVAs followed by Tukey *post-hoc* tests. A priori, demographic and learning variables were plotted and checked for normality of distribution by Kolmogorov-Smirnov tests. Variables showing non-parametric distribution were analyzed via Chi-square, Kruskal-Wallis and Mann-Whitney *U*-tests. A repeated measures ANOVA with Bonferroni *post hoc* tests was used to explore group differences in learning accuracy across the eight blocks, with group (control vs. patient) as the between-subjects variable and block (blocks 1–8) as the within-subjects variable.

IMAGING ACQUISITION

All patients and controls underwent the same imaging protocol with whole-brain T1 images acquired using 3T Philips MRI scanners with standard quadrature head coil (8 channels). The 3D T1-weighted sequences were acquired as follows: coronal orientation, matrix 256 × 256, 200 slices, 1 × 1 mm^2 in-plane resolution, slice thickness 1 mm, TE/TR = 2.6/5.8 ms.

VOXEL-BASED MORPHOMETRY (VBM) ANALYSIS

3D T1-weighted sequences were analyzed with FSL-VBM, a voxel-based morphometry analysis (Ashburner and Friston, 2000; Good et al., 2001) which is part of the FSL software package http://www.fmrib.ox.ac.uk/fsl/fslvbm/index.html (Smith et al., 2004). First, tissue segmentation was carried out using FMRIB's Automatic Segmentation Tool (FAST) (Zhang et al., 2001) from brain extracted images. The resulting gray matter partial volume maps were then aligned to the Montreal Neurological Institute standard space (MNI152) using the non-linear registration approach using FNIRT (Andersson et al., 2007a,b), which uses a b-spline representation of the registration warp field (Rueckert et al., 1999). The registered partial volume maps were then modulated (to correct for local expansion or contraction) by dividing them by the Jacobian of the warp field. The modulated images were then smoothed with an isotropic Gaussian kernel with a standard deviation of 3 mm (FWHM: 8 mm). A region-of-interest (ROI) mask for prefrontal and striatal brain regions was created by using the Harvard-Oxford cortical and subcortical structural atlas. The atlas regions that comprise the entire prefrontal cortex and striatum were included in the mask, these included frontal pole, superior frontal gyrus, middle frontal gyrus, inferior frontal gyrus, frontal medial cortex, subcallosal cortex, paracingulate gyrus, cingulate gyrus (anterior division), frontal orbital cortex, caudate, putamen, and nucleus accumbens. Finally, a voxelwise general linear model (GLM) was applied and permutation-based non-parametric testing was used to form clusters with the Threshold-Free Cluster Enhancement (TFCE) method (Smith and Nichols, 2009), tested for significance at $p < 0.05$, corrected for multiple comparisons via Family-wise Error (FWE) correction across space, unless otherwise stated.

RESULTS

DEMOGRAPHICS, CLINICAL CHARACTERISTICS AND NEUROPSYCHOLOGICAL ASSESSMENT

Demographics and general cognitive scores can be seen in **Table 1**. Participant groups did not differ in terms of age, education or MMSE score (p's > 0.1). Patients and controls did not differ in their Digit Span forwards score ($p > 0.6$), but patients were impaired relative to Controls for Digit Span backwards ($p < 0.05$). Groups were equivalent for Letter Fluency scores ($p > 0.2$) and although groups did not differ significantly on Trail Making B-A scores, there was a strong trend toward worse performance in the patients ($p = 0.06$). See **Table 1**.

LEARNING MEASURES

Overall accuracy scores on the discrimination learning task are shown in **Table 1** and learning accuracy across the eight blocks is shown in **Figure 1**. Overall accuracy across the 96 trials was not significantly different between the groups ($p > 0.1$). Results of the repeated measures ANOVA showed that there was no significant main effect of group [$F_{(1,\,26)} = 2.6, p > 0.1$]. Mauchly's test indicated that the assumption of sphericity had been violated [$\chi^2_{(27)} = 71.0, p < 0.001$] therefore degrees of freedom were corrected using Huynh-Feldt estimates of sphericity ($\varepsilon = 0.550$). The results show a significant main effect for block [$F_{(4.8,\,124.2)} = 20.3, p < 0.001$], which reflected that, irrespective of group, accuracy in blocks 6, 7, and 8 was significantly higher than in blocks 1, 2, and 3 (p-values < 0.05), accuracy in block 5 was significantly higher than in blocks 1 and 2 ($p < 0.05$), and accuracy in block 4 was higher than accuracy in block 1 ($p < 0.002$). There was no significant group by block interaction [$F_{(4.8,\,124.2)} = 1.6, p > 0.1$). *Post-hoc* between-group comparisons revealed that controls and PD patients only differed significantly on their accuracy in block 7 with controls having a higher accuracy score ($p < 0.05$), no significant difference were observed in other blocks ($p > 0.05$). Within-group *post-hoc* analysis showed that controls had consistent significant differences in accuracy between early and late blocks, with blocks 4, 5, 6, 7, and 8 all having higher accuracy than both blocks 1 and 2 (p-values < 0.05). PD patients showed a slightly less consistent pattern, with accuracy in blocks 5, 6, 7, and 8 higher than in block 1 (but not block 2) (p-values < 0.05); with all other block accuracies were equivalent, expect for blocks 7 and 8 being significantly higher than block 3 (p-values < 0.05).

Results of the learning rate and exploration parameters for the discrimination learning task, as derived from the computational model, are also shown in **Table 1**. Exploration parameters did not differ significantly between the groups ($p > 0.3$) and the small value of the parameter in both patients and controls suggested minimal exploration, which would be predicted based on the nature of the task. Learning Rate for the PD patients was significantly reduced relative to controls ($p = 0.001$) and these Learning Rate values were further analyzed in the VBM analysis. Results from the random responder model revealed the mean and standard deviation of pseudo-R^2 were 0.2901 and 0.173, respectively. This was significantly larger than zero, indicating our model performs better than chance at fitting individuals' data.

Participant groups did not differ in terms of explicit knowledge of Stimulus-Response-Outcome contingencies. The following mean (standard deviation) results on the three questionnaire sections were achieved, each section with a possible maximum score of 6 (i.e., 1 point per item). Stimulus-Response accuracy for controls was 5.6 (0.05) and for PD patients 5.3 (1.6); Response-Outcome accuracy for controls was 5.0 (1.2) and PD patients 4.6 (1.7); Stimulus-Outcome for controls was 3.5 (1.7) and PD patients 3.0 (2.2), with all p-values > 0.5. In a correlation analysis, none of the PD clinical variables (i.e., disease duration, Hoehn and Yahr stage, UPDRS III, DDE mg/day, BDI score) or the digits backward score, showed a significant relationship with the Learning Rate measure (p's > 0.1).

VBM ANALYSIS

The PD group was initially contrasted with controls to reveal overall patterns of brain atrophy in the fronto-striatal mask. PD patients showed gray matter atrophy bilaterally in the frontal orbital cortex and subcallosal cortex, extending back to the left ventral striatal (nucleus accumbens) territory; as well as in the inferior frontal gyri bilaterally (see Supplementary Table 1).

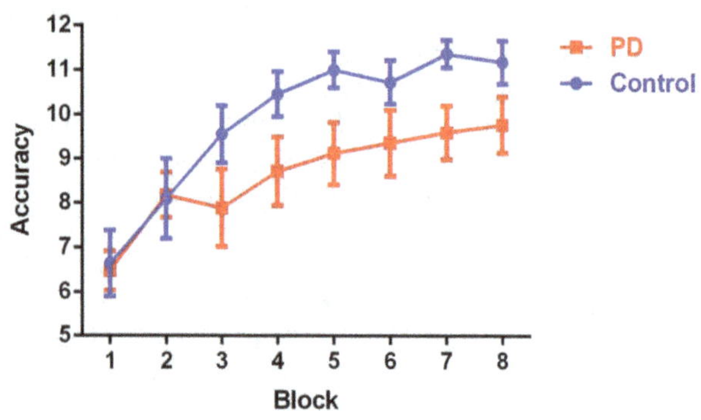

FIGURE 1 | Mean accuracy scores (with standard error bars) across the eight 12-trial blocks.

Learning rate was then entered as a covariate in the design matrix of the VBM analysis. For PD patients, Learning Rate score covaried with gray matter atrophy in the frontal medial cortex/frontal pole, the right inferior frontal gyrus and the left subcallosal cortex/left nucleus accumbens (see **Table 2** and **Figure 2**).

Finally, a partial correlation analysis was used to explore whether common damage to the ventromedial prefrontal cortex, right inferior frontal gyrus and left subcallosal cortex/nucleus

Table 2 | Region of interest Voxel-based morphometry (VBM) results showing areas of significant gray matter intensity decrease that covary with learning measures.

Regions	Hemisphere (L/R/B)	MNI coordinates			Number of voxels	*T*-score
		X	*Y*	*Z*		
LEARNING RATE						
Frontal medial cortex; Frontal pole	B	−6	46	−26	422	2.70
Inferior frontal gyrus	R	54	26	8	54	
Subcallosal/ extending back to L NAcc	L	−4	12	−14	46	

All results uncorrected at $p < 0.01$; only clusters with at least 40 contiguous voxels included.

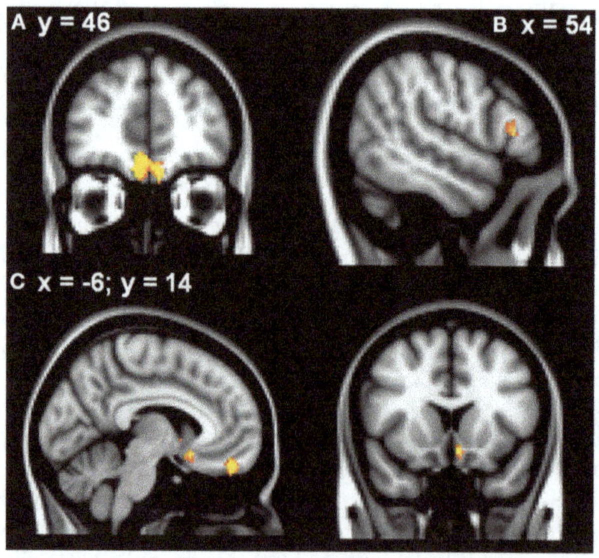

FIGURE 2 | VBM analysis showing the frontal and striatal regions that correlated with elevated learning rates in the patients in (A) frontal medial cortex (B) right inferior frontal gyrus (C) subcallosal/left nucleus accumbens. Clusters are overlaid on the MNI standard brain ($t > 2.50$). Cultured voxels show regions which were significant in the analyses for $p < 0.01$ uncorrected and a cluster threshold of 40 contiguous voxels.

accumbens explained the significant correlations with Learning Rate. The ventromedial prefrontal region still correlated significantly with Learning Rate ($p < 0.05$) when right inferior frontal gyrus and left subcallosal cortex/nucleus accumbens were taken into account. In contrast, neither right inferior frontal gyrus nor left subcallosal cortex/nucleus accumbens regions correlated significantly with Learning Rate when atrophy in the other regions was partialled out (p-values ≥ 0.2).

DISCUSSION

By employing a combined approach of computational modeling and VBM analysis, we show that PD patients have a learning acquisition deficit that is associated with volumetric reductions in discrete fronto-striatal regions. This is the first time that such learning deficits in PD have been probed via structural imaging techniques and our findings fit well with the broader learning literature, whilst highlighting a novel approach in order to further characterize discrimination learning in PD.

The nature of learning assessed in the current study reflects the formation of stimulus-response associations, which are learnt through incorporating feedback via a trial-and-error approach. Impaired learning acquisition rates on discrimination tasks have been demonstrated behaviorally in PD patients (Czernecki et al., 2002; Myers et al., 2003; de Wit et al., 2011; Shiner et al., 2012) and also in neurocomputational models of PD (Moustafa et al., 2010). Furthermore, Shohamy and colleagues (2004, 2006) have shown that in PD the feedback learning deficit is relatively specific, as patients are impaired when required to learn associations on the basis of feedback, but equivalent to controls when observational learning of the same associations was required.

Our results further confirm a feedback-based learning acquisition deficit in mild, non-demented PD. Patients and controls were equivalent in their exploration parameters, with both showing a minimal amount of exploration. This would be expected given the nature of the task wherein subjects are not encouraged to modify their responses as the stimulus-response-outcome contingencies do not change. Nevertheless, it further validates the utility of our model that it was able to identify this effect. Results from the analysis of learning accuracy across blocks indicated that deficient learning in the PD patients was mostly driven by poorer performance later in the task. We did not find a difference in explicit knowledge of stimulus: response-outcome contingencies, suggesting that despite a deficient learning rate the PD patients were ultimately able to attain a good level of knowledge of these contingencies (see also de Wit et al., 2011). The acquisition impairment did not correlate with any clinical disease variables; nor was a correlational relationship evident between learning rate and working memory (as assessed via the digit span backwards task), which was found to be mildly impaired. Importantly, on other executive domains assessed in the current study, the PD patients' performance was equivalent to controls, which supports the notion of a discrete discrimination learning deficit in this patient group.

The previous findings relating deficient feedback-based learning in PD to dopamine dysfunction have been somewhat equivocal, as comparisons between patients ON vs. OFF medication have found that performance on a variety of learning tasks is impaired in both scenarios (Czernecki et al., 2002; Ell et al., 2010; Moustafa and Gluck, 2011), or that performance differs based on task demands (Shohamy et al., 2006) or valence of feedback signals (Frank et al., 2004). A number of studies using feedback-based category learning in PD have suggested that respective demands on selective attention vs. working memory, which are differentially affected by dopamine therapy, may determine learning performance (Filoteo et al., 2005, 2007). Given that in the OFF state patients suffer severe depletion in dorsal striatum and its projection targets, whilst the ON state is associated with restoration of those levels and the possibility of dopaminergic "overdose" in ventral striatum and limbic regions (Cools et al., 2001), differential effects on discrimination learning would be expected. Nonetheless, the finding of similar effects arising from two ostensibly disparate conditions has been explained with respect to the "relative" rather than "absolute" levels of dopamine, as a reduced dynamic range of phasic dopamine activity can result from both the ON and OFF states (Frank, 2005).

In contrast to previous studies that have characterized discrimination learning deficits in PD with respect to dopaminergic dysfunction, our current results define these deficits with respect to the possible structural abnormalities that may be contributory. In addition to dopamine depletion, PD is also associated with gray matter loss and synaptic denervation in fronto-striatal regions essential to broad aspects of learning and feedback processing, including the striatum (Rosenberg-Katz et al., 2013), medial temporal regions (Filoteo et al., 2013) and ventromedial prefrontal cortex (O'Callaghan et al., 2013). More specifically, prefrontal volume loss has been identified in non-demented PD, in comparison to healthy controls (Song et al., 2011; Melzer et al., 2012). Our findings reveal that discrete fronto-striatal regions, namely ventromedial prefrontal cortex, right inferior frontal gyrus and nucleus accumbens, are directly associated with acquisition deficits during feedback-based discrimination learning. The presence of underlying gray matter loss contributing to learning deficits may to some degree explain why discrimination learning can be affected both ON and OFF medication, and thus indicate that dopamine imbalance may not be the sole explanation for learning deficits in PD.

Our findings potentially shed light on previous reports that disease severity in PD is associated with specific learning impairments (Owen et al., 1993; Swainson et al., 2006). In particular, Swainson et al. (2006) found that early-stage, unmedicated patients were not impaired on a complex discrimination learning task; whilst early-stage, medicated patients *were* impaired on the task, their performance was mediated by deficient perceptual categorization of the complex stimuli, rather than a learning deficit *per se*. In contrast, only patients with severe, medicated PD showed impaired learning in the absence of perceptual categorization deficits. This raises the possibility that some factor other than inappropriate dopamine levels may intervene in later-stage PD to produce learning impairments on the task. Interestingly, the comparison groups of Huntington's disease and frontal lobe lesion patients included in the study showed the same pattern of intact perceptual categorization, but impaired learning, suggesting that more extensive fronto-striatal dysfunction may underpin the learning impairments. Taken together with our findings, it may be that fronto-striatal atrophy is a contributing factor to those learning impairments seen in PD with disease progression.

The possibility that fronto-striatal atrophy can mediate learning performance is also relevant to previous studies that have identified considerable variation within their PD cohorts. For example, using a rule-based category learning task, Ashby et al. (2003) found that PD patients were impaired at the group level, however, this effect was driven by impaired performance in only half of the patients, with the remainder performing equivalent to controls. The authors interpreted this as evidence of distinctive PD sub-groups. Indeed, differences in the clinical phenotypes of PD are well recognized (Lewis et al., 2005) and evidence is accumulating that the presence of more widespread fronto-subcortical atrophy may be characteristic of certain sub-groups (Feldmann et al., 2008; Melzer et al., 2012; Rosenberg-Katz et al., 2013). An admixture of PD patients with and without prefrontal volume loss may contribute to within-group variation in learning performance.

Results from our partial correlation analysis suggest that atrophy in the ventromedial prefrontal region may be driving the association with acquisition deficits. Although previous research using functional MRI in healthy controls has identified striatal activity as crucial during the acquisition phase of learning tasks (Pessiglione et al., 2006; Foerde and Shohamy, 2011a), others have shown ventromedial prefrontal cortex activity during learning acquisition (de Wit et al., 2009). Whereas the gradual learning of stimulus-response associations is presumed to reflect "habit" learning that is mediated by basal ganglia dopamine signals (Shohamy et al., 2008), "goal-directed" learning, which involves a focus on stimulus-response-outcome associations, has been linked to medial prefrontal regions (Balleine and O'Doherty, 2009). The interplay between the habitual and goal-directed modes can be explained by the "dual-systems" account, whereby instrumental learning can be supported by either modality (Dickinson and Balleine, 1994; de Wit and Dickinson, 2009). In line with the possibility that acquisition of instrumental discriminations is partly supported by goal-directed learning, de Wit et al. (2009) showed that engagement of the ventromedial prefrontal cortex during discrimination learning was predictive of goal-directed performance during a subsequent test phase. During that "instructed outcome-devaluation" test phase, participants were told that some of the fruit outcomes were no longer worth points. Participants with relatively strong engagement of the ventromedial prefrontal cortex during learning were better able to direct their responses toward the still-valuable outcomes and away from the devalued ones. More recently, individual differences in the strength of the white-matter pathway between the ventromedial prefrontal cortex and caudate have also been implicated in goal-directed control, whilst connectivity between the posterior putamen and premotor cortex has been related to habit learning (de Wit et al., 2012). Given these previous investigations of the role of the ventromedial prefrontal cortex in action control, our results are in keeping with a deficit in goal-directed learning.

In the category learning literature, the Competition between Verbal and Implicit Systems model (COVIS; Ashby et al., 1998) has been proposed to explain the neural systems that mediate rule-based learning vs. procedural (information-integration) learning. Whilst both are inherently feedback-based, these learning mechanisms necessitate different strategies and depend on divergent systems. The former comprising of an explicit hypothesis-testing system underpinned by a broad network including prefrontal cortex, anterior cingulate, hippocampus and caudate head; and the latter, requiring perceptual information to be integrated at a pre-decisional level, is mediated by cortical-striatal synapses within the putamen and premotor cortex circuitry (Ashby and Maddox, 2011). However, there is growing consensus that prefrontal regions, in particular ventromedial prefrontal cortex, may play a role in both types of learning (Seger, 2008). Schnyer et al. (2009) explored this directly by contrasting ventromedial prefrontal cortex lesion patients on rule-based vs. information-integration learning and found that patients were impaired in both types of learning. Work by Seger and colleagues (Seger and Cincotta, 2005; Seger et al., 2010) has also highlighted the role of the ventral striatum in encoding feedback during unstructured category learning tasks. These findings suggest that the ventromedial prefrontal cortex and ventral striatum—important hubs in the cortico-striatal motivational loop—are critical for monitoring and integrating feedback, regardless of the learning strategy.

Ventromedial prefrontal regions and ventral striatum (particularly nucleus accumbens) are also more generally associated with reward processing (Kringelbach, 2005), which may further explain why these regions were implicated in acquisition learning deficits in our patients, as the feedback involved in the task was reward-oriented. Specific reward-learning deficits have previously been demonstrated in PD (Swainson et al., 2000; Housden et al., 2010), and based on the volumetric reductions we found in regions crucial to reward processing in our patient cohort, it is likely that deficient reward processing may have contributed to the acquisition deficits. Our finding that the right inferior frontal gyrus was also associated with the acquisition deficit may reflect the demands of more general cognitive control that is required in such a learning task. The right inferior frontal gyrus is well known to be implicated in inhibitory control of behavior (Aron et al., 2004), however, a broader interpretation of its action is that it is involved in the detection/monitoring of task-relevant cues (Hampshire et al., 2010) and in terms of learning processes, the region is recruited during reversal learning (Cools et al., 2002).

From a mechanistic account, the involvement of prefrontal regions in learning from trial-by-trial feedback is also emphasized in computational models that seek to integrate basal ganglia and prefrontal function with respect to higher level executive processes. In the computational accounts proposed by O'Reilly and Frank (2006), the prefrontal cortex is active in maintaining information, whereby task-relevant information is determined via basal ganglia-prefrontal interactions that serve as a gating mechanism (see also Hazy et al., 2007). In these models, basal ganglia dopamine-dependant learning systems are presumed to trigger updates of working memory representations in the prefrontal cortex, whilst simultaneously inhibiting task-irrelevant information—thus allowing intrinsic prefrontal cortical mechanisms to actively maintain the contents of working memory. Our results suggest that direct atrophy in prefrontal regions may interfere with the updating and maintenance of task-relevant information in these models, which may therefore contribute to deficient acquisition on learning tasks.

The VBM technique utilized in this study is not without limitations, including registration and normalization issues and imperfect gray-white matter segmentation, particularly in relation to already atypical brains (Mechelli et al., 2005). In addition, the analysis we conducted does not measure the particular morphological changes brain structures undergo in PD and in interpreting findings of reduced gray matter density, it must be borne in mind that the precise mechanisms of cell degeneration in PD are still a matter of debate (Obeso et al., 2010). Nevertheless, VBM provides an important tool to further characterize learning systems in PD.

Together, our findings suggest that discrete fronto-striatal regions contribute to the feedback-based learning deficits in PD. It is likely that gray matter loss in these regions interacts with dopaminergic dysfunction to produce these deficits, and that the ultimate behavioral manifestation reflects an interplay between neurotransmitter imbalance and underlying structural changes. Our findings have important implications for the development of learning theories based on PD as a model of dopaminergic dysfunction. Whereby current theories and computational approaches have tended to focus on dopamine imbalance in intra-basal ganglia circuitry, a broader appreciation of the more distributed brain changes, such as gray matter loss, and how these may also affect learning processes is crucial in order to continue to refine these theoretical models. These results highlight that dysfunction in dopaminergic systems may not be the sole explanation for feedback-based learning deficits in PD, but that gray matter loss may also contribute to these deficits.

AUTHOR CONTRIBUTIONS

Claire O'Callaghan contributed to the design and conceptualization of the study, data collection, analysis and interpretation of data, drafting and revision of the manuscript. Ahmed A. Moustafa carried out the computational modeling and contributed to interpretation of the data and revision of the manuscript. Sanne de Wit contributed to study conceptualization and manuscript revision. James M. Shine contributed to data collection and manuscript revision. Trevor W. Robbins was involved in revision of the manuscript. Simon J. G. Lewis contributed to interpretation of the data and revision of the manuscript. Michael Hornberger contributed to design and conceptualization of the study, analysis and interpretation of data, and revision of the manuscript.

ACKNOWLEDGMENTS

Claire O'Callaghan is supported by an Alzheimer's Australia Dementia Research Foundation PhD scholarship. Ahmed A. Moustafa is supported by UWS Competitive Research Grant (P00021210). Simon J. G. Lewis is supported by a National Health and Medical Research Council Practitioner Fellowship (1003007). Michael Hornberger is supported by an Australian Research Council Research Fellowship (DP110104202).

REFERENCES

Andersson, J. L. R., Jenkinson, M., and Smith, S. (2007a). *Non-linear Optimisation.* Available online at: www.fmrib.ox.ac.uk/analysis/techrep

Andersson, J. L. R., Jenkinson, M., and Smith, S. (2007b). *Non-linear Registration, aka Spatial Normalisation.* Available online at: www.fmrib.ox.ac.uk/analysis/techrep

Aron, A. R., Robbins, T. W., and Poldrack, R. A. (2004). Inhibition and the right inferior frontal cortex. *Trends Cogn. Sci.* 8, 170–175. doi: 10.1016/j.tics.2004.02.010

Ashburner, J., and Friston, K. J. (2000). Voxel-based morphometry–the methods. *Neuroimage* 11, 805–821. doi: 10.1006/nimg.2000.0582

Ashby, F. G., Alfonso-Reese, L. A., Turken, A. U., and Waldron, E. M. (1998). A neuropsychological theory of multiple systems in category learning. *Psychol. Rev.* 105, 442–481. doi: 10.1037/0033-295X.105.3.442

Ashby, F. G., and Maddox, W. T. (2011). Human category learning 2.0. *Ann. N.Y. Acad. Sci.* 1224, 147–161. doi: 10.1111/j.1749-6632.2010.05874.x

Ashby, F. G., Noble, S., Filoteo, J. V., Waldron, E. M., and Ell, S. W. (2003). Category learning deficits in Parkinson's disease. *Neuropsychology* 17, 115. doi: 10.1037/0894-4105.17.1.115

Balleine, B. W., and O'Doherty, J. P. (2009). Human and rodent homologies in action control: corticostriatal determinants of goal-directed and habitual action. *Neuropsychopharmacology* 35, 48–69. doi: 10.1038/npp.2009.131

Beck, A. T., Steer, R. A., and Brown, G. K. (1996). *Manual for the Beck Depression Inventory-II.* San Antonio, TX: Psychological Corporation.

Benton, A., Hamsher, K., and Sivan, A. (1994). *Multilingual Aphasia Examination.* San Antonio, TX: Psychological Corporation.

Bouton, M. E. (2007). *Learning and Behavior: A Contemporary Synthesis.* Sunderland, MA: Sinauer Associates.

Bromberg-Martin, E. S., Matsumoto, M., and Hikosaka, O. (2010). Dopamine in motivational control: rewarding, aversive, and alerting. *Neuron* 68, 815–834. doi: 10.1016/j.neuron.2010.11.022

Camerer, C., and Ho, T. H. (1999). Experience-weighted attraction learning in normal form games. *Econometrica* 67, 827–874. doi: 10.1111/1468-0262.00054

Cools, R., Barker, R. A., Sahakian, B. J., and Robbins, T. W. (2001). Enhanced or impaired cognitive function in parkinson's disease as a function of dopaminergic medication and task demands. *Cereb. Cortex* 11, 1136–1143. doi: 10.1093/cercor/11.12.1136

Cools, R., Clark, L., Owen, A. M., and Robbins, T. W. (2002). Defining the neural mechanisms of probabilistic reversal learning using event-related functional magnetic resonance imaging. *J. Neurosci.* 22, 4563–4567.

Czernecki, V., Pillon, B., Houeto, J. L., Pochon, J. B., Levy, R., and Dubois, B. (2002). Motivation, reward, and Parkinson's disease: influence of dopatherapy. *Neuropsychologia* 40, 2257–2267. doi: 10.1016/S0028-3932(02)00108-2

Daw, N. D., O'Doherty, J. P., Dayan, P., Seymour, B., and Dolan, R. J. (2006). Cortical substrates for exploratory decisions in humans. *Nature* 441, 876–879. doi: 10.1038/nature04766

de Wit, S., Barker, R. A., Dickinson, A. D., and Cools, R. (2011). Habitual versus goal-directed action control in Parkinson disease. *J. Cogn. Neurosci.* 23, 1218–1229. doi: 10.1162/jocn.2010.21514

de Wit, S., Corlett, P. R., Aitken, M. R., Dickinson, A., and Fletcher, P. C. (2009). Differential engagement of the ventromedial prefrontal cortex by goal-directed and habitual behavior toward food pictures in humans. *J. Neurosci.* 29, 11330–11338. doi: 10.1523/JNEUROSCI.1639-09.2009

de Wit, S., and Dickinson, A. (2009). Associative theories of goal-directed behaviour: a case for animal-human translational models. *Psychol. Res.* 73, 463–476. doi: 10.1007/s00426-009-0230-6

de Wit, S., Niry, D., Wariyar, R., Aitken, M. R., and Dickinson, A. (2007). Stimulus-outcome interactions during instrumental discrimination learning by rats and humans. *J. Exp. Psychol. Anim. Behav. Process.* 33, 1–11. doi: 10.1037/0097-7403.33.1.1

de Wit, S., Watson, P., Harsay, H. A., Cohen, M. X., van de Vijver, I., and Ridderinkhof, K. R. (2012). Corticostriatal connectivity underlies individual differences in the balance between habitual and goal-directed action control. *J. Neurosci.* 32, 12066–12075. doi: 10.1523/JNEUROSCI.1088-12.2012

Dickinson, A., and Balleine, B. (1994). Motivational control of goal-directed action. *Anim. Learn. Behav.* 22, 1–18. doi: 10.3758/BF03199951

Duncan, G. W., Firbank, M. J., O'Brien, J. T., and Burn, D. J. (2013). Magnetic resonance imaging: a biomarker for cognitive impairment in Parkinson's disease? *Mov. Disord.* 28, 425–438. doi: 10.1002/mds.25352

Ell, S. W., Weinstein, A., and Ivry, R. B. (2010). Rule-based categorization deficits in focal basal ganglia lesion and Parkinson's disease patients. *Neuropsychologia* 48, 2974–2986. doi: 10.1016/j.neuropsychologia.2010.06.006

Feldmann, A., Illes, Z., Kosztolanyi, P., Illes, E., Mike, A., Kover, F., et al. (2008). Morphometric changes of gray matter in Parkinson's disease with depression: a voxel-based morphometry study. *Mov. Disord.* 23, 42–46. doi: 10.1002/mds.21765

Filoteo, J. V., Maddox, W. T., Ing, A. D., Zizak, V., and Song, D. D. (2005). The impact of irrelevant dimensional variation on rule-based category learning in patients with Parkinson's disease. *J. Int. Neuropsychol. Soc.* 11, 503–513. doi: 10.1017/S1355617705050617

Filoteo, J. V., Maddox, W. T., and Song, D. D. (2007). Characterizing rule-based category learning deficits in patients with Parkinson's disease. *Neuropsychologia* 45, 305–320. doi: 10.1016/j.neuropsychologia.2006.06.034

Filoteo, J. V., Reed, J. D., Litvan, I., and Harrington, D. L. (2013). Volumetric correlates of cognitive functioning in nondemented patients with Parkinson's disease. *Mov. Disord.* doi: 10.1002/mds.25633. [Epub ahead of print].

Foerde, K., and Shohamy, D. (2011a). Feedback timing modulates brain systems for learning in humans. *J. Neurosci.* 31, 13157–13167. doi: 10.1523/JNEUROSCI.2701-11.2011

Foerde, K., and Shohamy, D. (2011b). The role of the basal ganglia in learning and memory: insight from Parkinson's disease. *Neurobiol. Learn. Mem.* 96, 624–636. doi: 10.1016/j.nlm.2011.08.006

Folstein, M. F., Folstein, S. E., and McHugh, P.R. (1975). Mini-Mental State: a practical method for grading the cognitive state of patients for the clinician. *J. Psychiatr. Res.* 12, 189–198. doi: 10.1016/0022-3956(75)90026-6

Frank, M. J. (2005). Dynamic dopamine modulation in the basal ganglia: a neurocomputational account of cognitive deficits in medicated and nonmedicated parkinsonism. *J. Cogn. Neurosci.* 17, 51–72. doi: 10.1162/0898929052880093

Frank, M. J., Moustafa, A. A., Haughey, H. M., Curran, T., and Hutchison, K. E. (2007). Genetic triple dissociation reveals multiple roles for dopamine in reinforcement learning. *Proc. Natl. Acad. Sci. U.S.A.* 104, 16311–16316. doi: 10.1073/pnas.0706111104

Frank, M. J., Seeberger, L. C., and O'Reilly, R. C. (2004). By carrot or by stick: cognitive reinforcement learning in parkinsonism. *Science* 306, 1940–1943. doi: 10.1126/science.1102941

Gibb, W. R. G., and Lees, A. J. (1988). A comparison of clinical and pathological features of young and old onset Parkinson's disease. *Neurology* 38, 1402–1406. doi: 10.1212/WNL.38.9.1402

Goetz, C. G., Tilley, B. C., Shaftman, S. R., Stebbins, G. T., Fahn, S., Martinez-Martin, P., et al. (2008). Movement Disorder Society-sponsored revision of the Unified Parkinson's Disease Rating Scale (MDS-UPDRS): Scale presentation and clinimetric testing results. *Mov. Disord.* 23, 2129–2170. doi: 10.1002/mds.22340

Gold, J. M., Waltz, J. A., Matveeva, T. M., Kasanova, Z., Strauss, G. P., Herbener, E. S., et al. (2012). Negative symptoms and the failure to represent the expected reward value of actions: behavioral and computational modeling evidence. *Arch. Gen. Psychiatry* 69, 129–138. doi: 10.1001/archgenpsychiatry.2011.1269

Good, C. D., Johnsrude, I. S., Ashburner, J., Henson, R. N., Friston, K. J., and Frackowiak, R. S. (2001). A voxel-based morphometric study of ageing in 465 normal adult human brains. *Neuroimage* 14, 21–36. doi: 10.1006/nimg.2001.0786

Hampshire, A., Chamberlain, S. R., Monti, M. M., Duncan, J., and Owen, A. M. (2010). The role of the right inferior frontal gyrus: inhibition and attentional control. *Neuroimage* 50, 1313–1319. doi: 10.1016/j.neuroimage.2009.12.109

Hazy, T. E., Frank, M. J., and O'Reilly, R. C. (2007). Towards an executive without a homunculus: computational models of the prefrontal cortex/basal ganglia system. *Philos. Trans. R. Soc. B Biol. Sci.* 362, 1601–1613. doi: 10.1098/rstb.2007.2055

Hoehn, M. M., and Yahr, M. D. (1967). Parkinsonism: onset, progression and mortality. *Neurology* 17, 427–422. doi: 10.1212/WNL.17.5.427

Housden, C. R., O'Sullivan, S. S., Joyce, E. M., Lees, A. J., and Rosier, J. P. (2010). Intact reward learning but elevated delay discounting in Parkinson's disease patients with impulsive-compulsive spectrum behaviors. *Neuropsychopharmacology* 35, 2155–2164. doi: 10.1038/npp.2010.84

Jellinger, K. A. (2001). The pathology of Parkinson's disease. *Adv. Neurol.* 86, 55–72.

Kringelbach, M. L. (2005). The human orbitofrontal cortex: linking reward to hedonic experinence. *Nat. Rev. Neurosci.* 6, 691–702. doi: 10.1038/nrn1747

Lewis, S. J., Foltynie, T., Blackwell, A. D., Robbins, T. W., Owen, A. M., and Barker, R. A. (2005). Heterogeneity of Parkinson's disease in the early clinical stages using a data driven approach. *J. Neurol. Neurosurg. Psychiatry* 76, 343–348. doi: 10.1136/jnnp.2003.033530

Mechelli, A., Price, C. J., Friston, K. J., and Ashburner, J. (2005). Voxel-based morphometry of the human brain: methods and applications. *Curr. Med. Imaging Rev.* 1, 105–113. doi: 10.2174/1573405054038726

Melzer, T. R., Watts, R., MacAskill, M. R., Pitcher, T. L., Livingston, L., Keenan, R. J., et al. (2012). Grey matter atrophy in cognitively impaired Parkinson's disease. *J. Neurol. Neurosurg. Psychiatry* 83, 188–194. doi: 10.1136/jnnp-2011-300828

Moustafa, A. A., and Gluck, M. A. (2011). A neurocomputational model of dopamine and prefrontal–striatal interactions during multicue category learning by Parkinson patients. *J. Cogn. Neurosci.* 23, 151–167. doi: 10.1162/jocn.2010.21420

Moustafa, A. A., Keri, S., Herzallah, M. M., Myers, C. E., and Gluck, M. A. (2010). A neural model of hippocampal–striatal interactions in associative learning and transfer generalization in various neurological and psychiatric patients. *Brain Cogn.* 74, 132–144. doi: 10.1016/j.bandc.2010.07.013

Myers, C. E., Shohamy, D., Gluck, M. A., Grossman, S., Kluger, A., Ferris, S., et al. (2003). Dissociating hippocampal versus basal ganglia contributions to learning and transfer. *J. Cogn. Neurosci.* 15, 185–193. doi: 10.1162/089892903321208123

Obeso, J. A., Rodriguez-Oroz, M. C., Goetz, C. G., Marin, C., Kordower, J. H., Rodriguez, M., et al. (2010). Missing pieces in the Parkinson's disease puzzle. *Nat. Med.* 16, 653–661. doi: 10.1038/nm.2165

O'Callaghan, C., Naismith, S. L., Hodges, J. R., Lewis, S. J. G., and Hornberger, M. (2013). Fronto-striatal atrophy correlates of inhibitory dysfunction in Parkinson's disease versus behavioural variant frontotemporal dementia. *Cortex* 49, 1833–1843. doi: 10.1016/j.cortex.2012.12.003

O'Reilly, R. C., and Frank, M. J. (2006). Making working memory work: a computational model of learning in the prefrontal cortex and basal ganglia. *Neural Comput.* 18, 283–328. doi: 10.1162/089976606775093909

Owen, A. M., Beksinska, M., James, M., Leigh, P. N., Summers, B. A., Marsden, C. D., et al. (1993). Visuospatial memory deficits at different stages of Parkinson's disease. *Neuropsychologia* 31, 627–644. doi: 10.1016/0028-3932(93)90135-M

Pessiglione, M., Seymour, B., Flandin, G., Dolan, R. J., and Frith, C. D. (2006). Dopamine-dependent prediction errors underpin reward-seeking behaviour in humans. *Nature* 442, 1042–1045. doi: 10.1038/nature05051

Price, A., Filoteo, J. V., and Maddox, W. T. (2009). Rule-based category learning in patients with Parkinson's disease. *Neuropsychologia* 47, 1213–1226. doi: 10.1016/j.neuropsychologia.2009.01.031

Reitan, R. M., and Wolfson, D. (1985). *The Halstead-Reitan Neuropsychological Test Battery.* Tucson, AZ: Neuropsychology Press.

Rosenberg-Katz, K., Herman, T., Jacob, Y., Giladi, N., Hendler, T., and Hausdorff, J. M. (2013). Gray matter atrophy distinguishes between Parkinson disease motor subtypes. *Neurology* 80, 1476–1484. doi: 10.1212/WNL.0b013e31828cfaa4

Rueckert, D., Sonoda, L. I., Hayes, C., Hill, D. L., Leach, M. O., and Hawkes, D. J. (1999). Nonrigid registration using free-form deformations: application to breast MR images. *IEEE Trans. Med. Imaging* 18, 712–721. doi: 10.1109/42.796284

Schnyer, D. M., Maddox, W. T., Ell, S., Davis, S., Pacheco, J., and Verfaellie, M. (2009). Prefrontal contributions to rule-based and information-integration category learning. *Neuropsychologia* 47, 2995–3006. doi: 10.1016/j.neuropsychologia.2009.07.011

Schultz, W. (2002). Getting formal with dopamine and reward. *Neuron* 36, 241–263. doi: 10.1016/S0896-6273(02)00967-4

Seger, C. A. (2008). How do the basal ganglia contribute to categorization? Their roles in generalization, response selection, and learning via feedback. *Neurosci. Biobehav. Rev.* 32, 265–278. doi: 10.1016/j.neubiorev.2007.07.010

Seger, C. A., and Cincotta, C. M. (2005). The roles of the caudate nucleus in human classification learning. *J. Neurosci.* 25, 2941–2951. doi: 10.1523/JNEUROSCI.3401-04.2005

Seger, C. A., Peterson, E. J., Cincotta, C. M., Lopez-Paniagua, D., and Anderson, C. W. (2010). Dissociating the contributions of independent corticostriatal systems to visual categorization learning through the use of reinforcement learning modeling and Granger causality modeling. *Neuroimage* 50, 644–656. doi: 10.1016/j.neuroimage.2009.11.083

Shiner, T., Seymour, B., Wunderlich, K., Hill, C., Bhatia, K. P., Dayan, P., et al. (2012). Dopamine and performance in a reinforcement learning task: evidence from Parkinson's disease. *Brain* 135, 1871–1883. doi: 10.1093/brain/aws083

Shohamy, D., Myers, C. E., Geghman, K. D., Sage, J., and Gluck, M. A. (2006). L-dopa impairs learning, but spares generalization, in Parkinson's disease. *Neuropsychologia* 44, 774. doi: 10.1016/j.neuropsychologia.2005.07.013

Shohamy, D., Myers, C. E., Kalanithi, J., and Gluck, M. A. (2008). Basal ganglia and dopamine contributions to probabilistic category learning. *Neurosci. Biobehav. Rev.* 32, 219–236. doi: 10.1016/j.neubiorev.2007.07.008

Shohamy, D., Myers, C., Grossman, S., Sage, J., Gluck, M., and Poldrack, R. (2004). Cortico-striatal contributions to feedback-based learning: converging data from neuroimaging and neuropsychology. *Brain* 127, 851–859. doi: 10.1093/brain/awh100

Smith, S. M., Jenkinson, M., Woolrich, M. W., Beckmann, C. F., Behrens, T. E., Johansen-Berg, H., et al. (2004). Advances in functional and structural MR image analysis and implementation as FSL. *Neuroimage* 23(Suppl. 1), S208–S219. doi: 10.1016/j.neuroimage.2004.07.051

Smith, S. M., and Nichols, T. E. (2009). Threshold-free cluster enhancement: addressing problems of smoothing, threshold dependence and localisation in cluster inference. *Neuroimage* 44, 83–98. doi: 10.1016/j.neuroimage.2008.03.061

Song, S. K., Lee, J. E., Park, H.-J., Sohn, Y. H., Lee, J. D., and Lee, P. H. (2011). The pattern of cortical atrophy in patients with Parkinson's disease according to cognitive status. *Mov. Disord.* 26, 289–296. doi: 10.1002/mds.23477

Sutton, R. S., and Barto, A. G. (1998). *Introduction to Reinforcement Learning.* Cambridge, MA: MIT Press.

Swainson, R., Rogers, R. D., Sahakian, B. J., Summers, B. A., Polkey, C. E., and Robbins, T. W. (2000). Probabilistic learning and reversal deficits in patients with Parkinson's disease or frontal or temporal lobe lesions: possible adverse effects of dopaminergic medication. *Neuropsychologia* 38, 596–612. doi: 10.1016/S0028-3932(99)00103-7

Swainson, R., SenGupta, D., Shetty, T., Watkins, L., Summers, B., Sahakian, B., et al. (2006). Impaired dimensional selection but intact use of reward feedback during visual discrimination learning in Parkinson's disease. *Neuropsychologia* 44, 1290–1304. doi: 10.1016/j.neuropsychologia.2006.01.028

Watkins, C. C. H., and Dayan, P. (1992). Q-learning. *Mach. Learn.* 8, 279–292. doi: 10.1007/BF00992698

Wechsler, D. (1997). *Wechsler Adult Intelligence Scale-III.* San Antonio, TX: The Psychological Corporation.

Zhang, Y., Brady, M., and Smith, S. (2001). Segmentation of brain MR images through a hidden Markov random field model and the expectation-maximization algorithm. *IEEE Trans. Med. Imaging* 20, 45–57. doi: 10.1109/42.906424

6

Haloperidol-Induced Changes in Neuronal Activity in the Striatum of the Freely Moving Rat

Dorin Yael[1†], Dagmar H. Zeef[2†], Daniel Sand[1], Anan Moran[3], Donald B. Katz[3], Dana Cohen[1], Yasin Temel[2] and Izhar Bar-Gad[1*]

[1] The Leslie & Susan Goldschmied (Gonda) Multidisciplinary Brain Research Center, Bar-Ilan University, Ramat-Gan, Israel
[2] Departments of Neuroscience and Neurosurgery, Maastricht University Medical Center, Maastricht, Netherlands
[3] Department of Psychology, Volen National Center for Complex Systems, Brandeis University, Waltham, MA, USA

Correspondence:
Izhar Bar-Gad, The Leslie & Susan Goldschmied (Gonda) Multidisciplinary Brain Research Center, Bar-Ilan University, Ramat-Gan 52900, Israel
e-mail: izhar.bar-gad@biu.ac.il
† These authors have contributed equally to this work.

The striatum is the main input structure of the basal ganglia, integrating input from the cerebral cortex and the thalamus, which is modulated by midbrain dopaminergic input. Dopamine modulators, including agonists and antagonists, are widely used to relieve motor and psychiatric symptoms in a variety of pathological conditions. Haloperidol, a dopamine D2 antagonist, is commonly used in multiple psychiatric conditions and motor abnormalities. This article reports the effects of haloperidol on the activity of three major striatal subpopulations: medium spiny neurons (MSNs), fast spiking interneurons (FSIs), and tonically active neurons (TANs). We implanted multi-wire electrode arrays in the rat dorsal striatum and recorded the activity of multiple single units in freely moving animals before and after systemic haloperidol injection. Haloperidol decreased the firing rate of FSIs and MSNs while increasing their tendency to fire in an oscillatory manner in the high voltage spindle (HVS) frequency range of 7–9 Hz. Haloperidol led to an increased firing rate of TANs but did not affect their non-oscillatory firing pattern and their typical correlated firing activity. Our results suggest that dopamine plays a key role in tuning both single unit activity and the interactions within and between different subpopulations in the striatum in a differential manner. These findings highlight the heterogeneous striatal effects of tonic dopamine regulation via D2 receptors which potentially enable the treatment of diverse pathological states associated with basal ganglia dysfunction.

Keywords: striatum, dopamine antagonist, extra cellular recording, neuronal subpopulations, oscillations

INTRODUCTION

The striatum is the main input structure of the basal ganglia, a group of sub-cortical nuclei involved in motor, limbic and associative behavior. The vast majority (>95%) of striatal neurons are the GABAergic projection neurons, which are traditionally termed medium spiny neurons (MSNs) (Rymar et al., 2004). MSNs can be divided into D1-receptor expressing MSNs projecting to the substantia nigra pars reticulata (SNr), and the entopeduncular nucleus (EP) and D2-receptor expressing MSNs projecting to the globus pallidus (GP) (Albin et al., 1989). MSNs are characterized by bursty firing in response to different movements and behaviors with a very low baseline firing rate (Wilson and Groves, 1981). Additionally, the striatum contains multiple small populations of interneurons (Tepper et al., 2004). Two of the most extensively studied interneuron populations are the GABAergic fast spiking interneurons (FSIs) and the cholinergic tonically active interneurons (TANs). FSIs, which comprise ~1% of the striatal cell population, receive inputs from the cortex and GP, project to surrounding MSNs, and exert a strong inhibitory modulation (Berke, 2011). Electrophysiologically, FSIs display narrow spike waveforms with a high baseline firing rate and resemble the FSIs found in the hippocampus and cerebral cortex (Somogyi and Klausberger, 2005; Berke, 2011). TANs, which make up 1–2% of the striatal population (Goldberg and Reynolds, 2011), have a tonic irregular firing pattern, lack burst activity, and are strongly influenced by both positive and aversive stimuli. TANs show wide and high amplitude extracellular spike waveforms, with a relatively long refractory period (Sharott et al., 2009).

Dopamine and dopamine receptors play a key role in controlling information processing during both normal and pathological states. Dopamine denervation is the pathological hallmark of Parkinson's disease, while a hyper-dopaminergic state has been associated with hyper-kinetic and hyper-behavioral disorders ranging from dyskinesia to schizophrenia. Within the striatum, dopamine modulates the activity of individual neurons as well as the dynamics within and between the neuronal subpopulations (Murer et al., 2002; Humphries et al., 2009). Phasic and tonic alterations of dopamine levels within the striatum lead to a variety of changes in neuronal activity. Reward related, phasic, release of dopamine from the midbrain leads to inhibition of the cholinergic interneurons (TANs) in both non-human primates and rats,

Abbreviations: BG, basal ganglia; FSI, fast spiking interneuron; GP, globus pallidus; HVS, high voltage spindle; MSN, medium spiny neuron; SNc, substantia nigra pars compacta; TAN, tonically active neuron.

and similar effects has been reported for aversive stimuli (Aosaki et al., 1994b; Raz et al., 1996; Ravel et al., 2003). Chronic depletion of dopamine, such as in the 6-OHDA rat model or MPTP treated primate model of PD leads to an increase in the firing rate of the TANs and the formation of oscillatory firing patterns (Raz et al., 1996; Kish et al., 1999). The effect of dopamine on MSNs has classically been divided into positive modulation via D1-receptors and negative modulation via the D2-receptors (Albin et al., 1989). This basic modulation of the direct (D1 receptor expressing) and indirect (D2 receptor expressing) MSNs is further dependent upon additional factors such as cortical input, as well as the behavioral state of the subject (Moyer et al., 2007; Gerfen and Surmeier, 2011). The FSIs neuronal firing rate has been shown to be dependent on dopamine in that it increases after agonist application and decreases after antagonist application (Wiltschko et al., 2010).

These pronounced motor and behavioral effects of dopamine are utilized in providing pharmacological treatment of multiple motor and psychiatric disorders. Antipsychotic drugs, which are widely used in psychiatric conditions such as psychosis and mania or hyperkinetic motor disorders such as tics and chorea, are classically divided into typical and atypical antipsychotics. Typical antipsychotics (e.g. haloperidol) have a high affinity for D2 receptors (Gardner et al., 2005). The D2 receptor is expressed in the indirect basal ganglia pathway and plays an important role in behavioral, cognitive as well as affective and motor pathologies (Cohen and Frank, 2009). The high affinity of typical antipsychotics for the D2 receptor is known to cause extrapyramidal side effects such as akinesia, dystonia, parkinsonism, and tardive dyskinesia, as well as cognitive and behavioral alterations (Strange, 2008).

The current study assessed the effects of haloperidol on multiple striatal neuron subtypes (MSNs, TANs, and FSIs) in freely moving rats. We used chronic multi-electrode recordings to characterize the changes at the single neuron level and discuss network dynamics within the striatum and their potential role in the cortico-basal ganglia pathway.

METHODS

ANIMALS

10 adult rats (five Sprague Dawley and five Long-Evans (Harlan) weighing 250–450 g) were used in this study. The animals were kept under controlled temperature, humidity, and lighting (12 h light/dark cycle) conditions and had free access to food and water. Experiments were performed during the light phase of the cycle. All procedures were approved and supervised by the Institutional Animal Care and Use Committee (IACUC) and were in accordance with the National Institute of Health Guide for the Care and Use of Laboratory Animals and the Bar-Ilan University Guidelines for the Use and Care of Laboratory Animals in Research. This study was approved by the National Committee for Experiments in Laboratory Animals at the Ministry of Health (permit number 6-01-11).

SURGICAL PROCEDURES

After arrival, the animals were housed in their home cage for at least 1 week before the operation. Animals were sedated with 5% isoflurane and then anesthetized with an intra-peritoneal injection of a mixture of ketamine HCl (100 mg/kg) and xylazine HCl (10 mg/kg) and an intra-muscular injection of atropine (0.1 mg). Anesthesia during the operation was maintained using isoflourane and supplementary injections of ketamine. The animals' scalp was shaved and cleaned, and anesthetic cream (2.5% lidocaine and 2.5% prilocaine) was applied into their ears to prevent discomfort during head fixation. The rats were placed in a stereotactic frame (Stoelting Co., Wood Dale, IL, USA) and their head was fixed. The scalp was sterilized and lidocaine (10 mg/ml) was locally injected into the skin around the incision location. A central incision was made and the skull was exposed. The head was then straightened by equalizing bregma-lambda height. Coordinates of the craniotomies were marked and holes were drilled. The dura was removed and 16 electrode arrays were slowly lowered unilaterally into the striatum and were grounded and fixed to the skull by screws and dental cement.

Two types of custom made multi-wire arrays were used. Four of the animals were implanted with non-movable 4 × 4 45 μm diameter isonel-coated tungsten microwire linear arrays (Yarom and Cohen, 2011) [AP +1.0, −0.5 ML 2.0, 4.0 DV 5.0 (Paxinos and Watson, 2007)] (**Figures 1A,C**). These arrays displayed higher probabilities of recording TANs. Six of the animals were implanted with movable bundles of 16 25 μm diameter formvar coated nichrome microwires (Grossman et al., 2008) [AP +1.0, −0.5 ML 2.0, 3.5 DV 4.0 (Paxinos and Watson, 2007)] (**Figures 1B,D**). These arrays displayed higher probabilities of recording MSNs and FSIs.

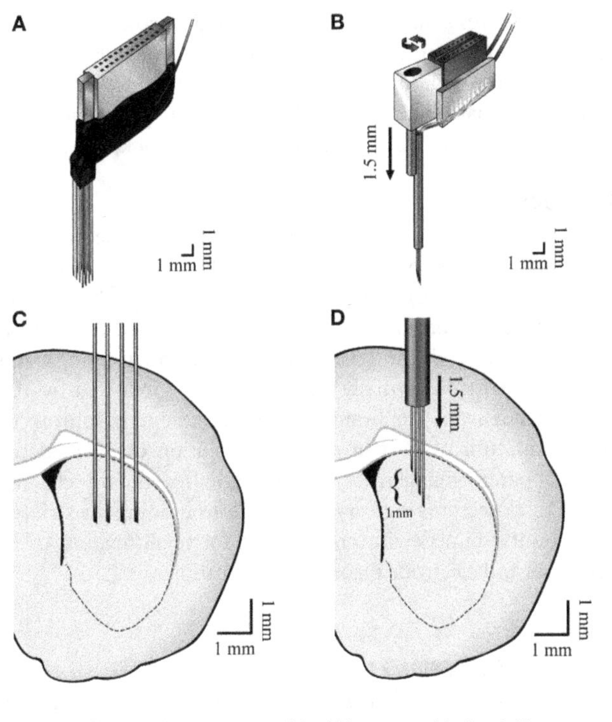

FIGURE 1 | Methods. Illustration of the **(A)** non-movable 4 × 4 45 μm diameter isonel-coated tungsten microwire linear arrays and the **(B)** movable bundles of 16 25 μm diameter formvar coated nichrome microwires and **(C,D)** their locations in the dorsal striatum.

EXPERIMENTAL SESSIONS

Experimental sessions began at least 7 days post-operation to allow full recovery of the animals. The animals were placed in the recording chamber, where they could move freely, and were connected to the recording system. The signal was continuously recorded throughout the session. The analog signal was amplified (*200), band-pass filtered (0.5–10000 Hz, 4 pole Butterworth filter) and digitized at a sampling rate of 44 KHz (Alpha-Lab SNR, Alpha-Omega Engineering, Nazareth, Israel). The digitized continuous raw signal was acquired to allow offline sorting and analysis. Sessions initiated with recordings in the naïve state, which was followed by recording of neuronal activity during and after a single subcutaneous haloperidol (0.05 mg) injection. Few experimental sessions were performed in some of the animals (2.5 ± 1.3 mean ± *SD*, sessions/animals), which were separated by prolonged periods (11.3 ± 7 mean ± *SD*, days between sessions) to avoid accumulation of Haloperidol effect. In order to minimize behavioral effects on the results, the electrophysiological recordings took place during resting state of the animals both before and after the injection. Notably, rest state following haloperidol injection included akinesia and rigidity which were not part of the pre-injection state.

DATA PREPROCESSING AND ANALYSIS

Spike sorting of multiple single units from the continuous raw signal was performed offline (Offline Sorter v2.8.8, Plexon, Dallas, TX). Offline sorting using a continuous signal instead of the more common segmented data makes it possible to obtain long overlapping windows (1.5–2 ms in our data) surrounding each spike, thereby increasing the fidelity and quality of the sorting. Only neurons that formed clear distinguishable clusters were included in the study. Neurons that did not display a stable wave-form throughout the recording session were eliminated from the database. All subsequent analyses were performed using custom-written MATLAB code (Mathworks, Natick, MA).

HISTOLOGY

After completion of the experimental sessions, the rats were deeply anesthetized with a mixture of ketamine (100 mg/kg), xylazine (10 mg/kg) and additional morphinhydroclorid (0.15 mg/kg). A current (–100 μA, 10 s) was passed through the tips of the electrodes to create small marker microlesions. Rats were perfused transcardially with 0.9% saline followed by 10% paraformaldehyde. The brains were removed and cryoprotected for a minimum of 48 h in a fixation solution of 30% sucrose in 10% paraformaldehyde. Brains were frozen and cut into 50 μm thick sections on a cryostat. Sections holding the striatum were counterstained with cresyl violet for identification of the structures and electrode placement verification.

RESULTS

EXPERIMENTAL SESSIONS

We continuously recorded extracellular activity in the dorsal striatum of freely moving rats in naïve and post-systemic haloperidol injection states using two types of 16 microwire arrays (25 and 45 μm wire diameter). The recordings were made in 10 rats over 22 separate recording sessions. Electrophysiological recordings in the naïve state began after an initial acclimatization period in which the animals were allowed to move freely and explore the recording cage. Recording in the naïve state lasted 30 min, continued throughout the injection time and for a post-injection period of 30 min. Injection of haloperidol induced observable akinesia and rigidity within a few minutes during all of the sessions. These behavioral effects could be modulated for short periods of time; for example, after moving the animals from the recording cage to their home cage, a short period of exploration could occur. An additional common phenomenon occurring after haloperidol injection was increased stereotypical behavior in the form of teeth chattering.

NEURONAL CLASSIFICATION

The recorded signal was offline sorted and the dataset of 87 single units was classified into three categories—MSNs (30/87, 34.5%), TANs (42/87, 48.3%), and FSIs (15/87, 17.2%) (**Figure 2A**). All the neurons presented well separated clusters which were stable throughout the whole recording session. The classification was first done subjectively using multiple parameters such as the mean waveform shape, inter-spike interval (ISI) histogram, firing rate and pattern, and was subsequently verified via clustering using three parameters: (1) mean firing rate during the naïve period, (2) peak to valley width of the mean spike waveform and (3) the ISI coefficient of variation (CV) where the different subpopulations formed three clearly separable clusters (**Figure 2B**). The mean firing rate was calculated using 600 s long segments taken from the naïve state recordings (ending at least 100 s prior to the haloperidol injection). MSNs typically displayed a low baseline firing rate of 1.9 ± 1.9 Hz (mean ± *SD*), TANs displayed a medium rate 4.2 ± 2.0 Hz (mean ± *SD*) and FSIs displayed the highest baseline rate 17.5 ± 10.3 Hz (mean ± *SD*). The CV was calculated using the same time windows by dividing the standard deviation of the 1st order ISIs by their mean. This measure varied across the striatal subpopulations: MSNs typically displayed a bursty firing pattern over low baseline activity and high CV value of 2.5 ± 0.7 (mean ± *SD*). FSIs displayed a bursty firing pattern over high baseline activity and a CV of 1.7 ± 0.6 (mean ± *SD*). TANs displayed a Poisson-like firing pattern and a CV value of 0.9 ± 0.3 (mean ± *SD*). Waveform peak to valley width was calculated using the waveforms of the whole recording periods. MSNs waveforms were typically wide and displayed a long positive second phase. FSIs displayed a narrow waveform, and TANs displayed wide waveform containing initial positive phase (**Figure 2C**).

HALOPERIDOL EFFECTS

Different statistics for comparison of the naïve, pre-haloperidol injection state and the post-haloperidol injection state were calculated using stable periods of continuous 600 s recordings from the naive state, ending at least 100 s prior to the haloperidol injection, and from the post-haloperidol injection state, starting at least 600 s after the haloperidol injection. This procedure produced stable periods and served to avoid transition periods.

The mean firing rates of the neurons during the stable windows of the naïve and post-haloperidol states were compared. Both MSNs and FSIs significantly lowered their firing rates after haloperidol injection (paired t-test, $p < 0.01$) from the mean

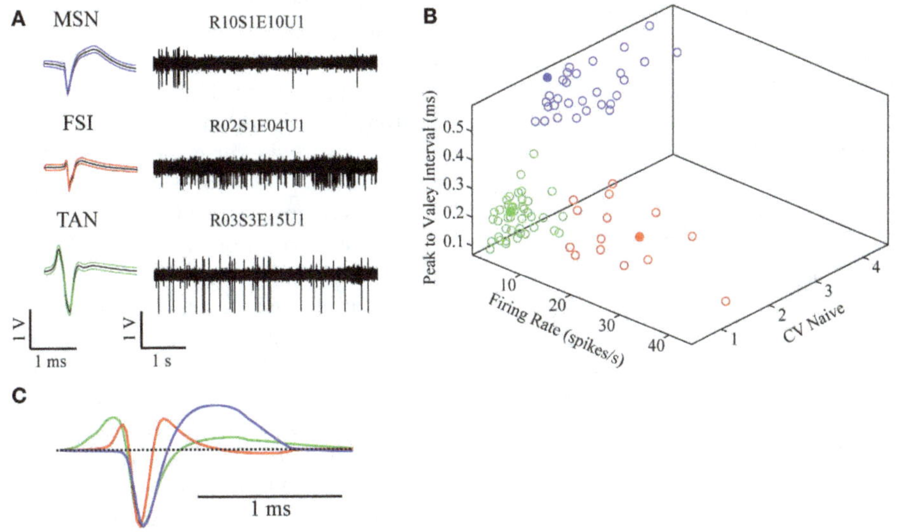

FIGURE 2 | Neuronal classification into striatal subtypes. (A) Examples of raw data (right) and spike waveform (left) of MSN, FSI, and TAN (black lines—mean, colored lines—mean ± *SD*). **(B)** Division of the classified neurons into three dimensional clusters by peak to valley width, firing rate and CV in the naïve state. Filled circles are the units presented in **(A)**. **(C)** Mean population waveform of MSN (blue), FSI (red), and TAN (green).

population baseline rates of 1.9 ± 0.4 Hz (mean ± s.e.m.) and 17.5 ± 2.6 Hz (mean± s.e.m.) to firing rates of 0.6 ± 0.2 Hz (mean ± s.e.m.) and 6.5 ± 1.4 Hz (mean ± s.e.m.), respectively (**Figure 3A**). To assess the behavior of individual neurons within each subtype comparisons were made of the distribution of firing rates of each neuron in 60 short (10 s) windows making up the stable periods. In a single unit analysis, 80% (24/30) of the MSNs (**Figure 3B**) and 100% (15/15) of the FSIs (**Figure 3C**) significantly lowered their firing rates after the haloperidol injection (*t*-test, $p < 0.01$). The TANs' firing rates were elevated after the haloperidol injection (paired *t*-test, $p < 0.01$) from a mean population baseline rate of 4.2 ± 0.3 Hz (mean ± s.e.m.) to a firing rate of 6.3 ± 0.4 Hz (mean ± s.e.m.) (**Figure 3A**). In a single unit analysis, 88% (37/42) of the TANs elevated their firing rate post-haloperidol injection in a significant manner (*t*-test, $p < 0.01$) (**Figure 3D**). The transition dynamics of firing rates following haloperidol were complex and dependent on the specific animal and session, however, the effects were clear across the population (**Figures 4A,B**). Despite the different dynamics across the sessions, simultaneously recorded neurons demonstrated the same dynamics in their transition phases and timing following the injection (**Figure 4C**).

The CV of the naïve and post-haloperidol states were calculated for single units during the same 600 s stable time frames by dividing the standard deviation of the ISIs by their mean. The MSNs significantly (paired *t*-test, $p < 0.01$) lowered their CVs following the haloperidol injection from a value of 2.53 ± 0.13 (mean ± s.e.m.) to a value of 1.95 ± 0.14 (mean ± s.e.m.) (**Figure 5A**). CV values of FSIs population did not change significantly (naïve 1.7 ± 0.2, post-haloperidol 1.9 ± 0.2, paired *t*-test $p > 0.01$) (**Figure 5B**). TANs significantly (paired *t*-test, $p < 0.01$) elevated their CV values from a baseline value of 0.90 ± 0.05 (mean ± s.e.m.) to a value of 0.99 ± 0.05 (mean ± s.e.m.)

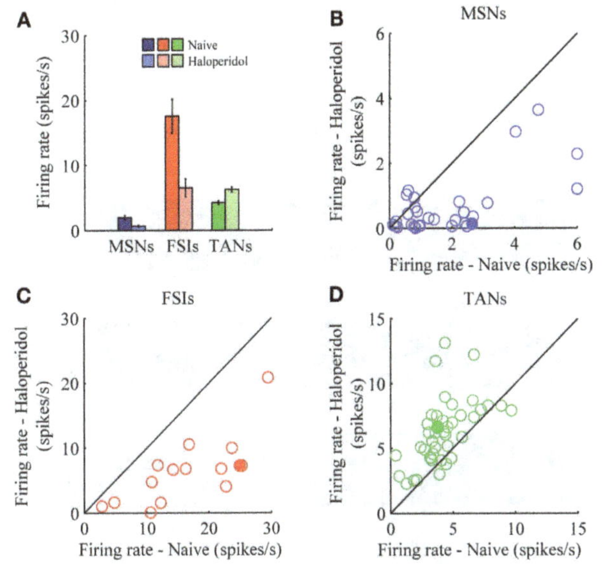

FIGURE 3 | Haloperidol-induced firing rate changes. (A) Population mean firing rates, before and after haloperidol injection. Error bars—s.e.m. Single neuron firing rates in the naïve and post-haloperidol injection states of **(B)** MSNs, **(C)** FSIs, and **(D)** TANs. Filled circles—the neurons shown in (**Figure 4A**).

post-haloperidol injection (**Figure 5C**). The changes in the TANs' CV values following the haloperidol injection might be explained by the shortening of their refractory period, which was clearly seen in their ISI histograms (**Figure 5D**) and autocorrelation functions (**Figure 5E**).

A total of 131 of TAN pairs were recorded simultaneously in the naïve and in the subsequent post-haloperidol injection state.

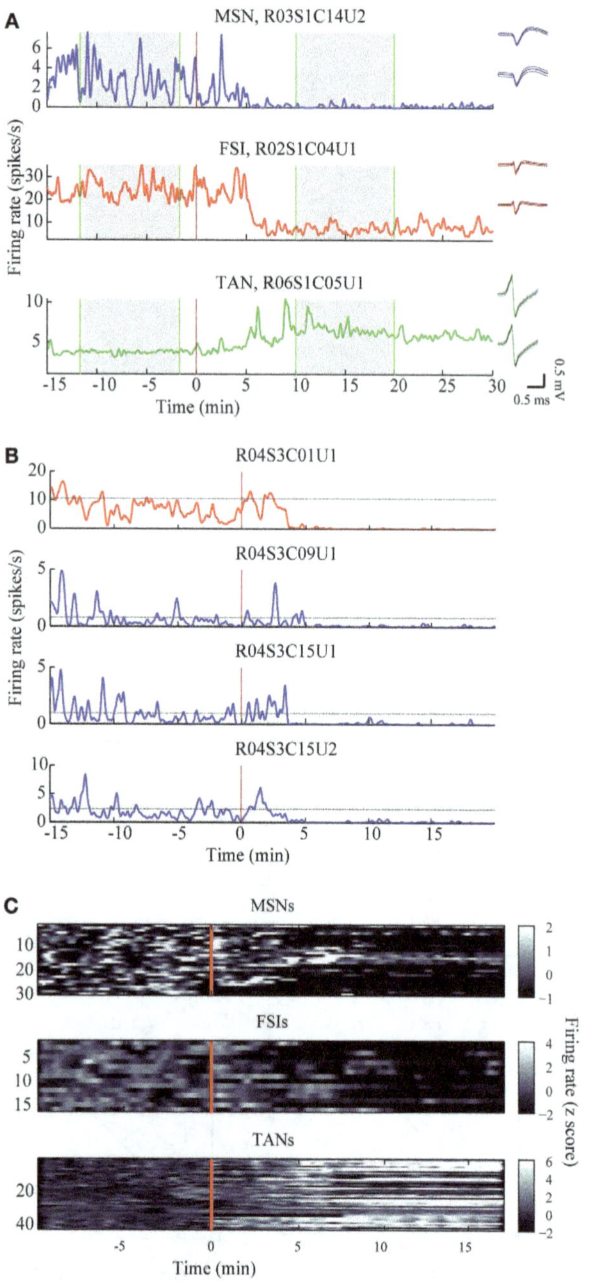

FIGURE 4 | Time course of firing rate modulations. (A) Examples of firing rate modulations of single MSN, FSI, and TAN. Red vertical lines—haloperidol injection times. Right panel—waveforms of the units before (top) and after (bottom) haloperidol injection (black lines—mean, colored lines mean ± *SD*). Green vertical lines—time frames used for stable states calculations. **(B)** Firing rate modulation of the whole neuronal population represented as z scores. **(C)** Example of haloperidol—induced firing rates modulations of one FSI (top) and three MSNs (bottom) recorded simultaneously.

In the naïve state many pairs exhibited significant ($p < 0.01$) positive correlations (62/131, 47.3%) and a smaller minority had significantly negative correlations (13/131, 9.9%). Following the haloperidol injection the asymmetry increased, in that the majority of the neurons displayed a significant positive correlation (85/131, 64.9%) and a smaller minority showed significant negatively correlations (6/131, 4.6%) (**Figure 6A**). The haloperidol injection changed the fraction of significantly correlated neurons in a significant manner (χ^2 test, $p < 0.01$). However, the mean pair-wise correlation, which was highly positive in both the naïve and post-haloperidol states, did not differ between the two states (**Figure 6B**). This correlation was calculated on the rate normalized correlation functions. Using the raw cross correlation functions yielded larger positive correlations, where the skew was due to the increased firing rate during the post-haloperidol state.

Oscillatory activity in the 7–9 Hz band could be observed in some of the LFP recordings in the naïve state. These oscillations, which are typical of high voltage spindles (HVS), occurred in 19/72 (26.4%) of the recordings and were typically short and intermittent. Following haloperidol injection the number of oscillatory LFPs increased significantly to 33/72 (45.8%) (χ^2 test, $p < 0.01$) and their duration and abundance increased (**Figures 7A,B**). The mean power of the LFP increased preferentially in the HVS frequency band and its harmonics (**Figure 7C**). This was accompanied by a smaller but significant peak in the HVS frequency and its first harmonic in the spiking activity of single neurons (**Figure 7D**). The number of neurons with a significant peak in the power spectrum increased from 7/87 (8.1%) in the naïve state to 21/87 (24.1%) during the post-haloperidol state (χ^2 test, $p < 0.01$).

The activity of single neurons during HVS varied greatly depending on the neuronal sub-type. Both FSIs and MSNs fired in an oscillatory manner in a fixed phase with the LFP. Oscillations of the LFP in the HSV frequency appeared prior to the injection but were increased notably following the haloperidol injection (**Figures 8A,B**). This was accompanied by equivalent oscillations in the neuronal spiking activity of MSNs and FSIs (FSI example—**Figures 8C,D**). The LFP and spike train signals were highly coherent following the haloperidol injection in the HVS base frequency and its harmonics (**Figures 8E,F**). In sharp contrast, TANs did not display spike train oscillatory activity during oscillations in the LFP (**Figures 9A–F**) and thus were not coherent with the LFP signal. This property was evident when observing the overall neuronal population, which demonstrated a roughly equal coherence of MSNs and FSIs with their background LFP with only a small coherence for the TAN population (**Figure 9G**).

DISCUSSION

In this study, we examined the effect of systemic haloperidol administration on the activity of neurons from different subpopulations within the striatum in freely moving rats. Our results demonstrate that neuronal sub-types within the striatum responded in a distinctly different fashion to the haloperidol application. MSNs and FSIs dramatically lowered their firing rate following haloperidol injection, whereas changes in the firing pattern were seen in the MSNs, which became more regular as a result of decreased bursting. In addition, the low frequency oscillations (7–9 Hz) that are typical of HVSs were evident following the haloperidol injection where the LFP signal became highly oscillatory and the firing pattern of both FSIs and MSNs

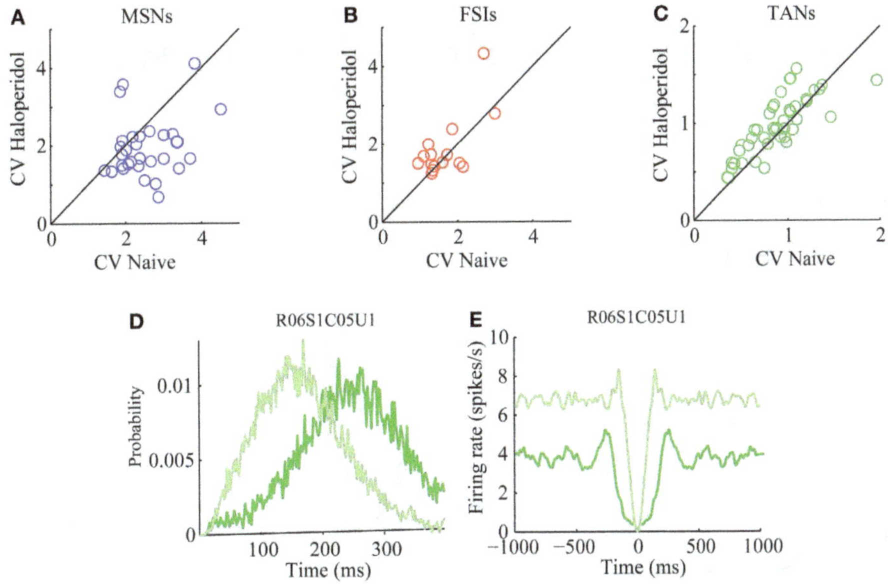

FIGURE 5 | Haloperidol—induced firing patterns modulations. Single neuron CVs in the naïve and post-haloperidol injection states of **(A)** MSNs, **(B)** FSIs, and **(C)** TANs. Example of **(D)** ISI histogram and **(E)** autocorrelation function of a single TAN (dark green—naïve state, light green—post-haloperidol state).

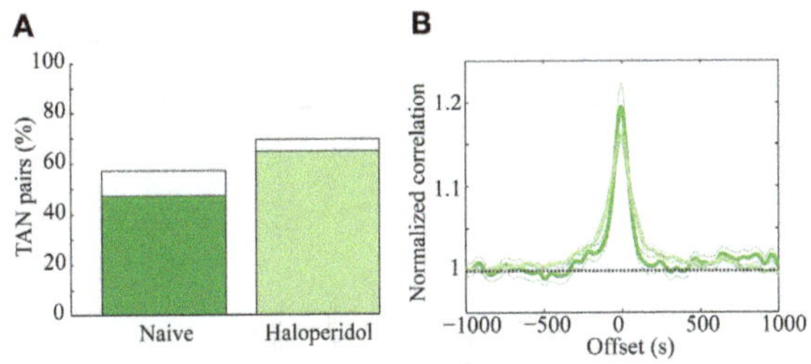

FIGURE 6 | Haloperidol modulation of TAN correlations. (A) Cross-correlation between TAN pairs, divided into significant ($p < 0.01$) positively correlated (green) and negatively correlated (white). **(B)** Mean correlation of the TAN pairs in the naïve (dark green) and post-haloperidol (light green). The narrow lines indicate one s.e.m. significance lines and the horizontal black dashed line indicates the normalized unity line. The scale is normalized to the mean rate of each pair.

became phase locked to these oscillations. The firing rate of TANs, on the other hand, showed a drug-induced increased firing rate, accompanied by a more irregular firing pattern resulting from a shortening of the relative refractory period. The TANs displayed a non-oscillatory firing pattern during periods of HVS and maintained the typical widely correlated activity within the sub-population.

The effects of dopamine modulation on both behavior and its underlying neuronal mechanisms have been studied extensively in the cortico-basal ganglia loop. Multiple techniques for dopamine modulation have been used in the study of movement and psychiatric disorders such as Parkinson's disease, Huntington's disease and Tourette syndrome, as well as in the study of normal processes such as plasticity, learning and reward. These techniques differ in such key aspects as (1) spread, (2) specificity, and (3) duration of the effect, which makes comparison across results complex. Dopamine denervation techniques range from widespread, non-specific chronic depletion of dopamine neurons, such as those observed following 6-OHDA injections or with genetic knockout models, to acute, focal, and specific antagonisms caused by localized dopamine antagonist microinjections or focal optogenetic modulations. In the current study we used systemic acute injections of the D2 antagonist haloperidol. In this case, spatially, the effect was widespread in the brain and did not only influence the striatal neurons. However, temporally, it had a limited duration, with minor impact on long term changes in the network function and structure. By contrast, chronic treatment with haloperidol has been shown to lead to significant plastic changes (Benes et al., 1985) and behavioral symptoms resembling tardive dyskinesia (Kinon et al., 1984). In addition, the dosage of haloperidol used in this study (0.05 mg) was lower by an order of magnitude than some recent studies (Burkhardt et al., 2007; Yang et al., 2013) that have examined its effect on the basal ganglia. The low dosage elicited the same behavioral symptoms to a large extent, while avoiding permanent damage such as potential apoptosis in the striatum and SNr (Mitchell et al., 2002) and resembling the dosage used in human patients.

Despite the differences between techniques, dopamine denervation mostly yields similar behavioral and neuronal results. Behaviorally, decreased dopamine levels have been shown to induce akinesia and parkinsonian-like symptoms such as rigidity. These outcomes are common to studies using localized 6-OHDA injection (Deumens et al., 2002), systemic injections of dopamine antagonists (Burkhardt et al., 2007) and tetrodotoxin (TTX) injections to the medial forebrain bundle (MFB) (Prosperetti

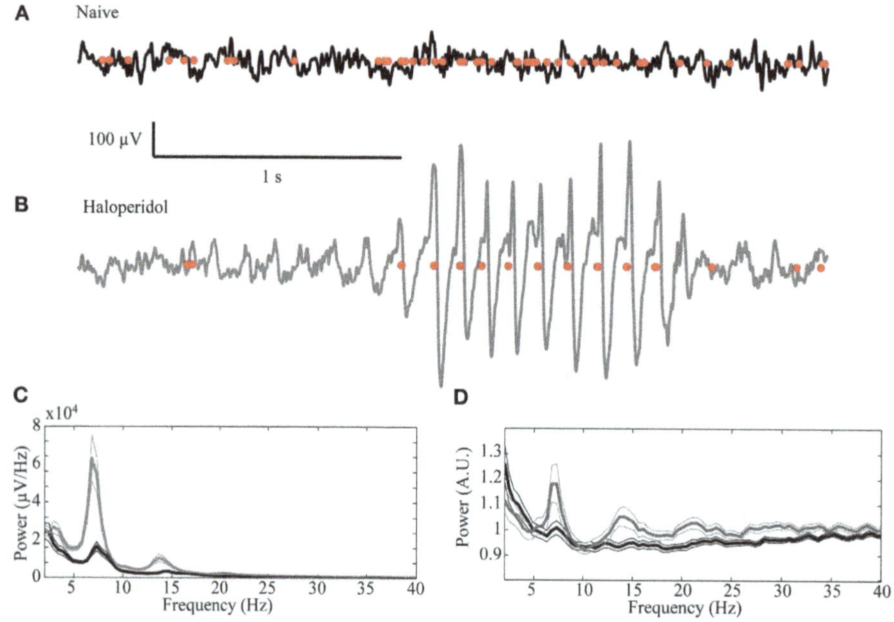

FIGURE 7 | High voltage spindles (HVSs) in the striatum. Example of a recording trace of the LFP (black line—naïve, gray—post-haloperidol injection) overlaid with the concurrent spikes (red dots) during the **(A)** naïve state and **(B)** post-haloperidol injection reflecting the HVSs. **(C,D)** Mean power of the **(C)** LFP recording ($n = 72$) and **(D)** spike trains ($n = 87$) during the naïve state (black) and post-haloperidol state (gray). The narrow lines indicate one s.e.m.

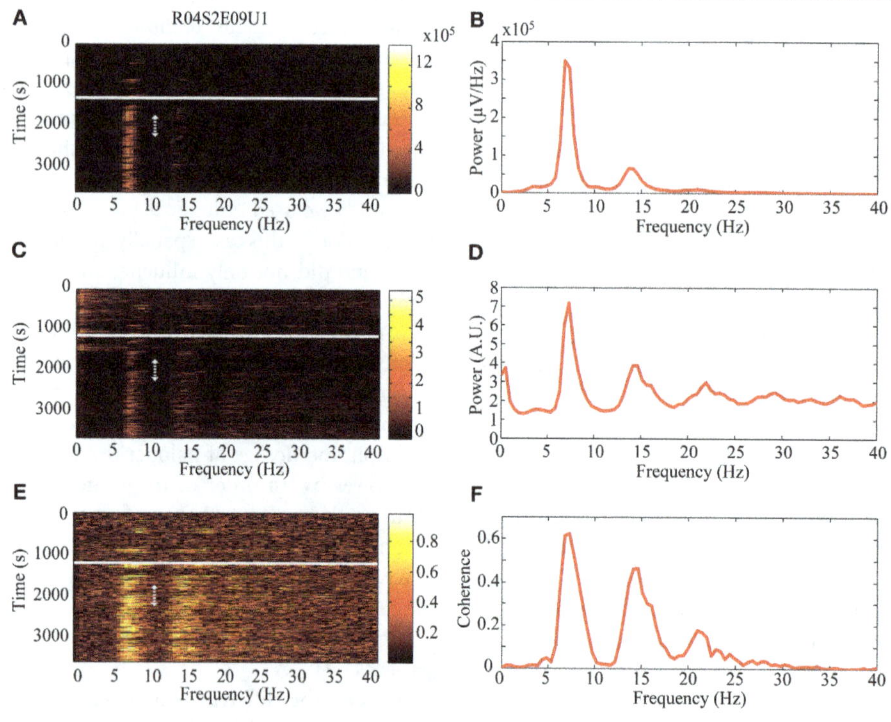

FIGURE 8 | Oscillatory neuronal activity during HVSs. The oscillatory activity is shown for a single recording of an FSI which spikes in an oscillatory manner during HVSs: **(A,B)** the LFP, **(C,D)** the spiking activity of a neuron sorted from the same electrode and **(E,F)** the coherence between the LFP and the spiking activity. The **(A,C)** spectrogram and **(E)** coherogram illustrate the changes in the oscillatory activity of the signals over 10 s windows throughout the session. The solid white line indicates the haloperidol injection time and the dotted white arrow indicates the stable post-haloperidol segment. The mean **(B,D)** power spectrum and **(F)** coherence are averaged over the stable post-haloperidol segment.

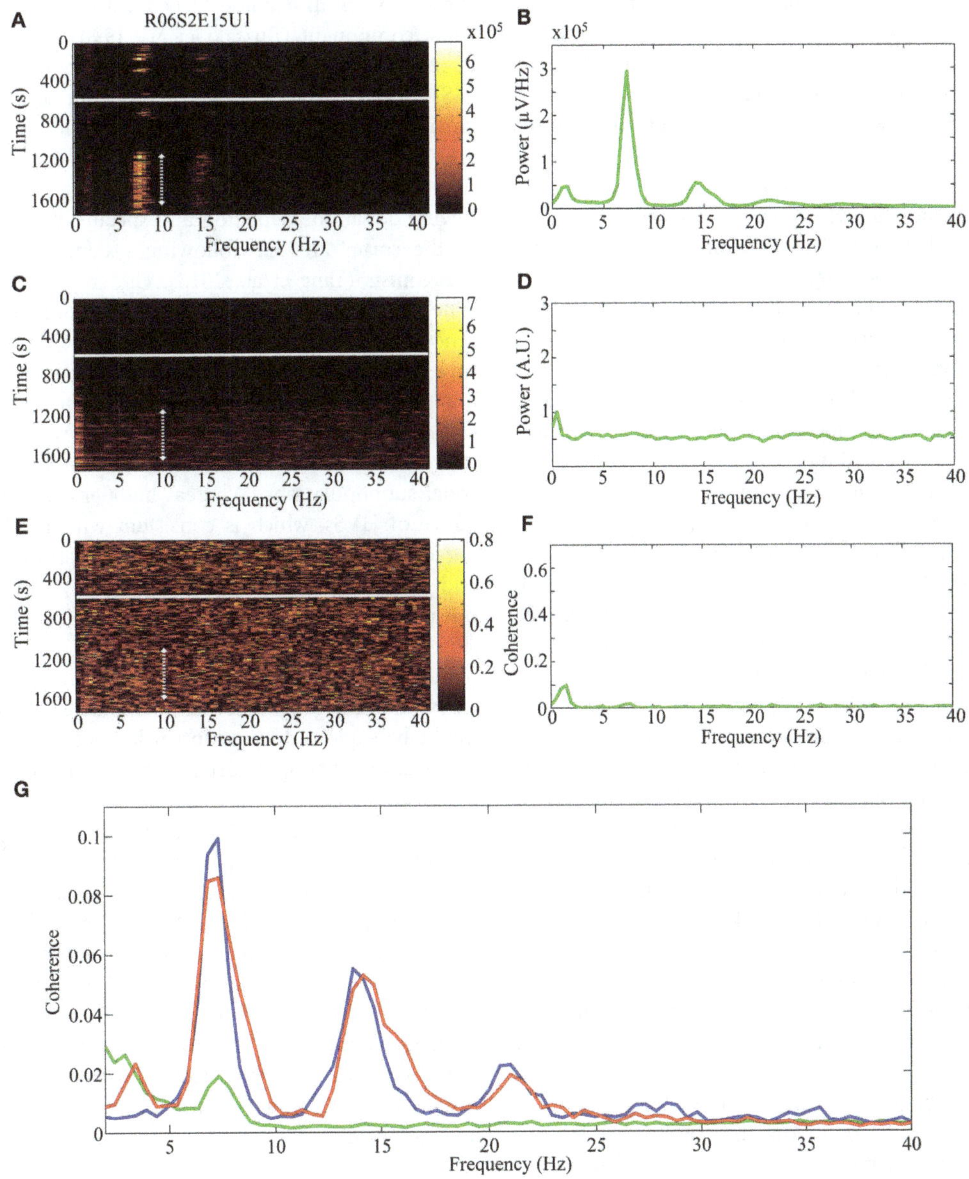

FIGURE 9 | Non-oscillatory neuronal activity during HVSs. The oscillatory activity is shown for a single recording of a TAN which does not spike in an oscillatory manner during HVSs: **(A,B)** the LFP, **(C,D)** the spiking activity of a neuron sorted from the same electrode and **(E,F)** the coherence between the LFP and the spiking activity. The **(A,C)** spectrogram and **(E)** coherogram illustrate the changes in the oscillatory activity of the signals over 10 s windows throughout the session. The solid white line indicates the haloperidol injection time and the dotted white arrow indicates the stable post-haloperidol segment. The mean **(B,D)** power spectrum and **(F)** coherence are averaged over the stable post-haloperidol segment. **(G)** Mean coherence between the LFP signal and the spiking activity of MSNs (blue), FSIs (red), and TANs (green) during the post-haloperidol segment.

et al., 2013). Neurophysiologically, striatal activity has been widely studied. However, the classification of striatal neurons into different populations has only recently become standardized, leaving multiple early studies hard to interpret as their data contain a myriad of cell types.

TANs in the dorsal striatum express both D2 and D5 receptors and receive dopaminergic input primarily from the SNc (Levey et al., 1993). *In vivo* intracellular recordings have shown that dopamine increase, via stimulation of the SNc, induces inhibition of the firing rate of TANs (Reynolds et al., 2004). Tonic dopamine depletion in 6-OHDA rats, on the other hand, increases their baseline discharge rate (Kish et al., 1999; Sanchez et al., 2011). Similarly, an acute block of the MFB by TTX also increases the firing rate (Prosperetti et al., 2013). Interestingly, while apomorphine likewise suppresses the firing rates of TANs (Fujita et al., 2013), D-Amphetamine, which increases the release of dopamine and inhibits its re-uptake, leads to an increased firing rate of TANs (Kish et al., 1999). In the non-human primate, no effect on spontaneous discharge rate of TANs by localized microinjections of either a D2 antagonist (sulpiride) or a D1 antagonist

(SCH23390) (Watanabe and Kimura, 1998), or by unilateral dopamine depletion by MPTP infusion to the caudate-putamen complex (Aosaki et al., 1994a), was observed in the striatum. Generally, the increased rate of TANs following haloperidol injection in our study is in line with most of the literature of dopamine modulation.

There are few studies of FSI modulation by dopamine given the nascent state of the field. However, the decreased firing rate of the FSIs following haloperidol application is consistent with *in vivo* studies reporting a decreased firing rate post eticlopride, a D2 receptor antagonist (Wiltschko et al., 2010).The effect of D2 on FSIs has been hypothesized to result from modulation of their GABAergic input (Bracci et al., 2002).

Unlike the general consistency between reports on TAN and FSI activity following dopamine modulations, previous studies of MSN activity paint a diverse and complex picture. The range of expression of dopamine receptors on MSNs is diverse: D1-like receptors have classically been assigned to the direct striato-nigral pathway and the D2-like receptors to the indirect striato-pallidal pathway and their activation increases and decreases the firing rate of MSNs, respectively (Albin et al., 1989). This might partially explain the heterogeneous results on the activity of MSNs following dopamine modulation in studies which do not break down MSNs into different subpopulations or use specific receptor modulation (Prosperetti et al., 2013). Chronically denervated animals tend to show an overall increase in firing rate (Kish et al., 1999; Chen et al., 2001), whereas acute denervation leads to increases and decreases in firing rate (Wiltschko et al., 2010; Prosperetti et al., 2013). Our data show contradictory results since most of our MSNs significantly lowered their firing rate following haloperidol administration. This is a surprising result in that the D2 receptor inactivation is expected to increase the MSN firing rate (Albin et al., 1989; DeLong, 1990), which may result from indirect network interactions.

The relationship between FSIs and MSNs firing following haloperidol injection did not follow their presumed interaction. A decrease in the firing rate of FSIs is expected to elevate the MSN firing rate, due to the strong inhibition that FSIs exert on MSNs (Koos and Tepper, 1999) whereas in our study both FSIs and MSNs lowered their firing rate. This discrepancy has been reported elsewhere, but the mechanism is still under debate (Lansink et al., 2010; Wiltschko et al., 2010). The most common suppositions are that in the dopamine depleted state, the FSIs reduce their sensitivity to cortical stimulation or the cortico-striatal input might have a larger influence post dopamine depletion (Kimura, 1990; Sharott et al., 2009; Berke, 2011).

HVSs appear in awake immobile rats and are characterized by a typical frequency of 5–13 Hz with a typical spike and wave shape (Klingberg and Pickenhain, 1968). HVSs have been studied extensively in multiple brain areas and have been observed in different parts of the cortico-basal ganglia loop. The origin of HVSs is still under debate and thalamic as well as cortical influences are thought to play an important role (Berke et al., 2004). Neurons in the striatum (presumably MSNs) were shown to fire in a phase locked with HVS, mostly within the spike component (Buzsaki et al., 1990). HVSs were shown to affect neuronal activity in the basal ganglia input (striatum—MSNs) and output (SNr) which are phase-locked to both the cortical and basal ganglia local field potentials (Dejean et al., 2007). Dopamine modulates HVSs, and recent studies have demonstrated the significant increase in these oscillations following dopamine depletion and specifically the LFP oscillations in the cortex and GP following systematic application of D2 antagonists (Yang et al., 2013). Under the dopamine depletion state in the 6-OHDA rat, the duration and frequency of occurrence of HVSs increased significantly (Dejean et al., 2008). This increase was also apparent following the injection of dopamine antagonists directly to the striatum (Deransart et al., 2000). Our results extend previously reported work by revealing that the effect of HVSs is not uniform across the different neuronal subpopulations. Whereas haloperidol increases the abundance of HVSs, which is consistent with the literature regarding dopaminergic reduction in the striatum and triggers FSIs and MSNs to show phase-locked activity to the LFP, TANs do not reveal this phenomenon and remain largely non-oscillatory. This contrasts with previous studies in the parkinsonian primate, which have found oscillatory activity that was coherent with basal ganglia oscillations (Raz et al., 1996, 2001).This might be explained by an intrinsic ability to generate spikes of TANs and/or stronger cortical or thalamocortical influences on MSNs and FSIs.

Haloperidol, given at amounts comparable to the dosage administered to human patients suffering from different movement and psychiatric disorders, produces profound behavioral and neuronal effects. Despite the clear behavioral effect, the underlying neuronal mechanism appears complex and diverse even within only the striatum itself. Different sub-populations of neurons are affected differentially and the effects include changes in neuronal rate, pattern, and interactions. This emphasizes the need to generate fine grain clustering of neurons to elucidate the mechanisms of action of pharmaceuticals on the brain as a whole and specifically on the striatum.

ACKNOWLEDGMENTS

We thank M. Dror for his help with the animals, K. Belelovsky and Y. Loewenstern for help with the histology. This work was supported by an Israel Science Foundation (ISF) grant (372/09), a National Institute for Psychobiology grant and a Tourette Syndrome Association (TSA) grant. D. H. Zeef was supported by a NENS Stipends grant.

REFERENCES

Albin, R. L., Young, A. B., and Penney, J. B. (1989). The functional anatomy of basal ganglia disorders. *Trends Neurosci.* 12, 366–375. doi: 10.1016/0166-2236(89)90074-X

Aosaki, T., Graybiel, A. M., and Kimura, M. (1994a). Effect of the nigrostriatal dopamine system on acquired neural responses in the striatum of behaving monkeys. *Science* 265, 412–415. doi: 10.1126/science.8023166

Aosaki, T., Tsubokawa, H., Ishida, A., Watanabe, K., Graybiel, A. M., and Kimura, M. (1994b). Responses of tonically active neurons in the primate's striatum undergo systematic changes during behavioral sensorimotor conditioning. *J. Neurosci.* 14, 3969–3984.

Benes, F. M., Paskevich, P. A., Davidson, J., and Domesick, V. B. (1985). The effects of haloperidol on synaptic patterns in the rat striatum. *Brain Res.* 329, 265–273. doi: 10.1016/0006-8993(85)90532-3

Berke, J. D. (2011). Functional properties of striatal fast-spiking interneurons. *Front. Syst. Neurosci.* 5:45. doi: 10.3389/fnsys.2011.00045

Berke, J. D., Okatan, M., Skurski, J., and Eichenbaum, H. B. (2004). Oscillatory entrainment of striatal neurons in freely moving rats. *Neuron* 43, 883–896. doi: 10.1016/j.neuron.2004.08.035

Bracci, E., Centonze, D., Bernardi, G., and Calabresi, P. (2002). Dopamine excites fast-spiking interneurons in the striatum. *J. Neurophysiol.* 87, 2190–2194. doi: 10.1152/jn.00754.2001

Burkhardt, J. M., Constantinidis, C., Anstrom, K. K., Roberts, D. C., and Woodward, D. J. (2007). Synchronous oscillations and phase reorganization in the basal ganglia during akinesia induced by high-dose haloperidol. *Eur. J. Neurosci.* 26, 1912–1924. doi: 10.1111/j.1460-9568.2007.05813.x

Buzsaki, G., Smith, A., Berger, S., Fisher, L. J., and Gage, F. H. (1990). Petit mal epilepsy and parkinsonian tremor: hypothesis of a common pacemaker. *Neuroscience* 36, 1–14. doi: 10.1016/0306-4522(90)90345-5

Chen, M. T., Morales, M., Woodward, D. J., Hoffer, B. J., and Janak, P. H. (2001). *In vivo* extracellular recording of striatal neurons in the awake rat following unilateral 6-hydroxydopamine lesions. *Exp. Neurol.* 171, 72–83. doi: 10.1006/exnr.2001.7730

Cohen, M. X., and Frank, M. J. (2009). Neurocomputational models of basal ganglia function in learning, memory and choice. *Behav. Brain Res.* 199, 141–156. doi: 10.1016/j.bbr.2008.09.029

Dejean, C., Gross, C. E., Bioulac, B., and Boraud, T. (2008). Dynamic changes in the cortex-basal ganglia network after dopamine depletion in the rat. *J. Neurophysiol.* 100, 385–396. doi: 10.1152/jn.90466.2008

Dejean, C., Gross, C. E., Bioulac, B., and Boraud, T. (2007). Synchronous high-voltage spindles in the cortex-basal ganglia network of awake and unrestrained rats. *Eur. J. Neurosci.* 25, 772–784. doi: 10.1111/j.1460-9568.2007.05305.x

DeLong, M. R. (1990). Primate models of movement disorders of basal ganglia origin. *Trends Neurosci.* 13, 281–285. doi: 10.1016/0166-2236(90)90110-V

Deransart, C., Riban, V., Le, B., Marescaux, C., and Depaulis, A. (2000). Dopamine in the striatum modulates seizures in a genetic model of absence epilepsy in the rat. *Neuroscience* 100, 335–344. doi: 10.1016/S0306-4522(00)00266-9

Deumens, R., Blokland, A., and Prickaerts, J. (2002). Modeling Parkinson's disease in rats: an evaluation of 6-OHDA lesions of the nigrostriatal pathway. *Exp. Neurol.* 175, 303–317. doi: 10.1006/exnr.2002.7891

Fujita, S., Kato, R., Cui, Y., Terakado, M., Suga, K., Koshikawa, N., et al. (2013). Apomorphine-induced modulation of neural activities in the ventrolateral striatum of rats. *Synapse* 67, 363–373. doi: 10.1002/syn.21644

Gardner, D. M., Baldessarini, R. J., and Waraich, P. (2005). Modern antipsychotic drugs: a critical overview. *CMAJ* 172, 1703–1711. doi: 10.1503/cmaj.1041064

Gerfen, C. R., and Surmeier, D. J. (2011). Modulation of striatal projection systems by dopamine. *Annu. Rev. Neurosci.* 34, 441–466. doi: 10.1146/annurev-neuro-061010-113641

Goldberg, J. A., and Reynolds, J. N. (2011). Spontaneous firing and evoked pauses in the tonically active cholinergic interneurons of the striatum. *Neuroscience* 198, 27–43. doi: 10.1016/j.neuroscience.2011.08.067

Grossman, S. E., Fontanini, A., Wieskopf, J. S., and Katz, D. B. (2008). Learning-related plasticity of temporal coding in simultaneously recorded amygdala-cortical ensembles. *J. Neurosci.* 28, 2864–2873. doi: 10.1523/JNEUROSCI.4063-07.2008

Humphries, M. D., Wood, R., and Gurney, K. (2009). Dopamine-modulated dynamic cell assemblies generated by the GABAergic striatal microcircuit. *Neural Netw.* 22, 1174–1188. doi: 10.1016/j.neunet.2009.07.018

Kimura, M. (1990). Behaviorally contingent property of movement-related activity of the primate putamen. *J. Neurophysiol.* 63, 1277–1296.

Kinon, B. J., Merson, D., and Kane, J. M. (1984). Effect of daily dose of chronic haloperidol and chronic apomorphine on behavioral hypersensitivity in the rat. *Psychopharmacology (Berl)* 84, 347–351. doi: 10.1007/BF00555211

Kish, L. J., Palmer, M. R., and Gerhardt, G. A. (1999). Multiple single-unit recordings in the striatum of freely moving animals: effects of apomorphine and D-amphetamine in normal and unilateral 6-hydroxydopamine-lesioned rats. *Brain Res.* 833, 58–70. doi: 10.1016/S0006-8993(99)01496-1

Klingberg, F., and Pickenhain, L. (1968) [Occurrence of "spindle discharges" in the rat in relation to behavior]. *Acta Biol. Med. Ger.* 20, 45–54.

Koos, T., and Tepper, J. M. (1999). Inhibitory control of neostriatal projection neurons by GABAergic interneurons. *Nat. Neurosci.* 2, 467–472. doi: 10.1038/8138

Lansink, C. S., Goltstein, P. M., Lankelma, J. V., and Pennartz, C. M. (2010). Fast-spiking interneurons of the rat ventral striatum: temporal coordination of activity with principal cells and responsiveness to reward. *Eur. J. Neurosci.* 32, 494–508. doi: 10.1111/j.1460-9568.2010.07293.x

Levey, A. I., Hersch, S. M., Rye, D. B., Sunahara, R. K., Niznik, H. B., Kitt, C. A., et al. (1993). Localization of D1 and D2 dopamine receptors in brain with subtype-specific antibodies. *Proc. Natl. Acad. Sci. U.S.A.* 90, 8861–8865. doi: 10.1073/pnas.90.19.8861

Mitchell, I. J., Cooper, A. C., Griffiths, M. R., and Cooper, A. J. (2002). Acute administration of haloperidol induces apoptosis of neurones in the striatum and substantia nigra in the rat. *Neuroscience* 109, 89–99. doi: 10.1016/S0306-4522(01)00455-9

Moyer, J. T., Wolf, J. A., and Finkel, L. H. (2007). Effects of dopaminergic modulation on the integrative properties of the ventral striatal medium spiny neuron. *J. Neurophysiol.* 98, 3731–3748. doi: 10.1152/jn.00335.2007

Murer, M. G., Tseng, K. Y., Kasanetz, F., Belluscio, M., and Riquelme, L. A. (2002). Brain oscillations, medium spiny neurons, and dopamine. *Cell. Mol. Neurobiol.* 22, 611–632. doi: 10.1023/A:1021840504342

Paxinos, G., and Watson, C. (2007). *The Rat Brain in Stereotaxic Coordinates.* Amsterdam: Elsevier.

Prosperetti, C., Di, G. G., Stefani, A., Moller, J. C., and Galati, S. (2013). Acute nigro-striatal blockade alters cortico-striatal encoding: an *in vivo* electrophysiological study. *Exp. Neurol.* 247, 730–736. doi: 10.1016/j.expneurol.2013.03.018

Ravel, S., Legallet, E., and Apicella, P. (2003). Responses of tonically active neurons in the monkey striatum discriminate between motivationally opposing stimuli. *J. Neurosci.* 23, 8489–8497.

Raz, A., Feingold, A., Zelanskaya, V., Vaadia, E., and Bergman, H. (1996). Neuronal synchronization of tonically active neurons in the striatum of normal and parkinsonian primates. *J. Neurophysiol.* 76, 2083–2088.

Raz, A., Frechter-Mazar, V., Feingold, A., Abeles, M., Vaadia, E., and Bergman, H. (2001). Activity of pallidal and striatal tonically active neurons is correlated in mptp-treated monkeys but not in normal monkeys. *J. Neurosci.* 21, RC128.

Reynolds, J. N., Hyland, B. I., and Wickens, J. R. (2004). Modulation of an afterhyperpolarization by the substantia nigra induces pauses in the tonic firing of striatal cholinergic interneurons. *J. Neurosci.* 24, 9870–9877. doi: 10.1523/JNEUROSCI.3225-04.2004

Rymar, V. V., Sasseville, R., Luk, K. C., and Sadikot, A. F. (2004). Neurogenesis and stereological morphometry of calretinin-immunoreactive GABAergic interneurons of the neostriatum. *J. Comp. Neurol.* 469, 325–339. doi: 10.1002/cne.11008

Sanchez, G., Rodriguez, M. J., Pomata, P., Rela, L., and Murer, M. G. (2011). Reduction of an afterhyperpolarization current increases excitability in striatal cholinergic interneurons in rat parkinsonism. *J. Neurosci.* 31, 6553–6564. doi: 10.1523/JNEUROSCI.6345-10.2011

Sharott, A., Moll, C. K., Engler, G., Denker, M., Grun, S., and Engel, A. K. (2009). Different subtypes of striatal neurons are selectively modulated by cortical oscillations. *J. Neurosci.* 29, 4571–4585. doi: 10.1523/JNEUROSCI.5097-08.2009

Somogyi, P., and Klausberger, T. (2005). Defined types of cortical interneurone structure space and spike timing in the hippocampus. *J. Physiol.* 562, 9–26. doi: 10.1113/jphysiol.2004.078915

Strange, P. G. (2008). Antipsychotic drug action: antagonism, inverse agonism or partial agonism. *Trends Pharmacol. Sci.* 29, 314–321. doi: 10.1016/j.tips.2008.03.009

Tepper, J. M., Koos, T., and Wilson, C. J. (2004). GABAergic microcircuits in the neostriatum. *Trends Neurosci.* 27, 662–669. doi: 10.1016/j.tins.2004.08.007

Watanabe, K., and Kimura, M. (1998) Dopamine receptor-mediated mechanisms involved in the expression of learned activity of primate striatal neurons. *J. Neurophysiol.* 79, 2568–2580.

Wilson, C. J., and Groves, P. M. (1981). Spontaneous firing patterns of identified spiny neurons in the rat neostriatum. *Brain Res.* 220, 67–80. doi: 10.1016/0006-8993(81)90211-0

Wiltschko, A. B., Pettibone, J. R., and Berke, J. D. (2010). Opposite effects of stimulant and antipsychotic drugs on striatal fast-spiking interneurons. *Neuropsychopharmacology* 35, 1261–1270. doi: 10.1038/npp.2009.226

Yang, C., Ge, S. N., Zhang, J. R., Chen, L., Yan, Z. Q., Heng, L. J., et al. (2013). Systemic blockade of dopamine D2-like receptors increases high-voltage spindles in the globus pallidus and motor cortex of freely moving rats. *PLoS ONE* 8:e64637. doi: 10.1371/journal.pone.0064637

Yarom, O., and Cohen, D. (2011). Putative cholinergic interneurons in the ventral and dorsal regions of the striatum have distinct roles in a two choice alternative association task. *Front. Syst. Neurosci.* 5:36. doi: 10.3389/fnsys.2011.00036

7

Mechanism of Parkinsonian Neuronal Oscillations in the Primate Basal Ganglia: Some Considerations Based on Our Recent Work

Atsushi Nambu[1,2]* and Yoshihisa Tachibana[1,2]

[1] *Division of System Neurophysiology, National Institute for Physiological Sciences, Okazaki, Japan*
[2] *Department of Physiological Sciences, Graduate University for Advanced Studies, Okazaki, Japan*

Correspondence:
Atsushi Nambu, Division of System Neurophysiology, National Institute for Physiological Sciences, 38 Nishigonaka, Myodaiji, Okazaki 444-8585, Japan
e-mail: nambu@nips.ac.jp

Accumulating evidence suggests that abnormal neuronal oscillations in the basal ganglia (BG) contribute to the manifestation of parkinsonian symptoms. In this article, we would like to summarize our recent work on the mechanism underlying abnormal oscillations in the parkinsonian state and discuss its significance in pathophysiology of Parkinson's disease. We recorded neuronal activity in the BG of parkinsonian monkeys treated with 1-methyl-4-phenyl-1,2,3,6-tetrahydropyridine. Systemic administration of L-DOPA alleviated parkinsonian motor signs and decreased abnormal neuronal oscillations (8–15 Hz) in the internal (GPi) and external (GPe) segments of the globus pallidus and the subthalamic nucleus (STN). Inactivation of the STN by muscimol ($GABA_A$ receptor agonist) injection also ameliorated parkinsonian signs and suppressed GPi oscillations. The blockade of glutamatergic inputs to the STN by local microinjection of a mixture of 3-(2-carboxypiperazin-4-yl)-propyl-1-phosphonic acid (glutamatergic NMDA receptor antagonist) and 1,2,3,4-tetrahydro-6-nitro-2,3-dioxo-benzo[f]quinoxaline-7-sulfonamide (glutamatergic AMPA/kainate receptor antagonist) suppressed neuronal oscillations in the STN. STN oscillations were also attenuated by the blockade of GABAergic neurotransmission from the GPe to the STN by muscimol inactivation of the GPe. These results suggest that cortical glutamatergic inputs to the STN and reciprocal GPe-STN interconnections are both important for the generation and amplification of the oscillatory activity of GPe and STN neurons in the parkinsonian state. The oscillatory activity in the STN is subsequently transmitted to the GPi and may contribute to manifestation of parkinsonian symptoms.

Keywords: Parkinson's disease, neuronal oscillation, globus pallidus, subthalamic nucleus, β-band, monkey, basal ganglia

INTRODUCTION

Parkinson's disease (PD) is a neurodegenerative disorder affecting motor and non-motor functions. Motor dysfunction in PD, including akinesia, tremor and rigidity is largely attributed to the progressive loss of dopaminergic (DAergic) neurons in the substantia nigra pars compacta. There are two hypotheses that explain the pathophysiology of PD. The "firing rate model" originally proposed that dopamine (DA) depletion reduces tonic excitation to striatal neurons projecting to the internal segment of the globus pallidus (GPi) (i.e., *direct* pathway) and tonic inhibition to striatal neurons projecting to the external segment of the globus pallidus (GPe) (*indirect* pathway) (DeLong, 1990; Mallet et al., 2006). Both of these changes are thought to increase average firing rates of GPi and substantia nigra pars reticulata neurons. This increased activity in the basal ganglia (BG) output nuclei induces decreased activity in thalamic and cortical neurons, resulting in akinesia. However, recent electrophysiological studies using 1-methyl-4-phenyl-1,2,3,6-tetrahydropyridine (MPTP)-induced PD monkeys have failed to detect an expected increase in GPi activity (Wichmann et al., 1999; Raz et al., 2000; Rivlin-Etzion et al., 2008).

The firing rate model has now been largely supplanted by the "firing pattern model" that emphasizes oscillatory and/or synchronized activity. Oscillatory and/or synchronized activity is frequently observed in the BG of patients with movement disorders and animal models, which may cause the disturbance of information processing in the BG (Bergman et al., 1998). Unit activity and local field potentials recorded from PD animals and patients have shown oscillatory and synchronized activity in the GPe, GPi and subthalamic nucleus (STN; Bergman et al., 1998; Levy et al., 2000; Raz et al., 2000; Brown et al., 2001; Brown, 2007). The frequency bands include the tremor (4–9 Hz) and β (10–30 Hz) bands. The β-band oscillation may be a primary cause of akinesia, since the treatment of akinesia with drugs effectively suppresses the β-band oscillation. Recent studies also reported β-band synchronized activity in STN neurons of PD patients (Moshel et al., 2013), and correlation between the high β-band activity and freezing gate in PD patients (Toledo et al., 2014). Deep brain stimulation (DBS), which has been widely accepted as an effective therapeutic option of PD, is suggested to improve motor symptoms by activation of efferent fibers (Hashimoto et al., 2003), changes of oscillatory activity (Vitek, 2008) and/or decoupling STN-GPi oscillations (Moran et al., 2012). By contrast, in the course of MPTP-treatment of monkeys, the appearance of PD motor symptoms preceded that of oscillatory activity (Leblois et al., 2007), seeming to contradict the firing pattern model.

In this article, we would like to summarize our recent work on the mechanism regulating the abnormal BG oscillations (Tachibana et al., 2011) and discuss its significance in PD pathophysiology.

OSCILLATORY ACTIVITY IN THE BG OF PD

The firing properties of BG neurons were compared between the normal and PD states of macaque monkeys. PD states were induced by MPTP treatment (2.4–2.5 mg/kg, carotid artery injection and additional intravenous injections). The average firing rates of GPe neurons were significantly decreased (normal, 65.2 ± 25.8 Hz; PD, 41.2 ± 22.5 Hz) and those of STN neurons were significantly increased (normal, 19.8 ± 9.7 Hz; PD, 27.6 ± 11.4 Hz) in the PD state, whereas the firing rate of GPi neurons were not changed (normal, 67.0 ± 24.3 Hz; PD, 63.1 ± 26.9 Hz). These data contradict the firing rate model. Burst strength (Levy et al., 2001a; Wichmann and Soares, 2006) was increased in the GPi/GPe and STN of the PD states. The mean power (Soares et al., 2004; Rivlin-Etzion et al., 2006) of the 8–15 Hz (low-β) oscillations was increased in the GPi/GPe and STN, whereas there were no consistent changes in the 3–8 Hz and 15–30 Hz (high-β) oscillations. Oscillatory bursts of GPi/GPe and STN neurons were observed as multiple peaks in the autocorrelograms (e.g., **Figures 1B1, 2B1, 3B1**). The peak frequency with a maximum power of the oscillatory bursts of GPi/GPe and STN neurons was around 14 Hz (**Figures 1B2, 2B2, 3B2**).

DA DEPENDENCE OF BG OSCILLATIONS

We first tested whether the abnormal BG oscillations depend on DAergic inputs. DA was administrated systemically to PD monkeys, and the effects on the neuronal activity of GPi/GPe and STN neurons were examined. The motor disability was ameliorated within 5 min after intravenous L-DOPA injections (2.5–3.5 mg/kg, iv). L-DOPA administration decreased 8–15 Hz oscillations in the GPi/GPe and STN. Approximately 30 min after L-DOPA injections, the monkeys returned to the PD states, and the abnormal oscillations reappeared. The overall firing rate was not changed throughout the injections. These results have demonstrated that abnormal burst firing and 8–15 Hz oscillatory activity of GPi/GPe and STN neurons are DA-dependent. They also suggest that neuronal oscillations in the GPi/GPe and STN, rather than their spontaneous firing rate changes, may be critical for PD symptoms, supporting the firing pattern model.

ORIGINS OF ABNORMAL GPi/GPe OSCILLATIONS

Then, the origins of 8–15 Hz GPi/GPe oscillations were examined. The GPi (Tachibana et al., 2008) and GPe (Kita et al., 2004) receive glutamatergic inputs from the STN and GABAergic inputs from the striatum and GPe (GPe-GPe projections via the intranuclear

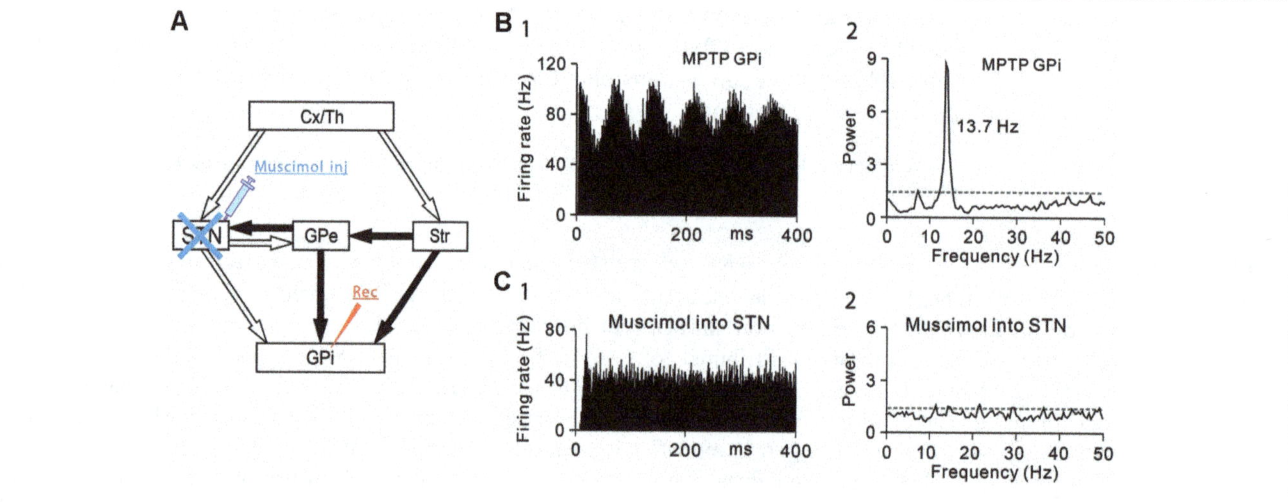

FIGURE 1 | Effects of subthalamic nucleus (STN) inactivation on neuronal activity of the internal segment of the globus pallidus (GPi) under the parkinsonian state. (A) A schematic diagram showing anatomical connections of the basal ganglia and the experimental method. Recording from GPi neurons was performed with muscimol injection into the STN to block STN inputs to the GPi. Open and filled arrows represent glutamatergic and GABAergic projections, respectively. Cx, cerebral cortex; GPe, external segment of the globus pallidus; Str, striatum; Th, thalamus. **(B)** A representative GPi neuron showing abnormal oscillations in the parkinsonian state. **(1)** Autocorrelograms calculated from a 50-s spike train and **(2)** power spectra of the same spike trains are shown. Gray dashed lines represent a confidence level of $P = 0.01$. **(C)** Muscimol inactivation of the STN decreased the firing rate and 8–15 Hz oscillatory activity of the GPi neuron. Modified from Tachibana et al. (2011).

axon collaterals). To determine which inputs contribute to abnormal 8–15 Hz GPi oscillations, each input was selectively blocked. Firstly, the STN was inactivated by injection of a $GABA_A$ receptor agonist, muscimol (4.4 mM, 0.5–1.0 μL) while GPi neuronal activity was simultaneously recorded (**Figure 1A**). Inactivation of the STN ameliorated PD motor signs, such as bradykinesia and rigidity, as previously reported (Bergman et al., 1990; Wichmann et al., 1994; Levy et al., 2001b) and decreased the 8–15 Hz oscillations (**Figures 1B, C**) and the firing rate.

Secondly, GABAergic inputs from the striatum and GPe were blocked, and the effects on the oscillatory activity of GPi/GPe neurons were examined. Microinjection of a $GABA_A$ receptor antagonist, gabazine (1 mM, 0.1–0.2 μL) in the vicinity of recorded GPi/GPe neurons increased the firing rate of GPi/GPe neurons, and augmented the 8–15 Hz GPi oscillations, but induced no changes in GPe oscillations. These results suggest that 8–15 Hz GPi/GPe oscillations are generated by glutamatergic inputs mainly from the STN, but not by GABAergic inputs from the striatum and GPe.

ORIGINS OF ABNORMAL STN OSCILLATIONS

Next, the origins of 8–15 Hz STN oscillations were examined. The STN receives glutamatergic inputs from the cerebral cortex and the thalamus, and GABAergic inputs from the GPe. Firstly, ionotropic glutamatergic inputs were blocked, and the effects on the oscillatory activity of STN neurons were examined (**Figure 2A**). Microinjection (0.1–0.2 μL) of a mixture of an *N*-methyl-D-aspartate receptor antagonist, 3-(2-carboxypiperazin-4-yl)-propyl-1-phosphonic acid (CPP, 1 mM) and an AMPA/kainate receptor antagonist, 1,2,3,4-tetrahydro-6-nitro-2,3-dioxo-benzo[f]quinoxaline-7-sulfonamide (NBQX, 1 mM) in the vicinity of recorded STN neurons decreased the 8–15 Hz oscillations (**Figures 2B, C**).

Secondly, GABAergic inputs from the GPe were blocked, and the effects on the oscillatory activity of STN neurons were examined (**Figure 3A**). Muscimol inactivation (1–2 μL) of the GPe attenuated the 8–15 Hz STN oscillations (**Figures 3B, C**) and increased the firing rate. However, the GPe inactivation induced no clear behavioral changes. These findings have shown that the 8–15 Hz STN oscillation are generated by glutamatergic inputs from the cortex and thalamus and GABAergic inputs from the GPe.

Previous studies reported the coherence between the electrocorticogram and the STN LFPs/STN unit activity in the PD state and have suggested that cortical glutamatergic inputs can drive STN oscillations in frequency bands below 30 Hz (Magill et al., 2000, 2001; Sharott et al., 2005; Mallet et al., 2008b). It is hypothesized that cortical β-rhythm is preferentially transmitted to the BG (Brittain and Brown, 2014). This idea is also supported by an optogenetic study that selective stimulation of cortico-STN projections ameliorated PD symptoms (Gradinaru et al., 2009). The other glutamatergic inputs to the primate STN may come from the intralaminar thalamic nuclei (Lanciego et al., 2009). The parafascicular thalamic nucleus (PF) neurons in PD rats showed oscillatory activity (0.5–2.5 Hz), but PF firings lagged STN firings (Parr-Brownlie et al., 2009).

Another origin of STN oscillations may be the GABAergic inputs from the GPe (Baufreton et al., 2005a). An *in vivo* rat study indicated that 15–30 Hz oscillations between GPe and STN neurons were developed during DA depletion (Mallet et al., 2008a). DAergic innervation in the GPe was decreased in PD monkeys (Schneider and Dacko, 1991), and the GPe-GPe GABAergic transmission was augmented (Watanabe et al., 2009). The oscillatory glutamatergic inputs mainly from the cortex and synchronized GABAergic inputs from the GPe may accelerate the

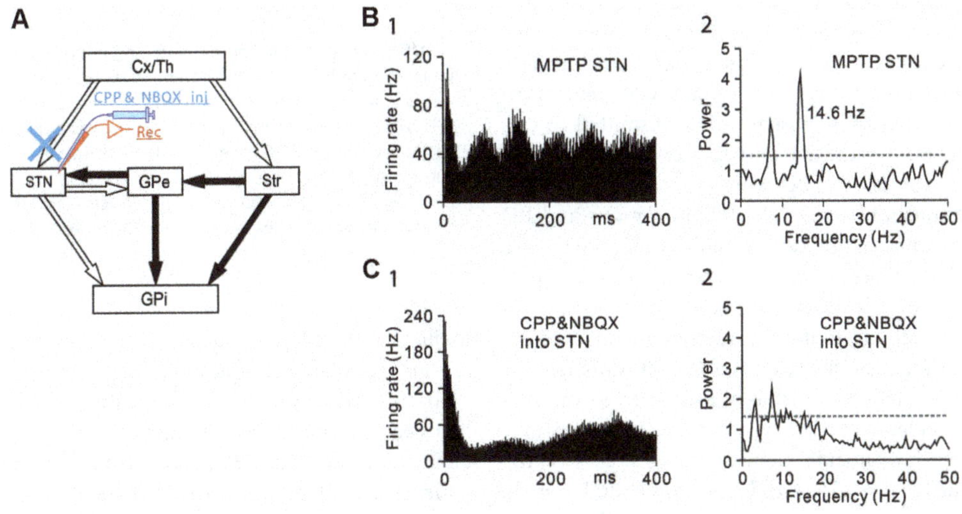

FIGURE 2 | Effects of the blockade of ionotropic glutamatergic inputs to STN neurons under the parkinsonian state. (A) Recording from STN neurons was performed with intrasubthalamic microinjection of CPP and NBQX to block glutamatergic inputs to the STN. **(B)** A representative STN neuron showing abnormal oscillatory activity under the parkinsonian state. **(C)** Intrasubthalamic microinjection of CPP and NBQX decreased 3–8 Hz and 8–15 Hz oscillations of the STN neuron. Modified from Tachibana et al. (2011).

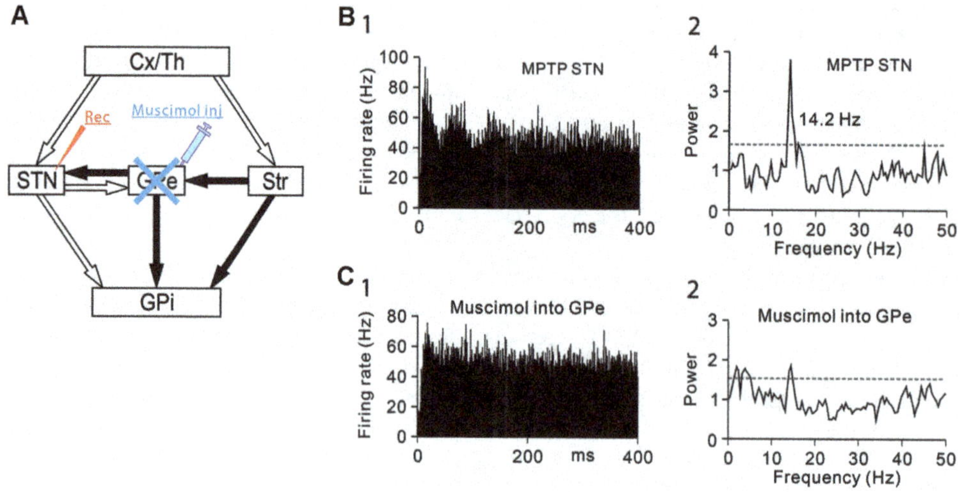

FIGURE 3 | Effects of GPe inactivation on STN neurons under the parkinsonian state. **(A)** Recording from STN neurons was performed with muscimol injection into the GPe to block GABAergic inputs from the GPe. **(B)** A representative STN neuron showing abnormal 8–15 Hz oscillations under the parkinsonian state. **(C)** Muscimol inactivation of the GPe decreased the 8–15 Hz oscillations and increased the firing rate of the STN neuron. Modified from Tachibana et al. (2011).

oscillatory activity in STN neurons (Shen and Johnson, 2000, 2005; Baufreton et al., 2005b; Baufreton and Bevan, 2008).

BG OSCILLATIONS AND PD PATHOPHYSIOLOGY

Our work shows the following results: (1) The loss of DA induced abnormal 8–15 Hz oscillations in GPi/GPe and STN neurons; (2) The abnormal 8–15 Hz GPi/GPe and STN oscillations were reversed by systemic DA administration; (3) The abnormal 8–15 Hz GPi/GPe oscillations were originated from the STN oscillations; and (4) The STN oscillations were driven by glutamatergic inputs mainly from the cortex and GABAergic inputs from the GPe. These findings support the firing pattern model and suggest the mechanism of BG oscillations: Glutamatergic inputs to the STN and reciprocal GPe-STN interconnections generate and amplify the oscillatory activity of STN and GPe neurons in PD. Such oscillatory activity is subsequently transmitted to GPi neurons, and finally reaches the thalamus, cortex and brain stem, contributing to the expression of PD symptoms (**Figure 4**).

The causal relationship between the BG oscillations and PD symptoms is a fundamental question. Leblois et al. (2007) have reported that oscillatory activity of BG neurons does not precede the appearance of PD motor symptoms in the course of chronic MPTP treatment of monkeys, questioning such causal relationship. Moreover, acute disruption of DA transmission did not develop oscillatory activity, which is distinct from chronically depleted animals (Mallet et al., 2008b). The BG oscillations may merely reflect other fundamental activity changes. In PD, the balance between the cortico-STN-GPi *hyperdirect* (Nambu et al., 2000), cortico-striato-GPi *direct* and cortico-striato-GPe *indirect* pathways was lost by the lack of DA in the striatum, and the "dynamic" network properties of the BG were changed (Nambu et al., 2005; Kita and Kita, 2011). It is suggested that the imbalance between the *hyperdirect* and *direct* pathways generates the BG oscillations (Leblois et al., 2006). Further studies are needed to solve this fundamental question.

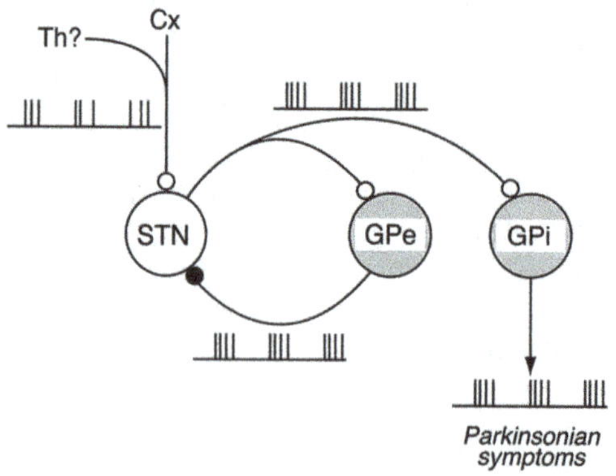

FIGURE 4 | Schematic diagram showing neural circuits involved in the generation of BG oscillations. Under the parkinsonian sate, glutamatergic inputs from the Cx (and also from the Th) to the STN and reciprocal GPe-STN interconnections can cooperatively generate and amplify the oscillatory activity of STN and GPe neurons. Such oscillatory activity is subsequently transmitted to the GPi, contributing to the expression of parkinsonian symptoms. Open and filled circles represent glutamatergic and GABAergic synapses, respectively. Modified from Tachibana et al. (2011).

In this article, we would like to emphasize a close relationship between the BG oscillations and PD symptoms. In fact, DAergic medication, STN-DBS, and voluntary movements in human patients are all reported to decrease the cortico-BG synchronization (Brown et al., 2001, 2004; Cassidy et al., 2002; Levy et al., 2002; Williams et al., 2002; Silberstein et al., 2005; Lafreniere-Roula et al., 2010). In a similar manner, the suppression of 8–15 Hz oscillations in the primate BG may be essential to ameliorate PD motor symptoms. These findings could shed light on the pathophysiology of PD and understanding the mechanisms of current therapies, and lead us to further rational treatments of PD.

REFERENCES

Baufreton, J., Atherton, J. F., Surmeier, D. J., and Bevan, M. D. (2005a). Enhancement of excitatory synaptic integration by GABAergic inhibitionin the subthalamic nucleus. *J. Neurosci.* 25, 8505–8517. doi: 10.1523/jneurosci.1163-05.2005

Baufreton, J., and Bevan, M. D. (2008). D2-like dopamine receptor-mediated modulation of activity-dependent plasticity at GABAergic synapses in the subthalamic nucleus. *J. Physiol.* 586, 2121–2142. doi: 10.1113/jphysiol.2008.151118

Baufreton, J., Zhu, Z. T., Garret, M., Bioulac, B., Johnson, S. W., and Taupignon, A. I. (2005b). Dopamine receptors set the pattern of activity generated in subthalamic neurons. *FASEB J.* 19, 1771–1777. doi: 10.1096/fj.04-3401hyp

Bergman, H., Feingold, A., Nini, A., Raz, A., Slovin, H., Abeles, M., et al. (1998). Physiological aspects of information processing in the basal ganglia of normal and parkinsonian primates. *Trends Neurosci.* 21, 32–38. doi: 10.1016/s0166-2236(97)01151-x

Bergman, H., Wichmann, T., and DeLong, M. R. (1990). Reversal of experimental parkinsonism by lesions of the subthalamic nucleus. *Science* 249, 1436–1438. doi: 10.1126/science.2402638

Brittain, J. S., and Brown, P. (2014). Oscillations and the basal ganglia: Motor control and beyond. *Neuroimage* 85, 637–647. doi: 10.1016/j.neuroimage.2013.05.084

Brown, P. (2007). Abnormal oscillatory synchronisation in the motor system leads to impaired movement. *Curr. Opin. Neurobiol.* 17, 656–664. doi: 10.1016/j.conb.2007.12.001

Brown, P., Mazzone, P., Oliviero, A., Altibrandi, M. G., Pilato, F., Tonali, P. A., et al. (2004). Effects of stimulation of the subthalamic area on oscillatory pallidal activity in Parkinson's disease. *Exp. Neurol.* 188, 480–490. doi: 10.1016/j.expneurol.2004.05.009

Brown, P., Oliviero, A., Mazzone, P., Insola, A., Tonali, P., and Di Lazzaro, V. (2001). Dopamine dependency of oscillations between subthalamic nucleus and pallidum in Parkinson's disease. *J. Neurosci.* 21, 1033–1038.

Cassidy, M., Mazzone, P., Oliviero, A., Insola, A., Tonali, P., Di Lazzaro, V., et al. (2002). Movement-related changes in synchronization in the human basal ganglia. *Brain* 125, 1235–1246. doi: 10.1093/brain/awf135

DeLong, M. R. (1990). Primate models of movement disorders of basal ganglia origin. *Trends Neurosci.* 13, 281–285. doi: 10.1016/0166-2236(90)90110-v

Gradinaru, V., Mogri, M., Thompson, K. R., Henderson, J. M., and Deisseroth, K. (2009). Optical deconstruction of parkinsonian neural circuitry. *Science* 324, 354–359. doi: 10.1126/science.1167093

Hashimoto, T., Elder, C. M., Okun, M. S., Patrick, S. K., and Vitek, J. L. (2003). Stimulation of the subthalamic nucleus changes the firing pattern of pallidal neurons. *J. Neurosci.* 23, 1916–1923.

Kita, H., and Kita, T. (2011). Cortical stimulation evokes abnormal responses in the dopamine-depleted rat basal ganglia. *J. Neurosci.* 31, 10311–10322. doi: 10.1523/JNEUROSCI.0915-11.2011

Kita, H., Nambu, A., Kaneda, K., Tachibana, Y., and Takada, M. (2004). Role of ionotropic glutamatergic and GABAergic inputs on the firing activity of neurons in the external pallidum in awake monkeys. *J. Neurophysiol.* 92, 3069–3084. doi: 10.1152/jn.00346.2004

Lafreniere-Roula, M., Darbin, O., Hutchison, W. D., Wichmann, T., Lozano, A. M., and Dostrovsky, J. O. (2010). Apomorphine reduces subthalamic neuronal entropy in parkinsonian patients. *Exp. Neurol.* 225, 455–458. doi: 10.1016/j.expneurol.2010.07.016

Lanciego, J. L., Lopez, I. P., Rico, A. J., Aymerich, M. S., Perez-Manso, M., Conte, L., et al. (2009). The search for a role of the caudal intralaminar nuclei in the pathophysiology of Parkinson's disease. *Brain Res. Bull.* 78, 55–59. doi: 10.1016/j.brainresbull.2008.08.008

Leblois, A., Boraud, T., Meissner, W., Bergman, H., and Hansel, D. (2006). Competition between feedback loops underlies normal and pathological dynamics in the basal ganglia. *J. Neurosci.* 26, 3567–3583. doi: 10.1523/jneurosci.5050-05.2006

Leblois, A., Meissner, W., Bioulac, B., Gross, C. E., Hansel, D., and Boraud, T. (2007). Late emergence of synchronized oscillatory activity in the pallidum during progressive Parkinsonism. *Eur. J. Neurosci.* 26, 1701–1713. doi: 10.1111/j.1460-9568.2007.05777.x

Levy, R., Ashby, P., Hutchison, W. D., Lang, A. E., Lozano, A. M., and Dostrovsky, J. O. (2002). Dependence of subthalamic nucleus oscillations on movement and dopamine in Parkinson's disease. *Brain* 125, 1196–1209. doi: 10.1093/brain/awf128

Levy, R., Dostrovsky, J. O., Lang, A. E., Sime, E., Hutchison, W. D., and Lozano, A. M. (2001a). Effects of apomorphine on subthalamic nucleus and globus pallidus internus neurons in patients with Parkinson's disease. *J. Neurophysiol.* 86, 249–260.

Levy, R., Hutchison, W. D., Lozano, A. M., and Dostrovsky, J. O. (2000). High-frequency synchronization of neuronal activity in the subthalamic nucleus of parkinsonian patients with limb tremor. *J. Neurosci.* 20, 7766–7775.

Levy, R., Lang, A. E., Dostrovsky, J. O., Pahapill, P., Romas, J., Saint-Cyr, J., et al. (2001b). Lidocaine and muscimol microinjections in subthalamic nucleus reverse Parkinsonian symptoms. *Brain* 124, 2105–2118. doi: 10.1093/brain/124.10.2105

Magill, P. J., Bolam, J. P., and Bevan, M. D. (2000). Relationship of activity in the subthalamic nucleus-globus pallidus network to cortical electroencephalogram. *J. Neurosci.* 20, 820–833.

Magill, P. J., Bolam, J. P., and Bevan, M. D. (2001). Dopamine regulates the impact of the cerebral cortex on the subthalamic nucleus–globus pallidus network. *Neuroscience* 106, 313–330. doi: 10.1016/s0306-4522(01)00281-0

Mallet, N., Ballion, B., Le Moine, C., and Gonon, F. (2006). Cortical inputs and GABA interneurons imbalance projection neurons in the striatum of parkinsonian rats. *J. Neurosci.* 26, 3875–3884. doi: 10.1523/jneurosci.4439-05.2006

Mallet, N., Pogosyan, A., Marton, L. F., Bolam, J. P., Brown, P., and Magill, P. J. (2008a). Parkinsonian beta oscillations in the external globus pallidus and their relationship with subthalamic nucleus activity. *J. Neurosci.* 28, 14245–14258. doi: 10.1523/JNEUROSCI.4199-08.2008

Mallet, N., Pogosyan, A., Sharott, A., Csicsvari, J., Bolam, J. P., Brown, P., et al. (2008b). Disrupted dopamine transmission and the emergence of exaggerated beta oscillations in subthalamic nucleus and cerebral cortex. *J. Neurosci.* 28, 4795–4806. doi: 10.1523/JNEUROSCI.0123-08.2008

Moran, A., Stein, E., Tischler, H., and Bar-Gad, I. (2012). Decoupling neuronal oscillations during subthalamic nucleus stimulation in the parkinsonian primate. *Neurobiol. Dis.* 45, 583–590. doi: 10.1016/j.nbd.2011.09.016

Moshel, S., Shamir, R. R., Raz, A., de Noriega, F. R., Eitan, R., Bergman, H., et al. (2013). Subthalamic nucleus long-range synchronization-an independent hallmark of human Parkinson's disease. *Front. Syst. Neurosci.* 7:79. doi: 10.3389/fnsys.2013.00079

Nambu, A., Tachibana, Y., Kaneda, K., Tokuno, H., and Takada, M. (2005). "Dynamic model of basal ganglia functions and Parkinson's disease," in *The Basal Ganglia VIII*, eds J. P. Bolam, C. A. Ingham and P. J. Magill (New York: Springer), 307–312.

Nambu, A., Tokuno, H., Hamada, I., Kita, H., Imanishi, M., Akazawa, T., et al. (2000). Excitatory cortical inputs to pallidal neurons via the subthalamic nucleus in the monkey. *J. Neurophysiol.* 84, 289–300.

Parr-Brownlie, L. C., Poloskey, S. L., Bergstrom, D. A., and Walters, J. R. (2009). Parafascicular thalamic nucleus activity in a rat model of Parkinson's disease. *Exp. Neurol.* 217, 269–281. doi: 10.1016/j.expneurol.2009.02.010

Raz, A., Vaadia, E., and Bergman, H. (2000). Firing patterns and correlations of spontaneous discharge of pallidal neurons in the normal and the tremulous 1-methyl-4-phenyl-1,2,3,6-tetrahydropyridine vervet model of parkinsonism. *J. Neurosci.* 20, 8559–8571.

Rivlin-Etzion, M., Marmor, O., Saban, G., Rosin, B., Haber, S. N., Vaadia, E., et al. (2008). Low-pass filter properties of basal ganglia cortical muscle loops in the normal and MPTP primate model of parkinsonism. *J. Neurosci.* 28, 633–649. doi: 10.1523/JNEUROSCI.3388-07.2008

Rivlin-Etzion, M., Ritov, Y., Heimer, G., Bergman, H., and Bar-Gad, I. (2006). Local shuffling of spike trains boosts the accuracy of spike train spectral analysis. *J. Neurophysiol.* 95, 3245–3256. doi: 10.1152/jn.00055.2005

Schneider, J. S., and Dacko, S. (1991). Relative sparing of the dopaminergic innervation of the globus pallidus in monkeys made hemi-parkinsonian by intracarotid MPTP infusion. *Brain Res.* 556, 292–296. doi: 10.1016/0006-8993(91)90318-p

Sharott, A., Magill, P. J., Harnack, D., Kupsch, A., Meissner, W., and Brown, P. (2005). Dopamine depletion increases the power and coherence of betaoscillations in the cerebral cortex and subthalamic nucleus of the awake rat. *Eur. J. Neurosci.* 21, 1413–1422. doi: 10.1111/j.1460-9568.2005.03973.x

Shen, K. Z., and Johnson, S. W. (2000). Presynaptic dopamine D2 and muscarine M3 receptors inhibit excitatory and inhibitory transmission to rat subthalamic neurones in vitro. *J. Physiol.* 525(Pt. 2), 331–341. doi: 10.1111/j.1469-7793.2000.00331.x

Shen, K. Z., and Johnson, S. W. (2005). Dopamine depletion alters responses to glutamate and GABA in the rat subthalamic nucleus. *Neuroreport* 16, 171–174. doi: 10.1097/00001756-200502080-00021

Silberstein, P., Pogosyan, A., Kuhn, A. A., Hotton, G., Tisch, S., Kupsch, A., et al. (2005). Cortico-cortical coupling in Parkinson's disease and its modulation by therapy. *Brain* 128, 1277–1291. doi: 10.1093/brain/awh480

Soares, J., Kliem, M. A., Betarbet, R., Greenamyre, J. T., Yamamoto, B., and Wichmann, T. (2004). Role of external pallidal segment in primate parkinsonism: comparison of the effects of 1-methyl-4-phenyl-1,2,3,6-tetrahydropyridine-induced parkinsonism and lesions of the external pallidal segment. *J. Neurosci.* 24, 6417–6426. doi: 10.1523/jneurosci.0836-04.2004

Tachibana, Y., Iwamuro, H., Kita, H., Takada, M., and Nambu, A. (2011). Subthalamo-pallidal interactions underlying parkinsonian neuronal oscillations in the primate basal ganglia. *Eur. J. Neurosci.* 34, 1470–1484. doi: 10.1111/j.1460-9568.2011.07865.x

Tachibana, Y., Kita, H., Chiken, S., Takada, M., and Nambu, A. (2008). Motor cortical control of internal pallidal activity through glutamatergic and GABAergic inputs in awake monkeys. *Eur. J. Neurosci.* 27, 238–253. doi: 10.1111/j.1460-9568.2007.05990.x

Toledo, J. B., López-Azcárate, J., Garcia-Garcia, D., Guridi, J., Valencia, M., Artieda, J., et al. (2014). High beta activity in the subthalamic nucleus and freezing of gait in Parkinson's disease. *Neurobiol. Dis.* 64, 60–65. doi: 10.1016/j.nbd.2013.12.005

Vitek, J. L. (2008). Deep brain stimulation: how does it work? *Cleve. Clin. J. Med.* 75(Suppl. 2), S59–S65. doi: 10.3949/ccjm.75.Suppl_2.S59

Watanabe, K., Kita, T., and Kita, H. (2009). Presynaptic actions of D2-like receptors in the rat cortico-striato-globus pallidus disynaptic connection in vitro. *J. Neurophysiol.* 101, 665–671. doi: 10.1152/jn.90806.2008

Wichmann, T., Bergman, H., and DeLong, M. R. (1994). The primate subthalamic nucleus. III. Changes in motor behavior and neuronal activity in the internal pallidum induced by subthalamic inactivation in the MPTP model of parkinsonism. *J. Neurophysiol.* 72, 521–530.

Wichmann, T., Bergman, H., Starr, P. A., Subramanian, T., Watts, R. L., and DeLong, M. R. (1999). Comparison of MPTP-induced changes in spontaneous neuronal discharge in the internal pallidal segment and in the substantia nigra pars reticulata in primates. *Exp. Brain Res.* 125, 397–409. doi: 10.1007/s002210050696

Wichmann, T., and Soares, J. (2006). Neuronal firing before and after burst discharges in the monkey basal ganglia is predictably patterned in the normal state and altered in parkinsonism. *J. Neurophysiol.* 95, 2120–2133. doi: 10.1152/jn.01013.2005

Williams, D., Tijssen, M., Van Bruggen, G., Bosch, A., Insola, A., Di Lazzaro, V., et al. (2002). Dopamine-dependent changes in the functional connectivity between basal ganglia and cerebral cortex in humans. *Brain* 125, 1558–1569. doi: 10.1093/brain/awf156

8

Global Actions of Nicotine on the Striatal Microcircuit

Víctor Plata, Mariana Duhne, Jesús Pérez-Ortega, Ricardo Hernández-Martinez, Pavel Rueda-Orozco, Elvira Galarraga, René Drucker-Colín and José Bargas*

División de Neurociencias, Instituto de Fisiología Celular, Universidad Nacional Autónoma de México, Mexico City, Mexico

***Correspondence:**
José Bargas, División de Neurociencias, Instituto de Fisiología Celular, Universidad Nacional Autónoma de México, Circuito ext s/n, México City DF 04510, México
e-mail: jbargas@ifc.unam.mx

The question to solve in the present work is: what is the predominant action induced by the activation of cholinergic-nicotinic receptors (nAChrs) in the striatal network given that nAChrs are expressed by several elements of the circuit: cortical terminals, dopamine terminals, and various striatal GABAergic interneurons. To answer this question some type of multicellular recording has to be used without losing single cell resolution. Here, we used calcium imaging and nicotine. It is known that in the presence of low micromolar N-Methyl-D-aspartate (NMDA), the striatal microcircuit exhibits neuronal activity consisting in the spontaneous synchronization of different neuron pools that interchange their activity following determined sequences. The striatal circuit also exhibits profuse spontaneous activity in pathological states (without NMDA) such as dopamine depletion. However, in this case, most pathological activity is mostly generated by the same neuron pool. Here, we show that both types of activity are inhibited during the application of nicotine. Nicotine actions were blocked by mecamylamine, a non-specific antagonist of nAChrs. Interestingly, inhibitory actions of nicotine were also blocked by the $GABA_A$-receptor antagonist bicuculline, in which case, the actions of nicotine on the circuit became excitatory and facilitated neuronal synchronization. We conclude that the predominant action of nicotine in the striatal microcircuit is indirect, via the activation of networks of inhibitory interneurons. This action inhibits striatal pathological activity in early Parkinsonian animals almost as potently as L-DOPA.

Keywords: striatal microcircuit, nicotine, nicotinic receptors, GABAergic interneurons

INTRODUCTION

The striatal microcircuit is composed of projection neurons and different classes of interneurons (e.g., Kawaguchi, 1993; Tepper and Bolam, 2004; Tepper et al., 2010). This circuit receives inputs from the cortex, the substantia nigra compacta (SNc) and the thalamus, among others, being a main entrance to the basal ganglia, a system of nuclei which encodes movement, associative learning, and procedural memory (Cools, 1980; DeLong, 1981; Aosaki et al., 1994; Kreitzer and Malenka, 2008; Do et al., 2012).

Although striatal projection neurons (SPNs) have low rates of basal firing in control conditions (e.g., Mink, 2003), uncorrelated excitatory drives such as N-Methyl-D-aspartate (2–5 μM NMDA) induces correlated neuronal activity in the control striatal microcircuit *in vitro* (Carrillo-Reid et al., 2008); similar to that produced during movement *in vivo* (Vautrelle et al., 2009). This activity consists in moments of recurrent and spontaneous synchronization in the firing of different neuron pools. This synchronous activity is alternated among the different neuron pools, generating the appearance of determined sequences, some of them being reverberant sequences or cycles (Carrillo-Reid et al., 2008, 2009a). These dynamics have been shown to be modulated by transmitters acting through G-protein coupled receptors and signaling pathways such as those activated by dopamine (DA) and acetyl-choline (ACh) (Carrillo-Reid et al., 2009a, 2011).

On the other hand, when deprived of DA supply, as in animal models of Parkinson's disease (PD), the striatal circuitry also generates a profuse spontaneous and synchronized activity without the addition of NMDA or any other excitatory drive. However, this pathological activity induced by DA-depletion differs from that found in control tissue: it is characterized by the loss of sequential activity and alternating dynamics. Almost all activity becomes generated by the same neuron pool with recurrent synchronization, resembling the repetitive oscillations found in Parkinsonian subjects (Jáidar et al., 2010). Here, we show that both control (with NMDA) and Parkinsonian activities are globally suppressed by nicotine administration.

The ACh present in the striatal microcircuit is released by local cholinergic interneurons and is the highest in any brain region together with the levels of choline acetyl-transferase, and choline-esterase (Mesulam et al., 1992; Contant et al., 1996; Goldberg et al., 2012). Cholinergic interneurons are autonomous pacemakers and ACh release is continuous and dynamic, thus, producing a varying tonic level of ACh in the whole striatum according to demand (Bennett and Wilson, 1999; Goldberg and Wilson, 2005).

The majority of the neurons (>90%) in the striatal circuit are SPNs which respond to ACh via muscarinic G-protein coupled receptors (Galarraga et al., 1999; Alcantara et al., 2001; Yan et al., 2001; Zhang et al., 2002). Known actions of these muscarinic receptors are facilitatory due in part to suppression of K^+-outward currents, directly or indirectly (Howe and Surmeier, 1995; Gabel and Nisenbaum, 1999; Galarraga et al., 1999; Lin et al., 2004; Olson et al., 2005; Pérez-Burgos et al., 2008; Pérez-Rosello et al., 2005; Shen et al., 2005).

However, much less is known about the nicotinic receptors present in this circuit (Goldberg et al., 2012). It is known that nAChRs are present in striatal dopaminergic terminals and promote DA release (e.g., Wonnacott et al., 2000; Grady et al., 2007; Keath et al., 2007; Livingstone and Wonnacott, 2009; Xiao et al., 2009; Cachope et al., 2012; Threlfell et al., 2012). It is also known that they are present in the terminals of cortical afferents and promote glutamate release (e.g., Marchi et al., 2002; Zhang and Warren, 2002; Campos et al., 2010). Finally, they are present in striatal GABAergic interneurons promoting GABA release that inhibits projection neurons (Koós and Tepper, 2002; Wilson, 2004; Kreitzer and Malenka, 2008; Livingstone and Wonnacott, 2009; Xiao et al., 2009; English et al., 2011; Ibáñez-Sandoval et al., 2011; Luo et al., 2013). Each of these actions has been studied directly and separately in cell-focused studies. However, it is not known which of them predominate in the microcircuit as a whole during nAChrs agonist administration.

Note that, if actions on glutamate afferents were predominant, we should see an enhancement of activity similar to that produced by NMDA alone, and a summation of effects would be evident. On the other hand, if the release of DA were the main action, mixed effects would appear: some interneurons are activated by DA, although their GABA release may be inhibited, being hard to foretell what is the net result (Bracci et al., 2002; Centonze et al., 2003). Activation of interneurons may enhance inhibition due to cholinergic activation. But at the network level, SPNs may be inhibited or excited by DA (e.g., Kiyatkin and Rebec, 1996), and both classes of DA-receptors, D_1 and D_2, increase synchronous firing (Carrillo-Reid et al., 2011). In addition, in the DA-depleted circuit, activity increases pathologically (Jáidar et al., 2010) while collateral inhibition is decreased (Taverna et al., 2008). In summary, a host of mixed and parallel actions makes hard to foretell what would be the global action of nicotinic receptors activation on the striatal microcircuit.

The importance of answering this question resides in the suspected neuro-protective action of nicotine in the prevention and development of PD (e.g., Costa et al., 2001; Quik et al., 2007; Kawamata et al., 2012). Although this postulate is still controversial (García-Montes et al., 2012), the hypothesis has its origin in epidemiological studies that claim less incidence of PD in smokers (Gorell et al., 1999; Herman et al., 2001; Driver et al., 2009), and in clinical studies that claim improvements of motor and cognitive symptoms in PD patients subjected to nicotine analogs (Fagerström et al., 1994; Villafane et al., 2007). From these arguments comes the importance of knowing with certainty what would be the end result of administering a tonic level of a nAChrs agonist in the striatal circuit, which in the present case is seen as a neuronal population of diverse elements capable to generate assembly dynamics (Carrillo-Reid et al., 2008) and involved in the generation of PD signs and symptoms.

MATERIALS AND METHODS

SLICE PREPARATION

Corticostriatal slices (300 μm) were obtained from PD20-40 male mice as previously described (Vergara et al., 2003). Animal experimentation followed the National Institutes of Health Guide for Care and Use of Laboratory Animals and the National University of Mexico guidelines. Slices were obtained with ice-cold saline (4°C) containing in mM: 123 NaCl, 3.5 KCl, 1 $MgCl_2$, 1.5 $CaCl_2$, 26 $NaHCO_3$, and 11 glucose (saturated with 95% O_2 and 5% CO_2). Slices remained in saline at room temperature (21–25°C) for at least 1 h before the experiments.

OPTICAL RECORDINGS OF NEURONAL POPULATIONS WITH SINGLE CELL RESOLUTION

Slices were incubated in the dark with 10 μM of the calcium indicator fluo-8 AM for about 20 min (Tef Labs, Austin, TX) in saline containing 0.1% dimethylsulphoxide (DMSO), equilibrated with 95% O_2 and 5% CO_2. We used an upright microscope equipped with a 10X, 0.95 NA water-immersion objective (E600FN Eclipse, Nikon, Melville, NY). To observe the changes in fluorescence we delivered pulses at 488 nm (50–100 ms exposure) to the preparation with a Lambda LS illuminator (Sutter instruments, Novato CA) connected to the microscope via fiber optics. The image field was 800 × 600 μm in size. Short movies (~180 s = epoch) were acquired at time intervals of 5–20 min during ≥60 min with a cooled digital camera (SenSys 1401E, Roper Scientific, Tucson, AZ) at 100–250 ms/frame.

Neurons active during the experiment (30 to 300 depending on number of epochs and age of animals; Carrillo-Reid et al., 2008) were identified due to their spontaneous calcium transients. They were recorded in control saline or during the application of NMDA and/or nicotine with or without ionotropic channel blockers such as: 6-cyano-2, 3-dihydroxy-7-nitro-quinoxaline disodium salt (10 μM CNQX), D-(-)-2-amino-5-phosphonovaleric acid (50 μM APV), bicuculline (10 μM) or gabazine (10 μM) (Sigma-Aldrich-RBI, St. Louis, MO). Stock solutions were prepared before experiments and added to the recording chamber in the final concentration indicated.

IMAGE PROCESSING

Neurons active in the field of view were selected automatically by a custom made program written in the LabView™ programming environment. The program processes the image sequence obtaining the fluorescence signals originated from action potentials discharge (Carrillo-Reid et al., 2008, 2009a). Briefly, a two dimensional coordinate was assigned for each cell. Each neuron was numbered and its precise location in the field of view was known. Calcium transients represent changes in fluorescence: $(F_i - F_o)/F_o$, where F_i denotes the fluorescence intensity at any frame and F_o denotes the basal fluorescence of each neuron. As it has been reported (Carrillo-Reid et al., 2008, 2009b; Jáidar et al., 2010) the first time derivative of the calcium transient reflects the time of electrical discharge of striatal neurons (>2.5 times the standard deviation of the noise value), in this way, the electrical activity of each neuron in the field of view could be followed along the experiment.

We constructed binary matrixes with the activity of dozens of neurons recorded simultaneously (raster plots). In each matrix, each row denotes an active neuron (numbered), while each column represents a time frame when an image was taken. Time axis represents the total number of frames making each movie converted into a minutes scale. For analysis, we considered calcium transients elicited by neurons only. Signals from neurons are much faster than signals from glial cells (Ikegaya et al., 2004; Sasaki et al., 2007; Carrillo-Reid et al., 2008). To visualize electrical activity from several active neurons, the binary matrix was plotted as a raster plot where neuronal firing is represented by dots. The activity histogram, shown below the raster plot, illustrates population activity of all neurons recorded during an experiment; it is obtained by the addition of all active neurons in each frame. Each spontaneous peak of synchronous activity denotes a pool of several neurons firing together (or having closely correlated activity). Note that each peak of synchronization is a neuronal column vector. Different colors denote that neuronal vectors are composed of different neuron pools.

STATISTICAL METHODS

Statistically significant peaks of co-active neurons were vectorized identified and counted (Carrillo-Reid et al., 2008), therefore, the level of correlated firing in the network can be quantitatively assessed and statistically compared. To assess the probability that a given peak of synchronization had appeared by chance, the points of the same matrix (raster plot) were used for MonteCarlo simulations with 10,000 replications. Thus, a level of significance is marked (dashed line) for all activity histograms. All the peaks of synchronization denoted by colors surpassed the significance level ($P < 0.05$). In control conditions without NMDA there are no significant peaks of synchronization. However, they appear in control tissue after adding NMDA. In addition they appear without NMDA when the tissue is depleted of dopamine (DA-depleted). If a treatment suppress NMDA-induced activity or DA-depletion induced activity, significant peaks of synchronization may go away in the activity histogram and the matrix only contains black dots denoting a decrease of network activity.

The sequence of peaks of synchronization in the activity histogram denotes the activity of the microcircuit along time, that is, a sequence of neuron pools synchronizing their firing and alternating their activity with other neuron pools. This type of circuit behavior has been called assembly dynamics (e.g., Carrillo-Reid et al., 2008). To know whether synchronization increased or decreased after a given treatment, the number of neuronal vectors was counted in each of several image sequences (epochs) at different times in the same experiment. Mean of averages from different slices were lumped together and a free-distribution statistic was employed (Mann-Whitney's U) for comparison. A Wilcoxon T-test was used to compare the same slice under different conditions. Note that each 3 min epoch commonly has dozens of individual cells. For comparison of epochs from different slices (**Figure 3**) the Kruskal-Wallis one way analysis of variance was used with *post hoc* Dunn tests.

These peaks of synchronization denote neuronal vectors that represent microcircuit activity in a multidimensional space, where the number of dimensions is given by the total number of active cells in each vector. Vectorization of network activity along the experiment allows the searching of recurrent patterns of activity, i.e., vectors being active repeatedly or different vectors alternating their activity (Schreiber et al., 2003; Ikegaya et al., 2004; Brown and Williams, 2005; Carrillo-Reid et al., 2008). The set of all these vectors connected by arrows represent the transitions between network states. To know whether the same vectors are active several times, similarity maps were constructed and all possible vector pairs were compared along time. The similarity index between any pair of vectors is defined by their normalized scalar product (Sasaki et al., 2007; Carrillo-Reid et al., 2008, 2009b): the cosine of the angle between the compared vectors. High similarity between vectors means that the activity of almost the same cells (same neuron pool) generated them at different times (Schreiber et al., 2003; Carrillo-Reid et al., 2008, 2009a; Jáidar et al., 2010). Different vectors (different neuron pools) are denoted by different colors in raster plots, activity histograms and locally linear embedding (LLE) graphs.

The method used to detect the dynamics of network states from multidimensional vectors has been published (Carrillo-Reid et al., 2008, 2009b; Jáidar et al., 2010). Briefly, dimensionality of population vectors representing network states was reduced by LLE, a dimensionality reduction technique that preserves the structure of non-linear multidimensional data (Roweis and Saul, 2000; Brown and Williams, 2005; Carrillo-Reid et al., 2008). Vectors are then projected into a two dimensional space. As a result, it is possible to visualize clusters of data points representing the recurrence of similar vectors with similar pools of neurons (network states) alternating their activity. Their sequences of activation may follow cycles or reverberation denoted by arrows (Schreiber et al., 2003; Sasaki et al., 2007; Carrillo-Reid et al., 2008, 2009b; Jáidar et al., 2010). To choose the optimal number of network states we used hard and fuzzy clustering algorithms and the Dunn's index as a validity function (Bezdek and Pal, 1998; Sasaki et al., 2007; Carrillo-Reid et al., 2008, 2009b).

Global neuronal activity over a given time was also represented by cumulative distributions of all cell activity in a given epoch. The rates of accumulation were approximated with *ad hoc* linear regressions. Their average slopes ± their estimation errors were compared for significant differences with non-paired Student's t tests, experiment by experiment. Average significance is reported. In addition, for sample comparisons of these parameters we used Wilcoxon's T statistic for paired samples and Mann-Whitney U statistic for non-paired samples (Plata et al., 2013).

THE 6-OHDA HEMI-PARKINSONIAN MODEL

Hemiparkinsonian animals, rats or BAC-mice, were obtained as previously reported (Jáidar et al., 2010). Briefly, animals were anesthetized with ketamine (85 mg/kg, i.p.) plus xylazine (15 mg/kg, i.p.) while immobilized on a stereotactic frame. Each animal received a unilateral injection of 6-OHDA (8 μg in 0.2 μl with 0.2 mg/ml of ascorbic acid) 0.1 μl/1 min in the substantia nigra pars compacta (SNc coordinates: 3.8 mm caudal, 1.8 mm lateral to bregma, and 7.1 mm ventral to the skull surface in rats and 2.6 mm caudal, 0.7 mm lateral to bregma and 4.5 mm ventral to the skull surface in post natal day 21 mice).

As described before (López-Huerta et al., 2012), the degree of DA deprivation was tested provoking turning behavior 8 days after the surgery using automated rotometers and amphetamine

(4 mg/kg, i.p.). Because these protocol has been extensively reported in several occasions (6-OHDA model; e.g., López-Huerta et al., 2012), here will not be reported in the Results, but only as a method to obtain hemiparkinsonian animals. Left and right full body turns were recorded for 90 min by a home-made computerized monitor. Animals showing >500 turns ipsilateral to the injected side were considered for further experiments.

RESULTS

CELL ASSEMBLY DYNAMICS IN THE STRIATAL MICROCIRCUIT

Figure 1A illustrates a raster plot or matrix showing the activity of >100 neurons in a field of view within a striatal slice in control conditions. Each row in the plot represents the electrical activity of one neuron across a series of images (columns) recorded by means of calcium-imaging using fluo-8 (see Materials and Methods). Leftmost frame shows 3 min of activity (an epoch) in control striatal tissue without NMDA: note the scarcity of spontaneous activity and the absence of significant peaks of synchronization. In the next three frames (3 epochs 3 min each) it is shown an increase in activity involving dozens of striatal individual neurons (single cell resolution) after adding 2 μM NMDA into the bath saline. All three epochs display the NMDA-induced activity. Colored dots denote neurons firing together and belonging to a pool of neurons. Different colors denote different neuron pools. The activity of these neurons is vectorized (column vectors). Note that neuronal vectors alternate their activity along time, that is, the network transits from one set of neurons to the other as indicated by different colors.

Activity histogram at bottom represents (**Figure 1B**) the summed neuronal activity of the matrix above, column by column, over time. Therefore, it represents a multicellular or population recording but with the possibility of locate and count each of the cells composing the peaks of synchronization (Carrillo-Reid et al., 2008, 2009a). The dashed horizontal line shows the level of statistical significance for the peaks of synchronization (obtained by Monte Carlo simulations, see above). Note that several peaks of neuronal synchronization, denoted by colors, cross this level, indicating that sets neurons synchronize their firing significantly and spontaneously and then alternate their activity with other synchronous neuron pools. Similarity index (**Figure 1C**) compares each neural vector with all others over time: a patchy appearance shows that similar and several vectors were in charge of activity through the time. Dimensionality reduction of neuronal vectors using LLE shows the same vectors projected into a two dimensional space with no units (**Figure 1D**; Carrillo-Reid et al., 2009a). Similar vectors group together (denoted by different colors) indicating various (3) network states in the circuit. Transitions between network states follow determined sequences or trajectories (arrows). Percentages give the probability of leaving a given network state. In this way, we can say that the group of neurons in the field of view shows cell assembly dynamics (Carrillo-Reid et al., 2008, 2009a). Note that in the control without NMDA (leftmost epoch in **Figure 1A**) there is no assembly dynamics. In the next three Figures, control activity indicates activity in the presence of 2 μM NMDA, that is, cell assembly dynamics or circuit activity. It is in this activity where we tested the global action of nicotine in the striatal circuitry.

GLOBAL ACTION OF NICOTINE IN THE ACTIVITY OF THE STRIATAL MICROCIRCUIT IS INHIBITORY

Raster plot in **Figure 2A** illustrates three epochs (3 min each separated by dashed vertical lines): the left epoch shows an activity similar to that described in **Figure 1A** in the continuous presence of 2 μM NMDA (arrow; NMDA was present all the time during this experiment): this activity reveals significant peaks of synchronization in the activity histogram below, the manifestation of assembly dynamics (**Figure 2B** colored). In NMDA presence, addition of 1 μM nicotine to the bath saline (middle epoch) drastically reduced the level of neuronal activity (horizontal bar indicates time of nicotine exposure). Nicotine reduced most circuit activity: less dots, absence of significant peaks synchronization. Note that the actions of nicotine were reversible upon washing (right epoch). Histogram of multicellular activity (**Figure 2B**; note significance level indicated by a dashed horizontal line) shows spontaneous and significant peaks of synchronization only in the presence of NMDA alone. Addition of nicotine abolished the peaks of synchronized activity even in the presence of NMDA (**Figure 2B**). Nonetheless, after nicotine was washed off, the peaks of synchronization begin to return (right epoch). By summating all activity from histogram in **Figure 2B** over time (all bars in the histogram for each epoch), we obtained a graph of cumulative cell activity (**Figure 2C**). It shows that total circuit activity in the presence of NMDA is much higher (*ad hoc* fitting of straight lines where slopes become the rate of accumulation along time ± estimation error). An average of a sample of experiments yields 479 ± 2 (act/min), which decays to 190 ± 1.5 (act/min) during nicotine ($n = 6$ slices; $P < 0.005$). **Figure 2D** shows the similarity matrix when nicotine is not present reassuring that assembly dynamics was present during NMDA. In addition, we counted the number of significant peaks of synchronization per epoch in the presence of NMDA and during nicotine in the continuous presence of NMDA (**Figure 2E**): an average of 3.3 ± 1.2 peaks/epoch in the control (NMDA) vs. 0.16 ± 0.4 peaks/epoch in the presence of nicotine ($n = 6$ slices; $n = 3$ epochs per slice; $^{**}P < 0.025$).

Figure 3 shows that actions of nicotine were blocked by 10 μM mecamylamine, a non-selective and non-competitive antagonist of nAChrs ($n = 4$). NMDA produced the usual increase in circuit activity with spontaneous and statistically significant peaks of synchronization (**Figures 3A,B** left epoch; NMDA was present during the whole experiment). This activity was greatly decreased when nicotine was added to the bath (middle epoch in **Figures 3A,B**), when significant peaks of synchronization disappeared, denoting that many individual neurons stopped firing (dots in the matrix). However, they partially returned when mecamylamine was added in the presence of both NMDA and nicotine (**Figures 3A,B** right epoch), suggesting that the actions of nicotine were receptor specific. A more complete characterization of the nicotinic receptors involved is out of the scope of the present report. Cumulative plots (**Figure 3C**) show that circuit activity is significantly lowered only when nicotine was added: an average of the sample of experiments yields 163 ±

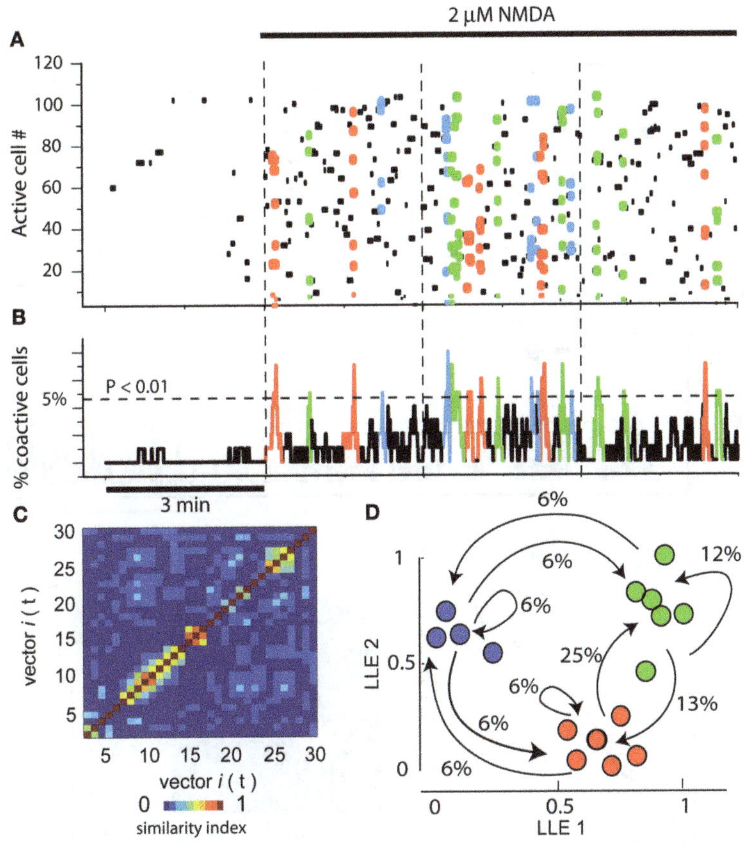

FIGURE 1 | Assembly dynamics in the control striatal circuitry after NMDA. (A) Raster plot showing the simultaneous activity of >100 neurons in a striatal slice using calcium-imaging. Each row in the matrix represents the activity of a single neuron across the series of images (columns). Left epoch shows 3 min of activity in control striatal tissue without NMDA. Note scarce activity and the absence of peaks of synchronization. In the next three epochs, separated by dashed vertical lines, 9 min of activity are shown after adding 2 μM NMDA into the bath saline (denoted by horizontal black line on top). Note that many more dots, some of them colored, populate the matrix. Colored dots denote the synchronized activity of several neurons in a given column or neighboring columns (a neuron pool is then represented as a column vector). Note that different neuron pools produce the circuit activity along time. **(B)** Activity histogram at bottom is the summed neuronal activity (multicellular activity) from the raster plot above column by column (frame by frame in a given movie). The dashed line shows the level of significance for the spontaneous peaks of synchronization denoted by colors (obtained by Monte Carlo simulations; statistically significant neuronal vectors; $n = 6$ slices). **(C)** A similarity index matrix compares each vector with all others along time: a patchy appearance shows that similar vectors were in charge of activity. **(D)** Dimensionality reduction using locally linear embedding (LLE) shows neuronal vectors projected in a two dimensional space with no units. Similar vectors grouped together (denoted by different colors) give raise to network states. The transitions among network states are denoted by arrows. Percentages give the probability to leave a given state. Colored dots and arrows represent the sequential activity of the circuit, that is, pools of neurons synchronized their firing and pass their activity from one pool of neurons to the other: cell assembly dynamics (Carrillo-Reid et al., 2008). Note reverberant trajectories in the sequence. Here and in the next figures, epochs (times of continuous image series) are separated by vertical dashed lines.

1.3 (act/min) in NMDA, which decays to 51 ± 0.7 (act/min) during nicotine ($n = 3$; average significance of $P < 0.01$). Note that subsequent addition of mecamylamine produced a return in the tendency of cumulative activity (green trace), even in the continuous presence of nicotine. The vectors similarity matrix reassured that NMDA-induced activity had assembly dynamics (**Figure 3D**). Histogram in **Figure 3E** shows average of synchronization peaks taken from several control slices in the presence of NMDA: 3.6 ± 0.34 peaks per epoch ($n = 10$ slices and $n = 10$ epochs). This average decreased significantly when nicotine was added to the superfusion: 0.2 ± 0.13 peaks per epoch ($^{***}P < 0.001$; $n = 10$ slices and $n = 10$ epochs). Note that when the non-selective nAChr antagonist, mecamylamine, was added to the bath saline, the peaks of synchronization returned gradually and significantly: 2.7 ± 0.33 peaks per epoch ($^{**}P < 0.01$; $n = 4$ slices; $n = 6$ epochs).

In summary, nicotine was capable to reduce circuit activity in the striatal network and its actions were both reversible (**Figure 2**) and blocked by mecamylamine (**Figure 3**). But nAChrs are ionotropic channels that carry inward currents that should excite, not inhibit circuit activity, just as NMDA-receptors. How it is possible that two ionotropic cationic receptors have opposite actions in the same circuit? According with some cell-focused studies, we hypothesized that the actions of nicotine were indirect via the activation of striatal GABAergic interneurons (e.g., English et al., 2011; Ibáñez-Sandoval et al., 2011; Luo et al., 2013).

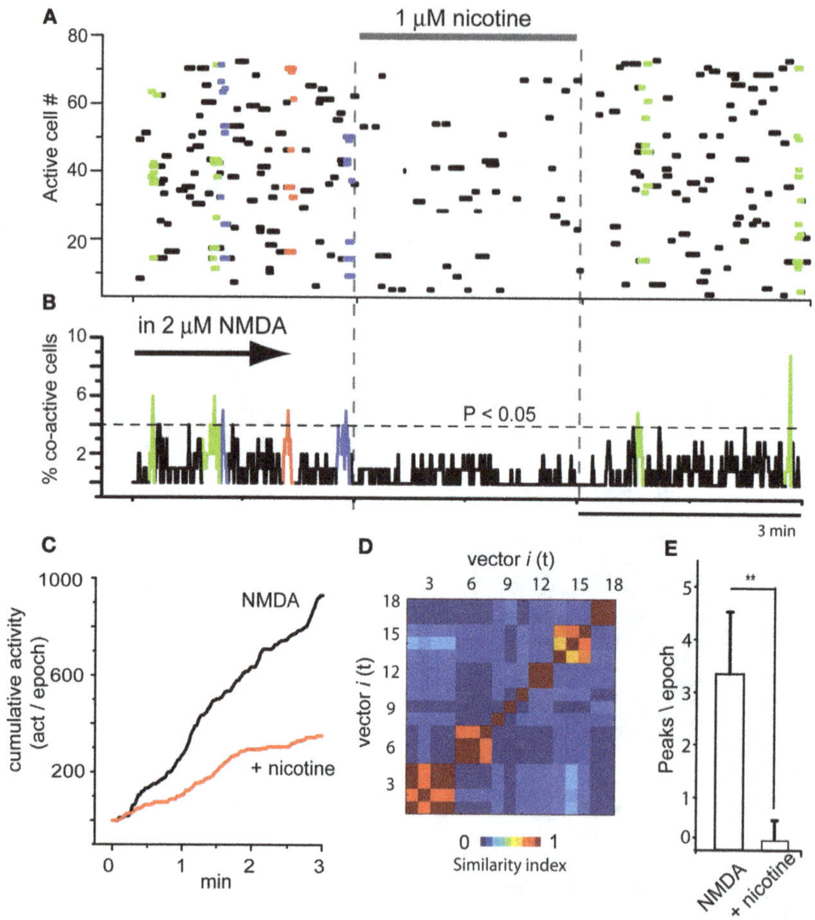

FIGURE 2 | Global actions of nicotine in the striatal circuit are inhibitory. **(A)** Raster plot illustrating three brief epochs (3 min each) taken from larger movies (as in **Figure 1A**). Left epoch: the simultaneous activity of 80 neurons in the continuous presence of NMDA (2 μM; denoted by an arrow, cf., **Figure 1**). The arrow denotes that NMDA is maintained all the time during this experiment. Colored dots show neuronal vectors indicating spontaneous synchronous activity of neuron pools. Middle epoch: nicotine (1 μM) is added to the bath saline in the presence of NMDA. Note that activity is decreased and the absence of colored dots indicates that spontaneous events of synchronization are now absent. Right epoch: a partial nicotine washing off, two significant peaks of synchronization appear indicating that nicotine actions were reversible. **(B)** Activity histogram displaying multicellular activity. Significant peaks of synchronization (colored) appear during NMDA but not after addition of nicotine even if NMDA is present. **(C)** Cumulative activity taken from histogram in **(B)** (addition of all bars in the histogram over time in a given epoch) shows that rate of accumulated activity was significantly higher in the absence of nicotine. Nicotine lowered the rate of cumulative activity significantly in all slices tested ($n = 6$ slices; $n = 3$ epochs per slice were taken). **(D)** Matrix of vectors similarity along time, without nicotine. **(E)** Histogram compares the appearance of peaks of synchronization per 3 min epoch in NMDA and in NMDA plus nicotine: it is clear that nicotine significantly abolished NMDA-induced synchronous activity. $^{**}P < 0.025$.

To see if this latter hypothesis was true we tried to block nicotine effects on the circuit with $GABA_A$-receptor antagonists.

INHIBITORY ACTION OF NICOTINE IN THE STRIATAL CIRCUIT IS BLOCKED BY $GABA_A$-RECEPTOR ANTAGONISTS

Figure 4A illustrates a raster plot with three epochs (separated by dashed vertical lines). At left, the usual neuronal activity found in striatal tissue after addition of 2 μM NMDA in the bath is shown (cf., **Figure 1**). Significant peaks of synchronization are present (**Figure 4B** left epoch; blue and red). At the middle epoch, 1 μM nicotine plus 10 μM bicuculline were added. In contrast with the action of bicuculline alone, where the activity of the circuit increases using the same pool of neurons over and over again (see Figure 8 in Carrillo-Reid et al., 2008 and Figure 5 in Jáidar et al., 2010), bicuculline together with nicotine, generated an activity of the circuit that displayed an increase of synchronization peaks (**Figures 4A,B** middle epoch). In these conditions, nicotine did not restrain circuit activity anymore and the induced activity consisted in a frenzy sequence of peaks coming from different neuron pools that alternate their activity without pace. 10 μM gabazine had the same results when administered with nicotine ($n = 3$; not shown but see: López-Huerta et al., 2012, 2013). Alternations among neuronal pools became frequent and rarely repeated.

In summary, bicuculline added alone increased activity based in a single or dominant peak of synchronization (see Carrillo-Reid et al., 2008; Jáidar et al., 2010), nicotine added alone, decreased the activity and peaks of synchronization disappeared

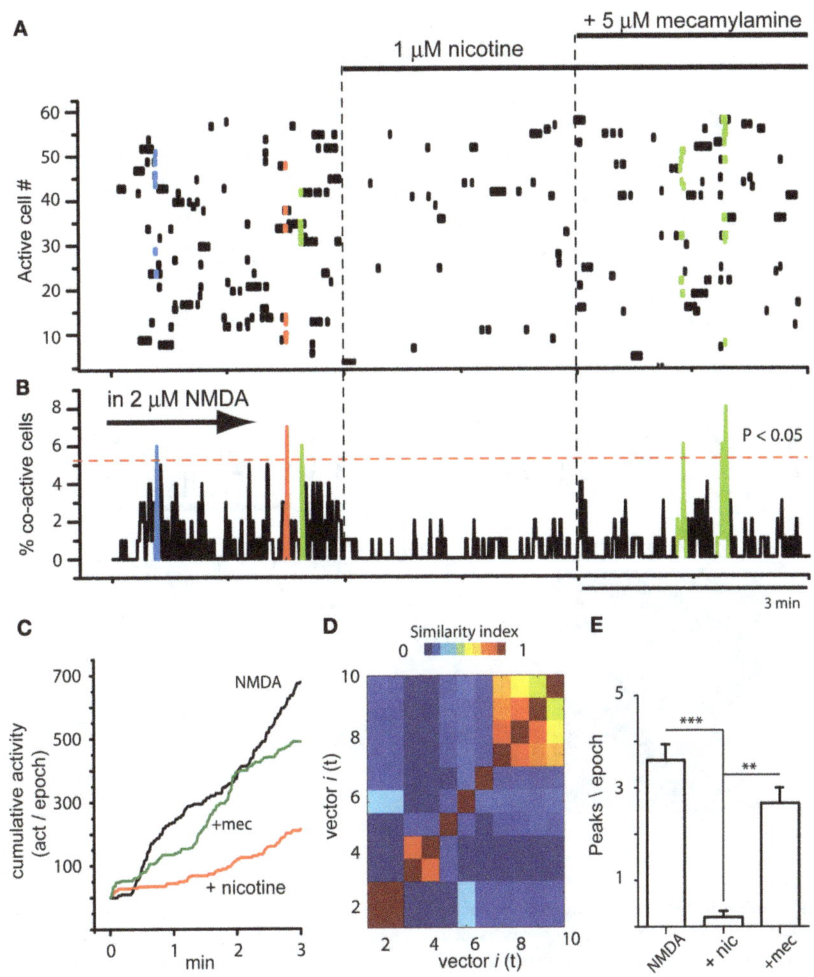

FIGURE 3 | Global actions of nicotine in the striatal circuit are blocked by mecamylamine. (A) Raster plot showing circuit activity in the presence of NMDA. Similarly to **Figure 2A**, left epoch shows activity with spontaneous synchronization of different neuron pools (colored dots). Middle epoch: nicotine (1 μM) added to the bath saline in the presence of NMDA induced a decrease in activity and the absence of color indicates that significant events of spontaneous synchronization are now absent. Right epoch: addition of 10 μM mecamylamine allowed the return of some peaks of synchronization showing that the activity of nicotine was receptor dependent ($n = 3$ slices; 6 epochs). **(B)** Activity histogram displaying multicellular activity from the raster plot above. Significant peaks of synchronization (colored) appear during NMDA. They disappeared when nicotine was added and reappeared after addition of mecamylamine to the bath saline. **(C)** Cumulative activity taken from histogram in **(B)** shows that rate of accumulated activity was significantly lower in the presence of nicotine plus NMDA than with NMDA alone. It is also shown that mecamylamine virtually restored the level of accumulated activity over time in the continuous presence of both NMDA and nicotine. **(D)** Matrix of vectors similarity along time reassured that activity in NMDA is due to network activity. **(E)** Histogram showing that the number of peaks of synchronization per epoch decreased significantly when nicotine was added in the presence of NMDA-induced activity (***$P < 0.001$) and then increased again, significantly (**$P < 0.01$), when mecamylamine was added in the presence of nicotine.

(**Figure 2**), but nicotine added with bicuculline increased activity based on an increase in the peaks of synchronization (**Figure 4**; cf., middle epoch with left and right epochs). The wash off of both drugs returned the circuit to usual levels in terms of activity during NMDA (**Figures 4A,B** right epoch). Similarity matrix includes vectors activity with bicuculline and nicotine (**Figure 4C**). Dimensionality reduction LLE compares circuit dynamics before (**Figure 4D** left; only two states red and blue) and after nicotine plus bicuculline (**Figure 4D** right; four states). Note that transitions between network states drastically augmented. This action was surprising in the sense that it suggests that several different sets of neurons are being activated by nicotine in spite of blocking $GABA_A$-receptor transmission, as in the case of DA D_2-receptor agonist action in the striatal circuit (cf., Figure 5B in Carrillo-Reid et al., 2011).

PARKINSONIAN ACTIVITY IN DOPAMINE DEPLETED STRIATUM IS REDUCED BY NICOTINE

A mice sample was lesioned unilaterally with 6-OHDA. The degree of DA deprivation in the striatal tissue was tested provoking turning behavior 8 days after the surgery using automated rotometers and amphetamine (4 mg/kg, i.p.). Animals showing >500 turns ipsilateral to the injected side were considered for further experiments (López-Huerta et al., 2012).

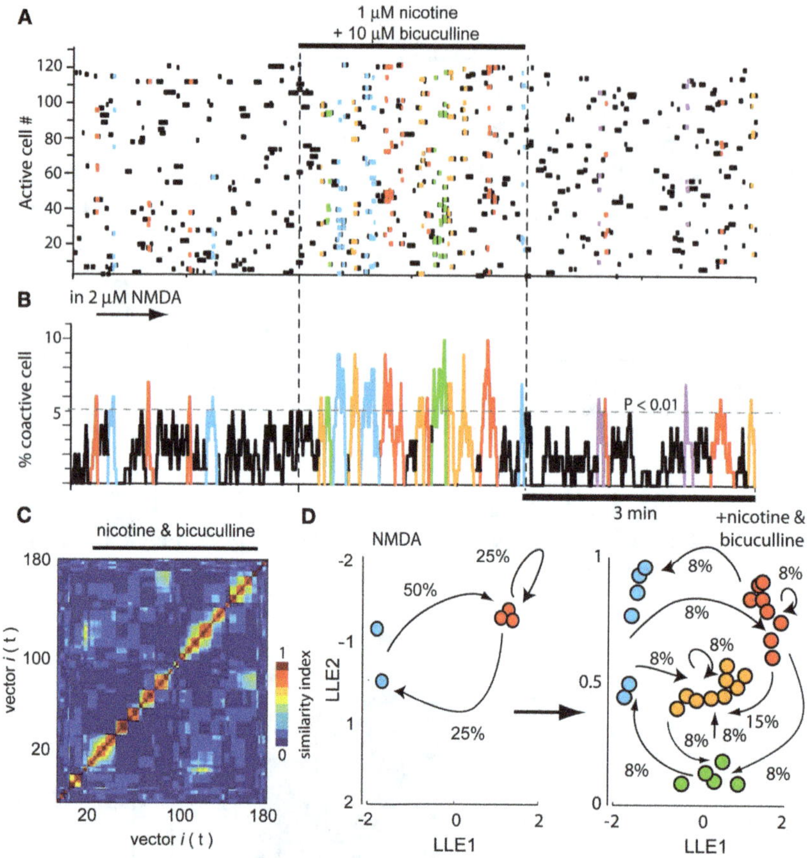

FIGURE 4 | Global actions of nicotine in the striatal circuit are blocked by bicuculline. (A) Raster plot showing again three different epochs of activity. At the left epoch, the typical activity of the striatal circuit with 2 μM NMDA is seen displaying two neuron pools with synchronized activity (red and blue). Middle epoch: neuronal activity is dramatically increased due to the addition of 1 μM nicotine plus 10 μM bicuculline into the bath saline. In contrast with what happens when bicuculline is administered alone (Carrillo-Reid et al., 2008), nicotine plus bicuculline showed a quite diverse set of synchronization peaks. Right epoch: nicotine plus bicuculline actions were reversible. **(B)** Activity histogram of summed multicellular activity showing that in control (left) there are five peaks of spontaneous synchronization belonging to two different neuron pools (blue and red). Peaks of synchronization increase in number and classes when both nicotine and bicuculline are added to the bath (middle epoch). When bicuculline is given alone, circuit activity is manifested by a highly recurrent peak of synchronization (Carrillo-Reid et al., 2008). Right epoch: activity begins to return to normal after the drugs were washed off. **(C)** Similarity matrix in the presence of both drugs. **(D)** LLE before (NMDA left) and after addition of nicotine plus bicuculline (right): note more network states and more transitions in circuit activity when both drugs are present.

As already reported (Jáidar et al., 2010), the DA depleted striatum exhibited spontaneous activity and peaks of statistically significant synchronization that appear spontaneously in the absence of NMDA or any other excitatory drive (**Figures 5A,B**; first three epochs). This pathological activity is different to the one recorded in the control striatum without NMDA (leftmost epoch in **Figure 1A**). It is also different than NMDA-induced activity in control tissue (Carrillo-Reid et al., 2008; Jáidar et al., 2010). First three epochs in the raster plot of **Figure 5A** show Parkinsonian activity followed by addition of nicotine in the last two epochs. In fact, nicotine was added after the beginning of the fourth epoch to appreciate the quick action of nicotine. Activity histogram (**Figure 5B**) shows that the DA-depleted microcircuit presents significant peaks of synchronization. Note however, that in this case the peaks are composed by the same pool of neurons (same color red), having recurrent activity once and again (Jáidar et al., 2010) as it is the case with bicuculline actions when it is given alone (Carrillo-Reid et al., 2008). In other words, DA-depletion produces an increased activity with no alternation. Interestingly, addition of 1 μM nicotine to the bath saline (last two frames) abolished Parkinsonian activity and the peaks of synchronization (last two epochs in **Figures 5A,B**). Cumulative activity clearly shows more activity over time for the Parkinsonian microcircuit (**Figure 5C**): average rate of activity over time in the DA deprived circuit was: 170 ± 1 (act/min) while it was 54 ± 0.4 (act/min) after nicotine ($n = 6$; $P < 0.006$), showing that nicotine significantly reduced pathological activity.

As previously reported (Jáidar et al., 2010), peaks of synchronization were made by similar neuronal vectors or the same network state having recurrent activity, according to similarity index and LLE analysis (**Figures 5D,E**; Jáidar et al., 2010). Note LLE (**Figure 5E**) showing the same network state recurring on itself absorbing all synchronized neurons, suggesting that this is the microcircuit correlate of Parkinsonian slow oscillations. It

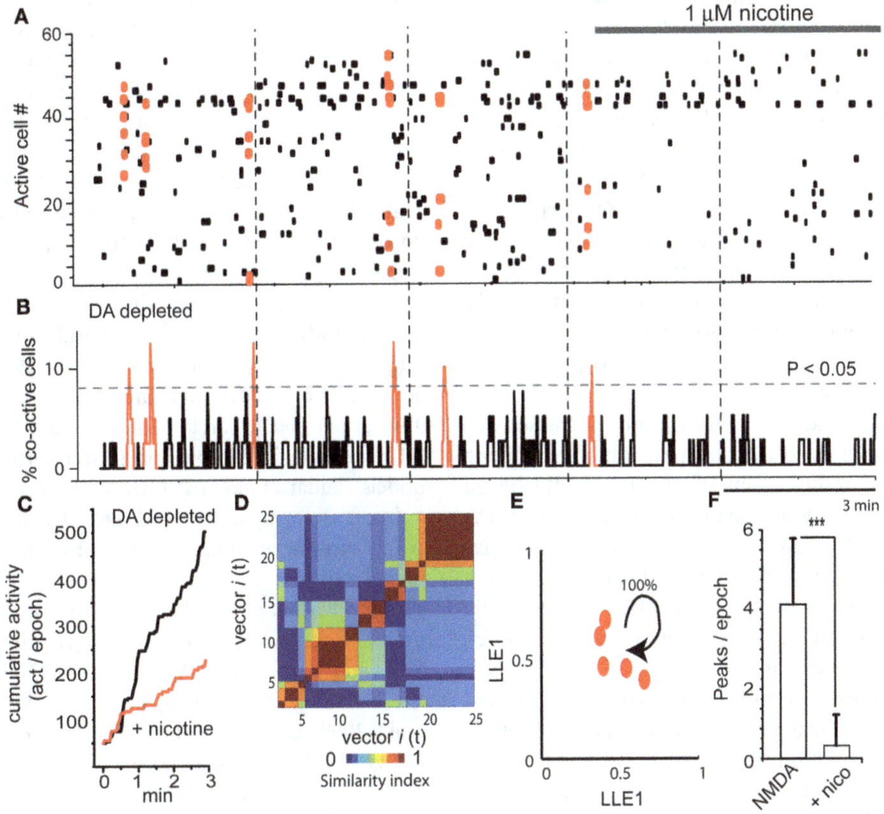

FIGURE 5 | Nicotine inhibits Parkinsonian activity in the dopamine depleted striatal microcircuit. (A) Raster plots showing five epochs of activity in a DA-depleted striatal circuit. There is spontaneous neuronal activity in the absence of NMDA (first three epochs shows activity in a 6-OHDA rodent model of hemi-Parkinsonism, see Materials and Methods). However, significant synchronization is composed of the same neuron pool. Last two epochs show that nicotine reduces this activity. **(B)** Note that activity during DA deprivation exhibits significant peaks of synchronization. However, all are depicted with the same color since similarity indexes indicate that these vectors are built with a similar set of neurons presenting correlated activity in a recurrent mode. Note that these peaks disappear during nicotine. **(C)** Cumulative activity is significantly higher during DA-depletion than during DA-depletion with nicotine. **(D)** Similarity matrix shows similar neuronal vectors dominating the activity through the time in the DA depleted microcircuit. **(E)** LLE shows that the same network state keeps repeating its firing over time in the DA depleted tissue (all dots are of the same group-color), as though the circuit could not leave this dominant network state (Jáidar et al., 2010). Nicotine was capable to suppress this recurrent network state significantly. **(F)** The histogram shows that peaks of spontaneous synchronization are virtually abolished by nicotine. $^{***}P < 0.005$.

was surprising that nicotine was capable to suppress the excess in activity and the dominant network state. Finally, we also quantified the number of synchronization peaks per epoch: it was an average of 4.2 ± 1.7 peaks/epoch ($n = 6$ slices; $n = 18$ epochs) in a sample of DA deprived slices and 0.3 ± 0.7 (peaks/epoch) in DA deprived slices during nicotine treatment (**Figure 5F**; $n = 6$ slices; $n = 12$ epochs; $^{***}P < 0.005$). In fact, the action of nicotine in this early Parkinsonian tissue is as potent as that of L-DOPA (cf., Plata et al., 2013).

DISCUSSION

Global action of nicotine in the striatal microcircuit reduced both the NMDA-induced neuronal activity in control tissue and the Parkinsonian pathological activity in the rodent 6-OHDA model of PD. However, nicotine, as NMDA, is an agonist of ligand-gated ionotropic channels whose role is to generate inward currents and depolarize target neurons. Nevertheless, each one of these agonists, NMDA and nicotine, has a completely different and even opposed action in the striatal circuit.

Cell-focused studies have disentangled an array of different actions of nicotine at the cellular and synaptic levels. First, nicotine activates nAChrs in incoming glutamate terminals inducing glutamate release (e.g., Marchi et al., 2002; Zhang and Warren, 2002; Campos et al., 2010). If this action were the predominant action at the microcircuit level, then it would be facilitatory of circuit activity and add to the activation produced by NMDA in the control circuit or to the pathological activity found in the DA-depleted circuit. This was not the case.

Second, nicotine also activates dopaminergic synapses inducing DA release (e.g., Wonnacott et al., 2000; Grady et al., 2007; Keath et al., 2007; Livingstone and Wonnacott, 2009; Xiao et al., 2009; Cachope et al., 2012; Threlfell et al., 2012). This action taken alone would lead to the induction of some kind of activity in the network (Carrillo-Reid et al., 2011) although this activity would be unpredictable solely based in cell-focused studies. On the one hand, DA induces firing in striatal interneurons. This action would favor inhibition of the circuit (Bracci et al., 2002). Nevertheless, besides postsynaptic activation of interneurons, DA also inhibits the release of GABA from the terminals of the same or different interneurons (Centonze et al., 2003). This, apparently, is a contradictory result. The end result of both actions taken together is hard to infer with cell-focused studies alone. This fact supports the need to observe actions of transmitters at the network level, and not only at the cellular level. Also, when seen at the circuit level, both classes of DA receptors, D_1 and D_2, induce an increase in spontaneous synchronized activity (Carrillo-Reid et al., 2011). Besides, individual SPNs may be inhibited or excited by DA (e.g., Kiyatkin and Rebec, 1996; Carrillo-Reid et al., 2011) depending on context. Taken one by one, it is difficult to make sense of all these actions and any inference about the end results is precluded. This fact supports the direct study of the global action in the microcircuit as a whole.

Furthermore, in case the activity of the circuit is increased due to DA-depletion (Jáidar et al., 2010), collateral inhibition among SPNs is decreased, and most actions of nicotine would be on GABAergic synapses made by interneurons. In such a case, DA analogs, such as L-DOPA, completely restore the control activity of the circuit, dramatically and reversible, being this action a neuronal correlate of behavioral and clinical trials (Plata et al., 2013). Accordingly, one question of the present work is how much nicotinic actions approximate that of L-DOPA.

Third, nAChrs actions have also been recorded in striatal GABAergic interneurons during cell-focused studies: nicotinic activation of several interneuron types such as fast-spiking (FS), low-threshold spiking (LTS), tonically firing neurogliaform cells, and others, release GABA upon nicotinic activation and inhibit projection neurons (Koós and Tepper, 2002; Wilson, 2004; Kreitzer and Malenka, 2008; Livingstone and Wonnacott, 2009; Xiao et al., 2009; English et al., 2011; Ibáñez-Sandoval et al., 2011; Luo et al., 2013). As the cell-focused studies described above, this appears to be another important action of nicotine when observed in isolation, cell by cell.

To conclude, cell-focused studies have revealed a host of mixed and parallel actions, some pointing to inhibitory and others to excitatory types of activity. Taken together, all these actions make hard to foretell what would be the global action of nicotinic receptors activation on the striatal microcircuit as a whole. The importance of answering this question is that clinical studies claim improvements of motor and cognitive symptoms in PD patients subjected to nicotine analogs (Fagerström et al., 1994; Villafane et al., 2007), that is, after systemic administration. Moreover, some epidemiological studies claim less incidence of PD in smokers (Gorell et al., 1999; Herman et al., 2001; Driver et al., 2009). Therefore, it is logical to question about what is the predominant action of nicotine in the striatal circuit when tonic concentrations are raised. To observe the answer to this matter directly at the microcircuit level, some type of multicell recording and therefore, a more sophisticated analysis, are required. However, the results surpassed any expectation about which of the mixed and parallel actions described in cell-focused studies predominates: nicotine readily and reversibly decreased control (with NMDA) and Parkinsonian activity. This observation gives raise to perhaps more important questions: what is the relation between nicotine actions and its supposed anti-Parkinsonian activity? Could it be used as an adjunct therapy in PD?

In summary, we demonstrate that the predominant action of a tonic elevation in nicotine concentration in the striatal microcircuit is the inhibition of network activity through the activation of GABAergic transmission, since inhibitory nicotinic action was blocked by $GABA_A$-receptor antagonists. Secondly, the inhibitory activity could be either on the assembly dynamics induced by an uncorrelated excitatory drive such as NMDA (Carrillo-Reid et al., 2008), or else, on the pathological activity derived from DA depletion (Jáidar et al., 2010) in early Parkinsonian animals models.

In the second case, nicotinic action is a microcircuit correlate of the already described anti-Parkinsonian actions of nicotine (Fagerström et al., 1994; Gorell et al., 1999; Costa et al., 2001; Herman et al., 2001; Villafane et al., 2007; Driver et al., 2009; Quik et al., 2007; García-Montes et al., 2012; Kawamata et al., 2012). Indeed, in comparison to our early Parkinsonian animal models (Jáidar et al., 2010), we show that the action of nicotine is almost as strong as that of L-DOPA (Plata et al., 2013). Such a strong anti-Parkinsonian action at the circuit level was certainly unexpected.

Many classes of striatal interneurons are known to express nAChrs and are capable to be activated by nicotinic analogs (Koós and Tepper, 2002; Wilson, 2004; Quik et al., 2007; Kreitzer and Malenka, 2008; Livingstone and Wonnacott, 2009; Xiao et al., 2009; English et al., 2011; Ibáñez-Sandoval et al., 2011; Luo et al., 2013). As a result, they release GABA and inhibit SPNs. This inhibition is blocked by $GABA_A$-receptor antagonists such as bicuculline (e.g., English et al., 2011; Ibáñez-Sandoval et al., 2011; Luo et al., 2013). Accordingly, here it is shown that global inhibitory nicotinic actions could be blocked with $GABA_A$-receptor antagonists such as bicuculline suggesting that the strong decrease in circuit activity, normal or pathological, is due to massive interneurons activation. In fact, the action of bicuculline alone in the circuit has been reported both in control activity (with NMDA; Carrillo-Reid et al., 2008) and in Parkinsonian activity (with DA-depletion; Jáidar et al., 2010). When administered alone, bicuculline produces an increase in activity, but similarly to Parkinsonian activity it is characterized by a dominant pool of neurons having spontaneous synchronization in a recurrent way (Carrillo-Reid et al., 2008). In the DA-depleted tissue, activity entrenches the dominant state produced by DA absence destroying the alternating dynamics that may remain (Jáidar et al., 2010). In contrast, when bicuculline was given in the presence of nicotine, a plural set of peaks of synchronization appeared, manifesting a strong assembly dynamics with abundant trajectories in the LLE plot. This behavior suggests that several classes of interneurons are being activated.

Further research is needed to find out which of the interneuron classes predominate over the others, since each element of the circuit may express a different nAChr. The importance of this future dissection about the mechanism of how these powerful nicotinic action may happen is that it is known that PD course with hypercholinergia (rev in: Pisani et al., 2005; Goldberg and Reynolds, 2011) and that some types of interneurons become hyperexcitable during DA depletion (Dehorter et al., 2009), a result that appear as counter-intuitive given the present data. Therefore, this action may involve the activation of a specific interneuron network (with a specific nAChr-class). A strong candidate is the neurogliaform interneuron which releases abundant GABA setting the stage for volume transmission (Ibáñez-Sandoval et al., 2011). Alternatively, nicotine may favor the synchronized network activity of an interneuron network united by gap junctions (Tepper et al., 2010). In both cases, activation of these neurons may be capable to inhibit the interneurons that are overactive during PD (Dehorter et al., 2009), including perhaps, the cholinergic ones. This future research may find that a specific receptor is involved, a necessary step to find selective ligands with potential therapeutic use. Finally, *in vivo* experiments are needed to answer another question: how such a potent inhibition would allow common motor tasks.

In any case, the present results highlight the possibility of using nicotine analogs as an adjunct to L-DOPA in PD therapy.

The increase in DA release induced by nicotine may have its own beneficial actions as long as some DA-terminals still remain (Wonnacott et al., 2000; Grady et al., 2007; Keath et al., 2007; Livingstone and Wonnacott, 2009; Xiao et al., 2009; Cachope et al., 2012; Threlfell et al., 2012). A possible difficulty is that DA and glutamate release are tied together, and have a reciprocal interaction and regulation. In any case, here, we present a bio-assay that allows the evaluation of control and pathological activity of the striatal microcircuit in which the actions of drugs with suspected therapeutic actions may be tested and compared with usual behavioral assays.

CONCLUSION

Calcium imaging techniques may serve to design bio-assays to test potential anti-Parkinsonian drugs in *in vitro* brain slices. Here, we tested nicotine, which has been suspected to possess anti-Parkinsonian activity for a long time. Indeed, it had an action similar to L-DOPA assayed in the same preparation (cf., Plata et al., 2013). However, both drugs were assayed in early Parkinsonian animals tested with turning behavior as a correlate of DA-deprivation. Further research is needed to test nicotine analogs in later stages of the disease, as for example, in dyskinesias.

In addition, we searched the mechanism of nicotinic actions which turned out to be indirect: the global effect of elevating the tonic concentration of nicotine in the striatal microcircuit was that of inhibiting the circuit in a way that was blocked by $GABA_A$-receptor antagonists, that is, most probably by activating a set of inhibitory interneurons. Further research is needed to find out which neurons and nAChRs are involved in these actions. But of the many parallel and sometimes contradictory actions that have been described separately in cell-focused studies, the activation of interneurons appeared to be the predominant one.

AUTHOR CONTRIBUTIONS

Víctor Plata, Mariana Duhne, Pavel Rueda-Orozco made most experiments, Ricardo Hernández-Martinez and Mariana Duhne lesioned animals with 6-OHDA and evaluated behavior, Víctor Plata and Jesús Pérez-Ortega made or modified acquisition and analysis software, Elvira Galarraga, René Drucker-Colín, and José Bargas had the original ideas, planned and reviewed the experiments, José Bargas and Víctor Plata wrote the article. Irakli Intskirveli reviewed the article.

ACKNOWLEDGMENTS

We thank A. Laville, G. X Ayala and A. Aparicio for technical support and advice and to Dr. C. Rivera for animal care. This work was supported by Consejo Nacional de Ciencia y Tecnología (CONACyT México) grants 98004 and 154131, and by grants from Dirección General de Asuntos del Personal Académico. Universidad Nacional Autónoma de México: IN-202914 and IN-202814 to Elvira Galarraga and José Bargas, respectively. Víctor Plata had a CONACyT doctoral fellowship and data in this work are part of his doctoral dissertation in the Posgrado en Ciencias Biomédicas de la Universidad Nacional Autónoma de México.

REFERENCES

Alcantara, A. A., Mrzljak, L., Jakab, R. L., Levey, A. I., Hersch, S. M., and Goldman-Rakic, P. S. (2001). Muscarinic m1 and m2 receptor proteins in local circuit and projection neurons of the primate striatum: anatomical evidence for cholinergic modulation of glutamatergic prefronto-striatal pathways. *J. Comp. Neurol.* 434, 445–460. doi: 10.1002/cne.1186

Aosaki, T., Subokawa, H., Ishida, A., Watanabe, K., Graybiel, M., and Kimura, M. (1994). Responses of tonically active neurons in the primate's striatum undergo systematic changes during behavioral sensorimotor conditioning. *J. Neurosci.* 14, 3969–3984.

Bennett, B. D., and Wilson, C. J. (1999). Spontaneous activity of neostriatal cholinergic interneurons *in vitro*. *J. Neurosci.* 19, 5586–5596.

Bezdek, J. C., and Pal, N. R. (1998). Some new indexes of cluster validity. *IEEE Trans. Syst. Man Cybern. B Cybern.* 28, 301–315. doi: 10.1109/3477.678624

Bracci, E., Centonze, D., Bernardi, G., and Calabresi, P. (2002). Dopamine excites fast-spiking interneurons in the striatum. *J. Neurophysiol.* 87, 2190–2194. doi: 0.1152/jn.00754.2001

Brown, P., and Williams, D. (2005). Basal ganglia local field potential activity: character and functional significance in the human. *Clin. Neurophysiol.* 116, 2510–2519. doi: 10.1016/j.clinph.2005.05.009

Cachope, R., Mateo, Y., Mathur, B. N., Irving, J., Wang, H. L., Morales, M., et al. (2012). Selective activation of cholinergic interneurons enhances accumbal phasic dopamine release: setting the tone for reward processing. *Cell Rep.* 2, 33–41. doi: 10.1016/j.celrep.2012.05.011

Campos, F., Alfonso, M., and Durán, R. (2010). *In vivo* modulation of alpha7 nicotinic receptors on striatal glutamate release induced by anatoxin-A. *Neurochem. Int.* 56, 850–855. doi: 10.1016/j.neuint.2010.03.010

Carrillo-Reid, L., Hernández-López, S., Tapia, D., Galarraga, E., and Bargas, J. (2011). Dopaminergic modulation of the striatal microcircuit: receptor-specific configuration of cell assemblies. *J. Neurosci.* 31, 14972–14983. doi: 10.1523/JNEUROSCI.3226-11.2011

Carrillo-Reid, L., Tecuapetla, F., Ibáñez-Sandoval, O., Hernández-Cruz, A., Galarraga, E., and Bargas, J. (2009a). Activation of the cholinergic system endows compositional properties to striatal cell assemblies. *J. Neurophysiol.* 101, 737–749. doi: 10.1152/jn.90975.2008

Carrillo-Reid, L., Tecuapetla, F., Vautrelle, N., Hernández, A., Vergara, R., Galarraga, E., et al. (2009b). Muscarinic enhancement of persistent sodium current synchronizes striatal medium spiny neurons. *J. Neurophysiol.* 102, 682–690. doi: 10.1152/jn.00134.2009

Carrillo-Reid, L., Tecuapetla, F., Tapia, D., Hernández-Cruz, A., Galarraga, E., Drucker-Colin, R., et al. (2008). Encoding network states by striatal cell assemblies. *J. Neurophysiol.* 99, 1435–1450. doi: 10.1152/jn.01131.2007

Centonze, D., Grande, C., Usiello, A., Gubellini, P., Erbs, E., Martin, A. B., et al. (2003). Receptor subtypes involved in the presynaptic and postsynaptic actions of dopamine on striatal interneurons. *J. Neurosci.* 23, 6245–6254.

Contant, C., Umbriaco, D., Garcia, S., Watkins, K. C., and Descarries, L. (1996). Ultrastructural characterization of the acetylcholine innervation in adult rat neostriatum. *Neuroscience* 71, 937–947. doi: 10.1016/0306-4522(95)00507-2

Cools, A. R. (1980). Role of the neostriatal dopaminergic activity in sequencing and selecting behavioural strategies: facilitation of processes involved in selecting the best strategy in a stressful situation. *Behav. Brain Res.* 1, 361–378. doi: 10.1016/0166-4328(80)90035-2

Costa, G., Abin-Carriquiry, J. A., and Dajas, F. (2001). Nicotine prevents striatal dopamine loss produced by 6-hydroxydopamine lesion in the substantia nigra. *Brain Res.* 888, 336–342. doi: 10.1016/S0006-8993(00)03087-0

Dehorter, N., Guigoni, C., Lopez, C., Hirsch, J., Eusebio, A., Ben-Ari, Y., et al. (2009). Dopamine- deprived striatal GABAergic interneurons burst and generate repetitive giganticIPSCs in medium spiny neurons. *J. Neurosci.* 29, 7776–7787. doi: 10.1523/JNEUROSCI.1527-09.2009

DeLong, M. R. (1981). Alzheimer disease: evidence for selective loss of cholinergic neurons in the nucleus basalis. *Ann. Neurol.* 10, 122–126. doi: 10.1002/ana.410100203

Do, J., Kim, J. I., Bakes, J., Lee, K., and Kaang, B. K. (2012). Functional roles of neurotransmitters and neuromodulators in the dorsal striatum. *Learn. Mem.* 20, 21–28. doi: 10.1101/lm.025015.111

Driver, J. A., Logroscino, G., Gaziano, J. M., and Kurth, T. (2009). Incidence and remaining life time risk of Parkinson disease in advanced age. *Neurology* 72, 432–438. doi: 10.1212/01.wnl.0000341769.50075.bb

English, D. F., Ibanez-Sandoval, O., Stark, E., Tecuapetla, F., Buzsáki, G., Deisseroth, K., et al. (2011). GABAergic circuits mediate the reinforcement-related signals of striatal cholinergic interneurons. *Nat. Neurosci.* 15, 123–130. doi: 10.1038/nn.2984

Fagerström, K. O., Pomerleau, O., Giordani, B., and Stelson, F. (1994). Nicotine may relieve symptoms of Parkinson's disease. *Psychopharmacology* 116, 117–119. doi: 10.1007/BF02244882

Gabel, L. A., and Nisenbaum, E. S. (1999). Muscarinic receptors differentially modulate the persistent potassium current in striatal spiny projection neurons. *J. Neurophysiol.* 81, 1418–1423.

Galarraga, E., Hernández-López, S., Reyes, A., Miranda, I., Bermudez-Rattoni, F., Vilchis, C., et al. (1999). Cholinergic modulation of neostriatal output: a functional antagonism between different types of muscarinic receptors. *J. Neurosci.* 19, 3629–3638.

García-Montes, J. R., Boronat-García, A., López-Colomé, A. M., Bargas, J., Guerra-Crespo, M., and Drucker-Colín, R. (2012). Is nicotine protective against Parkinson's disease? An experimental analysis. *CNS Neurol. Disord. Drug Targets* 11, 897–906. doi: 10.2174/1871527311201070897

Goldberg, J. A., Ding, J. B., and Surmeier, D. J. (2012). Muscarinic modulation of striatal function and circuitry. *Handb. Exp. Pharmacol.* 208, 223–241. doi: 10.1007/978-3-642-23274-9_10

Goldberg, J. A., and Reynolds, J. N. (2011). Spontaneous firing and evoked pauses in the tonically active cholinergic interneurons of the striatum. *Neuroscience* 198, 27–43. doi: 10.1016/j.neuroscience.2011.08.067

Goldberg, J. A., and Wilson, C. J. (2005). Control of spontaneous firing patterns by the selective coupling of calcium currents to calcium-activated potassium currents in striatal cholinergic interneurons. *J. Neurosci.* 25, 10230–10238. doi: 10.1523/JNEUROSCI.2734-05.2005

Gorell, J. M., Rybicki, B. A., Johnson, C. C., and Peterson, E. L. (1999). Smoking and Parkinson's disease: a dose-response relationship. *Neurology* 52, 115–119. doi: 10.1212/WNL.52.1.115

Grady, S. R., Salminen, O., Laverty, D. C., Whiteaker, P., McIntosh, J. M., Collins, A. C., et al. (2007). The subtypes of nicotinic acetylcholine receptors on dopaminergic terminals of mouse striatum. *Biochem. Pharmacol.* 74, 1235–1246. doi: 10.1016/j.bcp.2007.07.032

Herman, E. H., Vick, J. A., Strong, J. M., Parker, R. J., Geyer, H. M., Kramer, E. D., et al. (2001). Cardiovascular effects of buccal exposure to dermal nicotine patches in the dog: a comparative evaluation. *J. Toxicol. Clin. Toxicol.* 39, 135–142. doi: 10.1081/CLT-100103829

Howe, A. R., and Surmeier, D. J. (1995). Muscarinic receptors modulate N-, P-, and L-type Ca2+ currents in rat striatal neurons through parallel pathways. *J. Neurosci.* 15, 456–469.

Ibáñez-Sandoval, O., Tecuapetla, F., Unal, B., Shah, F., Koós, T., and Tepper, J. M. (2011). A novel functionally distinct subtype of striatal neuropeptide Y interneuron. *J. Neurosci.* 31, 16757–16769. doi: 10.1523/JNEUROSCI.2628-11.2011

Ikegaya, Y., Aaron, G., Cossart, R., Aronov, D., Lampl, I., Ferster, D., et al. (2004). Synfire chains and cortical songs: temporal modules of cortical activity. *Science* 304, 559–564. doi: 10.1126/science.1093173

Jáidar, O., Carrillo-Reid, L., Hernández, A., Drucker-Colín, R., Bargas, J., and Hernández-Cruz, A. (2010). Dynamics of the Parkinsonian striatal microcircuit: entrainment into a dominant network state. *J. Neurosci.* 30, 1326–1336. doi: 10.1523/JNEUROSCI.1380–1310.2010

Kawaguchi, Y. (1993). Physiological, morphological, and histochemical characterization of three classes of interneurons in rat neostriatum. *J. Neurosci.* 13, 4908–4923.

Kawamata, J., Suzuki, S., and Shimohama, S. (2012). α7 nicotinic acetylcholine receptor mediated neuroprotection in Parkinson's disease. *Curr. Drug Targets* 13, 623–630. doi: 10.2174/138945012800399026

Keath, J. R., Iacoviello, M. P., Barrett, L. E., Mansvelder, H. D., and McGehee, D. S. (2007). Differential modulation by nicotine of substantia nigra versus ventral tegmental area dopamine neurons. *J. Neurophysiol.* 98, 3388–3396. doi: 10.1152/jn.00760.2007

Kiyatkin, E. A., and Rebec, G. V. (1996). Dopaminergic modulation of glutamate-induced excitations of neurons in the neostriatum and nucleus accumbens of awake, unrestrained rats. *J. Neurophysiol.* 75, 142–153.

Koós, T., and Tepper, J. M. (2002). Dual cholinergic control of fast-spiking interneurons in the neostriatum. *J. Neurosci.* 22, 529–535.

Kreitzer, C., and Malenka, C. (2008). Striatal plasticity and basal ganglia circuit function. *Neuron* 60, 543–554. doi: 10.1016/j.neuron.2008.11.005

Lin, J. Y., Chung, K. K., de Castro, D., Funk, G. D., and Lipski, J. (2004). Effects of muscarinic acetylcholine receptor activation on membrane currents and intracellular messengers in medium spiny neurones of the rat striatum. *Eur. J. Neurosci.* 20, 1219–1230. doi: 10.1111/j.1460-9568.2004.03576.x

Livingstone, P. D., and Wonnacott, S. (2009). Nicotinic acetylcholine receptors and the ascending dopamine pathways. *Biochem. Pharmacol.* 78, 744–755. doi: 10.1016/j.bcp.2009.06.004

López-Huerta, V. G., Blanco-Hernández, E., Bargas, J., and Galarraga, E. (2012). Presynaptic modulation by somatostatin in the rat neostriatum is altered in a model of Parkinsonism. *J. Neurophysiol.* 108, 1032–1043. doi: 10.1152/jn.00244.2012

López-Huerta, V. G., Carrillo-Reid, L., Galarraga, E., Tapia, D., Fiordelisio, T., Drucker-Colin, R., et al. (2013). The balance of striatal feedback transmission is disrupted in a model of parkinsonism. *J. Neurosci.* 33, 4964–4975. doi: 10.1523/JNEUROSCI.4721-12.2013

Luo, R., Janssen, M. J., Partridge, J. G., and Vicini, S. (2013). Direct and GABA-mediated indirect effects of nicotinic ACh receptor agonists on striatal neurones. *J. Physiol.* 591, 203–217. doi: 10.1113/jphysiol.2012.241786

Marchi, M., Risso, F., Viola, C., Cavazzani, P., and Raiteri, M. (2002). Direct evidence that release-stimulating alpha7* nicotinic cholinergic receptors are localized on human and rat brain glutamatergic axon terminals. *J. Neurochem.* 80, 1071–1078. doi: 10.1046/j.0022-3042.2002.00805.x

Mesulam, M. M., Mash, D., Hersh, L., Bothwell, M., and Geula, C. (1992). Cholinergic innervation of the human striatum, globus pallidus, subthalamic nucleus. substantia nigra, and red nucleus. *J. Comp. Neurol.* 323, 252–268. doi: 10.1002/cne.903230209

Mink, J. W. (2003). "The Basal Ganglia," in *Fundamental Neuroscience*, 2nd Edn., eds L. R. Squire, F. E. Bloom, S. K. McConnell, J. L. Roberts, N. C. Spitzer, and M. J. Zigmond (New York, NY: Academic Press), 815–839.

Olson, P. A., Tkatch, T., Hernandez-López, S., Ulrich, S., Ilijic, E., Mugnaini, E., et al. (2005). G-protein-coupled receptor modulation of striatal CaV1.3 L-type Ca2+ channels is dependent on a Shank-binding domain. *J. Neurosci.* 25, 1050–1062. doi: 10.1523/JNEUROSCI.3327-04.2005

Pérez-Burgos, A., Pérez-Rosello, T., Salgado, H., Flores-Barrera, E., Prieto, G. A., Figueroa, A., et al. (2008). Muscarinic M(1) modulation of N and L types of calcium channels is mediated by protein kinase C in neostriatal neurons. *Neuroscience* 155, 1079–1097. doi: 10.1016/j.neuroscience.2008.06.047

Pérez-Rosello, T., Figueroa, A., Salgado, H., Vilchis, C., Tecuapetla, F., Guzmán, J. N., et al. (2005). Cholinergic control of firing pattern and neurotransmission in rat neostriatal projection neurons: role of CaV2.1 and CaV2.2 Ca2+ channels. *J. Neurophysiol.* 93, 2507–2519. doi: 10.1152/jn.00853.2004

Pisani, A., Centonze, D., Bernardi, G., and Calabresi, P. (2005). Striatal synaptic plasticity: implications for motor learning and Parkinson's disease. *Mov. Disord.* 20, 395–402. doi: 10.1002/mds.20394

Plata, V., Duhne, M., Pérez-Ortega, J., Barroso-Flores, J., Galarraga, E., and Bargas, J. (2013). Direct evaluation of L-DOPA actions on neuronal activity of Parkinsonian tissue *in vitro*. *BioMed. Res. Int.* 2013:519184. doi: 10.1155/2013/519184

Quik, M., Bordia, T., and O'Leary, K. (2007). Nicotinic receptors as CNS targets for Parkinson's disease. *Biochem. Pharmacol.* 74, 1224–1234. doi: 10.1016/j.bcp.2007.06.015

Roweis, S. T., and Saul, L. K. (2000). Nonlinear dimensionality reduction by locally linear embedding. *Science* 290, 2323–2326. doi: 10.1126/science.290.5500.2323

Sasaki, T., Matsuki, N., and Ikegaya, Y. (2007). Metastability of active CA3 networks. *J. Neurosci.* 27, 517–528. doi: 10.1523/JNEUROSCI.4514-06.2007

Schreiber, S., Fellous, J. M., Whitmer, D., Tiesinga, P., and Sejnowski, T. J. (2003). A new correlation-based measure of spike timing reliability. *Neurocomputing* 52, 925–931. doi: 10.1016/S0925-2312(02)00838-X

Shen, W., Hamilton, S. E., Nathanson, N. M., and Surmeier, D. J. (2005). Cholinergic suppression of KCNQ channel currents enhances excitability of striatal medium spiny neurons. *J. Neurosci.* 25, 7449–7458. doi: 10.1523/JNEUROSCI.1381-05.2005

Taverna, S., Ilijic, E., and Surmeier, D. J. (2008). Recurrent collateral connections of striatal medium spiny neurons are disrupted in models of Parkinson's disease. *J. Neurosci.* 28, 5504–5512. doi: 10.1523/JNEUROSCI.5493-07.2008

Tepper, J. M., and Bolam, J. (2004). Functional diversity and specificity of neostriatal interneurons. *Curr. Opin. Neurobiol.* 14, 685–692. doi: 10.1016/j.conb.2004.10.003

Tepper, J. M., Tecuapetla, F., Koós, T., and Ibáñez-Sandoval, O. (2010). Heterogeneity and diversity of striatal GABAergic interneurons. *Front. Neuroanat.* 4:150. doi: 10.3389/fnana.2010.00150

Threlfell, S., Lalic, T., Platt, N. J., Jennings, K. A., Deisseroth, K., and Cragg, S. J. (2012). Striatal dopamine release is triggered by synchronized activity in cholinergic interneurons. *Neuron* 75, 58–64. doi: 10.1016/j.neuron.2012.04.038

Vautrelle, N., Carrillo-Reid, L., and Bargas, J. (2009). "Diversity of up-state voltage transitions during different network states," in *Cortico-Subcortical Dynamics in Parkinson Disease*, ed K. Y. Tseng (New York, NY: Humana/Springer), 73–85. doi: 10.1007/978-1-60327-252-0_5

Vergara, R., Rick, C., Hernández-López, S., Laville, J. A., Guzman, J. N., Galarraga, E., et al. (2003). Spontaneous voltage oscillations in striatal projection neurons in a rat corticostriatal slice. *J. Physiol.* 553, 169–182. doi: 10.1113/jphysiol.2003.050799

Villafane, G., Cesaro, P., Rialland, A., Baloul, S., Azimi, S., Bourdet, C., et al. (2007). Chronic high dose transdermal nicotine in Parkinson's disease: an open trial. *Eur. J. Neurol.* 14, 1313–1316. doi: 10.1111/j.1468-1331.2007.01949

Wilson, C. J. (2004). "Basal Ganglia," in *The Synaptic Organization of the Brain*, 5th Edn. ed G. M. Shepherd (*Oxford: Oxford University Press*), 361–414. doi: 10.1093/acprof:0s0/9780195159561.003.0009

Wonnacott, S., Kaiser, S., Mogg, A., Soliakov, L., and Jones, I. W. (2000). Presynaptic nicotinic receptors modulating dopamine release in the rat striatum. *Eur. J. Pharmacol.* 393, 51–58. doi: 10.1016/S0014-2999(00)00005-4

Xiao, C., Nashmi, R., McKinney, S., Cai, H., McIntosh, J. M., and Lester, H. A. (2009). Chronic nicotine selectively enhances alpha4beta2 nicotinic acetylcholine receptors in the nigrostriatal dopamine pathway. *J. Neurosci.* 29, 12428–12439. doi: 10.1523/JNEUROSCI.2939-09.2009

Yan, Z., Flores-Hernandez, J., and Surmeier, D. J. (2001). Coordinated expression of muscarinic receptor messenger RNAs in striatal medium spiny neurons. *Neuroscience* 103, 1017–1024. doi: 10.1016/S0306-4522(01)00039-2

Zhang, L., and Warren, R. A. (2002). Muscarinic and nicotinic presynaptic modulation of EPSCs in the nucleus accumbens during postnatal development. *J. Neurophysiol.* 88, 3315–3330. doi: 10.1152/jn.01025.2001

Zhang, W., Yamada, M., Gomeza, J., Basile, A. S., and Wess, J. (2002). Multiple muscarinic acetylcholine receptor subtypes modulate striatal dopamine release, as studied with M1-M5 muscarinic receptor knock-out mice. *J. Neurosci.* 22, 6347–6352.

9

Disrupting Neuronal Transmission: Mechanism of DBS?

Satomi Chiken and Atsushi Nambu*

Division of System Neurophysiology, National Institute for Physiological Sciences and Department of Physiological Sciences, Graduate University for Advanced Studies, Myodaiji, Okazaki, Japan

Correspondence:
Atsushi Nambu, Division of System Neurophysiology, National Institute for Physiological Sciences and Department of Physiological Sciences, Graduate University for Advanced Studies, 38 Nishigonaka, Myodaiji, Okazaki 444-8585, Japan
e-mail: nambu@nips.ac.jp

Applying high-frequency stimulation (HFS) to deep brain structure, known as deep brain stimulation (DBS), has now been recognized an effective therapeutic option for a wide range of neurological and psychiatric disorders. DBS targeting the basal ganglia thalamo-cortical loop, especially the internal segment of the globus pallidus (GPi), subthalamic nucleus (STN) and thalamus, has been widely employed as a successful surgical therapy for movement disorders, such as Parkinson's disease, dystonia and tremor. However, the neurophysiological mechanism underling the action of DBS remains unclear and is still under debate: does DBS inhibit or excite local neuronal elements? In this review, we will examine this question and propose the alternative interpretation: DBS dissociates inputs and outputs, resulting in disruption of abnormal signal transmission.

Keywords: deep brain stimulation, basal ganglia, subthalamic nucleus, globus pallidus, cortico-basal ganglia loop, electrophysiology

INTRODUCTION

Applying high-frequency electrical stimulation (HFS) to a specific target in subcortical structures, known as deep brain stimulation (DBS), was introduced as a surgical treatment for movement disorders in early 1990s (Benabid et al., 1991, 1994; Siegfried and Lippitz, 1994a,b; Limousin et al., 1995). Since then, DBS has been widely accepted as an effective therapeutic option. DBS targeting the ventral thalamus dramatically alleviates essential and resting tremor (Benabid et al., 1991, 1996; Siegfried and Lippitz, 1994b; Koller et al., 1997; Rehncrona et al., 2003). DBS targeting the subthalamic nucleus (STN) and the internal segment of the globus pallidus (GPi) has been largely used for treatment of Parkinson's disease, and GPi-DBS has marked effects on improvement of dystonic symptoms (Limousin et al., 1995; Deep-Brain Stimulation for Parkinson's Disease Study Group, 2001; Coubes et al., 2004; Wichmann and Delong, 2006; Kringelbach et al., 2007; Ostrem and Starr, 2008; Vitek, 2008; Vidailhet et al., 2013). However, the exact mechanism of the effectiveness remains to be elucidated.

Since DBS gives rise to similar effects to those of lesions, it was originally considered to inhibit local neuronal elements. In fact, neuronal firings of neighboring neurons were inhibited by STN- or GPi-DBS (Boraud et al., 1996; Dostrovsky et al., 2000; Wu et al., 2001; Filali et al., 2004; Lafreniere-Roula et al., 2010). On the other hand, recent studies have emphasized activation of neuronal elements. Actually, STN-DBS increased activity of GPi neurons through the excitatory STN-GPi projections (Hashimoto et al., 2003; Galati et al., 2006; Reese et al., 2011), and GPi-DBS reduced activity of thalamic neurons through the inhibitory GPi-thalamic projections (Anderson et al., 2003; Pralong et al., 2003; Montgomery, 2006). In addition, recent studies reported multi-phasic responses consisting of excitation and inhibition in GPi neurons during GPi-DBS (Bar-Gad et al., 2004; Erez et al., 2009; McCairn and Turner, 2009; Leblois et al., 2010). In this article, we critically review recent studies, and discuss the possible mechanism of effectiveness of DBS.

DEEP BRAIN STIMULATION (DBS) INHIBITS LOCAL NEURONAL ELEMENTS

Both DBS and lesion were found to produce similar benefits on alleviation of symptoms. For example, STN-DBS has similar effects on Parkinsonian motor signs (Benazzouz et al., 1993; Benabid et al., 1994; Limousin et al., 1995) to the STN-lesion (Bergman et al., 1990; Aziz et al., 1991; Levy et al., 2001) and blockade of synaptic transmission from the STN to the GPi (Graham et al., 1990; Brotchie et al., 1991). Thus, DBS was originally assumed to inhibit local neuronal elements. Actually, the most common effect of STN- or GPi-HFS on neighboring neurons was reduction of the firing rates.

Distinct suppression of neuronal activity was recorded during STN-DBS around the stimulating sites in Parkinsonian patients during stereotactic surgery (Filali et al., 2004; Welter et al., 2004). Similar results were also obtained in animal models, such as Parkinsonian monkeys (Meissner et al., 2005; Moran et al., 2011) and rats (Tai et al., 2003; Shi et al., 2006). Stimulus artifacts hinder detection of spikes during 2–3 ms after stimulus pulses and some spikes may be obscured when neuronal activities are recorded nearby the stimulating electrodes. Recent studies enabled detection of spikes just after stimulus pulses by removal of stimulus artifacts using the template subtraction method (Wichmann, 2000; Hashimoto et al., 2002) and confirmed that STN-DBS decreased firing of neighboring neurons (Meissner et al., 2005; Moran et al., 2011). Although STN-HFS much decreased neuronal firing around the stimulation site, complete cessation of

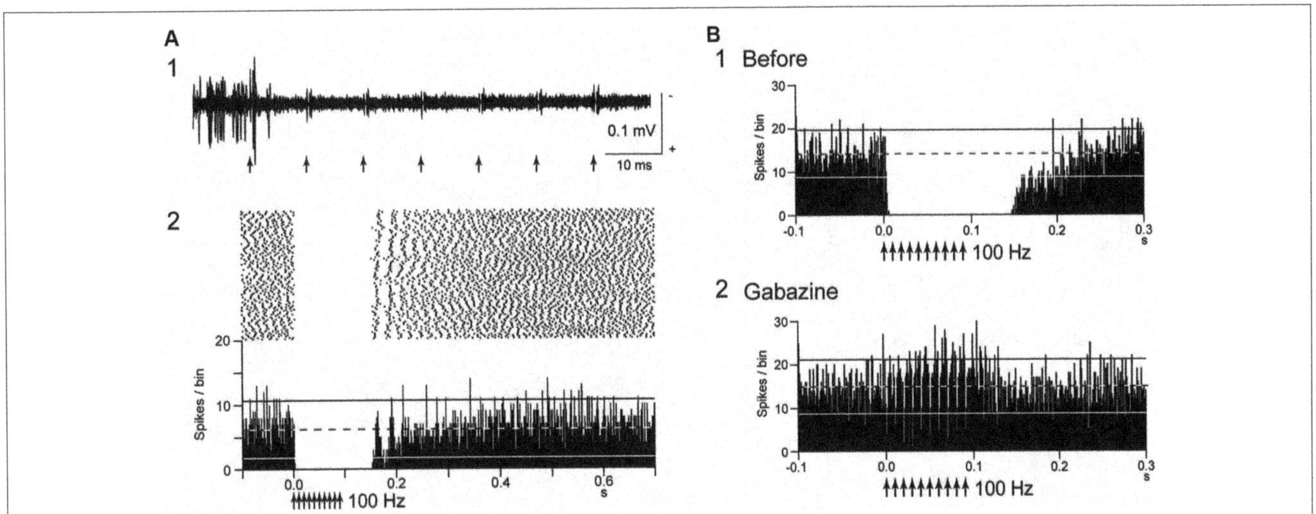

FIGURE 1 | Deep brain stimulation (DBS) inhibits local neuronal firing. **(A)** Responses of an internal pallidal (GPi) neuron to local GPi repetitive high-frequency stimulation (HFS; 30 μA, 100 Hz, 10 pulses) in a normal monkey. Raw traces of spike discharges after removing the stimulus artifacts by the template subtraction method **(1)** and raster and peristimulus time histogram (PSTHs; 100 trials; binwidth, 1 ms) **(2)** are shown. Arrows indicate the timing of local stimulation. Spontaneous discharges of the GPi neuron were completely inhibited by the stimulation. **(B)** Effect of local injection of gabazine ($GABA_A$ receptor antagonist) in the vicinity of the recorded GPi neuron on inhibition of spontaneous activity induced by GPi-HFS. The inhibition was abolished after gabazine injection. Modified from Chiken and Nambu (2013).

STN firing was observed in a limited number of neurons. STN-HFS at 140 Hz reduced mean firing rate of STN neurons by 77% in Parkinsonian patients, and among them, 71% of STN neurons exhibited residual neuronal activity, while only 29% of STN neurons exhibited total inhibition (Welter et al., 2004). Similar results were also observed in Parkinsonian monkeys (Meissner et al., 2005), and Parkinsonian and normal rats (Tai et al., 2003). Decreased abnormal oscillatory activity in the STN was also observed during STN-DBS in Parkinsonian monkeys (Meissner et al., 2005). Inhibitory effects sometimes outlasted the stimulus period (Tai et al., 2003; Filali et al., 2004; Welter et al., 2004).

Inhibitory effects of GPi-DBS on firing of the neighboring neurons were also reported (Boraud et al., 1996; Dostrovsky et al., 2000; Wu et al., 2001; McCairn and Turner, 2009). Complete inhibition of local neuronal firing was more commonly induced by GPi-DBS than by STN-DBS (**Figure 1A**). GPi-HFS at 100 Hz induced complete inhibition of 76% of neighboring neurons in normal monkeys (Chiken and Nambu, 2013), and the inhibition outlasted the stimulus period, sometimes over 100 ms after the end of stimulation. Similar post-train inhibition was also observed in Parkinsonian patients (Lafreniere-Roula et al., 2010).

To the contrary, multiphasic responses consisting of the excitation and inhibition during GPi-HFS were recently observed in GPi neurons of Parkinsonian monkeys (Bar-Gad et al., 2004; Erez et al., 2009; McCairn and Turner, 2009) and dystonic hamsters (Leblois et al., 2010). The discrepant results may be due to differences in stimulus parameters used in these experiments: larger axons are easily activated by electrical stimulation than smaller ones (Ranck, 1975), and continuous repetitive stimulation might cause failure of postsynaptic events due to receptor desensitization and/or transmitter depletion (Wang and Kaczmarek, 1998; Zucker and Regehr, 2002). Such multiphasic responses may normalize abnormal firings, such as bursting and oscillatory activity in Parkinson's disease and dystonia as described below.

MECHANISM OF INHIBITION

Several possible mechanisms account for the inhibitory responses have been proposed, including depolarization-block and inactivation of voltage-gated currents (Beurrier et al., 2001; Shin et al., 2007). However, these are less probable, because both single-pulse and low-frequency stimulation in the GPi evoked intense short latency inhibition in neighboring neurons (Dostrovsky et al., 2000; Dostrovsky and Lozano, 2002; Chiken and Nambu, 2013). Another possible mechanism is that the inhibition is caused by activation of GABAergic afferents in the stimulated nucleus (Boraud et al., 1996; Dostrovsky et al., 2000; Dostrovsky and Lozano, 2002; Meissner et al., 2005; Johnson et al., 2008; Liu et al., 2008; Deniau et al., 2010). A recent study confirmed that inhibitory responses induced by GPi-HFS were mediated by $GABA_A$ and $GABA_B$ receptors (Chiken and Nambu, 2013; **Figure 1B**). GABAergic inhibition is strong and inhibits even directly evoked spikes by GPi stimulation, which is characterized constant- and short latency (**Figures 2A, B**; Chiken and Nambu, 2013).

The GPi receives excitatory glutamatergic inputs from the STN as well as inhibitory GABAergic inputs from the striatum and GPe (Smith et al., 1994; Shink and Smith, 1995). Afferent axon terminals from the STN are also activated by the stimulation, but the glutamatergic excitation is probably overwhelmed because of predominance of GABAergic inputs in the GPi (Shink and Smith, 1995). On the other hand, many GPe neurons exhibited complex responses composed of both excitation and inhibition during GPe-HFS (Chiken and Nambu, 2013). The density of GPe terminals on GPi neurons is higher than those on GPe neurons

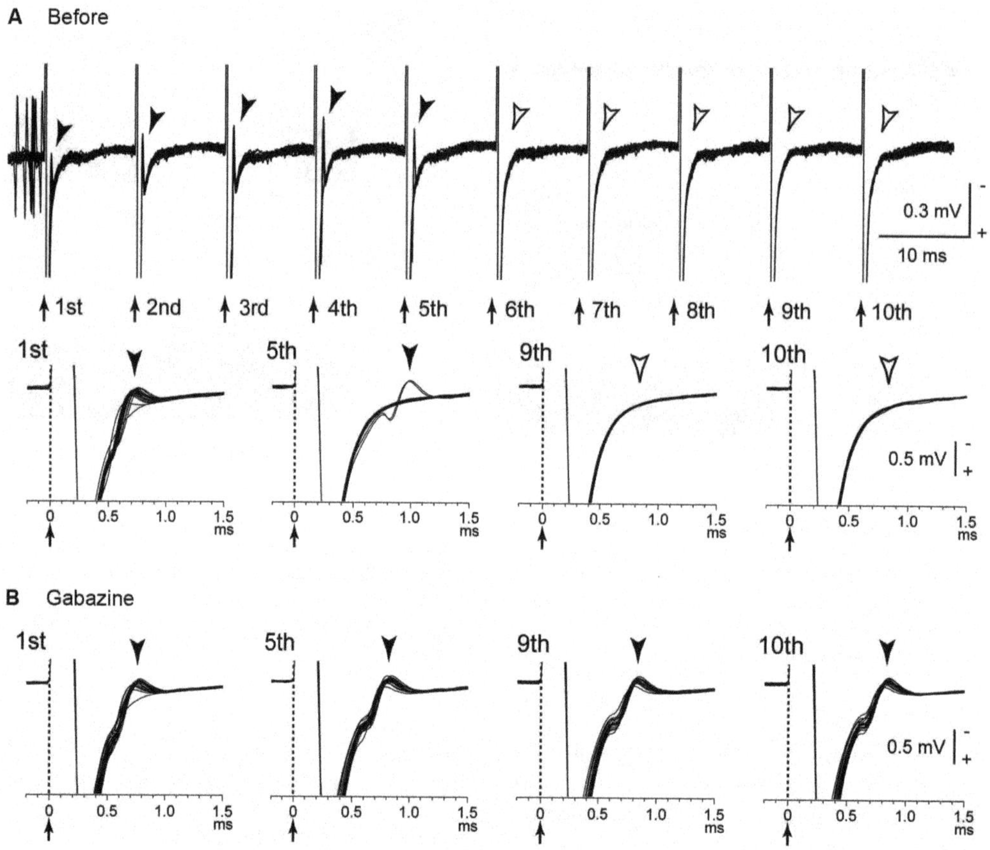

FIGURE 2 | Directly evoked spikes of GPi neurons were inhibited during GPi-HFS. (A) Raw traces showing directly evoked spikes of a GPi neuron by stimulus pulses during GPi-HFS (40 μA, 100 Hz, 10 pulses) in a normal monkey. Traces with long (top) and short (bottom) time scales are shown. Arrows with dotted lines indicate the timing of local stimulation (time 0 in the bottom traces). Filled arrowheads indicate directly evoked spikes. GPi-HFS failed to evoke spikes (open arrowheads; from 6th to 10th stimuli). **(B)** Effects of local gabazine injection on the inhibition of direct evoked GPi responses. Gabazine injection decreased failure rate, and each stimulus successfully evoked spikes (5th, 9th, and 10th stimuli). Modified from Chiken and Nambu (2013).

(Shink and Smith, 1995), and the balance between GABAergic and glutamatergic inputs may explain the different effects between GPe-HFS and GPi-HFS. Similarly, STN-HFS stimulated both glutamatergic and GABAergic afferents and generated both excitatory and inhibitory post-synaptic potentials (EPSPs and IPSPs) in the STN neurons (Lee et al., 2004). Thus, HFS activates afferent axons in the stimulated nucleus, and the effects vary depending on the composition of the inhibitory and excitatory axon terminals.

DEEP BRAIN STIMULATION (DBS) EXCITES LOCAL NEURONAL ELEMENTS

It is rational that local stimulation excites local neuronal elements. Actually, directly evoked spikes, which are characterized by short- and constant latency, are induced in GPi neurons by GPi-HFS (Johnson and McIntyre, 2008; McCairn and Turner, 2009). Such excitation may propagate through efferent projections. Thalamic activity was reduced during GPi-HFS through inhibitory GPi-thalamic projections in Parkinsonian monkeys (Anderson et al., 2003) and dystonia patients (Pralong et al., 2003; Montgomery, 2006). GPi activity was increased during STN-DBS through excitatory STN-GPi projections (Hashimoto et al., 2003; Galati et al., 2006; Reese et al., 2011). STN-DBS increased both glutamate and GABA levels in the substantia nigra pars reticulata (SNr) of normal rats in microdialysis studies (Windels et al., 2000; see also Windels et al., 2005). An intraoperative microdialysis study revealed that STN-DBS produced significant increase in extracellular concentration of cyclic guanosine monophosphate (cGMP) in the GPi (Stefani et al., 2005). Functional magnetic resonance imaging (MRI) and positron emission tomography (PET) studies in humans indicated that efferent outputs from the stimulated nucleus are excited during DBS (Jech et al., 2001; Hershey et al., 2003; Boertien et al., 2011). Changes of the firing rates and patterns of target nuclei may normalize abnormal firings, such as bursting and oscillatory activity, which are observes in the cortico-basal ganglia loop of Parkinson's disease and dystonia (Anderson et al., 2003; Hashimoto et al., 2003; Hammond et al., 2007; Johnson et al., 2008; Vitek, 2008; Deniau et al., 2010).

According to the modeling study (McIntyre et al., 2004), subthreshold HFS suppressed intrinsic firings in the cell bodies, while

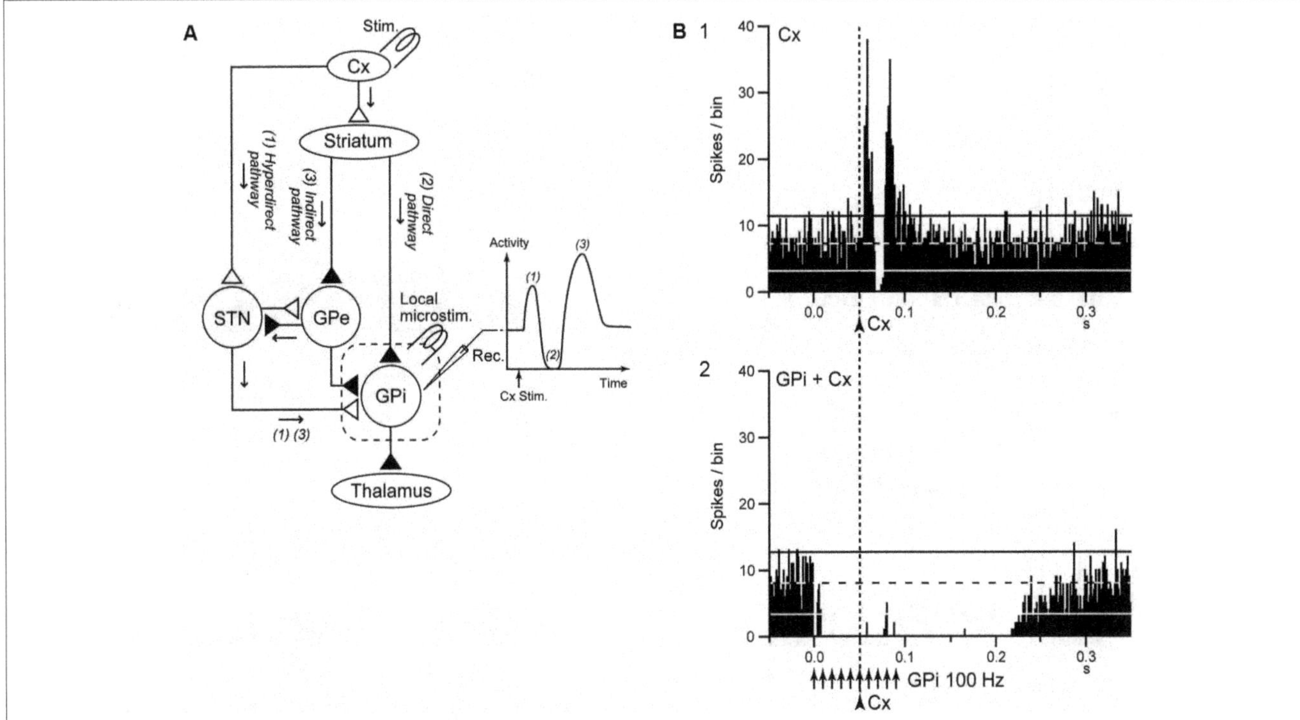

FIGURE 3 | GPi-DBS disrupts information flow through the GPi. (A) Schematic diagram showing the cortico-basal ganglia pathway and stimulating (Stim.) and recording (Rec.) sites in the electrophysiological experiments (left), along with a typical response pattern (right) in the (GPi) to cortical stimulation (Cx Stim.) with early excitation, inhibition, and late excitation, which are mediated by the **(1)** cortico-subthalamo (STN)-GPi *hyperdirect*, **(2)** striato-GPi *direct*, and **(3)** striato-external pallido (GPe)-STN-GPi *indirect* pathways, respectively. **(B)** Effects of local GPi-HFS on cortically evoked responses of a GPi neuron in a normal monkey. PSTH (100 trials) in response to the single pulse stimulation (arrowhead with dotted line) of the primary motor cortex (Cx) **(1)** and PSTH in response to Cx stimulation (arrowhead with dotted line) during GPi-HFS (arrows) **(2)** are shown. Cortical stimulation was applied 50 ms after the initiation of GPi-HFS. The cortically evoked responses were entirely inhibited during GPi-HFS. Modified from Chiken and Nambu (2013).

suprathreshold HFS generated efferent outputs at the stimulus frequency in the axon without representative activation of the cell bodies. Thus, although stimulation may fail to activate cell bodies of GPi neurons due to strong GABAergic inhibition, it can still excite the efferent axons and provide inhibitory inputs to the thalamus at the stimulus frequency.

DBS also antidromically excites afferent axons. Actually, antidromic activation of GPi neurons induced by STN-DBS was observed in Parkinsonian monkeys (Moran et al., 2011), and antidromic activation of thatamic (Vop) neurons induced by GPi-DBS was observed in Parkinsonian patients (Montgomery, 2006). Low intensity STN-HFS induced GABAergic inhibition in the SNr through antidromic activation of GPe neurons projecting to both the STN and SNr (Maurice et al., 2003; see also Moran et al., 2011), whereas higher intensity stimulation induced glutamatergic excitation in the SNr through activation of STN-SNr projections. STN-HFS also activated motor cortical neurons antidromically and suppressed abnormal low frequency synchronization including beta band oscillation in Parkinsonian rats (Li et al., 2007, 2012; Degos et al., 2013). Recent development of optogenetics has enabled selective stimulation of afferent inputs or efferent outputs, and contribute to analyzing the mechanism of effectiveness of DBS. A recent study has shown that selective stimulation of cortico-STN afferent axons can robustly ameliorate symptoms in Parkinsonian rats without activation of STN efferent axons (Gradinaru et al., 2009), suggesting that therapeutic effects of STN-DBS may be exclusively accounted for activation of cortico-STN afferent axons.

It is also probable that STN-DBS induces dopamine release through STN-SNc projections. STN-DBS induced dopamine release by activation of nigrostriatal dopaminergic neurons in rats (Meissner et al., 2003) and pigs (Shon et al., 2010), however it did not increase dopamine level of the striatum in human patients (Abosch et al., 2003; Hilker et al., 2003). DBS may also affect neurons whose axons pass nearby the stimulating site. A model-based study showed that clinically effective STN-DBS also activated the lenticular fasciculus, which is composed of GPi-thalamic fibers, in addition to STN neurons temselves (Miocinovic et al., 2006). Actually, STN-DBS induced direct excitation of GPi neurons through activation of the lenticular fasciculus (Moran et al., 2011).

Participation of non-neuronal glial tissues should also be considered as one of possible mechanisms of DBS effectiveness. DBS induced glutamate and adenosine triphosphate (ATP) release from astrocytes (Fellin et al., 2006; Tawfik et al., 2010). A recent study revealed that HFS applied to the thalamus induced abrupt increase in extracellular ATP and adenosine (Bekar et al., 2008).

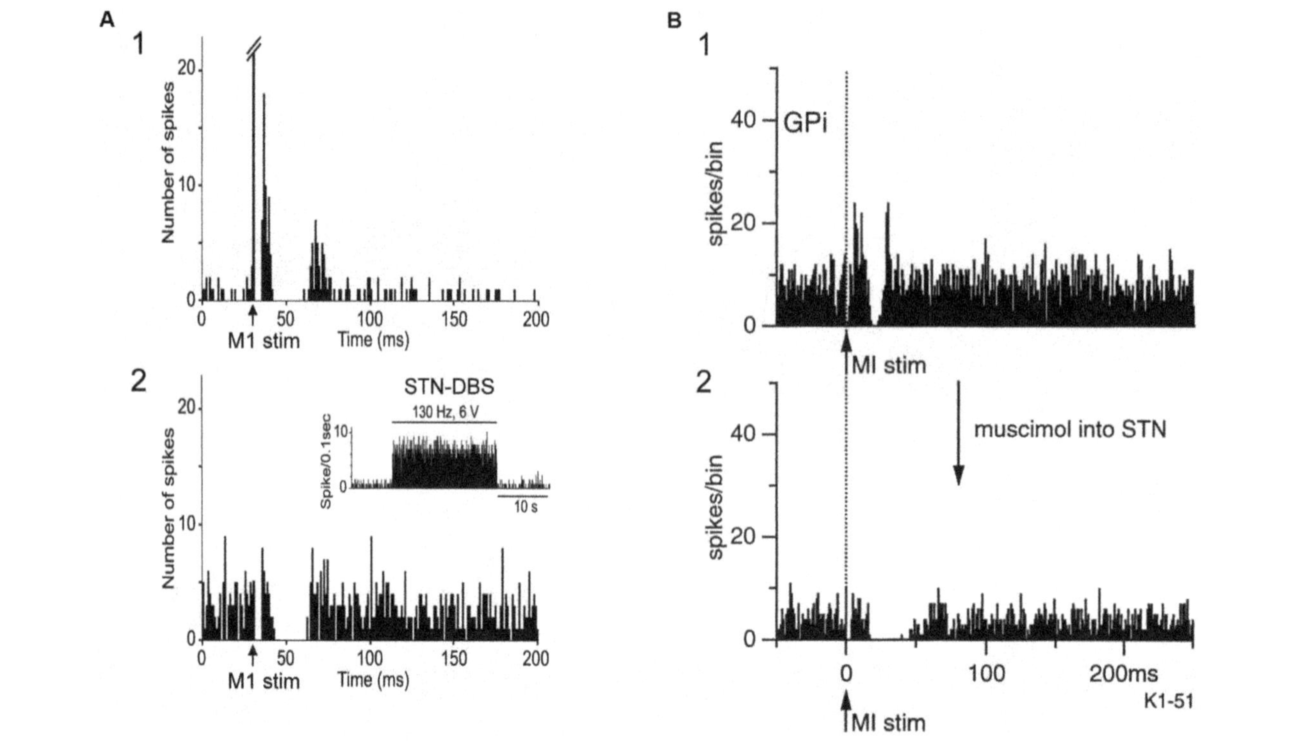

FIGURE 4 | Both STN-DBS and STN blocking disrupt information flow through the STN. (A) Effects of local STN-DBS on cortically evoked responses of a substantia nigra pars reticulata (SNr) neuron in a normal rat. PSTH (50 trials) in response to the single pulse stimulation of the Cx (arrow) **(1)** and PSTH in response to Cx stimulation during STN-DBS **(2)** are shown. The cortically evoked early and late excitation was abolished during STN-DBS, while cortically evoked inhibition was preserved. Modified from Maurice et al. (2003). **(B)** Effects of STN blocking on cortically evoked responses of a GPi neuron in a normal monkey. PSTH (100 trials) in response to the single pulse stimulation of the Cx (arrow with dotted line) **(1)** and PSTH in response to Cx stimulation after blocking STN activity by muscimol ($GABA_A$ receptor agonist) injection into the STN **(2)** are shown. The cortically evoked early and late excitation was abolished after injection of muscimol into the STN, while cortically evoked inhibition was preserved. Modified from Nambu et al. (2000). Note that the pattern of cortically evoked responses of a SNr neuron during STN-DBS is similar to that of a GPi neuron after STN blocking.

Adenosine activation of A1 receptors depressed excitatory transmission in the thalamus, and alleviated tremor in a mouse model. Thus, it is possible that ATP and glutamate are released from astrocytes triggered by DBS and modulate neuronal activity in the stimulated nucleus (Vedam-Mai et al., 2012; Jantz and Watanabe, 2013).

DEEP BRAIN STIMULATION (DBS) DISRUPTS NEURONAL TRANSMISSION

The striatum and STN are input stations of the basal ganglia and receive inputs from a wide area of the cerebral cortex (Mink, 1996; Nambu et al., 2002). The information is processed through the *hyperdirect*, *direct*, and *indirect* pathways and reaches the GPi/SNr, the output station of the basal ganglia (**Figure 3A**). During voluntary movements, neuronal signals originating in the cortex are considered to be transmitted through these pathways, reach the GPi/SNr and control movements (Mink, 1996; Nambu et al., 2002). Signal transmission through the *direct* pathway reduces GPi activity and facilitates movements by disinhibiting the thalamus, whereas the *hyperdirect* and *indirect* pathways increase GPi activity and suppress movements (Nambu et al., 2002; Nambu, 2007; Kravitz et al., 2010; Sano et al., 2013).

Chiken and Nambu (2013) recently examined responses of GPi neurons evoked by motor cortical stimulation during GPi-HFS in normal monkeys. In that study, both cortically evoked responses and spontaneous discharges were completely inhibited during GPi-HFS by strong GABAergic inhibition (**Figure 3B**), suggesting that GPi-HFS blocks information flow through the GPi. Since abnormal cortically evoked responses (Chiken et al., 2008; Kita and Kita, 2011; Nishibayashi et al., 2011) and abnormal bursts and oscillatory activity (Wichmann et al., 1994; Bergman et al., 1998; Starr et al., 2005; Brown, 2007; Chiken et al., 2008; Nishibayashi et al., 2011; Tachibana et al., 2011) were observed in GPi neurons in Parkinson's disease and dystonia, signal transmission of such abnormal activities to the thalamus and motor cortex would be responsible for motor symptoms. Thus, disruption of the abnormal information flow could suppress expression of motor symptoms. This mechanism may explain the paradox that GPi-DBS produces similar therapeutic effects to lesions of the GPi: both GPi-DBS and GPi-lesion interrupt abnormal information flow through the GPi.

STN-DBS may also interrupt neurotransmission of abnormal signals. Maurice et al. (2003) examined the effects of STN-DBS on cortically evoked responses of SNr neurons in normal rats.

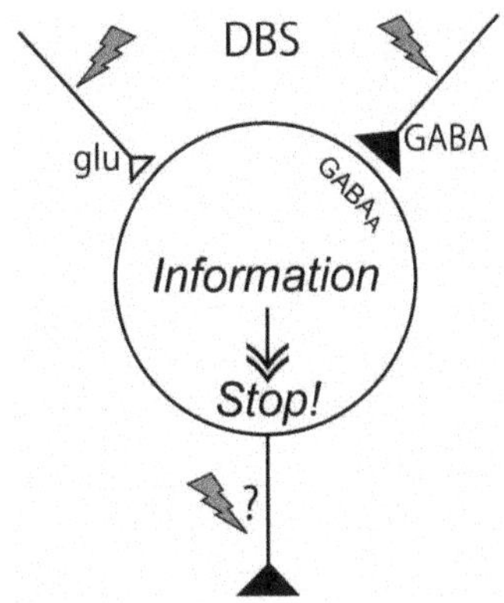

FIGURE 5 | Mechanism underling effectiveness of deep brain stimulation (DBS). DBS activates axon terminals in the stimulated nucleus and induces release of large amount of neurotransmitters, such as GABA and glutamate, and dissociates inputs and outputs in the stimulated nucleus, resulting in disruption of abnormal information flow through the cortico-basal ganglia loop.

Cortically evoked early and late excitation was totally abolished during high intensity STN-HFS, and much reduced during low intensity STN-DBS, while cortically evoked inhibition was preserved (**Figure 4A**), suggesting that information flow through the trans-STN pathway was blocked by STN-DBS without interrupting other pathways. The response patterns of SNr neurons during STN-DBS are similar to those of GPi neurons during STN blockade by muscimol in normal monkeys (Nambu et al., 2000; **Figure 4B**). Thus it is rational that STN-DBS has similar effect to lesion or silencing of the STN. In Parkinson's disease, due to the loss of dopaminergic modulation, the information flow through the striato-GPi *direct* pathway is weakened, whereas the information flow through the striato-GPe *indirect* pathway is facilitated. Both STN-DBS and STN lesioning may alter the balance of inhibitory inputs through the *direct* pathway and excitatory inputs through the *hyperdirect* and *indirect* pathways to the GPi by disrupting information flow through the STN, and effectively alleviate bradykinesia seen in Parkinson's disease. Similar idea, a functional disconnection of the stimulated elements, has also proposed by other groups (Anderson et al., 2006; Deniau et al., 2010; Moran et al., 2011).

CONCLUSION

DBS has variety of effects on neurons in the stimulated nucleus of the cortico-basal ganglia loop, though transmitter release, orthodromic activation of efferent axons, antidromic activation of afferent axons, and direct stimulation of passing axons nearby the stimulating electrode. The effects vary depending on the neural composition of the stimulated nucleus, and the effects extend much wider than originally expected. However, a common mechanism would underlie the effectiveness of DBS: DBS dissociates inputs and outputs in the stimulated nucleus and disrupts abnormal information flow through the cortico-basal ganglia loop (**Figure 5**). The mechanism may explain the paradox that DBS produces similar therapeutic effects to lesions or silencing of the nucleus.

ACKNOWLEDGMENTS

This work was supported by a Grant-in-Aid for Scientific Research (A) 21240039, the Core Research for Evolutional Science and Technology, Strategic Japanese-German Cooperative Programme, and Brain Machine Interface Development under the Strategic Research Program for Brain Sciences to Atsushi Nambu, and a Grant-in-Aid for Scientific Research (C) 25430021 to Satomi Chiken. We thank Kana Miyamoto, Shigeki Sato, Hitomi Isogai, and Keiko Matsuzawa for technical assistance.

REFERENCES

Abosch, A., Kapur, S., Lang, A. E., Hussey, D., Sime, E., Miyasaki, J., et al. (2003). Stimulation of the subthalamic nucleus in Parkinson's disease does not produce striatal dopamine release. *Neurosurgery* 53, 1095–1105. doi: 10.1227/01.neu.0000088662.69419.1b

Anderson, T. R., Hu, B., Iremonger, K., and Kiss, Z. H. (2006). Selective attenuation of afferent synaptic transmission as a mechanism of thalamic deep brain stimulation-induced tremor arrest. *J. Neurosci.* 26, 841–850. doi: 10.1523/jneurosci.3523-05.2006

Anderson, M. E., Postupna, N., and Ruffo, M. (2003). Effects of high-frequency stimulation in the internal globus pallidus on the activity of thalamic neurons in the awake monkey. *J. Neurophysiol.* 89, 1150–1160. doi: 10.1152/jn.00475.2002

Aziz, T. Z., Peggs, D., Sambrook, M. A., and Crossman, A. R. (1991). Lesion of the subthalamic nucleus for the alleviation of 1-methyl-4-phenyl-1,2,3,6-tetrahydropyridine (MPTP)-induced parkinsonism in the primate. *Mov. Disord.* 6, 288–292. doi: 10.1002/mds.870060404

Bar-Gad, I., Elias, S., Vaadia, E., and Bergman, H. (2004). Complex locking rather than complete cessation of neuronal activity in the globus pallidus of a 1-methyl-4-phenyl-1,2,3,6-tetrahydropyridine-treated primate in response to pallidal microstimulation. *J. Neurosci.* 24, 7410–7419. doi: 10.1523/jneurosci.1691-04.2004

Bekar, L., Libionka, W., Tian, G. F., Xu, Q., Torres, A., Wang, X., et al. (2008). Adenosine is crucial for deep brain stimulation-mediated attenuation of tremor. *Nat. Med.* 14, 75–80. doi: 10.1038/nm1693

Benabid, A. L., Pollak, P., Gao, D., Hoffmann, D., Limousin, P., Gay, E., et al. (1996). Chronic electrical stimulation of the ventralis intermedius nucleus of the thalamus as a treatment of movement disorders. *J. Neurosurg.* 84, 203–214. doi: 10.3171/jns.1996.84.2.0203

Benabid, A. L., Pollak, P., Gervason, C., Hoffmann, D., Gao, D. M., Hommel, M., et al. (1991). Long-term suppression of tremor by chronic stimulation of the ventral intermediate thalamic nucleus. *Lancet* 337, 403–406. doi: 10.1016/0140-6736(91)91175-t

Benabid, A. L., Pollak, P., Gross, C., Hoffmann, D., Benazzouz, A., Gao, D. M., et al. (1994). Acute and long-term effects of subthalamic nucleus stimulation in Parkinson's disease. *Stereotact. Funct. Neurosurg.* 62, 76–84. doi: 10.1159/000098600

Benazzouz, A., Gross, C., Féger, J., Boraud, T., and Bioulac, B. (1993). Reversal of rigidity and improvement in motor performance by subthalamic high-frequency stimulation in MPTP-treated monkeys. *Eur. J. Neurosci.* 5, 382–389. doi: 10.1111/j.1460-9568.1993.tb00505.x

Bergman, H., Feingold, A., Nini, A., Raz, A., Slovin, H., Abeles, M., et al. (1998). Physiological aspects of information processing in the basal ganglia of normal and parkinsonian primates. *Trends Neurosci.* 21, 32–38. doi: 10.1016/S0166-2236(97)01151-X

Bergman, H., Wichmann, T., and DeLong, M. R. (1990). Reversal of experimental parkinsonism by lesions of the subthalamic nucleus. *Science* 249, 1436–1438. doi: 10.1126/science.2402638

Beurrier, C., Bioulac, B., Audin, J., and Hammond, C. (2001). High-frequency stimulation produces a transient blockade of voltage-gated currents in subthalamic neurons. *J. Neurophysiol.* 85, 1351–1356.

Boertien, T., Zrinzo, L., Kahan, J., Jahanshahi, M., Hariz, M., Mancini, L., et al. (2011). Functional imaging of subthalamic nucleus deep brain stimulation in Parkinson's disease. *Mov. Disord.* 26, 1835–1843. doi: 10.1002/mds.23788

Boraud, T., Bezard, E., Bioulac, B., and Gross, C. (1996). High frequency stimulation of the internal globus pallidus (GPi) simultaneously improves parkinsonian symptoms and reduces the firing frequency of GPi neurons in the MPTP-treated monkey. *Neurosci. Lett.* 215, 17–20. doi: 10.1016/s0304-3940(96)12943-8

Brotchie, J. M., Mitchell, I. J., Sambrook, M. A., and Crossman, A. R. (1991). Alleviation of parkinsonism by antagonism of excitatory amino acid transmission in the medial segment of the globus pallidus in rat and primate. *Mov. Disord.* 6, 133–138. doi: 10.1002/mds.870060208

Brown, P. (2007). Abnormal oscillatory synchronisation in the motor system leads to impaired movement. *Curr. Opin. Neurobiol.* 17, 656–664. doi: 10.1016/j.conb.2007.12.001

Chiken, S., and Nambu, A. (2013). High-frequency pallidal stimulation disrupts information flow through the pallidum by GABAergic inhibition. *J. Neurosci.* 33, 2268–2280. doi: 10.1523/jneurosci.4144-11.2013

Chiken, S., Shashidharan, P., and Nambu, A. (2008). Cortically-evoked long-lasting inhibition of pallidal neurons in a transgenic mouse model of dystonia. *J. Neurosci.* 28, 13967–13977. doi: 10.1523/jneurosci.3834-08.2008

Coubes, P., Cif, L., El Fertit, H., Hemm, S., Vayssiere, N., Serrat, S., et al. (2004). Electrical stimulation of the globus pallidus internus in patients with primary generalized dystonia: long-term results. *J. Neurosurg.* 101, 189–194. doi: 10.3171/jns.2004.101.2.0189

Deep-Brain Stimulation for Parkinson's Disease Study Group. (2001). Deep-brain stimulation of the subthalamic nucleus or the pars interna of the globus pallidus in Parkinson's disease. *N. Engl. J. Med.* 345, 956–963. doi: 10.1056/nejmoa000827

Degos, B., Deniau, J. M., Chavez, M., and Maurice, N. (2013). Subthalamic nucleus high-frequency stimulation restores altered electrophysiological properties of cortical neurons in parkinsonian rat. *PLoS One* 8:e83608. doi: 10.1371/journal.pone.0083608

Deniau, J. M., Degos, B., Bosch, C., and Maurice, N. (2010). Deep brain stimulation mechanisms: beyond the concept of local functional inhibition. *Eur. J. Neurosci.* 32, 1080–1091. doi: 10.1111/j.1460-9568.2010.07413.x

Dostrovsky, J. O., Levy, R., Wu, J. P., Hutchison, W. D., Tasker, R. R., and Lozano, A. M. (2000). Microstimulation-induced inhibition of neuronal firing in human globus pallidus. *J. Neurophysiol.* 84, 570–574.

Dostrovsky, J. O., and Lozano, A. M. (2002). Mechanisms of deep brain stimulation. *Mov. Disord.* 17, S63–S68. doi: 10.1002/mds.10143

Erez, Y., Czitron, H., McCairn, K., Belelovsky, K., and Bar-Gad, I. (2009). Short-term depression of synaptic transmission during stimulation in the globus pallidus of 1-methyl-4-phenyl-1,2,3,6-tetrahydropyridine-treated primates. *J. Neurosci.* 29, 7797–7802. doi: 10.1523/jneurosci.0401-09.2009

Fellin, T., Pascual, O., and Haydon, P. G. (2006). Astrocytes coordinate synaptic networks: balanced excitation and inhibition. *Physiology (Bethesda)* 21, 208–215. doi: 10.1152/physiol.00161.2005

Filali, M., Hutchison, W. D., Palter, V. N., Lozano, A. M., and Dostrovsky, J. O. (2004). Stimulation-induced inhibition of neuronal firing in human subthalamic nucleus. *Exp. Brain Res.* 156, 274–281. doi: 10.1007/s00221-003-1784-y

Galati, S., Mazzone, P., Fedele, E., Pisani, A., Peppe, A., Pierantozzi, M., et al. (2006). Biochemical and electrophysiological changes of substantia nigra pars reticulata driven by subthalamic stimulation in patients with Parkinson's disease. *Eur. J. Neurosci.* 23, 2923–2928. doi: 10.1111/j.1460-9568.2006.04816.x

Gradinaru, V., Mogri, M., Thompson, K. R., Henderson, J. M., and Deisseroth, K. (2009). Optical deconstruction of parkinsonian neural circuitry. *Science* 324, 354–359. doi: 10.1126/science.1167093

Graham, W. C., Robertson, R. G., Sambrook, M. A., and Crossman, A. R. (1990). Injection of excitatory amino acid antagonists into the medial pallidal segment of a 1-methyl-4-phenyl-1,2,3,6-tetrahydropyridine (MPTP) treated primate reverses motor symptoms of parkinsonism. *Life Sci.* 47, PL91–PL97. doi: 10.1016/0024-3205(90)90376-3

Hammond, C., Bergman, H., and Brown, P. (2007). Pathological synchronization in Parkinson's disease: networks, models and treatments. *Trends Neurosci.* 30, 357–364. doi: 10.1016/j.tins.2007.05.004

Hashimoto, T., Elder, C. M., Okun, M. S., Patrick, S. K., and Vitek, J. L. (2003). Stimulation of the subthalamic nucleus changes the firing pattern of pallidal neurons. *J. Neurosci.* 23, 1916–1923.

Hashimoto, T., Elder, C. M., and Vitek, J. L. (2002). A template subtraction method for stimulus artifact removal in high-frequency deep brain stimulation. *J. Neurosci. Methods* 113, 181–186. doi: 10.1016/s0165-0270(01)00491-5

Hershey, T., Revilla, F. J., Wernle, A. R., McGee-Minnich, L., Antenor, J. V., Videen, T. O., et al. (2003). Cortical and subcortical blood flow effects of subthalamic nucleus stimulation in PD. *Neurology* 61, 816–821. doi: 10.1212/01.wnl.0000083991.81859.73

Hilker, R., Voges, J., Ghaemi, M., Lehrke, R., Rudolf, J., Koulousakis, A., et al. (2003). Deep brain stimulation of the subthalamic nucleus does not increase the striatal dopamine concentration in parkinsonian humans. *Mov. Disord.* 18, 41–48. doi: 10.1002/mds.10297

Jantz, J. J., and Watanabe, M. (2013). Pallidal deep brain stimulation modulates afferent fibers, efferent fibers and glia. *J. Neurosci.* 33, 9873–9875. doi: 10.1523/jneurosci.1471-13.2013

Jech, R., Urgosík, D., Tintera, J., Nebuzelský, A., Krásenský, J., Liscák, R., et al. (2001). Functional magnetic resonance imaging during deep brain stimulation: a pilot study in four patients with Parkinson's disease. *Mov. Disord.* 16, 1126–1132. doi: 10.1002/mds.1217

Johnson, M. D., and McIntyre, C. C. (2008). Quantifying the neural elements activated and inhibited by globus pallidus deep brain stimulation. *J. Neurophysiol.* 100, 2549–2563. doi: 10.1152/jn.90372.2008

Johnson, M. D., Miocinovic, S., McIntyre, C. C., and Vitek, J. L. (2008). Mechanisms and targets of deep brain stimulation in movement disorders. *Neurotherapeutics* 5, 294–308. doi: 10.1016/j.nurt.2008.01.010

Kita, H., and Kita, T. (2011). Cortical stimulation evokes abnormal responses in the dopamine-depleted rat basal ganglia. *J. Neurosci.* 31, 10311–10322. doi: 10.1523/jneurosci.0915-11.2011

Koller, W., Pahwa, R., Busenbark, K., Hubble, J., Wilkinson, S., Lang, A., et al. (1997). High-frequency unilateral thalamic stimulation in the treatment of essential and parkinsonian tremor. *Ann. Neurol.* 42, 292–299. doi: 10.1002/ana.410420304

Kravitz, A. V., Freeze, B. S., Parker, P. R. L., Kay, K., Thwin, M. T., Deisseroth, K., et al. (2010). Regulation of parkinsonian motor behaviours by optogenetic control of basal ganglia circuitry. *Nature* 466, 622–626. doi: 10.1038/nature09159

Kringelbach, M. L., Jenkinson, N., Owen, S. L., and Aziz, T. Z. (2007). Translational principles of deep brain stimulation. *Nat. Rev. Neurosci.* 8, 623–635. doi: 10.1038/nrn2196

Lafreniere-Roula, M., Kim, E., Hutchison, W. D., Lozano, A. M., Hodaie, M., and Dostrovsky, J. O. (2010). High-frequency microstimulation in human globus pallidus and substantia nigra. *Exp. Brain Res.* 205, 251–261. doi: 10.1007/s00221-010-2362-8

Leblois, A., Reese, R., Labarre, D., Hamann, M., Richter, A., Boraud, T., et al. (2010). Deep brain stimulation changes basal ganglia output nuclei firing pattern in the dystonic hamster. *Neurobiol. Dis.* 38, 288–298. doi: 10.1016/j.nbd.2010.01.020

Lee, K. H., Chang, S. Y., Roberts, D. W., and Kim, U. (2004). Neurotransmitter release from high-frequency stimulation of the subthalamic nucleus. *J. Neurosurg.* 101, 511–517. doi: 10.3171/jns.2004.101.3.0511

Levy, R., Lang, A. E., Dostrovsky, J. O., Pahapill, P., Romas, J., Saint-Cyr, J., et al. (2001). Lidocaine and muscimol microinjections in subthalamic nucleus reverse Parkinsonian symptoms. *Brain* 124, 2105–2118. doi: 10.1093/brain/124.10.2105

Li, S., Arbuthnott, G. W., Jutras, M. J., Goldberg, J. A., and Jaeger, D. (2007). Resonant antidromic cortical circuit activation as a consequence of high-frequency subthalamic deep-brain stimulation. *J. Neurophysiol.* 98, 3525–3537. doi: 10.1152/jn.00808.2007

Li, Q., Ke, Y., Chan, D. C., Qian, Z. M., Yung, K. K., Ko, H., et al. (2012). Therapeutic deep brain stimulation in Parkinsonian rats directly influences motor cortex. *Neuron* 76, 1030–1041. doi: 10.1016/j.neuron.2012.09.032

Limousin, P., Pollak, P., Benazzouz, A., Hoffmann, D., Le Bas, J. F., Broussolle, E., et al. (1995). Effect of parkinsonian signs and symptoms of bilateral subthalamic nucleus stimulation. *Lancet* 345, 91–95. doi: 10.1016/s0140-6736(95)90062-4

Liu, Y., Postupna, N., Falkenberg, J., and Anderson, M. E. (2008). High frequency deep brain stimulation: what are the therapeutic mechanisms? *Neurosci. Biobehav. Rev.* 32, 343–351. doi: 10.1016/j.neubiorev.2006.10.007

Maurice, N., Thierry, A. M., Glowinski, J., and Deniau, J. M. (2003). Spontaneous and evoked activity of substantia nigra pars reticulata neurons during high-frequency stimulation of the subthalamic nucleus. *J. Neurosci.* 23, 9929–9936.

McCairn, K. W., and Turner, R. S. (2009). Deep brain stimulation of the globus pallidus internus in the parkinsonian primate: local entrainment and suppression of low-frequency oscillations. *J. Neurophysiol.* 101, 1941–1960. doi: 10.1152/jn.91092.2008

McIntyre, C. C., Savasta, M., Walter, B. L., and Vitek, J. L. (2004). How does deep brain stimulation work? Present understanding and future questions. *J. Clin. Neurophysiol.* 21, 40–50. doi: 10.1097/00004691-200401000-00006

Meissner, W., Harnack, D., Reese, R., Paul, G., Reum, T., Ansorge, M., et al. (2003). High-frequency stimulation of the subthalamic nucleus enhances striatal dopamine release and metabolism in rats. *J. Neurochem.* 85, 601–609. doi: 10.1046/j.1471-4159.2003.01665.x

Meissner, W., Leblois, A., Hansel, D., Bioulac, B., Gross, C. E., Benazzouz, A., et al. (2005). Subthalamic high frequency stimulation resets subthalamic firing and reduces abnormal oscillations. *Brain* 128, 2372–2382. doi: 10.1093/brain/awh616

Mink, J. W. (1996). The basal ganglia: focused selection and inhibition of competing motor programs. *Prog. Neurobiol.* 50, 381–425. doi: 10.1016/s0301-0082(96)00042-1

Miocinovic, S., Parent, M., Butson, C. R., Hahn, P. J., Russo, G. S., Vitek, J. L., et al. (2006). Computational analysis of subthalamic nucleus and lenticular fasciculus activation during therapeutic deep brain stimulation. *J. Neurophysiol.* 96, 1569–1580. doi: 10.1152/jn.00305.2006

Montgomery, E. B. Jr. (2006). Effects of GPi stimulation on human thalamic neuronal activity. *Clin. Neurophysiol.* 117, 2691–2702. doi: 10.1016/j.clinph.2006.08.011

Moran, A., Stein, E., Tischler, H., Belelovsky, K., and Bar-Gad, I. (2011). Dynamic stereotypic responses of Basal Ganglia neurons to subthalamic nucleus high-frequency stimulation in the parkinsonian primate. *Front. Syst. Neurosci.* 5:21. doi: 10.3389/fnsys.2011.00021

Nambu, A. (2007). Globus pallidus internal segment. *Prog. Brain. Res.* 160, 135–150. doi: 10.1016/s0079-6123(06)60008-3

Nambu, A., Tokuno, H., and Takada, M. (2002). Functional significance of the cortico-subthalamo-pallidal 'hyperdirect' pathway. *Neurosci. Res.* 43, 111–117. doi: 10.1016/s0168-0102(02)00027-5

Nambu, A., Tokuno, H., Hamada, I., Kita, H., Imanishi, M., Akazawa, T., et al. (2000). Excitatory cortical inputs to pallidal neurons via the subthalamic nucleus in the monkey. *J. Neurophysiol.* 84, 289–300.

Nishibayashi, H., Ogura, M., Kakishita, K., Tanaka, S., Tachibana, Y., Nambu, A., et al. (2011). Cortically evoked responses of human pallidal neurons recorded during stereotactic neurosurgery. *Mov. Disord.* 26, 469–476. doi: 10.1002/mds.23502

Ostrem, J. L., and Starr, P. A. (2008). Treatment of dystonia with deep brain stimulation. *Neurotherapeutics* 5, 320–330. doi: 10.1016/j.nurt.2008.01.002

Pralong, E., Debatisse, D., Maeder, M., Vingerhoets, F., Ghika, J., and Villemure, J. G. (2003). Effect of deep brain stimulation of GPI on neuronal activity of the thalamic nucleus ventralis oralis in a dystonic patient. *Neurophysiol. Clin.* 33, 169–173. doi: 10.1016/j.neucli.2003.07.001

Ranck, J. B. Jr. (1975). Which elements are excited in electrical stimulation of mammalian central nervous system: a review. *Brain Res.* 98, 417–440. doi: 10.1016/0006-8993(75)90364-9

Reese, R., Leblois, A., Steigerwald, F., Potter-Nerger, M., Herzog, J., Mehdorn, H. M., et al. (2011). Subthalamic deep brain stimulation increases pallidal firing rate and regularity. *Exp. Neurol.* 229, 517–521. doi: 10.1016/j.expneurol.2011.01.020

Rehncrona, S., Johnels, B., Widner, H., Törnqvist, A. L., Hariz, M., and Sydow, O. (2003). Long-term efficacy of thalamic deep brain stimulation for tremor: double-blind assessments. *Mov. Disord.* 18, 163–170. doi: 10.1002/mds.10309

Sano, H., Chiken, S., Hikida, T., Kobayashi, K., and Nambu, A. (2013). Signals through the striatopallidal indirect pathway stop movements by phasic excitation in the substantia nigra. *J. Neurosci.* 33, 7583–7594. doi: 10.1523/jneurosci.4932-12.2013

Shi, L. H., Luo, F., Woodward, D. J., and Chang, J. Y. (2006). Basal ganglia neural responses during behaviorally effective deep brain stimulation of the subthalamic nucleus in rats performing a treadmill locomotion test. *Synapse* 59, 445–457. doi: 10.1002/syn.20261

Shin, D. S., Samoilova, M., Cotic, M., Zhang, L., Brotchie, J. M., and Carlen, P. L. (2007). High frequency stimulation or elevated K+ depresses neuronal activity in the rat entopeduncular nucleus. *Neuroscience* 149, 68–86. doi: 10.1016/j.neuroscience.2007.06.055

Shink, E., and Smith, Y. (1995). Differential synaptic innervation of neurons in the internal and external segments of the globus pallidus by the GABA- and glutamate-containing terminals in the squirrel monkey. *J. Comp. Neurol.* 358, 119–141. doi: 10.1002/cne.903580108

Shon, Y. M., Lee, K. H., Goerss, S. J., Kim, I. Y., Kimble, C., Van Gompel, J. J., et al. (2010). High frequency stimulation of the subthalamic nucleus evokes striatal dopamine release in a large animal model of human DBS neurosurgery. *Neurosci. Lett.* 475, 136–140. doi: 10.1016/j.neulet.2010.03.060

Siegfried, J., and Lippitz, B. (1994a). Bilateral chronic electrostimulation of ventroposterolateral pallidum: a new therapeutic approach for alleviating all parkinsonian symptoms. *Neurosurgery* 35, 1126–1130. doi: 10.1227/00006123-199412000-00016

Siegfried, J., and Lippitz, B. (1994b). Chronic electrical stimulation of the VL-VPL complex and of the pallidum in the treatment of movement disorders: personal experience since 1982. *Stereotact. Funct. Neurosurg.* 62, 71–75. doi: 10.1159/000098599

Smith, Y., Wichmann, T., and DeLong, M. R. (1994). Synaptic innervation of neurones in the internal pallidal segment by the subthalamic nucleus and the external pallidum in monkeys. *J. Comp. Neurol.* 343, 297–318. doi: 10.1002/cne.903430209

Starr, P. A., Rau, G. M., Davis, V., Marks, W. J. Jr., Ostrem, J. L., Simmons, D., et al. (2005). Spontaneous pallidal neuronal activity in human dystonia: comparison with Parkinson's disease and normal macaque. *J. Neurophysiol.* 93, 3165–3176. doi: 10.1152/jn.00971.2004

Stefani, A., Fedele, E., Galati, S., Pepicelli, O., Frasca, S., Pierantozzi, M., et al. (2005). Subthalamic stimulation activates internal pallidus: evidence from cGMP microdialysis in PD patients. *Ann. Neurol.* 57, 448–452. doi: 10.1002/ana.20402

Tachibana, Y., Iwamuro, H., Kita, H., Takada, M., and Nambu, A. (2011). Subthalamo-pallidal interactions underlying parkinsonian neuronal oscillations in the primate basal ganglia. *Eur. J. Neurosci.* 34, 1470–1484. doi: 10.1111/j.1460-9568.2011.07865.x

Tai, C. H., Boraud, T., Bezard, E., Bioulac, B., Gross, C., and Benazzouz, A. (2003). Electrophysiological and metabolic evidence that high-frequency stimulation of the subthalamic nucleus bridles neuronal activity in the subthalamic nucleus and the substantia nigra reticulata. *FASEB J.* 17, 1820–1830. doi: 10.1096/fj.03-0163com

Tawfik, V. L., Chang, S. Y., Hitti, F. L., Roberts, D. W., Leiter, J. C., Jovanovic, S., et al. (2010). Deep brain stimulation results in local glutamate and adenosine release: investigation into the role of astrocytes. *Neurosurgery* 67, 367–375. doi: 10.1227/01.neu.0000371988.73620.4c

Vedam-Mai, V., van Battum, E. Y., Kamphuis, W., Feenstra, M. G., Denys, D., Reynolds, B. A., et al. (2012). Deep brain stimulation and the role of astrocytes. *Mol. Psychiatry* 17, 124–131. doi: 10.1038/mp.2011.61

Vidailhet, M., Jutras, M. F., Roze, E., and Grabli, D. (2013). Deep brain stimulation for dystonia. *Handb. Clin. Neurol.* 116, 167–187. doi: 10.1016/B978-0-444-53497-2.00014-0

Vitek, J. L. (2008). Deep brain stimulation: how does it work? *Cleve. Clin. J. Med.* 75(Suppl. 2), S59–S65. doi: 10.3949/ccjm.75.suppl_2.s59

Wang, L. Y., and Kaczmarek, L. K. (1998). High-frequency firing helps replenish the readily releasable pool of synaptic vesicles. *Nature* 394, 384–388. doi: 10.1038/28645

Welter, M. L., Houeto, J. L., Bonnet, A. M., Bejjani, P. B., Mesnage, V., Dormont, D., et al. (2004). Effects of high-frequency stimulation on subthalamic neuronal activity in parkinsonian patients. *Arch. Neurol.* 61, 89–96. doi: 10.1001/archneur.61.1.89

Wichmann, T. (2000). A digital averaging method for removal of stimulus artifacts in neurophysiologic experiments. *J. Neurosci. Methods* 98, 57–62. doi: 10.1016/s0165-0270(00)00190-4

Wichmann, T., Bergman, H., and DeLong, M. R. (1994). The primate subthalamic nucleus. III. Changes in motor behavior and neuronal activity in the internal pallidum induced by subthalamic inactivation in the MPTP model of parkinsonism. *J. Neurophysiol.* 72, 521–530.

Wichmann, T., and Delong, M. R. (2006). Deep brain stimulation for neurologic and neuropsychiatric disorders. *Neuron* 52, 197–204. doi: 10.1016/j.neuron.2006.09.022

Windels, F., Bruet, N., Poupard, A., Urbain, N., Chouvet, G., Feuerstein, C., et al. (2000). Effects of high frequency stimulation of subthalamic nucleus on extracellular glutamate and GABA in substantia nigra and globus pallidus in the normal rat. *Eur. J. Neurosci.* 12, 4141–4146. doi: 10.1046/j.1460-9568.2000.00296.x

Windels, F., Carcenac, C., Poupard, A., and Savasta, M. (2005). Pallidal origin of GABA release within the substantia nigra pars reticulata during high-frequency stimulation of the subthalamic nucleus. *J. Neurosci.* 25, 5079–5086. doi: 10.1523/jneurosci.0360-05.2005

Wu, Y. R., Levy, R., Ashby, P., Tasker, R. R., and Dostrovsky, J. O. (2001). Does stimulation of the GPi control dyskinesia by activating inhibitory axons? *Mov. Disord.* 16, 208–216. doi: 10.1002/mds.1046

Zucker, R. S., and Regehr, W. G. (2002). Short-term synaptic plasticity. *Annu. Rev. Physiol.* 64, 355–405. doi: 10.1146/annurev.physiol.64.092501.114547

10

Time Representation in Reinforcement Learning Models of the Basal Ganglia

Samuel J. Gershman[1]*, Ahmed A. Moustafa[2] and Elliot A. Ludvig[3,4]

[1] Department of Brain and Cognitive Sciences, Massachusetts Institute of Technology, Cambridge, MA, USA
[2] School of Social Sciences and Psychology, Marcs Institute for Brain and Behaviour, University of Western Sydney, Sydney, NSW, Australia
[3] Princeton Neuroscience Institute and Department of Mechanical and Aerospace Engineering, Princeton University, Princeton, NJ, USA
[4] Department of Psychology, University of Warwick, Coventry, UK

***Correspondence:**
Samuel J. Gershman, Department of Brain and Cognitive Sciences, Massachusetts Institute of Technology, Room 46-4053, 77 Massachusetts Ave., Cambridge, MA 02139, USA
e-mail: sjgershm@mit.edu

Reinforcement learning (RL) models have been influential in understanding many aspects of basal ganglia function, from reward prediction to action selection. Time plays an important role in these models, but there is still no theoretical consensus about what kind of time representation is used by the basal ganglia. We review several theoretical accounts and their supporting evidence. We then discuss the relationship between RL models and the timing mechanisms that have been attributed to the basal ganglia. We hypothesize that a single computational system may underlie both RL and interval timing—the perception of duration in the range of seconds to hours. This hypothesis, which extends earlier models by incorporating a time-sensitive action selection mechanism, may have important implications for understanding disorders like Parkinson's disease in which both decision making and timing are impaired.

Keywords: reinforcement learning, basal ganglia, dopamine, interval timing, Parkinson's disease

INTRODUCTION

Computational models of reinforcement learning (RL) have had a profound influence on the contemporary understanding of the basal ganglia (Joel et al., 2002; Cohen and Frank, 2009). The central claim of these models is that the basal ganglia are organized to support prediction, learning and optimization of long-term reward. While this claim is now widely accepted, RL models have had little to say about the extensive research implicating the basal ganglia in interval timing—the perception of duration in the range of seconds to hours (Buhusi and Meck, 2005; Jones and Jahanshahi, 2009; Merchant et al., 2013). However, this is not to say that time is ignored by these models—on the contrary, time representation has been a pivotal issue in RL theory, particularly with regard to the role of dopamine (Suri and Schultz, 1999; Daw et al., 2006; Ludvig et al., 2008; Nakahara and Kaveri, 2010; Rivest et al., 2010).

In this review, we attempt a provisional synthesis of research on RL and interval timing in the basal ganglia. We begin by briefly reviewing RL models of the basal ganglia, with a focus on how they represent time. We then summarize the key data linking the basal ganglia with interval timing, drawing connections between computational approaches to timing and their relationship to RL models. Our central thesis is that by incorporating a time-sensitive action selection mechanism into RL models, a single computational system can support both RL and interval timing. This unified view leads to a coherent interpretation of decision making and timing deficits in Parkinson's disease.

REINFORCEMENT LEARNING MODELS OF THE BASAL GANGLIA

RL models characterize animals as agents that seek to maximize future reward (for reviews, see Maia, 2009; Niv, 2009; Ludvig et al., 2011). To do so, animals are assumed to generate a prediction of future reward and select actions according to a policy that maximizes that reward. More formally, suppose that at time t an agent occupies a state s_t (e.g., the agent's location or the surrounding stimuli) and receives a reward r_t. The agent's goal is to predict the *expected discounted future return*, or *value*, of visiting a sequence of states starting in state s_t (Sutton and Barto, 1998):

$$V(S_t) = E\left[\sum_{k=0} \gamma^k r_{t+k}\right], \tag{1}$$

where γ is a parameter that discounts distal rewards relative to proximal rewards, and E denotes an average over possibly stochastic sequences of states and rewards.

Typically, a state s_t is described by a set of D features, $\{x_t(1), \ldots, x_t(D)\}$, encoding sensory and cognitive aspects of an animal's current experience. Given this state representation, the value can be approximated by a weighted combination of the features:

$$\hat{V}(s_t) = \sum_d w_t(d)\, x_t(d)$$

where $\hat{V}$ is an estimate of the true value V. According to RL models of the basal ganglia, these features are represented by cortical inputs to the striatum, with the striatum itself encoding the estimated value (Maia, 2009; Niv, 2009; Ludvig et al., 2011). The strengths of these corticostriatal synapses are represented by a set of weights $\{w_t(1), \ldots, w_t(D)\}$.

These weights can be learned through a simple algorithm known as *temporal-difference (TD) learning,* which adjusts the weights on each time step based on the difference between received and predicted reward:

$$w_{t+1}(d) = w_t(d) + \alpha\delta_t e_t(d),$$

where α is a learning rate and δ_t is a prediction error defined as:

$$\delta_t = r_t + \gamma\hat{V}(s_{t+1}) - \hat{V}(s_t).$$

The *eligibility trace* $e_t(d)$ is updated according to:

$$e_{t+1}(d) = \gamma\lambda e_t(d) + x_t(d),$$

where λ is a decay parameter that determines the plasticity window of recent stimuli. The TD algorithm is a computationally efficient method that is known to converge to the true value function [see Equation (1) above] with enough experience and adequate features (Sutton and Barto, 1998).

The importance of this algorithm to neuroscience lies in the fact that the firing of midbrain dopamine neurons conforms remarkably well to the theoretical prediction error (Houk et al., 1995; Montague et al., 1996; Schultz et al., 1997; though see Redgrave et al., 2008 for a critique). For example, dopamine neurons increase their firing upon the delivery of an unexpected reward and pause when an expected reward is omitted (Schultz et al., 1997). The role of prediction errors in learning is supported by the observation that plasticity at corticostriatal synapses is gated by dopamine (Reynolds and Wickens, 2002; Steinberg et al., 2013), as well as a large body of behavioral evidence (Rescorla and Wagner, 1972; Sutton and Barto, 1990; Ludvig et al., 2012).

A fundamental question facing RL models is the choice of feature representation. Early applications of TD learning to the dopamine system assumed what is known as the *complete serial compound* (CSC; Moore et al., 1989; Sutton and Barto, 1990; Montague et al., 1996; Schultz et al., 1997), which represents every time step following stimulus onset as a separate feature. Thus, the first feature has a value of 1 for the first time step and 0 for all other time steps, the second feature has a value of 1 for the second time step and 0 for all other time steps, and so on. This CSC representation assumes a perfect clock, whereby the brain always knows exactly how many time steps have elapsed since stimulus onset.

The CSC is effective at capturing several salient aspects of the dopamine response to cued reward. A number of authors (e.g., Daw et al., 2006; Ludvig et al., 2008), however, have pointed out aspects of the dopamine response that appear inconsistent with the CSC. For example, the CSC predicts a large, punctate negative prediction error when an expected reward is omitted; the actual decrease in dopamine response is relatively small and temporally extended (Schultz et al., 1997; Bayer et al., 2007). Another problem with the CSC is that it predicts a large negative prediction error at the usual reward delivery time when a reward is delivered early. Contrary to this prediction, Hollerman and Schultz (1998) found that early reward evoked a large response immediately after the unexpected reward, but showed little change from baseline at the usual reward delivery time.

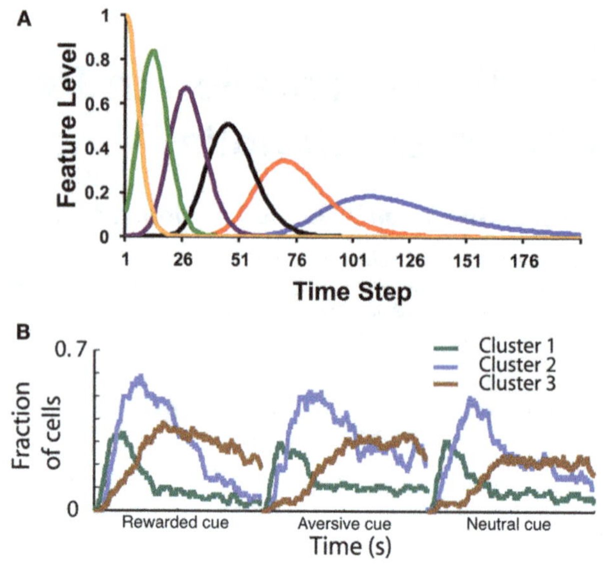

FIGURE 1 | (A) Example microstimuli. Each microstimulus acts as a dynamic feature, going up and then coming back down with a characteristic time course after the stimulus. **(B)** Fraction of medium spiny neurons recorded in the putamen with a significant response (both increases and decreases in firing rate) to cue events. In this task, a visual cue (fractal image) is presented at time 0, followed by an outcome (food, air puff, or neutral sound) 2 s later. Clusters correspond to groups of neurons with similar response profiles (see Adler et al., 2012 for details). Time courses are shown separately for cues that predict rewarding (food), aversive (air puff), or neutral (sound) outcomes. Note the similarity in the population response to the postulated time course of the theoretical microstimuli. Figure adapted from Adler et al. (2012) with permission from the publisher.

It is possible that these mismatches between theory and data reflect problems with a number of different theoretical assumptions. Indeed, several theoretical assumptions have been questioned by recent research (see Niv, 2009). We focus here on alternative time representations as one potential response to the findings mentioned above.

We will discuss two of these alternatives (see also Suri and Schultz, 1999; Nakahara and Kaveri, 2010; Rivest et al., 2010): (1) the microstimulus representation and (2) states with variable durations (a *semi-Markov* formalism) and only partial observability. For the former, Ludvig et al. (2008) proposed that when a stimulus is presented, it leaves a slowly decaying memory trace, which is encoded by a series of temporal receptive fields. Each feature (or "microstimulus") $x_t(d)$ represents the proximity between the trace and the center of the receptive field, producing a spectrum of features that vary with time, as illustrated in **Figure 1A**. Specifically, Ludvig et al. endowed each stimulus with microstimuli of the following form:

$$x_t(d) = \frac{y_t}{\sqrt{\sigma^2}} \exp\left(-\frac{\left(y_t - \frac{d}{D}\right)^2}{2\sigma^2}\right)$$

where D is the number of microstimuli, σ^2 controls the width of each receptive field, and y_t is the stimulus trace strength, which was set to 1 at stimulus onset and decreased exponentially with a decay rate of 0.985 per time step. Both cues and rewards elicit their own set of microstimuli. This feature representation is plugged into the TD learning equations described above.

The microstimulus representation is a temporally smeared version of the CSC: whereas in the CSC each feature encodes a single time point, in the microstimulus representation each feature encodes a temporal range (see also Grossberg and Schmajuk, 1989; Machado, 1997). With the CSC, as time elapses after a stimulus, there is one, unique feature active at each time point. Learned weights for that time point therefore all accrue to that one feature. In contrast, at any time point, a subset of the microstimuli is differentially activated. These serve as the features that can be used to generate a prediction of upcoming reward (values). Note how the temporal precision of the microstimuli decreases with time following stimulus onset, so that later microstimuli are more dispersed than earlier microstimuli.

Recent data from Adler et al. (2012) have provided direct evidence for microstimuli in the basal ganglia (**Figure 1B**). Recording from the putamen while a monkey was engaged in a classical conditioning task, Adler et al. found clusters of medium spiny neurons with distinct post-stimulus time courses (for both cues and outcomes). As postulated by Ludvig et al. (2008), the peak response time varied across clusters, with long latency peaks (i.e., late microstimuli) associated with greater dispersion. Recording from the caudate nucleus, Jin et al. (2009) also found clusters of neurons that encode time-stamps of different events. These neurons carry sufficient information to decode time from the population response. Early time points are decodable with higher fidelity compared to late time points, as would be expected if the dispersion of temporal receptive fields increases with latency.

A different solution to the limitations of the CSC was suggested by Daw et al. (2006). They proposed that dopaminergic prediction errors reflect a state space that is *partially observable* and *semi-Markov*. The partial-observability assumption means that the underlying state is inferred from sensory data (cues and rewards), rather than using the features as a proxy for the state. Thus, prediction errors are computed with respect to a *belief state*, a set of features encoding the probabilistic inference about the hidden state. The semi-Markov assumption means that each state is occupied for a random amount of time before transitioning. In the simulations of Daw et al. (2006), only two states were postulated: an interstimulus interval (ISI) state and an intertrial interval (ITI) state. Rewards are delivered upon transition from the ISI to the ITI state, and cues occur upon transition from the ITI to the ISI state. The learning rule in this model is more complex than the standard TD learning rule [which is used by the Ludvig et al. (2008) model]; however, the core idea of learning from prediction errors is preserved in this model.

It is instructive to compare how these two models account for the data on early reward presented by Hollerman and Schultz (1998). In the Ludvig et al. (2008) model, the weights for all the microstimuli are updated after every time step: the late microstimuli associated with the cue (i.e., those centered around the time of reward delivery) accrue positive weights, even after the time of reward delivery (a consequence of the temporal smearing). These post-reward positive predictions generate a negative prediction error, causing the early microstimuli associated with the reward to accrue negative weights. When reward is presented early, the net prediction is close to zero, because the positive weights on the late cue microstimuli compete with the negative weights on the early reward microstimuli. This interaction produces a negligible negative prediction error, consistent with the data of Hollerman and Schultz (1998). The account of Daw et al. (2006) is conceptually different: when reward is presented early, the model infers that a transition to the ITI state has occurred early, and consequently no reward is expected.

Thus far, we have discussed time representations in the service of RL and their implications for the timing of the dopamine response during conditioning. What do RL models have to say about interval timing *per se*? We will argue below that these are not really separate problems: interval timing tasks can be viewed fundamentally as RL tasks. Concomitantly, the role of dopamine and the basal ganglia in interval timing can be understood in terms of their computational contributions to RL. To elaborate this argument, we need to first review some of the relevant theory and data linking interval timing with the basal ganglia.

TIME REPRESENTATION IN THE BASAL GANGLIA: DATA AND THEORY

The role of the basal ganglia and dopamine in interval timing has been studied most extensively in the context of two procedures: the peak procedure (Catania, 1970; Roberts, 1981) and the bisection procedure (Church and Deluty, 1977). The peak procedure consists of two trial types: on fixed-interval trials, the subject is rewarded if a response is made after a fixed duration following cue presentation. On probe trials, the cue duration is extended, and no reward is delivered for responding. **Figure 2A** shows a typical response curve on probe trials: on average, the response rate peaks around the time of food presentation (20 or 40 s in the figure) is ordinarily available and then decreases. The peak time (a measure of the animal's interval estimate) is the time at which the response rate is maximal.

The other two curves in **Figure 2A** illustrate the standard finding that drugs (or genetic manipulations) that increase dopamine transmission, such as methamphetamine, shift the response curve leftward (Maricq et al., 1981; Matell et al., 2004, 2006; Cheng et al., 2007; Balci et al., 2010), whereas drugs that decrease dopamine transmission shift the response curve rightward (Drew et al., 2003; Macdonald and Meck, 2005).

In the bisection procedure, subjects are trained to respond differentially to short and long duration cues. Unreinforced probe trials with cue durations between these two extremes are occasionally presented. On these trials, typically, a psychometric curve is produced with greater selection of the long option (i.e.,

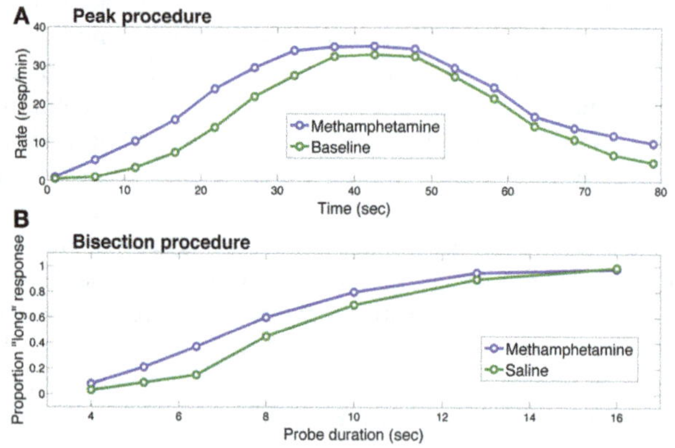

FIGURE 2 | Effects of methamphetamine on timing in (A) the peak procedure and (B) the bisection procedure in rats. Each curve in **(A)** represents response rate as a function of time, where time 0 corresponds to the trial onset. The methamphetamine curve corresponds to sessions in which rats were injected with methamphetamine; the baseline curve corresponds to sessions in which rats did not receive an injection. Each curve in **(B)** represents the proportion of trials on which the rat chose the "long" option as a function of probe cue duration. The saline curve corresponds to sessions in which the rat received a saline injection. In both procedures, methamphetamine leads to overestimation of the elapsing interval, producing early responding in the peak procedure and more "long" responses in the bisection procedure. Figure replotted from Maricq et al. (1981).

the option reinforced following long duration cues) with longer probes and greater selection of the short option with shorter probes and a gradual shift between the two (see **Figure 2B**). The indifference point or point of subjective equality is typically close to the geometric mean of the two anchor durations (Church and Deluty, 1977). Similar to the peak procedure, in the bisection procedure, **Figure 2B** shows how dopamine agonists usually produce a leftward shift in the psychometric curve—i.e., more "short" responses, whereas dopamine antagonists produce the opposite pattern (Maricq et al., 1981; Maricq and Church, 1983; Meck, 1986; Cheng et al., 2007). Under some circumstances, however, dopamine agonists induce temporal dysregulation with an overall flattening of the response curve and no shift in preference or peak times (e.g., Odum et al., 2002; McClure et al., 2005; Balci et al., 2008).

The most influential interpretation of these findings draws upon the class of pacemaker-accumulator models (Gibbon et al., 1997), according to which a pacemaker (an "internal clock") emits pulses that are accumulated by a counter to form a representation of subjective time intervals. The neurobiological implementation of this scheme might rely on populations of oscillating neurons (Miall, 1989; Matell and Meck, 2004), integration of ramping neural activity (Leon and Shadlen, 2003; Simen et al., 2011), or intrinsic dynamics of a recurrent network (Buonomano and Laje, 2010). Independent of the neural implementation, the idea is that drugs that increase dopamine speed up the internal clock, while drugs that decrease dopamine slow the internal clock down.

This interpretation is generally consistent with the findings from studies of patients with Parkinson's disease (PD), who have chronically low striatal dopamine levels. When off medication, these patients tend to underestimate the length of temporal intervals in verbal estimation tasks; dopaminergic medication alleviates this underestimation (Pastor et al., 1992; Lange et al., 1995). It should be noted, however, that some studies have found normal time perception in PD (Malapani et al., 1998; Spencer and Ivry, 2005; Wearden et al., 2008), possibly due to variations in disease severity (Artieda et al., 1992).

Pacemaker-accumulator models have been criticized on a number of grounds, such as lack of parsimony, implausible neurophysiological assumptions, and incorrect behavioral predictions (Staddon and Higa, 1999, 2006; Matell and Meck, 2004; Simen et al., 2013). Moreover, while the pharmacological data are generally consistent with the idea that dopamine modulates the speed of the internal clock, these data may also be consistent with other interpretations. One important alternative is the class of "distributed elements" models, which postulate a representation of time that is distributed over a set of elements; these elements come in various flavors, such as "behavioral states" (Machado, 1997), a cascade of leaky integrators (Staddon and Higa, 1999, 2006; Shankar and Howard, 2012), or spectral traces (Grossberg and Schmajuk, 1989). The effects of dopaminergic drugs might be explicable in terms of systematic changes in the pattern of activity across the distributed elements (see, for example, Grossberg and Schmajuk, 1989).

In fact, the microstimulus model of Ludvig et al. (2008) can be viewed as a distributed elements model embedded within the machinery of RL. This connection suggests a more ambitious theoretical synthesis: can we understand the behavioral and neurophysiological characteristics of interval timing in terms of RL?

TOWARD A UNIFIED MODEL OF REINFORCEMENT LEARNING AND TIMING

One suggestive piece of evidence for how RL models and interval timing can be integrated comes from the study of Fiorillo et al. (2008); (see also Kobayashi and Schultz, 2008). They trained monkeys on a variation of the peak procedure with classical contingencies (i.e., water was delivered independent of responding) while recording from dopamine neurons in the substantia nigra and ventral tegmental area with five different intervals spanning from 1 to 16 s. As shown in **Figure 3A**, they found that the dopamine response to the reward increased with the interval, and the dopamine response to the cue decreased with the interval.

Whereas the response to the cue can be explained in terms of temporal discounting, the response to the reward should not (according to the CSC representation) depend on the cue-reward interval. The perfect timing inherent in the CSC representation means that the reward can be equally well predicted at all time points. Thus, there should be no reward-prediction error, and no phasic dopamine response, at the time of reward regardless of the cue-reward interval. Alternatively, the dopamine response to reward can be understood as reflecting increasing uncertainty in the temporal prediction. **Figure 3B** shows how, using the microstimulus TD model as defined as in Ludvig et al. (2008), there is indeed an increase in the simulated reward prediction error as a function of interval. In the model, with longer intervals,

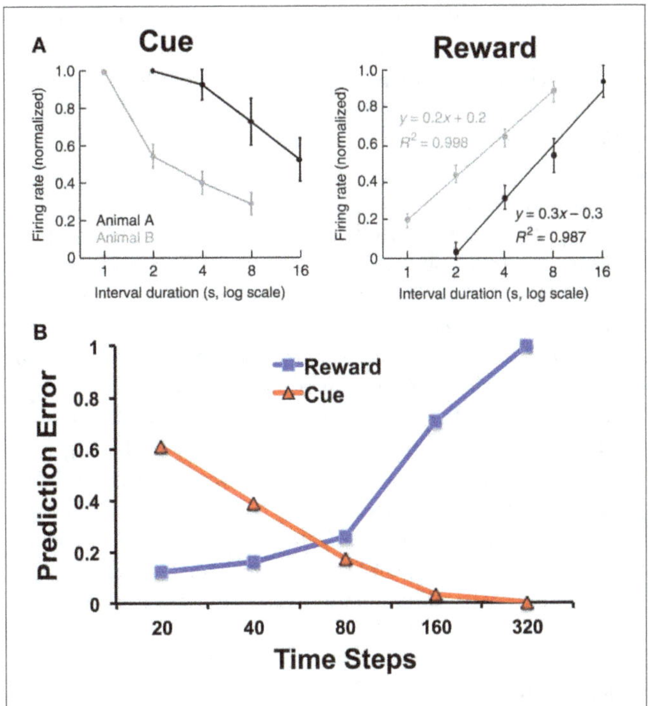

FIGURE 3 | (A) Firing rates of dopamine neurons in monkeys to cues and rewards as a function of cue-reward interval duration. Adapted from Fiorillo et al. (2008) with permission from the publisher. **(B)** Prediction errors to the reward and cue as a function of the interval duration for the microstimulus model. The simulations of the microstimulus model were run for 100 trials and used the same parameters specified in Ludvig et al. (2008): $\lambda = 0.95$, $\alpha = 0.01$, $\gamma = 0.98$, $D = 50$, $\sigma = 0.08$. We treated 20 time steps as a unit of 1 s, and each trial was separated by an interval of 500 time steps. Note the logarithmic scale on the x-axis.

the reward predictions are less temporally precise, and greater prediction errors persist upon reward receipt.

Interval timing procedures, such as the peak procedure, add an additional nuance to this problem by introducing instrumental contingencies. Animals must now not only predict the timing of reward, but also learn when to respond. To analyze this problem in terms of RL, we need to augment the framework introduced earlier to have actions. There are various ways to accomplish this (see Sutton and Barto, 1998). The Actor-Critic architecture (Houk et al., 1995; Joel et al., 2002) is one of the earliest and most influential approaches; it postulates a separate "actor" mechanism that probabilistically chooses an action a_t given the current state s_t. The action probabilities $p(s_t|a_t) \propto \exp\{f(s_t|a_t)\}$ are updated according to:

$$f(s_t|a_t) \leftarrow f(s_t|a_t) + \eta\delta_t[1 - p(s_t|a_t)],$$

where η is a learning rate parameter and δ_t is the is the prediction error defined earlier. The value estimation system plays the role of a "critic" that teaches the actor how to modify its action selection probabilities so as to reduce prediction errors.

When combined with the microstimulus representation, the actor-critic architecture naturally gives rise to timing behavior: in the peak procedure, on average, responding will tend to increase toward the expected reward time and decrease thereafter (see **Figure 2**). Importantly, the late microstimuli are less temporally precise than the early microstimuli, in the sense that their responses are more dispersed over time. As a consequence, credit for late rewards is assigned to a larger number of microstimuli. Under the assumption that response rate is proportion to predicted value, this dispersion of credit causes the timing of actions to be more spread out around the time of reward as the length of the interval increases, one of the central empirical regularities in timing behavior (Gibbon, 1977; see also Ludvig et al., 2012 for an exploration of this property in classical conditioning). As described above, an analog of this property has also been observed in the firing of midbrain dopamine neurons: response to reward increases linearly with the logarithm of the stimulus-reward interval, consistent with the idea that prediction errors are being computed with respect to a value signal whose temporal precision decreases over time (Fiorillo et al., 2008). To the best of our knowledge, pacemaker-accumulator models cannot account for the results presented in **Figure 3**, because they do not have reward-prediction errors in their machinery. Instead, they collect a distribution of past cue-reward intervals and draw from that distribution to create an estimate of the time to reward (e.g., Gibbon et al., 1984).

The partially observable semi-Markov model of Daw et al. (2006) can account for the findings of Fiorillo et al. (2008), but this account deviates from the normative RL framework. Daw et al. use an external timing signal with "scalar noise" (cf. Gibbon et al., 1984), implemented by adding Gaussian noise to the timing signal with standard deviation proportional to the interval. Scalar noise induces larger-magnitude prediction errors with increasing delays. However, these prediction errors are symmetric around 0 and hence cancel out on average. To account for the effects of cue-reward interval on the dopamine response, Daw et al. assume that negative prediction errors are rectified (see Bayer and Glimcher, 2005), resulting in a positive skew of the prediction error distribution. **Figure 4** shows how this asymmetric rectification results in average prediction errors that are increasingly positive for longer intervals. Note that rectification is not an intrinsic part of the RL framework, and in fact compromises the convergence of TD to the true value function. One potential solution to this problem is to posit a separate physiological channel for the signaling of negative prediction errors, possibly via serotonergic activity (Daw et al., 2002).

The microstimulus actor-critic model can also explain the effects of dopamine manipulations and Parkinson's disease. The key additional assumption is that early microstimuli (but not later ones) are primarily represented by the striatum. Timing in the milliseconds to seconds range depends on D2 receptors in the dorsal striatum (Rammsayer, 1993; Coull et al., 2011), suggesting that this region represents early microstimuli (whereas late microstimuli may be represented by other neural substrates, such as the hippocampus; see Ludvig et al., 2009). Because the post-synaptic effect of dopamine at D2 receptors is inhibitory, D2 receptor antagonists increase the firing of striatal neurons expressing D2 receptors, which mainly occur in the indirect or "NoGo" pathway and exert a suppressive influence on striatal output (Gerfen, 1992). Thus, the ultimate effect of D2 receptor

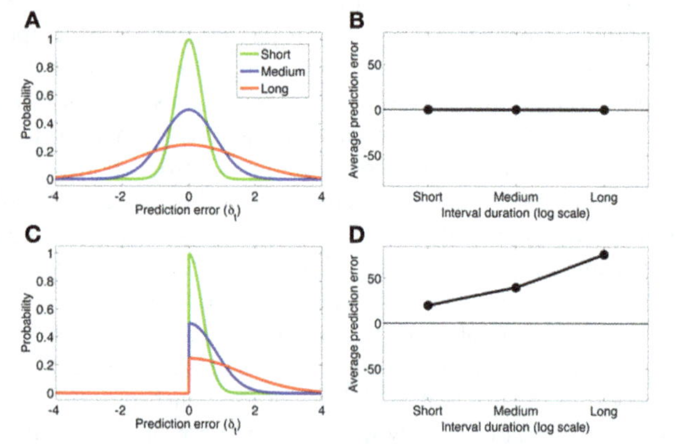

FIGURE 4 | (A) The distribution of prediction errors in the semi-Markov TD model (Daw et al., 2006) for three logarithmically spaced cue-reward interval durations (short, medium, long). The timing signal is corrupted by zero-mean Gaussian noise with standard deviation proportional to the interval duration. **(B)** The average prediction error under each distribution. A symmetric prediction error distribution implies that the average prediction error is invariant to the interval duration. **(C,D)** Same format as panels A and B, but where the prediction error distribution is rectified slightly below 0. This asymmetric distribution produces average prediction errors that scale approximately linearly with the log interval duration.

antagonists is to reduce striatal output, thereby attenuating the influence of early microstimuli on behavior. As a result, predictions of the upcoming reward will be biased later, and responses will occur later than usual (e.g., in the peak procedure). This fits with the observation that the rightward shift (overestimation) of estimated time following dopamine antagonist administration is proportional to the drug's binding affinity for D2 receptors (Meck, 1986). In contrast, dopamine agonists lead to a selective enhancement of the early microstimuli, producing earlier than usual responding (see **Figure 2A**).

A similar line of reasoning can explain some of the timing deficits in Parkinson's disease. The nigrostriatal pathway (the main source of dopamine to the dorsal striatum) is compromised in Parkinson's disease, resulting in reduced striatal dopamine levels. Because D2 receptors have a higher affinity for dopamine, Parkinson's disease leads to the predominance of D2-mediated activity and hence reduced striatal output (Wiecki and Frank, 2010). Our model thus predicts a rightward shift of estimated time, as is often observed experimentally (see above).

The linking of early microstimuli with the striatum in the model also leads to the prediction that low striatal dopamine levels will result in poorer learning of fast responses (which depend on the early microstimuli). In addition, responding will in general be slowed because the learned weights to the early microstimuli will be weak relative to those of late microstimuli. As a result, our model clearly predicts poorer learning of fast responses in Parkinson's disease. A study of temporal decision making in Parkinson's patients fits with this prediction (Moustafa et al., 2008). Patients were trained to respond at different latencies to a set of cues, with slow responses yielding more reward in an "increasing expected value" (IEV) condition and fast responses yielding more reward in a "decreasing expected value" (DEV) condition. It was found that the performance of medicated patients was better in the DEV condition, while performance of non-medicated patients was better in the IEV condition. If non-medicated patients have a paucity of short-timescale microstimuli (due to low striatal dopamine levels), then the model correctly anticipates that these patients will be impaired at learning about early events relative to later events.

Recently, Foerde et al. (2013) found that Parkinson's patients are impaired in learning from immediate, but not delayed, feedback in a probabilistic decision making task. This finding is also consistent with the idea that these patients lack a representational substrate for early post-stimulus events. Interestingly, they also found that patients with lesions of the medial temporal lobe show the opposite pattern, possibly indicating that this region (and in particular the hippocampus) is important for representing late microstimuli, as was suggested earlier by Ludvig et al. (2009). An alternative possibility is that the striatum and hippocampus both represent early and late microstimuli, but the stimulus trace decays more quickly in the striatum than in the hippocampus (Bornstein and Daw, 2012), which would produce a more graded segregation of temporal sensitivity between the two regions.

CONCLUSION

Timing and RL have for the most part been studied separately, giving rise to largely non-overlapping computational models. We have argued here, however, that these models do in fact share some important commonalities and reconciling them may provide a unified explanation of many behavioral and neural phenomena. While in this brief review we have only sketched such a synthesis, our goal is to plant the seeds for future theoretical unification.

One open question concerns how to reconcile the disparate theoretical ideas about time representation that were described in this paper. Our synthesis proposed a central role for a distributed elements representation of time such as the microstimuli of Ludvig et al. (2008). Could a representation deriving from the semi-Markov or pacemaker-accumulator models be used instead? This may be possible, but there are several reasons to prefer the microstimulus representation. First, microstimuli lend themselves naturally to the linear function approximation architecture that has been widely used in RL models of the basal ganglia. In contrast, the semi-Markov model requires additional computational machinery, and it is not obvious how to incorporate the pacemaker-accumulator model into RL theory. Second, the semi-Markov model accounts for the relationship between temporal precision and interval length at the expense of deviating from the normative RL framework. Third, as we noted earlier, pacemaker-accumulator models have a number of other weaknesses (see Staddon and Higa, 1999, 2006; Matell and Meck, 2004; Simen et al., 2013), such as lack of parsimony, implausible neurophysiological assumptions, and incorrect behavioral predictions. Nonetheless, it will be interesting to explore what aspects of these models can be successfully incorporated into the next generation of RL models.

ACKNOWLEDGMENTS

We thank Marc Howard and Nathaniel Daw for helpful discussions. Samuel J. Gershman was supported by IARPA via DOI contract D10PC2002 and by a postdoctoral fellowship from the MIT Intelligence Initiative. Ahmed A. Moustafa is partially supported by a 2013 internal UWS Research Grant Scheme award P00021210. Elliot A. Ludvig was partially supported by NIH Grant #P30 AG024361 and the Princeton Pyne Fund.

REFERENCES

Adler, A., Katabi, S., Finkes, I., Israel, Z., Prut, Y., and Bergman, H. (2012). Temporal convergence of dynamic cell assemblies in the striato-pallidal network. *J. Neurosci.* 32, 2473–2484. doi: 10.1523/JNEUROSCI.4830-11.2012

Artieda, J., Pastor, M. A., Lacruz, F., and Obeso, J. A. (1992). Temporal discrimination is abnormal in Parkinson's disease. *Brain* 115, 199–210. doi: 10.1093/brain/115.1.199

Balci, F., Ludvig, E. A., Abner, R., Zhuang, X., Poon, P., and Brunner, D. (2010). Motivational effects on interval timing in dopamine transporter (DAT) knockdown mice. *Brain Res.* 1325, 89–99. doi: 10.1016/j.brainres.2010.02.034

Balci, F., Ludvig, E. A., Gibson, J. M., Allen, B. D., Frank, K. M., Kapustinski, B. J., et al. (2008). Pharmacological manipulations of interval timing using the peak procedure in male C3H mice. *Psychopharmacology (Berl.)* 201, 67–80. doi: 10.1007/s00213-008-1248-y

Bayer, H. M., and Glimcher, P. W. (2005). Midbrain dopamine neurons encode a quantitative reward prediction error signal. *Neuron* 47, 129–141. doi: 10.1016/j.neuron.2005.05.020

Bayer, H. M., Lau, B., and Glimcher, P. W. (2007). Statistics of midbrain dopamine neuron spike trains in the awake primate. *J. Neurophysiol.* 98, 1428–1439. doi: 10.1152/jn.01140.2006

Bornstein, A. M., and Daw, N. D. (2012). Dissociating hippocampal and striatal contributions to sequential prediction learning. *Eur. J. Neurosci.* 35, 1011–1023. doi: 10.1111/j.1460-9568.2011.07920.x

Buhusi, C. V., and Meck, W. H. (2005). What makes us tick? Functional and neural mechanisms of interval timing. *Nat. Rev. Neurosci.* 6, 755–765. doi: 10.1038/nrn1764

Buonomano, D. V., and Laje, R. (2010). Population clocks: motor timing with neural dyanmics. *Trends Cogn. Sci.* 14, 520–527. doi: 10.1016/j.tics.2010.09.002

Catania, R. A. (1970). "Reinforcement schedules and psychophysical judgements," in *The Theory of Reinforcement Schedules*, ed W. N. Schoenfeld (New York, NY: Appleton-Century Crofts), 1–42.

Cheng, R. K., Ali, Y. M., and Meck, W. H. (2007). Ketamine "unlocks" the reduced clock-speed effects of cocaine following extended training: evidence for dopamine-glutamate interactions in timing and time perception. *Neurobiol. Learn. Mem.* 88, 149–159. doi: 10.1016/j.nlm.2007.04.005

Church, R. M., and Deluty, H. Z. (1977). The bisection of temporal intervals. *J. Exp. Psychol. Anim. Behav. Process.* 3, 216–228. doi: 10.1037/0097-7403.3.3.216

Cohen, M. X., and Frank, M. J. (2009). Neurocomputational models of basal ganglia function in learning, memory and choice. *Behav. Brain Res.* 199, 141–156. doi: 10.1016/j.bbr.2008.09.029

Coull, J. T., Cheng, R. K., and Meck, W. H. (2011). Neuroanatomical and neurochemical substrates of timing. *Neuropsychopharmacology* 36, 3–25. doi: 10.1038/npp.2010.113

Daw, N. D., Courville, A. C., and Touretzky, D. S. (2006). Representation and timing in theories of the dopamine system. *Neural Comput.* 18, 1637–1677. doi: 10.1162/neco.2006.18.7.1637

Daw, N. D., Kakade, S., and Dayan, P. (2002). Opponent interactions between serotonin and dopamine. *Neural Netw.* 15, 603–616. doi: 10.1016/S0893-6080(02)00052-7

Drew, M. R., Fairhurst, S., Malapani, C., Horvitz, J. C., and Balsam, P. D. (2003). Effects of dopamine antagonists on the timing of two intervals. *Pharmacol. Biochem. Behav.* 75, 9–15. doi: 10.1016/S0091-3057(03)00036-4

Fiorillo, C. D., Newsome, W. T., and Schultz, W. (2008). The temporal precision of reward prediction in dopamine neurons. *Nat. Neurosci.* 11, 966–973. doi: 10.1038/nn.2159

Foerde, K., Race, E., Verfaellie, M., and Shohamy, D. (2013). A role for the medial temporal lobe in feedback-driven learning: evidence from amnesia. *J. Neurosci.* 33, 5698–5704. doi: 10.1523/JNEUROSCI.5217-12.2013

Gerfen, C. R. (1992). The neostriatal mosaic: multiple levels of compartmental organization in the basal ganglia. *Annu. Rev. Neurosci.* 15, 285–320. doi: 10.1146/annurev.ne.15.030192.001441

Gibbon, J. (1977). Scalar expectancy theory and Weber's law in animal timing. *Psychol. Rev.* 84, 279–325. doi: 10.1037/0033-295X.84.3.279

Gibbon, J., Church, R. M., and Meck, W. H. (1984). "Scalar timing in memory," in *Annals of the New York Academy of Sciences: Timing and Time Perception*, Vol. 423, eds J. Gibbon and L. G. Allan (New York, NY: New York Academy of Sciences), 52–77.

Gibbon, J., Malapani, C., Dale, C. L., and Gallistel, C. R. (1997). Towards a neurobiology of temporal cognition: advances and challenges. *Curr. Opin. Neurobiol.* 7, 170–184. doi: 10.1016/S0959-4388(97)80005-0

Grossberg, S., and Schmajuk, N. A. (1989). Neural dynamics of adaptive timing and temporal discrimination during associative learning. *Neural Netw.* 2, 79–102. doi: 10.1016/0893-6080(89)90026-9

Hollerman, J. R., and Schultz, W. (1998). Dopamine neurons report an error in the temporal prediction of reward during learning. *Nat. Neurosci.* 1, 304–309. doi: 10.1038/1124

Houk, J. C., Adams, J. L., and Barto, A. G. (1995). "A model of how the basal ganglia generate and use neural signals that predict reinforcement," in *Models of information Processing in the Basal Ganglia*, eds J. C. Houk, J. L. Davis, and D. G. Beiser (Cambridge, MA: MIT Press), 249–270.

Jin, D. Z., Fujii, N., and Graybiel, A. M. (2009). Neural representation of time in cortico-basal ganglia circuits. *Proc. Natl. Acad. Sci. U.S.A.* 106, 19156–19161. doi: 10.1073/pnas.0909881106

Joel, D., Niv, Y., and Ruppin, E. (2002). Actor-critic models of the basal ganglia: new anatomical and computational perspectives. *Neural Netw.* 15, 535–547. doi: 10.1016/S0893-6080(02)00047-3

Jones, C. R., and Jahanshahi, M. (2009). The substantia nigra, the basal ganglia, dopamine and temporal processing. *J. Neural Transm. Suppl.* 73, 161–171. doi: 10.1007/978-3-211-92660-4_13

Kobayashi, S., and Schultz, W. (2008). Influence of reward delays on responses of dopamine neurons. *J. Neurosci.* 28, 7837–7846. doi: 10.1523/JNEUROSCI.1600-08.2008

Lange, K. W., Tucha, O., Steup, A., Gsell, W., and Naumann, M. (1995). Subjective time estimation in Parkinson's disease. *J. Neural Transm. Suppl.* 46, 433–438.

Leon, M. I., and Shadlen, M. N. (2003). Representation of time by neurons in the posterior parietal cortex of the macaque. *Neuron* 38, 317–327. doi: 10.1016/S0896-6273(03)00185-5

Ludvig, E. A., Bellemare, M. G., and Pearson, K. G. (2011). "A primer on reinforcement learning in the brain: psychological, computational, and neural perspectives," in *Computational Neuroscience for Advancing Artificial Intelligence: Models, Methods and Applications*, eds E. Alonso and E. Mondragon (Hershey, PA: IGI Global), 111–144.

Ludvig, E. A., Sutton, R. S., and Kehoe, E. J. (2008). Stimulus representation and the timing of reward-prediction errors in models of the dopamine system. *Neural Comput.* 20, 3034–3054. doi: 10.1162/neco.2008.11-07-654

Ludvig, E. A., Sutton, R. S., and Kehoe, E. J. (2012). Evaluating the TD model of classical conditioning. *Learn. Behav.* 40, 305–319. doi: 10.3758/s13420-012-0082-6

Ludvig, E. A., Sutton, R. S., Verbeek, E. L., and Kehoe, E. J. (2009). A computational model of hippocampal function in trace conditioning. *Adv. Neural Inf. Process. Syst.* 21, 993–1000.

Macdonald, C. J., and Meck, W. H. (2005). Differential effects of clozapine and haloperidol on interval timing in the supraseconds range. *Psychopharmacology (Berl.)* 182, 232–244. doi: 10.1007/s00213-005-0074-8

Machado, A. (1997). Learning the temporal dynamics of behavior. *Psychol. Rev.* 104, 241–265. doi: 10.1037/0033-295X.104.2.241

Maia, T. (2009). Reinforcement learning, conditioning, and the brain: successes and challenges. *Cogn. Affect. Behav. Neurosci.* 9, 343–364. doi: 10.3758/CABN.9.4.343

Malapani, C., Rakitin, B., Levy, R., Meck, W. H., Deweer, B., Dubois, B., et al. (1998). Coupled temporal memories in Parkinson's disease: a dopamine-related dysfunction. *J. Cogn. Neurosci.* 10, 316–331. doi: 10.1162/089892998562762

Maricq, A. V., and Church, R. M. (1983). The differential effects of haloperidol and methamphetamine on time estimation in the rat. *Psychopharmacology (Berl.)* 79, 10–15. doi: 10.1007/BF00433008

Maricq, A. V., Roberts, S., and Church, R. M. (1981). Methamphetamine and time estimation. *J. Exp. Psychol. Anim. Behav. Process.* 7, 18–30. doi: 10.1037//0097-7403.7.1.18

Matell, M. S., Bateson, M., and Meck, W. H. (2006). Single-trials analyses demonstrate that increases in clock speed contribute to the methamphetamine-induced horizontal shifts in peak-interval timing functions. *Psychopharmacology (Berl.)* 188, 201–212. doi: 10.1007/s00213-006-0489-x

Matell, M. S., King, G. R., and Meck, W. H. (2004). Differential modulation of clock speed by the administration of intermittent versus continuous cocaine. *Behav. Neurosci.* 118, 150–156. doi: 10.1037/0735-7044.118.1.150

Matell, M. S., and Meck, W. H. (2004). Cortico-striatal circuits and interval timing: coincidence detection of oscillatory processes. *Cogn. Brain Res.* 21, 139–170. doi: 10.1016/j.cogbrainres.2004.06.012

McClure, E. A., Saulsgiver, K. A., and Wynne, C. D. L. (2005). Effects of d-amphetamine on temporal discrimination in pigeons. *Behav. Pharmacol.* 16, 193–208. doi: 10.1097/01.fbp.0000171773.69292.bd

Meck, W. H. (1986). Affinity for the dopamine D2 receptor predicts neuroleptic potency in decreasing the speed of an internal clock. *Pharmacol. Biochem. Behav.* 25, 1185–1189. doi: 10.1016/0091-3057(86)90109-7

Merchant, H., Harrington, D. L., and Meck, W. H. (2013). Neural basis of the perception and estimation of time. *Annu. Rev. Neurosci.* 36, 313–336. doi: 10.1146/annurev-neuro-062012-170349

Miall, C. (1989). The storage of time intervals using oscillating neurons. *Neural Comput.* 1, 359–371. doi: 10.1162/neco.1989.1.3.359

Montague, P. R., Dayan, P., and Sejnowski, T. J. (1996). A framework for mesencephalic dopamine systems based on predictive Hebbian learning. *J. Neurosci.* 16, 1936–1947.

Moore, J. W., Desmond, J. E., and Berthier, N. E. (1989). Adaptively timed conditioned responses and the cerebellum: a neural network approach. *Biol. Cybern.* 62, 17–28. doi: 10.1007/BF00217657

Moustafa, A. A., Cohen, M. X., Sherman, S. J., and Frank, M. J. (2008). A role for dopamine in temporal decision making and reward maximization in Parkinsonism. *J. Neurosci.* 28, 12294–12304. doi: 10.1523/JNEUROSCI.3116-08.2008

Nakahara, H., and Kaveri, S. (2010). Internal-time temporal difference model for neural value-based decision making. *Neural Comput.* 22, 3062–3106. doi: 10.1162/NECO_a_00049

Niv, Y. (2009). Reinforcement learning in the brain. *J. Math. Psychol.* 53, 139–154. doi: 10.1016/j.jmp.2008.12.005

Odum, A. L., Lieving, L. M., and Schaal, D. W. (2002). Effects of D-amphetamine in a temporal discrimination procedure: selective changes in timing or rate dependency? *J. Exp. Anal. Behav.* 78, 195–214. doi: 10.1901/jeab.2002.78-195

Pastor, M. A., Artieda, J., Jahanshahi, M., and Obeso, J. A. (1992). Time estimation and reproduction is abnormal in Parkinson's disease. *Brain* 115, 211–225. doi: 10.1093/brain/115.1.211

Rammsayer, T. H. (1993). On dopaminergic modulation of temporal information processing. *Biol. Psychol.* 36, 209–222. doi: 10.1016/0301-0511(93)90018-4

Redgrave, P., Gurney, K., and Reynolds, J. (2008). What is reinforced by phasic dopamine signals? *Brain Res. Rev.* 58, 322–339. doi: 10.1016/j.brainresrev.2007.10.007

Rescorla, R. A., and Wagner, A. R. (1972). "A theory of Pavlovian conditioning: variations in the effectiveness of reinforcement and nonreinforcement," in *Classical Conditioning II: Current Research and Theory*, eds A. H. Black and W. F. Prokasy (New York, NY: Appleton-Century Crofts), 64–69.

Reynolds, J. N. J., and Wickens, J. R. (2002). Dopamine-dependent plasticity of corticostriatal synapses. *Neural Netw.* 15, 507–521. doi: 10.1016/S0893-6080(02)00045-X

Rivest, F., Kalaska, J. F., and Bengio, Y. (2010). Alternative time representation in dopamine models. *J. Comput. Neurosci.* 28, 107–130. doi: 10.1007/s10827-009-0191-1

Roberts, S. (1981). Isolation of an internal clock. *J. Exp. Psychol. Anim. Behav. Process.* 7, 242–268. doi: 10.1037/0097-7403.7.3.242

Schultz, W., Dayan, P., and Montague, P. R. (1997). A neural substrate of prediction and reward. *Science* 275, 1593–1599. doi: 10.1126/science.275.5306.1593

Shankar, K. H., and Howard, M. W. (2012). A scale-invariant internal representation of time. *Neural Comput.* 24, 134–193. doi: 10.1162/NECO_a_00212

Simen, P., Balci, F., deSouza, L., Cohen, J. D., and Holmes, P. (2011). A model of interval timing by neural integration. *J. Neurosci.* 31, 9238–9253. doi: 10.1523/JNEUROSCI.3121-10.2011

Simen, P., Rivest, F., Ludvig, E. A., Balci, F., and Killeen, P. (2013). Timescale invariance in the pacemaker-accumulator family of timing models. *Timing Time Percept.* 1, 159–188. doi: 10.1163/22134468-00002018

Spencer, R. M., and Ivry, R. B. (2005). Comparison of patients with Parkinson's disease or cerebellar lesions in the production of periodic movements involving event-based or emergent timing. *Brain Cogn.* 58, 84–93. doi: 10.1016/j.bandc.2004.09.010

Staddon, J. E. R., and Higa, J. J. (1999). Time and memory: towards a pacemaker-free theory of interval timing. *J. Exp. Anal. Behav.* 71, 215–251. doi: 10.1901/jeab.1999.71-215

Staddon, J. E. R., and Higa, J. J. (2006). Interval timing. *Nat. Rev. Neurosci.* 7. doi: 10.1038/nrn1764-c1

Steinberg, E. E., Keiflin, R., Bolvin, J. R., Witten, I. B., Deisseroth, K., and Janak, P. H. (2013). A causal link between prediction errors, dopamine neurons and learning. *Nat. Neurosci.* 16, 966–973. doi: 10.1038/nn.3413

Suri, R. E., and Schultz, W. (1999). A neural network model with dopamine-like reinforcement signal that learns a spatial delayed response task. *Neuroscience* 91, 871–890. doi: 10.1016/S0306-4522(98)00697-6

Sutton, R. S. and Barto, A. G. (1990). "Time-derivative models of Pavlovian reinforcement," in *Learning and Computational Neuroscience: Foundations of Adaptive Networks*, eds M. Gabriel and J. Moore (Cambridge, MA: MIT Press), 497–537.

Sutton, R. S., and Barto, A. G. (1998). *Reinforcement Learning: An Introduction.* Cambridge, MA: MIT Press.

Wearden, J. H., Smith-Spark, J. H., Cousins, R., Edelstyn, N. M., Cody, F. W., and O'Boyle, D. J. (2008). Stimulus timing by people with Parkinson's disease. *Brain Cogn.* 67, 264–279. doi: 10.1016/j.bandc.2008.01.010

Wiecki, T. V., and Frank, M. J. (2010). Neurocomputational models of motor and cognitive deficits in Parkinson's disease. *Prog. Brain Res.* 183, 275–297. doi: 10.1016/S0079-6123(10)83014-6

11

Hemispheric Differences in the Mesostriatal Dopaminergic system

Ilana Molochnikov and Dana Cohen*

The Leslie and Susan Gonda Multidisciplinary Brain Research Center, Bar-Ilan University, Ramat-Gan, Israel

Correspondence:
Dana Cohen, The Gonda Brain Research Center, Bar Ilan University, Building number 901, Ramat Gan 52900, Israel
e-mail: danacoh@gmail.com

The mesostriatal dopaminergic system, which comprises the mesolimbic and the nigrostriatal pathways, plays a major role in neural processing underlying motor and limbic functions. Multiple reports suggest that these processes are influenced by hemispheric differences in striatal dopamine (DA) levels, DA turnover and its receptor activity. Here, we review studies which measured the concentration of DA and its metabolites to examine the relationship between DA imbalance and animal behavior under different conditions. Specifically, we assess evidence in support of endogenous, inter-hemispheric DA imbalance; determine whether the known anatomy provides a suitable substrate for this imbalance; examine the relationship between DA imbalance and animal behavior; and characterize the symmetry of the observed inter-hemispheric laterality in the nigrostriatal and the mesolimbic DA systems. We conclude that many studies provide supporting evidence for the occurrence of experience-dependent endogenous DA imbalance which is controlled by a dedicated regulatory/compensatory mechanism. Additionally, it seems that the link between DA imbalance and animal behavior is better characterized in the nigrostriatal than in the mesolimbic system. Nonetheless, a variety of brain and behavioral manipulations demonstrate that the nigrostriatal system displays symmetrical laterality whereas the mesolimbic system displays asymmetrical laterality which supports hemispheric specialization in rodents. The reciprocity of the relationship between DA imbalance and animal behavior (i.e., the capacity of animal training to alter DA imbalance for prolonged time periods) remains controversial, however, if confirmed, it may provide a valuable non-invasive therapeutic means for treating abnormal DA imbalance.

Keywords: dopamine, laterality, striatum, side preference, VTA, nucleus accumbens

INTRODUCTION

There is a general consensus regarding cerebral dominance and hemispheric specialization in the human brain in which the right hemisphere is dominant for analyzing complex visuo-spatial relationships and for the perception and expression of emotions, whereas language is represented in the left hemisphere (Kimura and Archibald, 1974; Gazzaniga, 1995; Davidson and Kenneth, 2004; Fox and Reed, 2008; Gotts et al., 2013). Healthy subjects display asymmetries in the DA system, which in humans have been associated, for example, with lateralized motor performance and hand preference (Bracha et al., 1987; De La Fuente-Fernandez et al., 2000; Mohr and Bracha, 2004). Pathological DA asymmetries occur in neuropsychiatric and neurodegenerative disorders such as schizophrenia, depression, and Parkinson's disease (Peterson et al., 1993; Seibyl et al., 1995; Gruzelier, 1999; Hietala et al., 1999; Van Dyck et al., 2002; Hsiao et al., 2003, 2013). Inter-hemispheric imbalance in DA concentration and its metabolites has been described in the rodent mesostriatal system and in related structures such as prefrontal cortex (PFC), Entorhinal cortex (EC) and the hippocampus (Glick et al., 1982; Schneider et al., 1982; Denenberg and Rosen, 1983; Drew et al., 1986; Fride and Weinstock, 1987; Nowak, 1989; Rodriguez et al., 1994; Becker, 1999; Hietala et al., 1999; Thiel and Schwarting, 2001; Van Dyck et al., 2002; Silva et al., 2007; Vernaleken et al., 2007; Cannon et al., 2009; Martin-Soelch et al., 2011; Hsiao et al., 2013). This DA imbalance in the mesostriatal system has been associated with a variety of motor and cognitive aspects of behavior among which are spatial performance such as side preference in a T maze or during lever-press (Zimmerberg et al., 1974; Glick et al., 1981; Castellano et al., 1987), locomotor activity (Glick and Ross, 1981; Glick et al., 1988; Cabib et al., 1995; Nielsen et al., 1997; Budilin et al., 2008), difference in sensitivity to intracranial self-stimulation, motivation, responsiveness to stress, and appetitive and aversive stimuli (Glick et al., 1981; Carlson et al., 1991, 1993; Besson and Louilot, 1995; Sullivan and Gratton, 1998; Berridge et al., 1999; Sullivan and Dufresne, 2006; Fox and Reed, 2008; Tomer et al., 2008, 2014; Laplante et al., 2013).

In this review, we address the midbrain DA system functionality by examining the laterality of the mesostriatal system in populations of animals as reflected in DA imbalance across hemispheres. To do so, we specify the type, origin and destination of primarily midbrain DA neurons, review evidence supporting DA related hemispheric laterality as assessed by measuring DA levels and its metabolite dihydroxyphenylacetic acid (DOPAC), examine correlations between DA imbalance and spatial and cognitive biases in animal behavior, and finally, we discuss the ways in which these correlations are altered in response to unilateral and systemic biochemical intervention and behavioral manipulation. We particularly ask whether or not manipulations generate a symmetrical effect across hemispheres (i.e., whether a unilaterally applied manipulation generates a mirror image of the effect generated by applying that manipulation to the other hemisphere). The search for papers was done using relevant key words such as asymmetry, laterality, DA, ventral tegmental area (VTA), substantia nigra (SN), striatum, nucleus accumbens (NAc), PFC, medial forebrain bundle (MFB), 6-hydroxydopamine (6-OHDA), unilateral, left, right, inter hemispheric, mesostriatal, mesolimbic, nigrostriatal, affective, limbic, etc. Papers were selected irrespective of results if reported data comprised left/right information without collapsing them across hemispheres.

ANATOMY AND CONNECTIVITY

The two prime dopaminergic fiber groups, the A9 and A10, are located in the ventral midbrain (Dahlstroem and Fuxe, 1964). The A10 group is the largest group of DAergic cells in the ventral midbrain tegmentum which is located for the most part in the VTA. The A10 group represents about two thirds (~65%) of VTA cell population. In addition, the VTA comprises a sizable population of GABAergic inhibitory neurons (~30%) and excitatory glutamatergic neurons (~5%) (Nauta et al., 1978; Johnson and North, 1992). This DAergic group gives rise to the mesolimbic DA system projecting through the MFB primarily to the ventral striatum (NAc) (Dahlstroem and Fuxe, 1964). The A9 group is the most densely packed group of DAergic cells, which is located in the substantia nigra pars compacta (SNc) and accounts for about 90% of the neuronal population in this relatively homogenous structure, in addition to a small population of GABAergic inhibitory neurons (10%). The A9 group constitutes the nigrostriatal DAergic pathway which projects through the MFB to the dorsal striatum (dStr) composed of the caudate and putamen. Another small group of DAergic cells in rodents and primates is the A8 group, located in the midbrain reticular formation.

The DAergic signal arising from these midbrain structures enables basal ganglia (BG) control of motor planning and action selection (Wurtz and Hikosaka, 1986; Berns and Sejnowski, 1998; Gurney et al., 2001) by two parallel pathways diverging in the striatum and separating the BG loop into the direct, striatonigral pathway, and the indirect, striatopallidal pathway, via medium-sized spiny projection neurons (MSNs) expressing D1 receptors and D2 receptors, respectively (Alexander and Crutcher, 1990; Gerfen et al., 1990). The subthalamic nucleus which is a part of the indirect pathway also receives direct cortical input via the hyper-direct fast pathway that bypasses the striatum and is therefore independent of striatal DA input (Kita, 1992; Nambu et al., 2000, 2002). The balance between the direct and indirect pathways is thought to be essential for proper BG function (Albin et al., 1989; Wichmann and Delong, 1996; Delong and Wichmann, 2007). The MSNs, which are GABAergic neurons, make up the vast majority (90–95%) of striatal neurons in rodents and primates (Kemp and Powell, 1971; Mensah and Deadwyler, 1974; Wilson and Groves, 1980; Graveland and Difiglia, 1985). The MSNs relay information via the direct and indirect pathways to the two major output stations of the BG, the substantia nigra pars reticulata (SNr) and the globus pallidus internal segment (or the entopeduncular nucleus in rodents) which are both primarily GABAergic (Van Der Kooy and Wise, 1980; Oertel and Mugnaini, 1984; Bolam et al., 1985, 1993; Parent and Hazrati, 1995).

CONNECTIVITY WITHIN THE MESOSTRIATAL SYSTEMS

The DA neurons in the SNc project predominantly to the striatum, which also receives a small percentage of DA inputs from the SNr and VTA (Van Der Kooy and Wise, 1980). Overall, at least 85% of the fibers reaching the striatum from the midbrain arise from the DA mesostriatal neurons. Of the 15% of the non-DA carrying fibers reaching the striatum, about 2% arrive from the VTA, 3–4% from the SNc, and 8–9% arrive from the SNr (Van Der Kooy et al., 1981; Swanson, 1982; Fallon et al., 1983; Gerfen et al., 1987). In turn, neurons located in the striatal patches (Gerfen, 1984, 1985) project back to the DAergic neurons in the SNc (Gerfen et al., 1987). The two types of SNc neurons also project onto the NAc and comprise about 38% of its midbrain input (Swanson, 1982). The NAc projections back to the nigral complex are substantially larger than the nigrostriatal fibers it receives (Nauta et al., 1978).

All three types of VTA neurons project onto the NAc and comprise 40% of its midbrain input (Phillipson, 1979; Swanson, 1982). Of these NAc afferents, 85% are primarily DAergic and the remaining 15% arise from GABA or glutamate releasing neurons (Swanson, 1982; Gerfen et al., 1987; Gonzalez-Hernandez et al., 2004, p. 23; Stuber et al., 2012; Ishikawa et al., 2013). In turn, the NAc sends inhibitory projections back to VTA GABAergic neurons including those that innervated it, thus enabling reciprocal information transfer (Nauta et al., 1978; Phillipson, 1979; Kalivas et al., 1993). In addition, the VTA DAergic neurons are inhibited by GABAergic interneurons located in the VTA (Stuber et al., 2012; Van Zessen et al., 2012).

Approximately 1–3% of the DA fibers reaching the striatum come from the contralateral SNc, the VTA and the posterior lateral hypothalamic area (Veening et al., 1980; Gerfen et al., 1982; Swanson, 1982; Altar et al., 1983; Fallon et al., 1983; Consolazione et al., 1985; Lieu and Subramanian, 2012). Less than 10% of the VTA efferents cross the midline to the contralateral side (Swanson, 1982) where they give rise to about 8% of the fibers reaching the NAc and about 1–3% of the fibers reaching the dStr (Carter and Fibiger, 1977; Altar et al., 1983; Douglas et al., 1987). This inter-hemispheric communication does not pass through the corpus callosum (Fass and Butcher, 1981) and instead decussates before the fibers reach the lateral hypothalamic area, close to the VTA (Altar et al., 1983; Douglas et al., 1987). It has been shown that VTA and SN neurons project either ipsilaterally or contralaterally but not bilaterally (Loughlin and Fallon, 1982).

CONNECTIVITY BETWEEN THE MESOSTRIATAL SYSTEMS AND RELATED STRUCTURES

The cortical targets of the SN include the PFC, the motor cortex and the EC (Loughlin and Fallon, 1984). All major regions of the cerebral cortex communicate with the striatum bilaterally, however, with ipsilateral predominance (Veening et al., 1980; Fisher et al., 1986; McGeorge and Faull, 1989; Brog et al., 1993; Totterdell and Meredith, 1997; Alloway et al., 2006; Lieu and Subramanian, 2012). Importantly, a single SN neuron sends collaterals to limbic, striatal, and cortical structures, unlike VTA neurons that can project solely to one terminal field (Loughlin and Fallon, 1984).

Projection neurons in the VTA arrive at the PFC and synapse on pyramidal neurons that project to the contralateral PFC (Carr and Sesack, 2000; Hnasko et al., 2012; Stuber et al., 2012) suggesting that the PFC is ideally suited to modulate inter-hemispheric information flow between itself and the BG. Additionally, the PFC sends excitatory glutamatergic projections onto VTA GABAergic neurons which innervate the NAc, and also onto VTA DAergic neurons which project back to the PFC (Carr and Sesack, 2000).

The VTA neurons also project to the EC of which 46% of the projections are DAergic. The EC in turn sends glutamatergic projections to the striatum, mainly to the NAc core (Krayniak et al., 1981; Finch et al., 1995; Moser et al., 2010). Similar to the VTA-NAc connectivity, the majority of the fibers (92%) arrive at the ipsilateral EC whereas the remaining fibers reach the contralateral EC (Swanson, 1982). In addition to the bidirectional communication between the VTA and the NAc, and the VTA-EC-NAc circuit, these structures are also part of a complex loop engaging the hippocampus. Specifically, DAergic neurons in the VTA project to the hippocampus which through the subiculum, NAc and the ventral pallidum releases DA neurons in the VTA from tonic inhibitory ventral pallidum influence (Lisman and Grace, 2005). In addition, the glutamatergic neurons in the VTA project back to the ventral pallidum (Hnasko et al., 2012).

Observation of the mesostriatal and mesolimbic DA pathways reveals a symmetrical connectivity with a primary influence in the ipsilateral side and a minor influence in the contralateral side (illustrated in **Figure 1**). Symmetrical fiber connectivity entails that unilateral manipulations of the DA system will affect mainly the manipulated side and that the outcome of left vs. right manipulations will be symmetrical as long as physiological factors are not taken into account. Inter-hemispheric communication allowing bilateral influence of unilateral manipulation is supported primarily by the PFC without breaking the symmetry. It is noteworthy that information is lacking regarding fiber distribution differences in the left vs. right hemispheres. If fiber distribution differences exist, they may yield asymmetrical, bi-lateral response to a variety of unilateral manipulations.

ENDOGENOUS ASYMMETRY IN THE DAergic SYSTEM

Endogenous differences in the DA system of population of animals were observed in adulthood by many groups. These differences were expressed in DA level and metabolites, D1 and D2 receptor concentration, binding potential of the receptors and DA transporters measured in the neocortex, striatum and NAc. However, reports by different laboratories do not always concur in occurrence site, magnitude and the directionality of the observed imbalance (Glick et al., 1982; Schneider et al., 1982; Denenberg and Rosen, 1983; Drew et al., 1986; Fride and

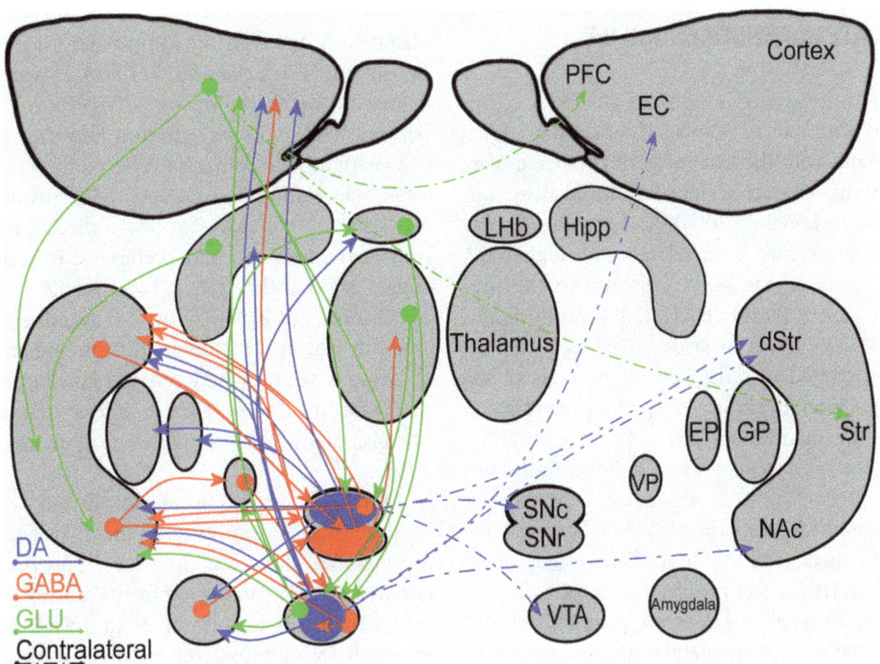

FIGURE 1 | A schematic diagram of the connectivity within and between the mesostriatal pathways and related structures. Shown are the ipsilateral (solid lines) and contralateral (dashed lines) projections of fibers containing DA (blue), GABA (red), or glutamate (green). Abbreviations: PFC, Prefrontal Cortex; EC, Entorhinal cortex; Hipp, Hippocampus; LHb, Lateral Habenula; Str, Striatum; dStr, Dorsal Striatum; NAc, Nucleus Accumbens; GP, Globus pallidus; EP, Entopeduncular nucleus; VP, Ventral Pallidum; SNc, Substantia Nigra Pars Compacta; SNr, Substantia Nigra Pars Reticulata; VTA, Ventral Tegmental Area.

Weinstock, 1987; Nowak, 1989; Rodriguez et al., 1994; Giardino, 1996; Becker, 1999; Thiel and Schwarting, 2001; Van Dyck et al., 2002; Silva et al., 2007; Vernaleken et al., 2007; Cannon et al., 2009; Martin-Soelch et al., 2011; Hsiao et al., 2013). Examination of the results and experimental conditions reveals, in addition to methodology of measurement, differences in animals' age, gender ratio, and in the species and strains of animals used. A clue for reconciling this discrepancy may be found in reports describing an inter-hemispheric regulatory/compensatory process which acts differentially in both hemispheres to restore DAergic balance. Such a process has been suggested to be active during development (Rodriguez et al., 1994; Giardino, 1996; Frohna et al., 1997; Vernaleken et al., 2007) and following tissue damage (Altar et al., 1983; Pritzel et al., 1983; Carlson et al., 1996; Roedter et al., 2001; Blesa et al., 2011). This regulatory/compensatory process which is time-dependent utilizes mechanisms of action such as controlling the ratio of D1/D2 receptors (Joyce, 1991a,b), changing the number of synaptic terminals (Jaeger et al., 1983; Lawler et al., 1995; Meshul et al., 1999; Gittis et al., 2011; Golden et al., 2013), and enhancing DA turnover and release from the available fibers (Ikegami et al., 2006). If the influence of this regulatory process on the expression of DA imbalance is experience dependent the discrepancy across laboratories could be reconciled because the variance in animals' experience is likely to be smaller within a laboratory than across laboratories. Hence, observation of hemispheric chemical imbalance may be obscured by the animal's unique experience and therefore studying DA imbalance in relation to animal behavior, preferably during a well-defined task, may minimize the influence of experience and could potentially reveal a robust effect that is consistent across laboratories.

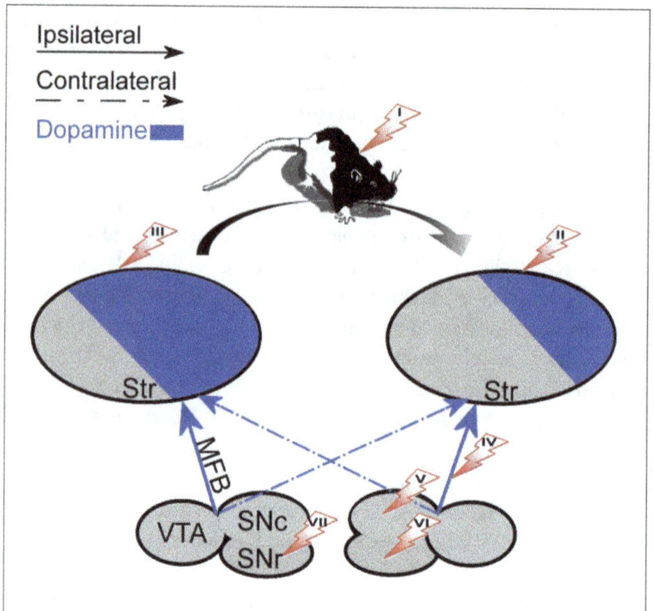

FIGURE 2 | The effect of unilateral biochemical manipulations. The specified manipulations were placed on the side that induced rotation in the right direction (marked with an arrow). The direction of rotation was always contralateral to the striatum with a high DA concentration (left). (I) systemic administration of d-amphetamine (enhances natural asymmetry). (II) 6-OHDA lesion of the striatum. (III) DA agonists, Acetylcholine antagonists or NMDA administered to the striatum. (IV) 6-OHDA lesion of the MFB. (V) 6-OHDA lesion or DA administration to the SNc. (VI) GABA antagonists administered to the SNr. (VII) DA agonists, Acetylcholine agonists or GABA agonists administered to the SNr.

BEHAVIORAL CORRELATES OF ENDOGENOUS DA ASYMMETRY

The degree of right hand preference in humans positively correlates with left putamen dominance, whereas right caudate dominance positively correlates with the level of performance during simultaneous bimanual movements in right-handed healthy subjects (De La Fuente-Fernandez et al., 2000). Rodents also display paw preference yet this preference is correlated with higher DA and DOPAC concentrations in the NAc ipsilateral to the preferred limb (Cabib et al., 1995; Budilin et al., 2008). Additionally, lateralization of DOPAC/DA ratios in favor of the right ventral striatum was positively related to right-side thigmotaxis (Thiel and Schwarting, 2001). Generally, however, spatial preference in rodents appears to be the manifestation of difference in activity occurring between the nigrostriatal systems. Specifically, rats forced to select a side (left or right) in a T maze displayed significantly higher DA content in the striatum contralateral to the preferred side than to the ipsilateral striatum (Zimmerberg et al., 1974). Similarly, the preferred direction of rotation was directly linked to the asymmetry in baseline DA (see **Figure 2**): the preferred direction of rotation was contralateral to the striatum with higher DA (Glick et al., 1988). Further support for this observation comes from intracranial self-stimulation experiments showing that the side having a lower threshold for stimulation was contralateral to the direction of spontaneous rotations (Glick et al., 1981). Opposite to DA levels, lower DOPAC values were observed in the striatum contralateral to the preferred direction of rotation (Glick et al., 1977, 1988). However, haloperidol, which decreases the activation of DA receptors, inversed the relation between DOPAC concentration and direction of rotation without changing the animal's preferred direction (Jerussi and Taylor, 1982), suggesting that DOPAC concentration by itself may be a less reliable predictor of rotation direction. The preferred direction of rotation and paw preference in rodents are uncorrelated suggesting that they reflect two distinct processes (Nielsen et al., 1997) each correlated with DA asymmetry in a different striatal sub-region. This distinction in rodents contrasts with data showing a relation between human handedness and preferred direction of rotation; right-handers preferred left-sided turning and non-right-handers preferred right-sided turning (Mohr et al., 2003).

Other brain areas were also linked with spatial preference in rodents. For example, in the two-lever operant conditioning task rats showed a right lever bias that was correlated with enhanced activity in the left frontal cortex (Glick and Ross, 1981). Additionally, enhanced activity in the left PFC was observed during right rotation preference. These findings are consistent with reports of PFC-striatum interactions. Specifically, phasic activation of the PFC has been shown to increase DA release in the ipsilateral NAc (Taber and Fibiger, 1995) probably via glutamate-induced activation of DA neurons in the VTA (Karreman and Moghaddam, 1996).

As opposed to the motor and sensory modalities displaying characteristic laterality, limbic entities such as stressors and natural rewards (food, liquid, or pleasure) lack laterality. Nonetheless, several studies suggest that endogenous DA asymmetry can be correlated with affective behaviors as well. For example, human baseline asymmetry in D2 receptor availability in the left relative to the right striatum was associated with greater positive incentive motivation (Tomer et al., 2008; Martin-Soelch et al., 2011). Moreover, human subjects with higher D2 binding in the left hemisphere were sensitive to learning from positive reinforcement whereas those with higher D2 binding in the right hemisphere were sensitive to learning from negative reinforcement (Tomer et al., 2014). Additionally, right-biased rats were significantly more active and had a stronger side preference than left-biased rats (Glick and Ross, 1981) which also may suggest attention/motivation influence.

THE INFLUENCE OF BRAIN MANIPULATION ON ANIMAL BEHAVIOR

In the previous section we reviewed evidence showing correlations between endogenous DA imbalance and natural behavior. In the following section we examine how systemic and unilateral artificial alteration of the inter-hemispheric DA imbalance influences animals' behavior.

MANIPULATIONS IN THE NIGROSTRIATAL SYSTEM

Systemic biochemical manipulations

Systemic application of d-amphetamine, which enhances DA concentration at the DAergic terminals was found to enhance the rate of rotations in the preferred direction prior to the injection (Jerussi and Glick, 1976), as well as the inter-hemispheric difference in striatal DA content in a dose dependent manner (Glick et al., 1981). Moreover, d-amphetamine application further lowered the threshold for MFB activation and consequently further biased the side preference of self-stimulation (Glick et al., 1981). Apomorphine, which is a non-selective DA agonist, induced rotational behavior in rats similar to d-amphetamine. The induced rotation increased with apomorphine dosage until reaching a plateau (Jerussi and Glick, 1975). Conversely, apomorphine administration significantly decreased the number of times rats chose their preferred arm in a T-Maze but did not alter the side preference observed prior to drug application (Castellano et al., 1987) which may indicate drug spread into limbic regions. Inhibition of catecholamine synthesis by Alpha-methyl-para-tyrosine (AMPT) markedly reduced or completely abolished d-amphetamine induced rotation (Jerussi and Glick, 1976), but did not affect rotation elicited by apomorphine (Jerussi and Glick, 1975), suggesting that these two drugs operate differently. Haloperidol prevented the rotation elicited by both d-amphetamine and apomorphine (Jerussi and Glick, 1976), indicating its robust influence.

Local biochemical manipulations

A more selective way to induce DA imbalance in the nigrostriatal pathway is by unilaterally injecting DA agonists and antagonists into the dStr or the SN. **Figure 2** summarizes the results obtained following unilateral manipulations. Local injection of DA into the SNc induced weak ipsiversive or mixed ipsiversive and contraversive rotation probably due to DA autoreceptors which locally inhibit DA neurons (Jang et al., 2011). Injection of DA into the SNr only induced contraversive circling (Kelly et al., 1984). Local injection of apomorphine to the SNr or SNc had a mild influence on the tendency of the rats to rotate (Kelly et al., 1984), suggesting activation of other neuronal mechanisms that counteract the influence of apomorphine on DAergic neurons. Unilateral injections of apomorphine into the dStr induced contraversive turning as did injections of d-amphetamine, NMDA (Ossowska and Wolfarth, 1995), and atropine which is a muscarinic acetylcholine receptor antagonist (Jerussi and Glick, 1976).

GABA-related drugs and GABA antagonists applied intranigrally also facilitated rotational behavior; GABA, $GABA_A$ agonist (e.g., muscimol) and $GABA_B$ agonists (e.g., γ-hydroxybutyric acid and baclofen) injected unilaterally into the SNr of rats elicited contraversive turning by disinhibiting the SNr influence on the striatum and enhancing DA activation ipsilaterally to the injection site, whereas unilateral injections of $GABA_A$ antagonist (e.g., bicuculline) produced ipsiversive turning by enhancing SNr inhibition of the striatum (Olpe et al., 1977; Scheel-Kruger et al., 1977).

Unilateral optical stimulation of MSNs in the direct or the indirect striatal pathways concurred with previously described manipulations which unilaterally enhanced or attenuated DA level; direct pathway activation led to contraversive rotation, whereas indirect pathway activation yielded ipsiversive rotation (Kravitz et al., 2010). Such a selective activation of the two pathways validates the influence of DA hemispheric imbalance on preferred rotation direction in the absence of a compensatory mechanism influence.

Unilateral lesions using 6-hydroxydopamine

6-hydroxydopamine (6-OHDA) is a neurotoxic compound that selectively destroys catecholamine neurons by penetrating their membrane via the DA or noradrenaline reuptake transporters (Simola et al., 2007). The 6-OHDA injection site determines the extent of damage caused by the neurotoxin and its specificity. Unilateral injection in the MFB has been shown to lesion both the uncrossed and crossed projections of the A9 and A10 cell groups converging on the ipsilateral dStr, and produces extensive catecholamine neuron destruction of about 97% of the cells primarily in the ipsilateral SNc and VTA. The contralateral SNc and VTA are less affected by the neurotoxin injection (Altar et al., 1983) because only a small percentage of their efferents (1% and 8% in the SNc and VTA, respectively) pass through the injection site (Iwamoto et al., 1976; Altar et al., 1983; Torres and Dunnett, 2012).

A more specific lesion can be produced by injecting the neurotoxin into the SNc, which leads to the destruction of only the nigrostriatal (A9) pathway, and more focal damage can be created by lesioning sub-regions of the dStr complex, which induces cell death of 50–99% of the SNc neurons depending on the affected dStr volume (reviewed in Deumens et al., 2002). These three procedures serve as classic animal models for Parkinson's disease (Ungerstedt and Arbuthnott, 1970; Simola et al., 2007). All of these lesions produce a biochemical imbalance in which lower

DA levels are measured in the ipsilateral-to-lesion dStr than in the contralateral dStr. This biochemical imbalance is correlated with behavioral alterations such as the development of motor slowness and a turning preference bias toward the side of the lesion (Roedter et al., 2001; Simola et al., 2007). Specifically, 6-OHDA lesions of either the SNc, MFB, or the dStr induce ipsiversive-to-lesion rotation (Jerussi and Glick, 1976; Glick et al., 1977; Carman et al., 1991; Annett et al., 1992; Deumens et al., 2002). The lesion-induced turning behavior ceases within the first post-operative week (Pritzel et al., 1983) thus setting an upper bound on the time required for the compensatory processes to become evident.

It is interesting to note that unilateral optical activation of MSNs in the direct/indirect pathway induced contraversive/ipsiversive rotations similar to that induced by 6-OHDA lesions. This finding suggests that alterations in DA concentrations influence the balance in activation of the direct vs. indirect pathways; reduced DA concentration tips the scale toward activation of the striatopallidal pathway whereas enhanced DA concentration emphasizes the striatonigral pathway.

Unilateral lesions and systemic biochemical manipulations

Systemic administration of pharmacological agents influenced the direction of turning evoked by the 6-OHDA lesion by enhancing or reducing the lesion-induced biochemical imbalance. d-amphetamine produced ipsilateral circling behavior whereas haloperidol and pimozide, which decrease the activation of DA receptors, produced contralateral circling behavior in rats with 6-OHDA lesion in the SNc (Iwamoto et al., 1976). Electrolytic lesions of the SNc induced a rotation preference similar to that induced by 6-OHDA (Arbuthnott and Crow, 1971; Iwamoto et al., 1976). Systemic administration of apomorphine generated a more complex outcome depending on the type and extent of the resulting tissue damage; apomorphine yielded contraversive circling following 6-OHDA lesions (Iwamoto et al., 1976; Glick et al., 1977; Meshul and Allen, 2000) and the number of rotations depended on the extent of tissue damage. By contrast, apomorphine led to ipsiversive circling following electrolytic lesion (Iwamoto et al., 1976).

Overall, artificial enhancement of striatal DA imbalance in rodents produces circling behavior in the direction toward the side with depleted DA concentration (see **Figure 2**). The outcome of this category of manipulations which ultimately influence striatal DA processing and transmission is consistent regardless of which component in the circuit has been manipulated and whether the manipulation enhanced or attenuated activity.

MANIPULATIONS IN THE MESOLIMBIC SYSTEM

Application of 6-OHDA to the mesolimbic system produced characteristic behavioral deficits different in nature from those produced by lesioning the nigrostriatal system. Unilateral injection of 6-OHDA to the right VTA or SN impaired acquisition of operant tasks (Hritcu et al., 2008). Bilateral small 6-OHDA lesions of the VTA produced a significant increase in spontaneous locomotor activity whereas large 6-OHDA lesions of the VTA or the NAc produced hypoactivity in the open field, a complete blockade of the locomotor stimulating effects of d-amphetamine, and a profound supersensitive response to apomorphine expressed as enhanced locomotion (Koob et al., 1981). Interestingly, a radiofrequency-VTA lesion caused a greater increase in spontaneous activity relative to the VTA 6-OHDA lesion, suggesting the presence of a powerful inhibitory influence of the mesolimbic DA system within the VTA (Koob et al., 1981).

Manipulations of structures interacting with the mesolimbic system

Experiments described thus far support the view that the relationship between the manipulation-induced DA imbalance and the animal's induced rotation direction is symmetric across hemispheres (see **Figure 2**). Experiments directly assessing the existence and function of DA imbalance in the mesolimbic pathway are lacking. However, some of the information can be deduced from experiments addressing the issue indirectly, for example, by applying pharmacological intervention in structures which interact with the mesolimbic system such as the PFC, EC, and hippocampus. Such experiments reveal that despite the apparent anatomical symmetry of the fibers unilateral manipulations influence the DA system asymmetrically. The results of these experiments are summarized in **Table 1**.

The effect of PFC manipulations on the mesolimbic DA system

The PFC represents information in the short term working memory (Kolb et al., 1994; Kesner et al., 1996; Goldman-Rakic, 2011) and is crucial for spatial and emotional response selection which are influenced by mesocortical DA (Thierry et al., 1976; Delatour and Gisquet-Verrier, 1999; Sullivan, 2004). As previously mentioned the interaction between mesostriatal DA and PFC is reciprocal (Carr and Sesack, 2000; Hnasko et al., 2012; Stuber et al., 2012). 6-OHDA lesions of the mesocortical DA innervating the right mPFC and anterior cingulate induced a significant bilateral reduction in DA content and an increase in DA turnover in the striatum (Sullivan and Szechtman, 1995). Similar lesions to the left mPFC and anterior cingulate did not affect striatal DA. Moreover, similar to unilateral lesion of the right PFC, bilateral lesions also reduced DA content and increased DA turnover but the response was limited to the right NAc (Sullivan and Szechtman, 1995). Evidence for the asymmetrical influence exerted by the PFC on the striatum also comes from studies performed on human subjects. For example, application of a continuous TMS theta burst stimulation (cTBS) to the left dorsolateral PFC of healthy young right-handed adults inhibited DA release bilaterally in the caudate and ipsilaterally in the putamen, whereas right dorsolateral PFC cTBS did not influence binding potential in the striatum (Ko et al., 2008).

A few studies correlated DA imbalance following chemical manipulations of the PFC with behavior. For example, correlations were observed between DA depletion induction in the right medial PFC (mPFC) and rats exhibiting the most severe stress-induced gastric pathology—ulcers (Sullivan and Szechtman, 1995). Additionally, unilateral injection of DA (D1/D2) antagonist into the mPFC significantly enhanced the restraint stress-induced increases in corticotrophin and corticosterone in non-handled rats (Sullivan and Dufresne, 2006). However, similar experiments in handled rats showed that only

Table 1 | The reported directionality of DA imbalance in the mesolimbic system following biochemical and behavioral manipulations.

	Manipulation type \ Manipulated side	Left	Right	Bilateral	References
Local biochemical manipulations	6-OHDA mPFC	No effect	DA Str	DA NAc	Sullivan and Szechtman, 1995
			DOPAC/DA Str	DOPAC/DA NAc	
	TMS dorsolateral PFC	DA Caudate	No effect		Ko et al., 2008
		DA Putamen			
	Lidocaine mPFC and methamphetamine	DA NAc			Uehara et al., 2007
	Lidocaine mPFC, Exitotoxic EC, and methamphetamine	DA NAc			
	Exitotoxic EC	DA dStr and NAc	DOPAC/DA NAc		Uehara et al., 2000
		DA mPFC			
		DOPAC/DA NAc			
	6-OHDA EC	DA NAc	DOPAC/DA NAc		Louilot and Choulli, 1997
		DOPAC/DA NAc			
		DOPAC NAc			
	D2 antagonist EC	DOPAC NAc	No effect		Louilot and Le Moal, 1994
	D2 agonist EC	DOPAC NAc	No effect		
	D2 antagonist VH	DOPAC NAc	DOPAC NAc		
	D2 agonist VH	DOPAC NAc	DOPAC NAc		
	TTX EC	DOPAC NAc	DOPAC NAc		
Behavioral	Appetitive odor			DA NAc	Besson and Louilot, 1995
	Aversive conditioning			DA NAc	
	Tail pinch			DA NAc	Laplante et al., 2013
				DA mPFC	Sullivan and Gratton, 1998
	Repetitive restraint and handling			DOPAC mPFC	Sullivan and Dufresne, 2006
	Repetitive restraint without handling			DOPAC mPFC	
	15 min restraint			HVA/DA mPFC	Carlson et al., 1991
	60 min restraint			DA mPFC	
	Bright novel environment without distraction			DOPAC/DA PFC	Berridge et al., 1999

A circle denotes the spatial distribution of the manipulation outcome. Colored area indicates a significant increase (red) or decrease (blue) in DA or its metabolites in the corresponding hemisphere. Data were included from different species, ages, and measurement techniques.

right side DA receptor blockade induced elevation of peak stress hormone levels (Sullivan and Dufresne, 2006). These data provide supporting evidence for the asymmetrical relationship between DA imbalance in the mesolimbic system and the animals' affective behavior, and further emphasize that the animals' experience may hamper attempts to characterize this relationship.

The effect of EC and hippocampus manipulations on the mesolimbic DA system

The EC and the ventral hippocampus (VH) receive DAergic projections from the VTA, and depending on event novelty (Lisman and Grace, 2005) act upon the VTA to regulate the DAergic transmission to the NAc (Louilot and Le Moal, 1994; Kurachi et al., 2000). Inter-hemispheric comparison of changes in DA and DOPAC concentration in the NAc and related regions following pharmacological intervention in the EC or VH revealed a time-dependent process with complex lateralization. Excitotoxic lesion of the left EC decreased DOPAC levels in the NAc and the mPFC 2 weeks post lesion (Kurachi et al., 2000). Moreover, measurements performed in adolescence following excitotoxic lesion of the left EC in newborn rats showed bilateral enhancement of DA concentration in the NAc and dStr, and a unilateral decrease in the right mPFC. The NAc also displayed a bilateral decrease in DOPAC/DA concentration ratio whereas the dStr did not. None of these alterations in the DA system was detected in the newborns (Uehara et al., 2000). When the left EC of adult rats was lesioned with 6-OHDA the outcome was reversed; DA tissue content decreased whereas DOPAC tissue content and the resultant DOPAC/DA ratio increased in the NAc (Louilot and Choulli, 1997). It remains to be seen whether the differences in outcome are due to the age at which the lesion was made or due to the lesion type. A similar lesion to the right EC caused elevation in DOPAC/DA ratio only in the left NAc (Louilot and Choulli, 1997). A more specific intervention by manipulation of both D1 and D2 receptors in the EC and VH significantly influenced DOPAC concentrations in the NAc such that the effect of the D2 manipulation was more pronounced than that of D1 (Louilot and Le Moal, 1994). Specifically, administration of a D2 receptor antagonist in the left EC increased DOPAC concentration in both NAc whereas administration of a D2 agonist caused the opposite effect (i.e., decreased DOPAC concentration in both NAc). Injection of a D2 antagonist or agonist into the right EC did not influence DOPAC levels in the NAc. Injections of a D2 antagonist and agonist into the VH evoked similar responses as left EC injections but the response was limited to the side ipsilateral to the injected hemisphere (Louilot and Le Moal, 1994). Moreover, injection of the neurotoxic compound Tetrodotoxin (TTX) into the left EC decreased DOPAC in both NAc whereas TTX in the right EC increased DA transmission in the ipsilateral NAc and decreased DOPAC in the contralateral NAc (Louilot and Le Moal, 1994). Unilateral TTX injections into the VH decreased DOPAC in the NAc of both hemispheres irrespective of injection side (Louilot and Le Moal, 1994). These side-dependent alterations in NAc DA release and its metabolites support the existence of an asymmetrical functional interdependence between midbrain DAergic pathways reaching the EC and the NAc (Louilot and Choulli, 1997).

Consistent with altered mesolimbic DAergic transmission, a left EC excitotoxic lesion in adult rats enhanced spontaneous and methamphetamine induced locomotor activity (Sumiyoshi et al., 2004; Kopniczky et al., 2006). Interestingly, the methamphetamine-induced normalized DA release in the ipsilateral NAc or dStr did not change in comparison to sham-operated animals possibly due to enhanced postsynaptic sensitivity rather than presynaptic alteration in DA levels (Uehara et al., 2000; Sumiyoshi et al., 2004). When the excitotoxic lesion to the left EC was combined with ipsilateral inactivation of the mPFC by lidocaine (a non-selective blocker of axonal fibers of passage as well as neurons) the methamphetamine-induced DA release in the ipsilateral NAc was substantially enhanced (Uehara et al., 2007). By contrast, ipsilateral inactivation of the mPFC by lidocaine alone reduced the methamphetamine-induced DA release in the NAc, which is consistent with previous data. Overall, inactivation of the mPFC together with structural abnormalities in the EC leads to deregulation of DAergic neurotransmission in limbic regions (Uehara et al., 2007).

The results described thus far strengthen assumptions concerning the lateralized involvement of the PFC, the EC, and the VH in the modulation and possibly regulation of mesostriatal DA asymmetry (Glick and Ross, 1981; Glick and Carlson, 1989; Fox and Reed, 2008). Overall, it seems that the nigrostriatal system displays symmetrical laterality (i.e., the outcome of different manipulations applied to one hemisphere is a mirror image of the outcome obtained when the manipulation is applied to other hemispheres), whereas the DA mesolimbic system and related structures display asymmetrical laterality (i.e., the outcome of different unilateral manipulations is not a mirror image of the same manipulation applied to the other hemisphere), The occurrence of an asymmetrical laterality supports the notion of specialized hemispheric function (Sullivan, 2004; Fox and Reed, 2008).

THE INFLUENCE OF ANIMAL TRAINING ON DA IMBALANCE IN THE NIGROSTRIATAL SYSTEM

Thus, far we have described how endogenous DA imbalance in the nigrostriatal system correlates with animal behavior and how accentuation of this biochemical imbalance can alter behavior. Below we address the opposite question of whether utilizing different behavioral tasks can induce or influence the basal DA imbalance.

Prior to training on an electrified T-maze (Zimmerberg et al., 1974) a relatively small percentage (about 54–59%) of animals displayed side preference (Castellano et al., 1987). After training the vast majority (85.71%) of the rats displayed a side preference with a strong bias toward the right arm (80%—right arm preference; 20%—left arm preference) (Castellano et al., 1987). Unilateral lesions using 6-OHDA ipsilaterally to the preferred side did not change preference parameters, whereas contralateral lesion massively and persistently decreased the choice of the side preferred preoperatively (Castellano et al., 1987). A similar outcome was observed when rats were trained to circle for a sucrose reward in a randomly assigned direction. Prior to training, caudate and NAc DA and DOPAC levels were the same in both hemispheres. By contrast, following training a significant increase occurred in both DA and DOPAC concentrations in the caudate and NAc contralateral to the turning direction whereas these concentrations did not change in the ipsilateral caudate compared to control animals (Yamamoto and Freed, 1982, 1984a). Amphetamine administration further enhanced turning in the trained direction regardless of the animals' previous circling preference. As in naive animals, amphetamine-induced circling led to increased DA concentrations in the caudate contralateral to the trained circling direction (Yamamoto and Freed, 1984b). These findings are congruent with the previously described relationship between DA imbalance and side preference.

Similar experiments (Szostak et al., 1986, 1988, 1989; Glick and Carlson, 1989) in which water-deprived animals were trained on circling behavior failed to replicate the results described by Yamamoto et al. (Yamamoto and Freed, 1982, 1984a,b). In particular, circling did not produce a biochemical imbalance in the nigrostriatal and the mesolimbic DA system; rats trained to circle using a continuous schedule of reinforcement did not exhibit any change in concentrations of striatal DA or DOPAC although alterations in DA and DA turnover were detected in the mPFC (Szostak et al., 1986; Glick and Carlson, 1989). Changing the reward schedule induced enhanced DAergic activity in both the NAc and the dStr (Szostak et al., 1986). A plausible explanation arises from a report which showed that different regions of the striatum exhibit different DA and DOPAC concentrations, thus suggesting striatal region specialization (Szostak et al., 1989). Importantly, the use of a water deprivation protocol without circling training was sufficient to induce a bilateral decrease in DOPAC/DA ratio in the NAc and mPFC (Glick and Carlson, 1989).

The following experiments further strengthen the relationship between DA imbalance and rotation direction. Unilateral 6-OHDA lesions of the MFB of rats trained to circle in their preferred direction for water reinforcement revealed a complex scenario that fits relatively well with the chemical imbalance described in control animals. Specifically, rats with a lesion contralateral to their trained direction stopped turning in that direction and often turned in the untrained direction. By contrast, rats lesioned ipsilaterally to the direction of reinforced circling exhibited only a 50% decrease in the rate of reinforced responding. These findings also highlight the effect of training on DA hemispheric imbalance. Following these procedures the experimental contingencies were reversed such that all rats had to turn in the untrained direction. After the reversal, the contralaterally lesioned group had to turn toward the lesion and consequently easily acquired the reversal, however, reinforced rates of responding did not reach preoperative rates possibly due to altered motivation (Mogenson et al., 1980; Smith et al., 2002; Wise, 2002; Solstad et al., 2008). Conversely, the ipsilaterally lesioned group had to turn away from the lesion and consequently was unable to acquire the reversal and continued to turn in the originally trained direction (Szostak et al., 1988). These findings are in line with the previously described rotation direction induced by 6-OHDA lesions. Moreover, these experiments suggest a causal relationship between DA imbalance and rotation direction because they imply that the direction of circling cannot be altered by training as long as the biochemical imbalance cannot be reversed.

Overall, by considering that alterations in DA/DOPAC concentrations resulting from training appear to be sensitive to variations in the training protocol such as reward schedule, severity and type of deprivation (food or water), type of reward delivered (sucrose, water, or food) and level of performance reached following training, the question whether DA imbalance may be effectively manipulated by training, which is a simple non-invasive procedure and as such may have a therapeutic capacity, remains controversial. These findings also raise the question whether the observed behavioral bias is a byproduct of the current DA imbalance or whether the regulatory mechanism promotes actions aimed to attenuate the inherent hemispheric laterality by overworking the less active regions.

THE INFLUENCE OF ANIMAL TRAINING ON DA IMBALANCE IN THE MESOLIMBIC SYSTEM

The question whether behavioral manipulations can induce or influence DA imbalance in the mesolimbic system has been addressed by utilizing different behavioral paradigms involving stress. Stress induction lacks laterality and therefore in all of the experiments emergent results reflect internal network properties. In this section we focus primarily on experiments showing DA measures in the NAc and PFC in attempt to identify whether laterality appears. A summary of the results is shown in **Table 1**.

DA responses to a naturally attractive olfactory stimulus were elevated in both NAc, most markedly in the right core. However, conditioned taste aversion following LiCl treatment resulted in elevation in DA levels in the left but not right NAc core which further expanded to the left shell upon a second presentation of the now aversive stimulus (Besson and Louilot, 1995). Different results were obtained when instead of presenting aversive stimulus physical stress was applied. The amplitude of DA release following tail pinch was higher in the right NAc compared to the left (Laplante et al., 2013) whereas in the mPFC DA release increased bilaterally (Sullivan and Gratton, 1998). Moreover, the duration of DA response in the left mPFC was significantly longer than that in the right mPFC (Sullivan and Gratton, 1998).

DA measures in the right mPFC correlated with reduced stress levels following 5 repetitions of restraint stress induction in both handled and non-handled animals (Sullivan and Dufresne, 2006). However, in handled rats DA turnover in the right mPFC was significantly higher than the left whereas in non-handled rats DA turnover in the left mPFC was significantly higher relative to the right mPFC (Sullivan and Dufresne, 2006). It should be noted however, that these results are incongruent with earlier findings regarding the cortical lateralization of emotional regulation which is facilitated by early postnatal handling stimulation, and fails to occur in the absence of postnatal handling (Denenberg, 1981; Sullivan and Dufresne, 2006). DA turnover in the right mPFC was higher than the left also in animals that received a foot shock without being able to terminate it (Carlson et al., 1993). When animals could control foot shock termination, DA turnover increased in the mPFC bilaterally (Carlson et al., 1993). Similarly, when rats and mice were exposed to a brightly lit novel environment (novelty stress) DA turnover in the right PFC was significantly higher than the left PFC in animals that weren't given the option of engaging in a non-escape behavior (e.g., chewing an inedible object), compared to those who did (Berridge et al., 1999). Thus, once animals are able to attenuate the physiological stress by controlling stressor termination or by engaging in a coping or displacement behavior the stress-induced DA response in the right PFC is attenuated (Berridge et al., 1999).

DA concentration measurements following different durations of restraint stress provide additional support for the correlation observed between stress level and DA imbalance in the mPFC. DA concentration increased in the right mPFC and reached significance relative to the left mPFC after the animals were kept restraint for an hour, and DA turnover was significantly higher in the left relative to the right mPFC following 15 min of restraint stress but not following prolonged restraint duration. These experiments suggest an alternative hypothesis in which a left to right shift in the mesocortical DA activation occurs with prolonged exposure to stress (Carlson et al., 1991).

The lack of agreement between these reports suggests that laterality in the mesolimbic DA system depends on factors such as the type of induced stress, stress duration and animal's previous experience (Denenberg, 1981; Fox and Reed, 2008). Therefore, these experiments do not allow addressing the question of whether causality exists between DA imbalance in the mesolimbic system and behavior; whether DA imbalance can reduce stress levels or alternatively that DA imbalance is determined by the animals' sensitivity to stress induction should be addressed by utilizing different experimental methods. In any case, despite the absence of a consistent link between behavioral manipulations lacking directionality and DA imbalance in the mesolimbic system these experiments support an asymmetrical processing characteristic of a specialized left vs. right network.

DISCUSSION

DA imbalance across brain hemispheres is inherent in newborns. With development, this imbalance decreases due to an inter-hemispheric time-dependent regulatory mechanism which differentially influences the DA system in each hemisphere (Rodriguez et al., 1994; Giardino, 1996; Frohna et al., 1997; Vernaleken et al., 2007). This mechanism also compensates for alterations in the endogenous DA imbalance following brain lesion and possibly neurodegenerative processes. The existence of such a mechanism raises the question whether there is a way to influence DA imbalance by utilizing specially designed behavioral manipulations that directly or indirectly activate the mechanism. Although controversial, studies in the nigrostriatal system suggest this possibility is feasible whereas in the mesolimbic system the feasibility of this approach remains to be explored. If successful, this approach can influence the development of novel non-invasive therapeutic means for the treatment of various disorders affected by alterations in DA imbalance.

The EC, the hippocampus, and PFC are part of a network which modulates NAc responses to DA arriving from the VTA. This network seems to display asymmetric left-right laterality rather than displaying the symmetric laterality observed in the nigrostriatal system. This difference in laterality is consistent with the roles played by each BG circuit: the sensorimotor and associative regions (dStr) display laterality which matches the laterality of their sensory inputs, whereas the limbic regions (NAc) which process abstract inputs supposedly lacking laterality are sensitive to the laterality of prefrontal and temporal lobe structures. Such laterality fits well with the concept of hemispheric specialization described in the PFC in relation to various behaviors (Clark et al., 2003; Sullivan, 2004; Goel et al., 2007; Fox and Reed, 2008; Lupinsky et al., 2010). Additional studies are required to determine whether the observed left-right laterality in the mesolimbic system has functional implications for information processing in subcortical structures (e.g., BG) or does it merely reflect the asymmetric functionality in structures such as the EC and the PFC.

The DA system plays a major role in the planning and execution of movements and in acquisition and expression of learned appetitive behaviors which allow the organism to adapt to its surrounding and thus essential for animals survival. To enable comprehensive understanding of the structure and function of this system, it is essential to plan and execute experiments which in addition to factors such as age, gender, and previous experience, take into account the existence of hemispheric specialization, the endogenous DA imbalance and its influence on behavior, and the way in which behavior can influence this imbalance.

ACKNOWLEDGMENT

This study was financed in part by a REALNET (FP7-ICT270434) grant from the European Commission.

REFERENCES

Albin, R. L., Young, A. B., and Penney, J. B. (1989). The functional anatomy of basal ganglia disorders. *Trends Neurosci.* 12, 366–375. doi: 10.1016/0166-2236(89)90074-X

Alexander, G. E., and Crutcher, M. D. (1990). Functional architecture of basal ganglia circuits: neural substrates of parallel processing. *Trends Neurosci.* 13, 266–271. doi: 10.1016/0166-2236(90)90107-L

Alloway, K. D., Lou, L., Nwabueze-Ogbo, F., and Chakrabarti, S. (2006). Topography of cortical projections to the dorsolateral neostriatum in rats: multiple overlapping sensorimotor pathways. *J. Comp. Neurol.* 499, 33–48. doi: 10.1002/cne.21039

Altar, A., Neve, K. A., Loughlin, S. E., Marshall, J. F., and Fallon, J. H. (1983). The crossed mesostriatal projection: neurochemistry and developmental response to lesion. *Brain Res.* 279, 1–8. doi: 10.1016/0006-8993(83)90157-9

Annett, L. E., Rogers, D. C., Hernandez, T. D., and Dunnett, S. B. (1992). Behavioural analysis of unilateral monoamine depletion in the marmoset. *Brain* 115(Pt 3), 825–856. doi: 10.1093/brain/115.3.825

Arbuthnott, G. W., and Crow, T. J. (1971). Relation of contraversive turning to unilateral release of dopamine from the nigrostriatal pathway in rats. *Exp. Neurol.* 30, 484–491. doi: 10.1016/0014-4886(71)90149-X

Becker, J. B. (1999). Gender differences in dopaminergic function in striatum and nucleus accumbens. *Pharmacol. Biochem. Behav.* 64, 803–812. doi: 10.1016/S0091-3057(99)00168-9

Berns, G. S., and Sejnowski, T. J. (1998). A computational model of how the basal ganglia produce sequences. *J. Cogn. Neurosci.* 10, 108–121. doi: 10.1162/089892998563815

Berridge, C. W., Mitton, E., Clark, W., and Roth, R. H. (1999). Engagement in a non-escape (displacement) behavior elicits a selective and lateralized suppression of frontal cortical dopaminergic utilization in stress. *Synapse* 32, 187–197. doi: 10.1002/(SICI)1098-2396(19990601)32:3<187::AID-SYN5>3.0.CO;2-9

Besson, C., and Louilot, A. (1995). Asymmetrical involvement of mesolimbic dopaminergic neurons in affective perception. *Neuroscience* 68, 963–968. doi: 10.1016/0306-4522(95)00255-H

Blesa, J., Juri, C., Garcia-Cabezas, M. A., Adanez, R., Sanchez-Gonzalez, M. A., Cavada, C., et al. (2011). Inter-hemispheric asymmetry of nigrostriatal dopaminergic lesion: a possible compensatory mechanism in Parkinson's disease. *Front. Syst. Neurosci.* 5:92. doi: 10.3389/fnsys.2011.00092

Bolam, J. P., Powell, J. F., Wu, J. Y., and Smith, A. D. (1985). Glutamate decarboxylase-immunoreactive structures in the rat neostriatum: a correlated light and electron microscopic study including a combination of Golgi impregnation with immunocytochemistry. *J. Comp. Neurol.* 237, 1–20. doi: 10.1002/cne.902370102

Bolam, J. P., Smith, Y., Ingham, C. A., Von Krosigk, M., and Smith, A. D. (1993). Convergence of synaptic terminals from the striatum and the globus pallidus onto single neurones in the substantia nigra and the entopeduncular nucleus. *Prog. Brain Res.* 99, 73–88. doi: 10.1016/S0079-6123(08)61339-4

Bracha, H. S., Seitz, D. J., Otemaa, J., and Glick, S. D. (1987). Rotational movement (circling) in normal humans: sex difference and relationship to hand, foot and eye preference. *Brain Res.* 411, 231–235. doi: 10.1016/0006-8993(87)91074-2

Brog, J. S., Salyapongse, A., Deutch, A. Y., and Zahm, D. S. (1993). The patterns of afferent innervation of the core and shell in the "accumbens" part of the rat ventral striatum: immunohistochemical detection of retrogradely transported fluoro-gold. *J. Comp. Neurol.* 338, 255–278. doi: 10.1002/cne.903380209

Budilin, S. Y., Midzyanovskaya, I. S., Shchegolevskii, N. V., Ioffe, M. E., and Bazyan, A. S. (2008). Asymmetry in dopamine levels in the nucleus accumbens and motor preference in rats. *Neurosci. Behav. Physiol.* 38, 991–994. doi: 10.1007/s11055-008-9082-6

Cabib, S., D'Amato, F. R., Neveu, P. J., Deleplanque, B., Le Moal, M., and Puglisi-Allegra, S. (1995). Paw preference and brain dopamine asymmetries. *Neuroscience* 64, 427–432. doi: 10.1016/0306-4522(94)00401-P

Cannon, D. M., Klaver, J. M., Peck, S. A., Rallis-Voak, D., Erickson, K., and Drevets, W. C. (2009). Dopamine type-1 receptor binding in major depressive disorder assessed using positron emission tomography and [11C]NNC-112. *Neuropsychopharmacology* 34, 1277–1287. doi: 10.1038/npp.2008.194

Carlson, J. N., Fitzgerald, L. W., Keller, R. W. Jr., and Glick, S. D. (1991). Side and region dependent changes in dopamine activation with various durations of restraint stress. *Brain Res.* 550, 313–318. doi: 10.1016/0006-8993(91)91333-V

Carlson, J. N., Fitzgerald, L. W., Keller, R. W. Jr., and Glick, S. D. (1993). Lateralized changes in prefrontal cortical dopamine activity induced by controllable and uncontrollable stress in the rat. *Brain Res.* 630, 178–187. doi: 10.1016/0006-8993(93)90655-7

Carlson, J. N., Visker, K. E., Keller, R. W. Jr., and Glick, S. D. (1996). Left and right 6-hydroxydopamine lesions of the medial prefrontal cortex differentially alter subcortical dopamine utilization and the behavioral response to stress. *Brain Res.* 711, 1–9. doi: 10.1016/0006-8993(95)01290-7

Carman, L. S., Gage, F. H., and Shults, C. W. (1991). Partial lesion of the substantia nigra: relation between extent of lesion and rotational behavior. *Brain Res.* 553, 275–283. doi: 10.1016/0006-8993(91)90835-J

Carr, D. B., and Sesack, S. R. (2000). Projections from the rat prefrontal cortex to the ventral tegmental area: target specificity in the synaptic associations with mesoaccumbens and mesocortical neurons. *J. Neurosci.* 20, 3864–3873.

Carter, D. A., and Fibiger, H. C. (1977). Ascending projections of presumed dopamine-containing neurons in the ventral tegmentum of the rat as demonstrated by horseradish peroxidase. *Neuroscience* 2, 569–576. doi: 10.1016/0306-4522(77)90052-5

Castellano, M. A., Diaz-Palarea, M. D., Rodriguez, M., and Barroso, J. (1987). Lateralization in male rats and dopaminergic system: evidence of right-side population bias. *Physiol. Behav.* 40, 607–612. doi: 10.1016/0031-9384(87)90105-3

Clark, L., Manes, F., Antoun, N., Sahakian, B. J., and Robbins, T. W. (2003). The contributions of lesion laterality and lesion volume to decision-making impairment following frontal lobe damage. *Neuropsychologia* 41, 1474–1483. doi: 10.1016/S0028-3932(03)00081-2

Consolazione, A., Bentivoglio, M., Goldstein, M., and Toffano, G. (1985). Evidence for crossed catecholaminergic nigrostriatal projections by combining wheat germ agglutinin-horseradish peroxidase retrograde transport and tyrosine hydroxylase immunocytochemistry. *Brain Res.* 338, 140–143. doi: 10.1016/0006-8993(85)90256-2

Dahlstroem, A., and Fuxe, K. (1964). Evidence for the existence of monoamine-containing neurons in the central nervous system. I. Demonstration of monoamines in the cell bodies of brain stem neurons. *Acta Physiol. Scand. Suppl.* Suppl. 232, 231–255.

Davidson, R. J., and Kenneth, H. (2004). *The Asymmetrical Brain.* Cambridge, MA: MIT Press.

De La Fuente-Fernandez, R., Kishore, A., Calne, D. B., Ruth, T. J., and Stoessl, A. J. (2000). Nigrostriatal dopamine system and motor lateralization. *Behav. Brain Res.* 112, 63–68. doi: 10.1016/S0166-4328(00)00165-0

Delatour, B., and Gisquet-Verrier, P. (1999). Lesions of the prelimbic-infralimbic cortices in rats do not disrupt response selection processes but induce delay-dependent deficits: evidence for a role in working memory? *Behav. Neurosci.* 113, 941–955. doi: 10.1037/0735-7044.113.5.941

Delong, M. R., and Wichmann, T. (2007). Circuits and circuit disorders of the basal ganglia. *Arch. Neurol.* 64, 20–24. doi: 10.1001/archneur.64.1.20

Denenberg, V. H. (1981). Hemispheric laterality in animals and the effects of early experience. *Behav. Brain Sci.* 4, 1–49. doi: 10.1017/S0140525X00007330

Denenberg, V. H., and Rosen, G. D. (1983). Interhemispheric coupling coefficients: sex differences in brain neurochemistry. *Am. J. Physiol.* 245, R151–R153.

Deumens, R., Blokland, A., and Prickaerts, J. (2002). Modeling Parkinson's disease in rats: an evaluation of 6-OHDA lesions of the nigrostriatal pathway. *Exp. Neurol.* 175, 303–317. doi: 10.1006/exnr.2002.7891

Douglas, R., Kellaway, L., Mintz, M., and Van Wageningen, G. (1987). The crossed nigrostriatal projection decussates in the ventral tegmental decussation. *Brain Res.* 418, 111–121. doi: 10.1016/0006-8993(87)90967-X

Drew, K. L., Lyon, R. A., Titeler, M., and Glick, S. D. (1986). Asymmetry in D-2 binding in female rat striata. *Brain Res.* 363, 192–195. doi: 10.1016/0006-8993(86)90678-5

Fallon, J. H., Wang, C., Kim, Y., Canepa, N., Loughlin, S., and Seroogy, K. (1983). Dopamine- and cholecystokinin-containing neurons of the crossed mesostriatal projection. *Neurosci. Lett.* 40, 233–238. doi: 10.1016/0304-3940(83)90044-7

Fass, B., and Butcher, L. L. (1981). Evidence for a crossed nigrostriatal pathway in rats. *Neurosci. Lett.* 22, 109–113. doi: 10.1016/0304-3940(81)90072-0

Finch, D. M., Gigg, J., Tan, A. M., and Kosoyan, O. P. (1995). Neurophysiology and neuropharmacology of projections from entorhinal cortex to striatum in the rat. *Brain Res.* 670, 233–247. doi: 10.1016/0006-8993(94)01279-Q

Fisher, R. S., Boylan, M. K., Hull, C. D., Buchwald, N. A., and Levine, M. S. (1986). Branched projections of cat sensorimotor cortex: multiple retrograde labeling via commissural corticocortical, decussated corticostriatal and undecussated corticostriatal axons. *Brain Res.* 384, 395–400. doi: 10.1016/0006-8993(86)91180-7

Fox, N. A., and Reed, B. C. (2008). "Cortical Asymmetry-effects of early experience on the development of cerebral asymmetry and approach-withdrawal" in *Handbook of Approach and Avoidance Motivation*, ed A. J. Elliot (New York, NY: Psychology Press), 35–49.

Fride, E., and Weinstock, M. (1987). Increased interhemispheric coupling of the dopamine systems induced by prenatal stress. *Brain Res. Bull.* 18, 457–461. doi: 10.1016/0361-9230(87)90020-7

Frohna, P. A., Neal-Beliveau, B. S., and Joyce, J. N. (1997). Delayed plasticity of the mesolimbic dopamine system following neonatal 6-OHDA lesions. *Synapse* 25, 293–305. doi: 10.1002/(SICI)1098-2396(199703)25:3<293::AID-SYN9>3.0.CO;2-6

Gazzaniga, M. S. (1995). Principles of human brain organization derived from split-brain studies. *Neuron* 14, 217–228. doi: 10.1016/0896-6273(95)90280-5

Gerfen, C. R. (1984). The neostriatal mosaic: compartmentalization of corticostriatal input and striatonigral output systems. *Nature* 311, 461–464. doi: 10.1038/311461a0

Gerfen, C. R. (1985). The neostriatal mosaic. I. Compartmental organization of projections from the striatum to the substantia nigra in the rat. *J. Comp. Neurol.* 236, 454–476. doi: 10.1002/cne.902360404

Gerfen, C. R., Engber, T. M., Mahan, L. C., Susel, Z., Chase, T. N., Monsma, F. J., et al. (1990). D1 and D2 dopamine receptor-regulated gene expression of striatonigral and striatopallidal neurons. *Science* 250, 1429–1432. doi: 10.1126/science.2147780

Gerfen, C. R., Herkenham, M., and Thibault, J. (1987). The neostriatal mosaic: II. Patch- and matrix-directed mesostriatal dopaminergic and non-dopaminergic systems. *J. Neurosci.* 7, 3915–3934.

Gerfen, C. R., Staines, W. A., Arbuthnott, G. W., and Fibiger, H. C. (1982). Crossed connections of the substantia nigra in the rat. *J. Comp. Neurol.* 207, 283–303. doi: 10.1002/cne.902070308

Giardino, L. (1996). Right-left asymmetry of D1- and D2-receptor density is lost in the basal ganglia of old rats. *Brain Res.* 720, 235–238. doi: 10.1016/0006-8993(96)00144-8

Gittis, A. H., Hang, G. B., Ladow, E. S., Shoenfeld, L. R., Atallah, B. V., Finkbeiner, S., et al. (2011). Rapid target-specific remodeling of fast-spiking inhibitory circuits after loss of dopamine. *Neuron* 71, 858–868. doi: 10.1016/j.neuron.2011.06.035

Glick, S. D., and Carlson, J. N. (1989). Regional changes in brain dopamine and serotonin metabolism induced by conditioned circling in rats: effects of water deprivation, learning and individual differences in asymmetry. *Brain Res.* 504, 231–237. doi: 10.1016/0006-8993(89)91362-0

Glick, S. D., Carlson, J. N., Baird, J. L., Maisonneuve, I. M., and Bullock, A. E. (1988). Basal and amphetamine-induced asymmetries in striatal dopamine release and metabolism: bilateral *in vivo* microdialysis in normal rats. *Brain Res.* 473, 161–164. doi: 10.1016/0006-8993(88)90329-0

Glick, S. D., Jerussi, T. P., and Zimmerberg, B. (1977). "Behavioral and neuropharmacological correlates of nigrostriatal asymmetry in rats," in *Lateralization in the Nervous System*, ed S. Harnad (Oxford: Elsevier Science), 213–249. doi: 10.1016/B978-0-12-325750-5.50020-8

Glick, S. D., and Ross, D. A. (1981). Right-sided population bias and lateralization of activity in normal rats. *Brain Res.* 205, 222–225. doi: 10.1016/0006-8993(81)90737-X

Glick, S. D., Ross, D. A., and Hough, L. B. (1982). Lateral asymmetry of neurotransmitters in human brain. *Brain Res.* 234, 53–63. doi: 10.1016/0006-8993(82)90472-3

Glick, S. D., Weaver, L. M., and Meibach, R. C. (1981). Amphetamine enhancement of reward asymmetry. *Psychopharmacology (Berl.)* 73, 323–327. doi: 10.1007/BF00426459

Goel, V., Tierney, M., Sheesley, L., Bartolo, A., Vartanian, O., and Grafman, J. (2007). Hemispheric specialization in human prefrontal cortex for resolving certain and uncertain inferences. *Cereb. Cortex* 17, 2245–2250. doi: 10.1093/cercor/bhl132

Golden, J. P., Demaro, J. A. 3rd., Knoten, A., Hoshi, M., Pehek, E., Johnson, E. M., et al. (2013). Dopamine-dependent compensation maintains motor behavior in mice with developmental ablation of dopaminergic neurons. *J. Neurosci.* 33, 17095–17107. doi: 10.1523/JNEUROSCI.0890-13.2013

Goldman-Rakic, P. S. (2011). Circuitry of primate prefrontal cortex and regulation of behavior by representational memory. *Compr. Physiol.* 373–417. doi: 10.1002/cphy.cp010509

Gonzalez-Hernandez, T., Barroso-Chinea, P., and Rodriguez, M. (2004). Response of the GABAergic and dopaminergic mesostriatal projections to the lesion of the contralateral dopaminergic mesostriatal pathway in the rat. *Mov. Disord.* 19, 1029–1042. doi: 10.1002/mds.20206

Gotts, S. J., Jo, H. J., Wallace, G. L., Saad, Z. S., Cox, R. W., and Martin, A. (2013). Two distinct forms of functional lateralization in the human brain. *Proc. Natl. Acad. Sci. U.S.A.* 110, E3435–E3444. doi: 10.1073/pnas.1302581110

Graveland, G. A., and Difiglia, M. (1985). The frequency and distribution of medium-sized neurons with indented nuclei in the primate and rodent neostriatum. *Brain Res.* 327, 307–311. doi: 10.1016/0006-8993(85)91524-0

Gruzelier, J. H. (1999). Functional neuropsychophysiological asymmetry in schizophrenia: a review and reorientation. *Schizophr. Bull.* 25, 91–120. doi: 10.1093/oxfordjournals.schbul.a033370

Gurney, K., Prescott, T. J., and Redgrave, P. (2001). A computational model of action selection in the basal ganglia. I. A new functional anatomy. *Biol. Cybern.* 84, 401–410. doi: 10.1007/PL00007984

Hietala, J., Syvalahti, E., Vilkman, H., Vuorio, K., Rakkolainen, V., Bergman, J., et al. (1999). Depressive symptoms and presynaptic dopamine function in neuroleptic-naive schizophrenia. *Schizophr. Res.* 35, 41–50. doi: 10.1016/S0920-9964(98)00113-3

Hnasko, T. S., Hjelmstad, G. O., Fields, H. L., and Edwards, R. H. (2012). Ventral tegmental area glutamate neurons: electrophysiological properties and projections. *J. Neurosci.* 32, 15076–15085. doi: 10.1523/JNEUROSCI.3128-12.2012

Hritcu, L., Ciobica, A., and Artenie, V. (2008). Effects of right-unilateral 6-hydroxydopamine infusion-induced memory impairment and oxidative stress: relevance for Parkinson's disease. *Cent. Eur. J. Biol.* 3, 250–257. doi: 10.2478/s11535-008-0023-8

Hsiao, M. C., Lin, K. J., Liu, C. Y., and Schatz, D. B. (2013). The interaction between dopamine transporter function, gender differences, and possible laterality in depression. *Psychiatry Res.* 211, 72–77. doi: 10.1016/j.pscychresns.2012.06.004

Hsiao, M. C., Lin, K. J., Liu, C. Y., Tzen, K. Y., and Yen, T. C. (2003). Dopamine transporter change in drug-naive schizophrenia: an imaging study with 99mTc-TRODAT-1. *Schizophr. Res.* 65, 39–46. doi: 10.1016/S0920-9964(03)00006-9

Ikegami, M., Ichitani, Y., Takahashi, T., and Iwasaki, T. (2006). Compensatory increase in extracellular dopamine in the nucleus accumbens of adult rats with neonatal 6-hydroxydopamine treatment. *Nihon Shinkei Seishin Yakurigaku Zasshi* 26, 111–117.

Ishikawa, M., Otaka, M., Huang, Y. H., Neumann, P. A., Winters, B. D., Grace, A. A., et al. (2013). Dopamine triggers heterosynaptic plasticity. *J. Neurosci.* 33, 6759–6765. doi: 10.1523/JNEUROSCI.4694-12.2013

Iwamoto, E. T., Loh, H. H., and Way, E. L. (1976). Circling behavior in rats with 6-hydroxydopamine or electrolytic nigral lesions. *Eur. J. Pharmacol.* 37, 339–356. doi: 10.1016/0014-2999(76)90042-X

Jaeger, C. B., Joh, T. H., and Reis, D. J. (1983). The effect of forebrain lesions in the neonatal rat: survival of midbrain dopaminergic neurons and the crossed nigrostriatal projection. *J. Comp. Neurol.* 218, 74–90. doi: 10.1002/cne.902180105

Jang, J. Y., Jang, M., Kim, S. H., Um, K. B., Kang, Y. K., Kim, H. J., et al. (2011). Regulation of dopaminergic neuron firing by heterogeneous dopamine autoreceptors in the substantia nigra pars compacta. *J. Neurochem.* 116, 966–974. doi: 10.1111/j.1471-4159.2010.07107.x

Jerussi, T. P., and Glick, S. D. (1975). Apomorphine-induced rotation in normal rats and interaction with unilateral caudate lesions. *Psychopharmacologia* 40, 329–334. doi: 10.1007/BF00421471

Jerussi, T. P., and Glick, S. D. (1976). Drug-induced rotation in rats without lesions: behavioral and neurochemical indices of a normal asymmetry in nigro-striatal function. *Psychopharmacology (Berl.)* 47, 249–260. doi: 10.1007/BF00427609

Jerussi, T. P., and Taylor, C. A. (1982). Bilateral asymmetry in striatal dopamine metabolism: implications for pharmacotherapy of schizophrenia. *Brain Res.* 246, 71–75. doi: 10.1016/0006-8993(82)90143-3

Johnson, S. W., and North, R. A. (1992). Two types of neurone in the rat ventral tegmental area and their synaptic inputs. *J. Physiol.* 450, 455–468.

Joyce, J. N. (1991a). Differential response of striatal dopamine and muscarinic cholinergic receptor subtypes to the loss of dopamine. I. Effects of intranigral or intracerebroventricular 6-hydroxydopamine lesions of the mesostriatal dopamine system. *Exp. Neurol.* 113, 261–276. doi: 10.1016/0014-4886(91)90016-6

Joyce, J. N. (1991b). Differential response of striatal dopamine and muscarinic cholinergic receptor subtypes to the loss of dopamine. II. Effects of 6-hydroxydopamine or colchicine microinjections into the VTA or reserpine treatment. *Exp. Neurol.* 113, 277–290. doi: 10.1016/0014-4886(91)90017-7

Kalivas, P. W., Churchill, L., and Klitenick, M. A. (1993). GABA and enkephalin projection from the nucleus accumbens and ventral pallidum to the ventral tegmental area. *Neuroscience* 57, 1047–1060. doi: 10.1016/0306-4522(93)90048-K

Karreman, M., and Moghaddam, B. (1996). The prefrontal cortex regulates the basal release of dopamine in the limbic striatum: an effect mediated by ventral tegmental area. *J. Neurochem.* 66, 589–598. doi: 10.1046/j.1471-4159.1996.66020589.x

Kelly, E., Jenner, P., and Marsden, C. D. (1984). Behavioural effects mediated by unilateral nigral dopamine receptor stimulation in the rat. *Exp. Brain Res.* 55, 243–252. doi: 10.1007/BF00237275

Kemp, J. M., and Powell, T. P. (1971). The structure of the caudate nucleus of the cat: light and electron microscopy. *Philos. Trans. R. Soc. Lond. B Biol. Sci.* 262, 383–401. doi: 10.1098/rstb.1971.0102

Kesner, R. P., Hunt, M. E., Williams, J. M., and Long, J. M. (1996). Prefrontal cortex and working memory for spatial response, spatial location, and visual object information in the rat. *Cereb. Cortex* 6, 311–318. doi: 10.1093/cercor/6.2.311

Kimura, D., and Archibald, Y. (1974). Motor functions of the left hemisphere. *Brain* 97, 337–350. doi: 10.1093/brain/97.1.337

Kita, H. (1992). Responses of globus pallidus neurons to cortical stimulation: intracellular study in the rat. *Brain Res.* 589, 84–90. doi: 10.1016/0006-8993(92)91164-A

Ko, J. H., Monchi, O., Ptito, A., Bloomfield, P., Houle, S., and Strafella, A. P. (2008). Theta burst stimulation-induced inhibition of dorsolateral prefrontal cortex reveals hemispheric asymmetry in striatal dopamine release during a set-shifting task: a TMS-[(11)C]raclopride PET study. *Eur. J. Neurosci.* 28, 2147–2155. doi: 10.1111/j.1460-9568.2008.06501.x

Kolb, B., Buhrmann, K., McDonald, R., and Sutherland, R. J. (1994). Dissociation of the medial prefrontal, posterior parietal, and posterior temporal cortex for spatial navigation and recognition memory in the rat. *Cereb. Cortex* 4, 664–680. doi: 10.1093/cercor/4.6.664

Koob, G. F., Stinus, L., and Le Moal, M. (1981). Hyperactivity and hypoactivity produced by lesions to the mesolimbic dopamine system. *Behav. Brain Res.* 3, 341–359. doi: 10.1016/0166-4328(81)90004-8

Kopniczky, Z., Dochnal, R., Macsai, M., Pal, A., Kiss, G., Mihaly, A., et al. (2006). Alterations of behavior and spatial learning after unilateral entorhinal ablation of rats. *Life Sci.* 78, 2683–2688. doi: 10.1016/j.lfs.2005.10.014

Kravitz, A. V., Freeze, B. S., Parker, P. R., Kay, K., Thwin, M. T., Deisseroth, K., et al. (2010). Regulation of parkinsonian motor behaviours by optogenetic control of basal ganglia circuitry. *Nature* 466, 622–626. doi: 10.1038/nature09159

Krayniak, P. F., Meibach, R. C., and Siegel, A. (1981). A projection from the entorhinal cortex to the nucleus accumbens in the rat. *Brain Res.* 209, 427–431. doi: 10.1016/0006-8993(81)90165-7

Kurachi, M., Sumiyoshi, T., Shibata, R., Sun, Y. J., Uehara, T., Tanii, Y., et al. (2000). Changes in limbic dopamine metabolism following quinolinic acid lesions of the left entorhinal cortex in rats. *Psychiatry Clin. Neurosci.* 54, 83–89. doi: 10.1046/j.1440-1819.2000.00641.x

Laplante, F., Dufresne, M. M., Ouboudinar, J., Ochoa-Sanchez, R., and Sullivan, R. M. (2013). Reduction in cholinergic interneuron density in the nucleus accumbens attenuates local extracellular dopamine release in response to stress or amphetamine. *Synapse* 67, 21–29. doi: 10.1002/syn.21612

Lawler, C. P., Gilmore, J. H., Watts, V. J., Walker, Q. D., Southerland, S. B., Cook, L. L., et al. (1995). Interhemispheric modulation of dopamine receptor interactions in unilateral 6-OHDA rodent model. *Synapse* 21, 299–311. doi: 10.1002/syn.890210404

Lieu, C. A., and Subramanian, T. (2012). The interhemispheric connections of the striatum: implications for Parkinson's disease and drug-induced dyskinesias. *Brain Res. Bull.* 87, 1–9. doi: 10.1016/j.brainresbull.2011.09.013

Lisman, J. E., and Grace, A. A. (2005). The hippocampal-VTA loop: controlling the entry of information into long-term memory. *Neuron* 46, 703–713. doi: 10.1016/j.neuron.2005.05.002

Loughlin, S. E., and Fallon, J. H. (1982). Mesostriatal projections from ventral tegmentum and dorsal raphe: cells project ipsilaterally or contralaterally but not bilaterally. *Neurosci. Lett.* 32, 11–16. doi: 10.1016/0304-3940(82)90221-X

Loughlin, S. E., and Fallon, J. H. (1984). Substantia nigra and ventral tegmental area projections to cortex: topography and collateralization. *Neuroscience* 11, 425–435. doi: 10.1016/0306-4522(84)90034-4

Louilot, A., and Choulli, M. K. (1997). Asymmetrical increases in dopamine turnover in the nucleus accumbens and lack of changes in locomotor responses following unilateral dopaminergic depletions in the entorhinal cortex. *Brain Res.* 778, 150–157. doi: 10.1016/S0006-8993(97)01050-0

Louilot, A., and Le Moal, M. (1994). Lateralized interdependence between limbicotemporal and ventrostriatal dopaminergic transmission. *Neuroscience* 59, 495–500. doi: 10.1016/0306-4522(94)90171-6

Lupinsky, D., Moquin, L., and Gratton, A. (2010). Interhemispheric regulation of the medial prefrontal cortical glutamate stress response in rats. *J. Neurosci.* 30, 7624–7633. doi: 10.1523/JNEUROSCI.1187-10.2010

Martin-Soelch, C., Szczepanik, J., Nugent, A., Barhaghi, K., Rallis, D., Herscovitch, P., et al. (2011). Lateralization and gender differences in the dopaminergic response to unpredictable reward in the human ventral striatum. *Eur. J. Neurosci.* 33, 1706–1715. doi: 10.1111/j.1460-9568.2011.07642.x

McGeorge, A. J., and Faull, R. L. (1989). The organization of the projection from the cerebral cortex to the striatum in the rat. *Neuroscience* 29, 503–537. doi: 10.1016/0306-4522(89)90128-0

Mensah, P., and Deadwyler, S. (1974). The caudate nucleus of the rat: cell types and the demonstration of a commissural system. *J. Anat.* 117, 281–293.

Meshul, C. K., and Allen, C. (2000). Haloperidol reverses the changes in striatal glutamatergic immunolabeling following a 6-OHDA lesion. *Synapse* 36, 129–142. doi: 10.1002/(SICI)1098-2396(200005)36:2<129::AID-SYN6>3.0.CO;2-4

Meshul, C. K., Emre, N., Nakamura, C. M., Allen, C., Donohue, M. K., and Buckman, J. F. (1999). Time-dependent changes in striatal glutamate synapses following a 6-hydroxydopamine lesion. *Neuroscience* 88, 1–16. doi: 10.1016/S0306-4522(98)00189-4

Mogenson, G. J., Jones, D. L., and Yim, C. Y. (1980). From motivation to action: functional interface between the limbic system and the motor system. *Prog. Neurobiol.* 14, 69–97. doi: 10.1016/0301-0082(80)90018-0

Mohr, C., and Bracha, H. S. (2004). Compound measure of hand-foot-eye preference masked opposite turning behavior in healthy right-handers and non-right-handers: technical comment on Mohr et al. (2003). *Behav. Neurosci.* 118, 1145–1146. doi: 10.1037/0735-7044.118.5.1145

Mohr, C., Landis, T., Bracha, H. S., and Brugger, P. (2003). Opposite turning behavior in right-handers and non-right-handers suggests a link between handedness and cerebral dopamine asymmetries. *Behav. Neurosci.* 117, 1448–1452. doi: 10.1037/0735-7044.117.6.1448

Moser, E. I., Witter, M. P., and Moser, M. B. (2010). "Entorhinal cortex" in *Handbook of Brain Microcircuits*, eds S. M. Gordon and S. Grillner (New York, NY: Oxford University Press), 175–192.

Nambu, A., Tokuno, H., Hamada, I., Kita, H., Imanishi, M., Akazawa, T., et al. (2000). Excitatory cortical inputs to pallidal neurons via the subthalamic nucleus in the monkey. *J. Neurophysiol.* 84, 289–300.

Nambu, A., Tokuno, H., and Takada, M. (2002). Functional significance of the cortico-subthalamo-pallidal 'hyperdirect' pathway. *Neurosci. Res.* 43, 111–117. doi: 10.1016/S0168-0102(02)00027-5

Nauta, W. J., Smith, G. P., Faull, R. L., and Domesick, V. B. (1978). Efferent connections and nigral afferents of the nucleus accumbens septi in the rat. *Neuroscience* 3, 385–401. doi: 10.1016/0306-4522(78)90041-6

Nielsen, D. M., Visker, K. E., Cunningham, M. J., Keller, R. W. Jr., Glick, S. D., and Carlson, J. N. (1997). Paw preference, rotation, and dopamine function in Collins HI and LO mouse strains. *Physiol. Behav.* 61, 525–535. doi: 10.1016/S0031-9384(96)00496-9

Nowak, G. (1989). Lateralization of neocortical dopamine receptors and dopamine level in normal Wistar rats. *Pol. J. Pharmacol. Pharm.* 41, 133–137.

Oertel, W. H., and Mugnaini, E. (1984). Immunocytochemical studies of GABAergic neurons in rat basal ganglia and their relations to other neuronal systems. *Neurosci. Lett.* 47, 233–238. doi: 10.1016/0304-3940(84)90519-6

Olpe, H. R., Schellenberg, H., and Koella, W. P. (1977). Rotational behavior induced in rats by intranigral application of GABA-related drugs and GABA antagonists. *Eur. J. Pharmacol.* 45, 291–294. doi: 10.1016/0014-2999(77)90012-7

Ossowska, K., and Wolfarth, S. (1995). Stimulation of glutamate receptors in the intermediate/caudal striatum induces contralateral turning. *Eur. J. Pharmacol.* 273, 89–97. doi: 10.1016/0014-2999(94)00671-S

Parent, A., and Hazrati, L. N. (1995). Functional anatomy of the basal ganglia. I. The cortico-basal ganglia-thalamo-cortical loop. *Brain Res. Brain Res. Rev.* 20, 91–127. doi: 10.1016/0165-0173(94)00007-C

Peterson, B. S., Riddle, M. A., Cohen, D. J., Katz, L. D., Smith, J. C., and Leckman, J. F. (1993). Human basal ganglia volume asymmetries on magnetic resonance images. *Magn. Reson. Imaging* 11, 493–498. doi: 10.1016/0730-725X(93)90468-S

Phillipson, O. T. (1979). Afferent projections to the ventral tegmental area of Tsai and interfascicular nucleus: a horseradish peroxidase study in the rat. *J. Comp. Neurol.* 187, 117–143. doi: 10.1002/cne.901870108

Pritzel, M., Huston, J. P., and Sarter, M. (1983). Behavioral and neuronal reorganization after unilateral substantia nigra lesions: evidence for increased interhemispheric nigrostriatal projections. *Neuroscience* 9, 879–888. doi: 10.1016/0306-4522(83)90276-2

Rodriguez, M., Martin, L., and Santana, C. (1994). Ontogenic development of brain asymmetry in dopaminergic neurons. *Brain Res. Bull.* 33, 163–171. doi: 10.1016/0361-9230(94)90246-1

Roedter, A., Winkler, C., Samii, M., Walter, G. F., Brandis, A., and Nikkhah, G. (2001). Comparison of unilateral and bilateral intrastriatal 6-hydroxydopamine-induced axon terminal lesions: evidence for interhemispheric functional coupling of the two nigrostriatal pathways. *J. Comp. Neurol.* 432, 217–229. doi: 10.1002/cne.1098

Scheel-Kruger, J., Arnt, J., and Magelund, G. (1977). Behavioural stimulation induced by muscimol and other GABA agonists injected into the substantia nigra. *Neurosci. Lett.* 4, 351–356. doi: 10.1016/0304-3940(77)90183-5

Schneider, L. H., Murphy, R. B., and Coons, E. E. (1982). Lateralization of striatal dopamine (D2) receptors in normal rats. *Neurosci. Lett.* 33, 281–284. doi: 10.1016/0304-3940(82)90385-8

Seibyl, J. P., Marek, K. L., Quinlan, D., Sheff, K., Zoghbi, S., Zea-Ponce, Y., et al. (1995). Decreased single-photon emission computed tomographic [123I]beta-CIT striatal uptake correlates with symptom severity in Parkinson's disease. *Ann. Neurol.* 38, 589–598. doi: 10.1002/ana.410380407

Silva, M. A., Topic, B., Lamounier-Zepter, V., Huston, J. P., Tomaz, C., and Barros, M. (2007). Evidence for hemispheric specialization in the marmoset (*Callithrix penicillata*) based on lateralization of behavioral/neurochemical correlations. *Brain Res. Bull.* 74, 416–428. doi: 10.1016/j.brainresbull.2007.07.012

Simola, N., Morelli, M., and Carta, A. R. (2007). The 6-hydroxydopamine model of Parkinson's disease. *Neurotox. Res.* 11, 151–167. doi: 10.1007/BF03033565

Smith, A. D., Amalric, M., Koob, G. F., and Zigmond, M. J. (2002). Effect of bilateral 6-hydroxydopamine lesions of the medial forebrain bundle on reaction time. *Neuropsychopharmacology* 26, 756–764. doi: 10.1016/S0893-133X(01)00420-1

Solstad, T., Boccara, C. N., Kropff, E., Moser, M. B., and Moser, E. I. (2008). Representation of geometric borders in the entorhinal cortex. *Science* 322, 1865–1868. doi: 10.1126/science.1166466

Stuber, G. D., Britt, J. P., and Bonci, A. (2012). Optogenetic modulation of neural circuits that underlie reward seeking. *Biol. Psychiatry* 71, 1061–1067. doi: 10.1016/j.biopsych.2011.11.010

Sullivan, R. M. (2004). Hemispheric asymmetry in stress processing in rat prefrontal cortex and the role of mesocortical dopamine. *Stress* 7, 131–143. doi: 10.1080/102538900410001679310

Sullivan, R. M., and Dufresne, M. M. (2006). Mesocortical dopamine and HPA axis regulation: role of laterality and early environment. *Brain Res.* 1076, 49–59. doi: 10.1016/j.brainres.2005.12.100

Sullivan, R. M., and Gratton, A. (1998). Relationships between stress-induced increases in medial prefrontal cortical dopamine and plasma corticosterone levels in rats: role of cerebral laterality. *Neuroscience* 83, 81–91. doi: 10.1016/S0306-4522(97)00370-9

Sullivan, R. M., and Szechtman, H. (1995). Asymmetrical influence of mesocortical dopamine depletion on stress ulcer development and subcortical dopamine systems in rats: implications for psychopathology. *Neuroscience* 65, 757–766. doi: 10.1016/0306-4522(94)00531-9

Sumiyoshi, T., Tsunoda, M., Uehara, T., Tanaka, K., Itoh, H., Sumiyoshi, C., et al. (2004). Enhanced locomotor activity in rats with excitotoxic lesions of the entorhinal cortex, a neurodevelopmental animal model of schizophrenia: behavioral and *in vivo* microdialysis studies. *Neurosci. Lett.* 364, 124–129. doi: 10.1016/j.neulet.2004.04.027

Swanson, L. W. (1982). The projections of the ventral tegmental area and adjacent regions: a combined fluorescent retrograde tracer and immunofluorescence study in the rat. *Brain Res. Bull.* 9, 321–353. doi: 10.1016/0361-9230(82)90145-9

Szostak, C., Jakubovic, A., Phillips, A. G., and Fibiger, H. C. (1986). Bilateral augmentation of dopaminergic and serotonergic activity in the striatum and nucleus accumbens induced by conditioned circling. *J. Neurosci.* 6, 2037–2044.

Szostak, C., Jakubovic, A., Phillips, A. G., and Fibiger, H. C. (1989). Neurochemical correlates of conditioned circling within localized regions of the striatum. *Exp. Brain Res.* 75, 430–440. doi: 10.1007/BF00247949

Szostak, C., Porter, L., Jakubovic, A., Phillips, A. G., and Fibiger, H. C. (1988). Conditioned circling in rats: bilateral involvement of the mesotelencephalic dopamine system demonstrated following unilateral 6-hydroxydopamine lesions. *Neuroscience* 26, 395–401. doi: 10.1016/0306-4522(88)90157-1

Taber, M. T., and Fibiger, H. C. (1995). Electrical stimulation of the prefrontal cortex increases dopamine release in the nucleus accumbens of the rat: modulation by metabotropic glutamate receptors. *J. Neurosci.* 15, 3896–3904.

Thiel, C. M., and Schwarting, R. K. (2001). Dopaminergic lateralisation in the forebrain: relations to behavioural asymmetries and anxiety in male Wistar rats. *Neuropsychobiology* 43, 192–199. doi: 10.1159/000054889

Thierry, A. M., Tassin, J. P., Blanc, G., and Glowinski, J. (1976). Selective activation of mesocortical DA system by stress. *Nature* 263, 242–244. doi: 10.1038/263242a0

Tomer, R., Goldstein, R. Z., Wang, G. J., Wong, C., and Volkow, N. D. (2008). Incentive motivation is associated with striatal dopamine asymmetry. *Biol. Psychol.* 77, 98–101. doi: 10.1016/j.biopsycho.2007.08.001

Tomer, R., Slagter, H. A., Christian, B. T., Fox, A. S., King, C. R., Murali, D., et al. (2014). Love to win or hate to lose? Asymmetry of dopamine D2 receptor binding predicts sensitivity to reward versus punishment. *J. Cogn. Neurosci.* 26, 1039–1048. doi: 10.1162/jocn_a_00544

Torres, E. M., and Dunnett, S. B. (2012). "6-OHDA lesion models of Parkinson's disease in the rat" in *Animal Models of Movement Disorders*, Vol. 2, eds E. L. Lane and S. B. Dunnett (New York, NY: Humana Press), 267–279. doi: 10.1007/978-1-61779-301-1

Totterdell, S., and Meredith, G. E. (1997). Topographical organization of projections from the entorhinal cortex to the striatum of the rat. *Neuroscience* 78, 715–729. doi: 10.1016/S0306-4522(96)00592-1

Uehara, T., Sumiyoshi, T., Matsuoka, T., Itoh, H., and Kurachi, M. (2007). Effect of prefrontal cortex inactivation on behavioral and neurochemical abnormalities in rats with excitotoxic lesions of the entorhinal cortex. *Synapse* 61, 391–400. doi: 10.1002/syn.20383

Uehara, T., Tanii, Y., Sumiyoshi, T., and Kurachi, M. (2000). Neonatal lesions of the left entorhinal cortex affect dopamine metabolism in the rat brain. *Brain Res.* 860, 77–86. doi: 10.1016/S0006-8993(00)01985-5

Ungerstedt, U., and Arbuthnott, G. W. (1970). Quantitative recording of rotational behavior in rats after 6-hydroxy-dopamine lesions of the nigrostriatal dopamine system. *Brain Res.* 24, 485–493. doi: 10.1016/0006-8993(70)90187-3

Van Der Kooy, D., Coscina, D. V., and Hattori, T. (1981). Is there a non-dopaminergic nigrostriatal pathway? *Neuroscience* 6, 345–357. doi: 10.1016/0306-4522(81)90128-7

Van Der Kooy, D., and Wise, R. A. (1980). Retrograde fluorescent tracing of substantia nigra neurons combined with catecholamine histofluorescence. *Brain Res.* 183, 447–452. doi: 10.1016/0006-8993(80)90479-5

Van Dyck, C. H., Seibyl, J. P., Malison, R. T., Laruelle, M., Zoghbi, S. S., Baldwin, R. M., et al. (2002). Age-related decline in dopamine transporters: analysis of striatal subregions, nonlinear effects, and hemispheric asymmetries. *Am. J. Geriatr. Psychiatry* 10, 36–43. doi: 10.1097/00019442-200201000-00005

Van Zessen, R., Phillips, J. L., Budygin, E. A., and Stuber, G. D. (2012). Activation of VTA GABA neurons disrupts reward consumption. *Neuron* 73, 1184–1194. doi: 10.1016/j.neuron.2012.02.016

Veening, J. G., Cornelissen, F. M., and Lieven, P. A. (1980). The topical organization of the afferents to the caudatoputamen of the rat. A horseradish peroxidase study. *Neuroscience* 5, 1253–1268. doi: 10.1016/0306-4522(80)90198-0

Vernaleken, I., Weibrich, C., Siessmeier, T., Buchholz, H. G., Rosch, F., Heinz, A., et al. (2007). Asymmetry in dopamine D(2/3) receptors of caudate nucleus is lost with age. *Neuroimage* 34, 870–878. doi: 10.1016/j.neuroimage.2006.10.013

Wichmann, T., and Delong, M. R. (1996). Functional and pathophysiological models of the basal ganglia. *Curr. Opin. Neurobiol.* 6, 751–758. doi: 10.1016/S0959-4388(96)80024-9

Wilson, C. J., and Groves, P. M. (1980). Fine structure and synaptic connections of the common spiny neuron of the rat neostriatum: a study employing intracellular inject of horseradish peroxidase. *J. Comp. Neurol.* 194, 599–615. doi: 10.1002/cne.901940308

Wise, R. A. (2002). Brain reward circuitry: insights from unsensed incentives. *Neuron* 36, 229–240. doi: 10.1016/S0896-6273(02)00965-0

Wurtz, R. H., and Hikosaka, O. (1986). Role of the basal ganglia in the initiation of saccadic eye movements. *Prog. Brain Res.* 64, 175–190. doi: 10.1016/S0079-6123(08)63412-3

Yamamoto, B. K., and Freed, C. R. (1982). The trained circling rat: a model for inducing unilateral caudate dopamine metabolism. *Nature* 298, 467–468. doi: 10.1038/298467a0

Yamamoto, B. K., and Freed, C. R. (1984a). Asymmetric dopamine and serotonin metabolism in nigrostriatal and limbic structures of the trained circling rat. *Brain Res.* 297, 115–119. doi: 10.1016/0006-8993(84)90547-X

Yamamoto, B. K., and Freed, C. R. (1984b). Reversal of amphetamine-induced circling preference in trained circling rats. *Life Sci.* 34, 675–682. doi: 10.1016/0024-3205(84)90232-7

Zimmerberg, B., Glick, S. D., and Jerussi, T. P. (1974). Neurochemical correlate of a spatial preference in rats. *Science* 185, 623–625. doi: 10.1126/science.185.4151.623

12

The Emergence of Two Anti-Phase Oscillatory Neural Populations in a Computational Model of the Parkinsonian Globus Pallidus

Robert Merrison-Hort[1]* and Roman Borisyuk[1,2]

[1] Centre for Robotics and Neural Systems, School of Computing and Mathematics, The University of Plymouth, Plymouth, UK
[2] Neural Networks Laboratory, Institute of Mathematical Problems in Biology, Russian Academy of Sciences, Pushchino, Russia

Correspondence:
Robert Merrison-Hort, Centre for Robotics and Neural Systems, School of Computing and Mathematics, The University of Plymouth, A221 Portland Square, Drake Circus, Plymouth PL4 8AA, UK
e-mail: robert.merrison@plymouth.ac.uk

Experiments in rodent models of Parkinson's disease have demonstrated a prominent increase of oscillatory firing patterns in neurons within the Parkinsonian globus pallidus (GP) which may underlie some of the motor symptoms of the disease. There are two main pathways from the cortex to GP: via the striatum and via the subthalamic nucleus (STN), but it is not known how these inputs sculpt the pathological pallidal firing patterns. To study this we developed a novel neural network model of conductance-based spiking pallidal neurons with cortex-modulated input from STN neurons. Our results support the hypothesis that entrainment occurs primarily via the subthalamic pathway. We find that as a result of the interplay between excitatory input from the STN and mutual inhibitory coupling between GP neurons, a homogeneous population of GP neurons demonstrates a self-organizing dynamical behavior where two groups of neurons emerge: one spiking in-phase with the cortical rhythm and the other in anti-phase. This finding mirrors what is seen in recordings from the GP of rodents that have had Parkinsonism induced via brain lesions. Our model also includes downregulation of Hyperpolarization-activated Cyclic Nucleotide-gated (HCN) channels in response to burst firing of GP neurons, since this has been suggested as a possible mechanism for the emergence of Parkinsonian activity. We found that the downregulation of HCN channels provides even better correspondence with experimental data but that it is not essential in order for the two groups of oscillatory neurons to appear. We discuss how the influence of inhibitory striatal input will strengthen our results.

Keywords: Parkinson's disease, globus pallidus, oscillation, synchronization, HCN, downregulation, deep-brain stimulation

1. INTRODUCTION

Parkinson's disease is a neurodegenerative disorder which (amongst other symptoms) causes a range of movement-related disturbances such as tremor and slowness (bradykinesia). The primary pathology of the disease is the death of dopaminergic neurons in the basal ganglia (BG), specifically those in the substantia nigra pars compacta (SNc). Since the dopaminergic neurons in the SNc provide widespread innervation to the other regions of the basal ganglia, it is not surprising that their loss results in profound changes to neuronal activity in these regions. What is not yet understood is the precise mechanism by which abnormal neuronal activity arises as a result of dopamine loss—and how this activity relates to motor symptoms. One very successful hypothesis for this was the so-called "rate" hypothesis (DeLong, 1990), which held that motor areas of the basal ganglia are divided into two feed-forward pathways that transfer information from the cortex to the thalamus: a pro-kinetic "direct" and an anti-kinetic "indirect" pathway. According to this model, loss of dopamine input to the striatum upsets the balance of these two pathways, resulting in movement abnormalities. While the rate hypothesis makes predictions that have resulted in successful treatments, such as lesioning of hyperactive nuclei on the indirect pathway (Lozano et al., 1995; Gill and Heywood, 1997), more recent electrophysiological studies have demonstrated that the changes in neuronal activity that underlie Parkinsonian motor impairment are likely to be considerably more complex than those implied by the rate model [see Rubin et al. (2012) for review].

One aspect of pathological activity in the Parkinsonian basal ganglia that is under active investigation is the increase in synchronous oscillatory firing. Local field potential (LFP) recordings from the subthalamic nucleus (STN) of patients with Parkinson's disease show a clear increase in power in the β frequency band (10–30 Hz) when patients are off medication [reviewed in Eusebio and Brown (2009)], and the size of the reduction in β power that occurs with dopamine-replacement medication is positively correlated with the concomitant improvement in severity of anti-kinetic symptoms (Kühn et al., 2006). There are a number of reasons why widespread pathological oscillations may cause motor deficits, for example they may impair the ability to relay information (Mallet et al., 2008b). It has also been proposed that, in health, sporadic β oscillations act as a global signal for maintenance of the current motor activity (Jenkinson and Brown, 2011).

What is the neural basis for the exaggerated oscillatory activity of the Parkinsonian basal ganglia? One possibility is that the reciprocally-connected neurons of the excitatory STN and inhibitory globus pallidus (GP; homologous to the external globus pallidus in primates) act as a neural oscillator. Several computational studies have suggested that this is a plausible mechanism (Gillies et al., 2002; Terman et al., 2002; Holgado et al., 2010). *In vitro* work in slices containing only STN and GP neurons have also shown that oscillatory firing is indeed possible (Plenz and Kital, 1999), though only at frequencies much lower than the β band.

Another possible explanation for exaggerated BG β oscillations in Parkinson's disease is that dopamine acts to modulate the effects of rhythmic cortical activity on cortical-basal ganglia pathways, such that in conditions of reduced dopamine this network becomes pathologically entrained to cortical rhythms. Evidence for this comes from studies that have used signal processing techniques to attempt determine whether β band coherence between the cortex and basal ganglia is directed from cortex to STN or vice versa. Such studies have shown that, in patients with Parkinson's disease (Litvak et al., 2011) or Parkinsonian rodents (Sharott et al., 2005), the oscillations arise in the cortex and drive STN activity. Computational studies that investigate the synchronization of basal ganglia neurons in Parkinson's disease often consider the neurons to be phase oscillators, which either synchronize themselves Popovych and Tass (2012) or become synchronized through common external inputs Wilson et al. (2011).

Experiments using rodent models of Parkinson's disease provide compelling evidence that under Parkinsonian conditions the activity of neurons in the GP are much more susceptible to entrainment by cortical rhythms than in the healthy case. Under conditions of urethane anaesthesia, neurons in the GP of healthy rodents show uncorrelated tonic firing. However, in animals where Parkinsonism has been induced, either through chronic lesioning of the SNc with 6-hydroxydopamine (OHDA) (Ni et al., 2000; Magill et al., 2001) or acute inactivation of SNc projection fibers (Galati et al., 2009), the spiking activity of the majority of GP neurons becomes significantly correlated with cortical "slow wave activity" (SWA); this is the major cortical rhythm in the anaesthetized state and has a frequency of approximately 1 Hz. These experiments also reveal that, in the chronic lesioned case at least, the neurons in GP are split into two major groups, distinguished by whether they preferentially fire during the active phase (ECoG peaks) or inactive phase (ECoG troughs) of SWA in dopamine-deprived conditions. These will be referred to as the TA and TI groups, respectively. The underlying basis for this division is unknown, but the same division is seen in respect to cortico-pallidal synchronization that occurs transiently at β frequencies in response to sensory stimulation in OHDA lesioned rodents (Mallet et al., 2008a), which suggests that the same mechanism may be responsible for pathological entrainment in both behavioral states/frequency bands. If this is the case, then understanding this mechanism may lead to improved treatments for Parkinson's disease. Unfortunately we do not currently know the route through which oscillatory cortical input entrains the GP, although it is likely to involve the two major sources of synaptic input to GP neurons: the inhibitory medium spiny projection neurons of the striatum and excitatory STN neurons. Both receive widespread cortical inputs and both show increased firing during the peaks of SWA under Parkinsonian conditions in rodents (Magill et al., 2001; Tseng et al., 2001). Given that the majority of GP neurons belong to the TI group it has been suggested that cortical oscillations are most effectively relayed via the inhibitory striatum (Walters et al., 2007), but this view is challenged by the fact that the entrainment of GP neurons to SWA appears to be critically dependent on a functioning STN (Ni et al., 2000; Galati et al., 2009).

In this paper we test the hypothesis that the inhibitory network of GP neurons allows two anti-phase groups of oscillatory neurons to appear in response to rhythmic excitatory STN input only. To do this we consider a small neural network model of interconnected conductance-based GP neurons. Although the parameters of the neurons in this population are homogeneous, our simulations reveal a mechanism by which the two oscillatory groups can appear. This collective behavior is the result of a self-organization process that depends on the GP neurons' inhibitory dynamics and rhythmic STN modulation. We study the neural network model under healthy and Parkinsonian conditions and demonstrate a good correspondence between simulation results and experimental recordings. Special attention has been paid to studying the possible role of downregulation of hyperpolarization-activated cyclic nucleotide-gated (HCN) channels in this network, based on the effect that these channels appear to have on GP neurons' responses to synaptic input (Chan et al., 2004; Boyes et al., 2007) and the suggestion that oscillatory activity may not appear immediately after dopamine lesion and might instead depend on slower adaptive processes (Degos et al., 2009).

The structure of this paper is as follows. Section 2 describes our model including the cellular properties of model GP neurons, how STN neuron activity was generated, the nature of synaptic connectivity and our proposed model for HCN downregulation. Section 3 describes the results of simulations and demonstrates that model GP neurons behave realistically both in isolation and as part of a network. It also shows how the network's activity changes under simulated Parkinsonian conditions in a way that is similar to the results of previous biological experiments. Section 4 examines results in the context of what has been seen in animal models of Parkinson's disease and discusses what the results might mean in terms of potential improvements to treatments for the disease.

2. MATERIALS AND METHODS

Figure 1 shows a simple representation of the neural network model which includes a population of 100 interconnected GP neurons (right panel, blue) which receive excitatory synaptic input from 50 STN neurons (left panel, red). Each GP neuron is described by a detailed single compartment conductance based model of the Hodgkin–Huxley type with inhibitory connections from other GP neurons. The STN neurons are described by a simple enhanced leaky integrate-and-fire model. Neurons in the STN population are not connected to each other but they are modulated by a common cortical slow-wave rhythm and make excitatory synapses onto GP neurons.

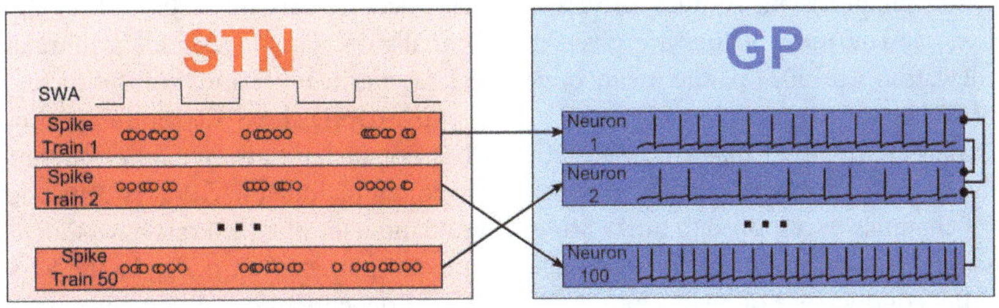

FIGURE 1 | An overview of the model. Integrate-and-fire STN neurons, modulated by an approximately 1 Hz rhythm, provide excitatory synaptic input to a population of GP neurons. Inhibitory local synaptic connections between GP neurons have random connectivity.

2.1. MODEL GP NEURONS

The model GP neurons are of standard Hodgkin–Huxley type, with a single compartment per neuron. We included ten voltage-gated ionic channels as in the multicompartmental modeling work of Günay et al. (2008): fast and slow delayed rectifying K_+ (Kv3 and Kv2, respectively), fast and slow A-type K_+ ($Kv4_{fast}$, $Kv4_{slow}$), M-type K_+ (KCNQ), fast spike-producing Na_+ (NaF), persistent pacemaking Na_+ (NaP), hyper-polarization activated Ca_{2+} (HVA), and fast and slow mixed-conductance hyperpolarization-activated channels (HCN_{fast}, HCN_{slow}). For simplicity our model does not include calcium-gated potassium "SK" channels, as these channels' most significant effect on the activity of GP neurons appears to be a lengthening of spike afterhyperpolarization (AHP) (Deister et al., 2009), and we were able achieve physiologically realistic AHPs without this channel. Equation 1 describes how the membrane potential (V) of a model GP neuron evolves in time.

$$C\frac{dV}{dt} = g_{leak}(E_{leak} - V) + I_{naf} + I_{nap} + I_{kv2} + I_{kv3} + I_{kv4f} + I_{kv4s} + I_{kcnq} + I_{hva} + I_{hcnf} + I_{hcns} + I_{syn} + I_{ext} \quad (1)$$

Here C and g_{leak} are the total membrane capacitance and leak conductance and E_{leak} is the reversal potential of the leak channels. Values for these parameters are given in **Table 1**. I_{syn} is the total synaptic current received by the neuron (see below). I_{ext} is an externally applied current that was only non-zero when testing the response of individual GP neurons to current injections. The remaining currents correspond to the voltage-dependent channels, each of which has an activation gate (represented by the state variable m) and, for most channels, an inactivation gate (state variable h). Two channels have slow inactivation gates (s) in addition to their activation and inactivation gates. Equation 2 shows the current due to a channel with all three gates:

$$I = m^{\mu} h^{\rho} s^{\phi} g_X (E_X - V) \quad (2)$$

Here E_X is the reversal potential of the channel, g_X is the maximum conductance of the channel, and μ, ρ and ϕ are integers that give the relative numbers of gating molecules. **Table 2** shows which channels contain each gate type and the corresponding values of μ, ρ and ϕ. Note that the parameters governing the dynamics of each gate vary from channel to channel. Since we use the same equations and parameters for channel gates as Günay et al. (2008) we do not reproduce these here and instead refer to the supplementary material of that paper where they are listed.

We could not directly use the channel maximum conductance parameters from Günay et al. (2008), since this was a multicompartmental model and the conductances varied widely between the different compartments. Instead we adjusted the channel conductances so that our model neurons exhibited intrinsic pacemaking and displayed realistic responses to depolarizing and hyperpolarizing current injections. The chosen conductances are shown in **Table 1**. In order to generate a range of intrinsic pacemaking frequencies we applied Gaussian noise to

Table 1 | Passive membrane parameters and channel conductances for the model GP neurons.

Parameter	Value	Units
C	141.6	pF
g_{leak}	4.012	nS
E_{leak}	−60.0	nS
g_{naf}	5900.0	nS
g_{nap}	17.7	nS
$g_{kv2,3,4f,4s}$	590.0	nS
g_{kcnq}	1.77	nS
g_{hva}	1.77	nS
$g_{hcaf,s}$	177.0	nS
E_k	−80.0	mV
E_{na}	55.0	mV
E_{ca}	120.0	mV
E_{hcn}	−30.0	mV

Table 2 | The relative proportion of gating molecules of each type for each channel in the model GP neurons.

Channel	μ	ρ	ϕ
NaF	3	1	1
NaP	3	1	1
$Kv2,3,4_{fast}$, 4_{slow}	4	1	–
KCNQ	4	–	–
HVA	1	–	–
HCN_{fast}, HCN_{slow}	1	–	–

the maximum conductances of the persistent sodium and HCN channels (g_{nap}, g_{hcnf}, and g_{hcns}). The mean values are given in **Table 1** and the standard deviation was 50% of the mean value for NaP and 30% for both HCN channels.

It has been proposed (Chan et al., 2011) that a homeostatic mechanism may reduce the intrinsic firing rate of GP neurons via downregulation of HCN channels in response to burst firing. Our model includes a possible mechanism for this downregulation by allowing the maximum conductance of HCN channels to decrease. This occurs during periods of elevated firing rate, which are indicated by high intracellular calcium concentration ($[Ca]$). In order to model the dynamics of this calcium concentration we use the equations from Terman et al. (2002). The rate of change of intracellular calcium is given by Equation 3:

$$\frac{d[Ca]}{dt} = \epsilon(I_{hva} - k_{Ca}[Ca]) \tag{3}$$

Here ϵ represents calcium buffering and has the value $10^{-4}\frac{Ms}{CL}$, while k_{Ca} is the calcium pump rate and has the value $15.0\frac{CL}{Ms}$ [parameter values from Rubin and Terman (2004)]. I_{hva} represents the instantaneous current due to HVA channels (these are the only Ca_{+} channels in the model). The maximum conductance of HCN channels remains constant during time steps and is adjusted between steps when $[Ca] > T_{HCN}$, where T_{HCN} is the threshold above which downregulation occurs. The amount by which the conductance is adjusted takes the form of a sigmoid curve and is given in Equation 4.

$$g_{HCN}(t + \Delta t) = max\left[0, g_{HCN}(t) - \frac{k_{HCN}\Delta t}{1 + exp(\frac{\theta - [Ca](t+\Delta t)}{\sigma})}\right] \tag{4}$$

Here k_{HCN} is the maximum conductance change that can occur in one step, θ is the level of intracellular calcium that gives half the maximum change, and σ is the slope of the sigmoid. We do not have any data from biological experiments to suggest values for the downregulation parameters. Since we hypothesize that downregulation mostly only occurs during fast burst firing under Parkinsonian conditions, we chose parameters such that, in healthy conditions, downregulation only occurred in the very fastest firing GP neurons. The values of k_{HCN} and σ that we chose give a fairly rapid reduction in maximum HCN conductance in response to elevated firing rates. The downregulation parameters that we chose are: $T_{HCN} = 0.2$, $k_{HCN} = 6 \times 10^{-4}$, $\sigma = 0.1$, $\theta = 0.5$.

Note that our model GP neurons are supposed to represent those in the rodent GP. This nucleus is usually considered to be equivalent to the so-called "external" pallidus (GPe) in primates.

2.2. MODEL STN NEURONS

Since the aim of this study is to investigate the effects of rhythmic STN input upon the neurons of the GP, we did not model STN neurons to the same level of biological detail as GP neurons. Instead, to simulate the SWA-modulated bursting of STN neurons that occurs under urethane anaesthesia we use an enhanced integrate-and-fire generator of neural activity, as described in Borisyuk (2002). The STN neurons include an exponentially decaying threshold, accumulation of membrane potential, stochastic noise and an absolute refractory period. Aside from approximating the SWA modulation of STN activity our model does not include any synaptic inputs to the STN. In particular we do not include the GP-STN projection because experiments in urethane-anaesthetized rats have shown that the changes in firing rate and pattern that occur in the STN following OHDA-lesion are not dependent on synaptic input from the GP (Hassani et al., 1996).

During urethane anaesthesia STN neurons display uncorrelated bursting activity that is modulated by a slow rhythm (Magill et al., 2001) which, for the purposes of this paper, we assume arises from excitatory cortical inputs. Since firing is uncorrelated, each STN spike train is generated independently using a procedure that results in spiking activity that is similar to the spiking activity of real neurons. The generated spike trains contain activity that is oscillatory with a period of 1300 ms (≈0.8 Hz), where cycle is made up of an 800 ms "inactive" phase and a 500 ms "active" phase. The spike trains are constructed by alternately sampling from two intermediate spike trains, one with slow irregular firing and one with fast irregular firing (for the inactive and active periods, respectively). The average firing rates are 0.5 Hz for the inactive period and 30 Hz for the active period; under simulated Parkinsonian conditions the firing frequency during the active phase is increased to 60 Hz. **Figure 2** shows cross-correlations between two STN spike trains which demonstrate that within the active bursting period activity is not correlated (A), but that there is strong common modulation at 0.8 Hz (B). **Figures 2C,D** are raster plots of the generated spiking activity of 50 STN neurons in healthy and Parkinsonian conditions, respectively, demonstrating a clear increase in firing frequency during the active phase in the Parkinsonian case.

2.3. SYNAPTIC CONNECTIVITY

Each model neuron contains two variables, $o(t)$ and $c(t)$, which represent synaptic opening and closing, respectively. When a neuron spikes (defined by the membrane potential crossing 0 mV in the positive direction), both variables are step-increased by 1. Following this, the variables decay exponentially to zero according to different time constants τ_o and τ_c, respectively (Eq. 5). Since $\tau_o < \tau_c$, a transient synaptic current arises in all post-synaptic neurons following a spike, according to Eq. 6:

$$\frac{do}{dt} = -\frac{1}{\tau_o}o \qquad \frac{dc}{dt} = -\frac{1}{\tau_c}c \tag{5}$$

$$I_{syn} = (c - o)g_{Syn}(e_{rev} - V) \tag{6}$$

Here e_{rev} is the reversal potential of the synapse (mV) and V is the membrane potential of the post-synaptic neuron (mV). The value of parameters e_{rev}, τ_c and τ_o vary based on the type of the neuron (glutamatergic STN or GABAergic GP). g_{Syn} denotes the maximum unitary conductance of a synapse (nS) and its value for a particular synapse is drawn from a Gaussian distribution. The mean of this distribution was g_{SG} for STN-GP synapses and g_{GG} for intra-GP synapses and the standard deviation was 30% of the mean in both cases.

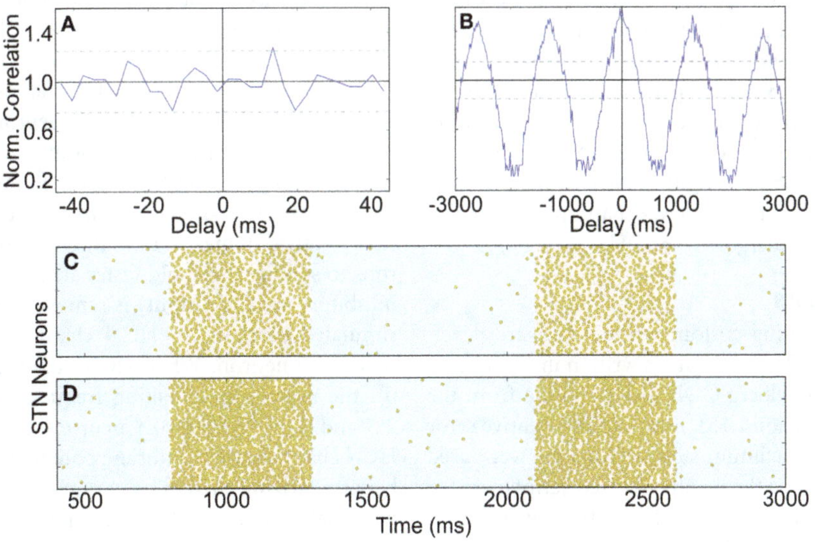

FIGURE 2 | Properties and spiking activity of STN neurons. (A) Example cross-correlation between two STN neuron spike trains on a short time window (30 bins, 3 ms each) shows independent firing. **(B)** Longer time window reveals slow (1300 ms) oscillations (400 bins, 20 ms each). **(C)** Spiking activity of STN neurons under healthy conditions. **(D)** Increased intensity of active-phase firing under Parkinsonian conditions. In **(C,D)** the background is shaded to show the active (pink) and inactive (blue) phases of the SWA cycles. **(A,B)** are normalized using the procedure described in Brillinger (1976): if X_i is the unscaled spike count in histogram bin i then the scaled value X_i' is given by: $X_i' = \frac{TX_i}{2hN_A N_B}$, where T is the total simulation time, h is half the width of a cross-correlation bin and N_A and N_B are the total spike counts for each spike train. A normalized value of 1 indicates that there is no correlation at a particular delay, while deviations from 1 indicate positive or negative correlations. The horizontal bars show the 95% confidence interval for significant correlations (Brillinger, 1976).

For the intra-GP inhibitory synapses we used synaptic time constants $\tau_o = 5$ ms and $\tau_c = 40$ ms from unpublished current-clamp recordings of GP-GP IPSPs taken from slices containing rat GP, cortex and striatum [Alon Korngreen, personal communication]. Similarly, we chose $g_{GG} = 0.5$ nS which gives a peak IPSP of 0.5 mV (measured as deflection away from a holding potential of -65 mV during injection of hyperpolarizing current) to match the same experimental recordings. We used a standard GABA reversal potential of -80 mV. Connectivity between GP neurons was uniformly random, with each neuron inhibiting 20 others (no self-connections).

Anatomical data regarding the structure of the STN-GP projection is currently lacking. However, it is clear that there are many fewer STN neurons than GP neurons and that each GP neuron only samples the activity of a small proportion of STN neurons (Jaeger and Kita, 2011). We therefore arbitrarily chose to model 50 STN neurons, each of which makes excitatory synapses onto two randomly selected GP neurons. The time constants of STN-GP synapses in the model are $\tau_o = 0.2$ ms and $\tau_c = 60$ ms, based on the recordings shown in Loucif et al. (2005). The average maximum synaptic conductance (g_{SG}) used for the healthy case was chosen to be just low enough such that the majority of GP neurons didn't show significant entrainment to the SWA rhythm and we investigated the effects of increasing the value in the Parkinsonian case.

2.4. MODELING OF PARKINSONISM

We simulate the OHDA-lesioned (Parkinsonian) rat basal ganglia by making three changes to the model's parameters: (i) faster STN firing during the active phase of SWA (**Figure 2D**) (ii) increased STN-GP synapse strength and (iii) increased intra-GP inhibition strength. Although the changes that occur to functional connectivity in the basal ganglia in Parkinson's disease are currently under active investigation, there is experimental support for facilitation of both GP-GP (Johnson and Napier, 1997) and STN-GP (Johnson and Napier, 1997; Hernández et al., 2006) synapses. Similarly, under urethane anaesthesia it has been shown that spiking in the STN continues to be modulated by the cortical SWA rhythm, but that its firing becomes more intense during the active period (Magill et al., 2001; Galati et al., 2009).

2.5. CATERGORIZATION OF NEURON ACTIVITY

We used a simple method to catergorize GP neurons as being of type TA (in-phase with active SWA), TI (in-phase with inactive SWA), NM (not modulated by SWA) or QU (quiet). Each spike fired by the neuron to be catergorized is represented by a complex number that indicates its phase in relation to SWA. The sum of these complex numbers then gives an indication of the average phase, ω, as shown in Eq. 7.

$$\omega_k = \sum_{s \in S_k} e^{i\theta(s)} \tag{7}$$

Here S_k is the set of spike times for neuron k ($0 \leq k < 100$) and $\theta(s)$ is the phase of SWA at time s ($0 \leq \theta(s) < 2\pi$). The argument of the complex number ω_k indicates the average SWA phase at which neuron k fires, while its modulus provides an indication of how strongly SWA-modulated the firing is. Normalizing the modulus by the number of spikes gives a confidence measure $c_k = \frac{|\omega_k|}{|S_k|}$, where $c_k = 0$ indicates that spikes did not fire preferentially at any one phase and $c_k = 1$ indicates that every spike occurred at exactly the same phase. After visual inspection of spike trains, we decided to catergorize neurons with confidence $c < 0.1$ as NM. We catergorized neurons with $c \geq 0.1$ as either TA or TI based on whether the average phase was during the active or inactive part of the SWA cycle. Neurons that fired fewer than one spike every SWA cycle on average were catergorized as QU.

2.6. IMPLEMENTATION DETAILS

We simulated the model using custom written software developed by R Merrison-Hort. This software is written in C and uses the adaptive Runge-Kutta-Felberg ODE solver routine from the GNU Scientific Library (version 1.15). Absolute and relative error tolerances of 10^{-5} and a maximum step size of 1 ms were used for all simulations. To analyse the results we used scripts written in the Python (2.7) programming language with routines from the NumPy (1.6.2) and SciPy (0.11.0rc1) libraries. For each set of parameters twelve simulations were performed, with different random neural connectivity, STN spike trains and parameter noise (as described above) in each simulation.

All reported mean values are given with their standard deviation.

3. RESULTS

3.1. MODEL GP NEURONS BEHAVE REALISTICALLY UNDER HEALTHY CONDITIONS

The characteristics of the model GP neurons qualitatively match that those of real rodent GP neurons in a number of key ways and are illustrated in **Figure 3A**. When no synaptic or injected currents are present (dark blue trace in **Figure 3A**), most model neurons (96%; 481/500) pacemake at a range of frequencies (23.6 Hz ± 4.0). Depolarizing current injections increase the frequency of firing (green trace), with very high frequencies possible (up to approximately 200 Hz). Hyperpolarizing current injections result in a prominent and transient "sag" in membrane potential (red, cyan and pink traces). The first spike after hyperpolarizing current is removed occurs after a similar delay regardless of the size of the injected current. These properties match those seen in experiments with slices of rodent GP (Chan et al., 2004; Bugaysen et al., 2010).

The mixed-conductance HCN channels play an important role in the activity of the model GP neurons and their response to hyperpolarizing input. The combination of a reasonably depolarized reversal potential (−30 mV) (Lüthi and McCormick, 1998) and activation at hyperpolarized membrane potentials (lower than −60 mV) means that these channels act to return neurons to spiking threshold faster after hyperpolarizing current (or inhibitory synaptic input) is removed. **Figure 3B** shows how the simulated blockade of HCN channels affects the activity of a model GP neuron. When HCN channels are removed ($g_{hcnf,s} = 0$), the average pacemaking frequency decreases to 15.8 Hz ± 2.5 and 12% (58/500) of neurons do not pacemake. Without HCN channels the membrane potential sag is no longer seen, and hyperpolarizing current has a much stronger effect on membrane potential. The time between the removal of hyperpolarizing current and the return of spiking is also much longer, and much more sensitive to the hyperpolarization level. These results agree with previous work that has investigated the role of HCN channels using mouse GP slices and multicompartmental simulations (Chan et al., 2004).

3.2. HEALTHY NETWORK ACTIVITY

Whilst we were able to base STN firing rate and the conductance of GP-GP synapses directly on experimental evidence, we could only do this indirectly with the STN-GP synaptic conductance (g_{SG}). We chose a value of 0.1 nS for this parameter in the healthy case as this gives similar proportions of neurons in the TI, TA and NM groups as seen in experiments. **Figure 4A** shows this distribution [cf. Figure 2A in Mallet et al. (2008b)] and **Figure 4B** shows the spiking activity of the TI, TA and NM neurons in one trial. A small proportion of neurons (9.9% ± 2.1) are catergorized as QU because they fire spikes rarely or not at all; we are not sure if this is a biologically accurate result as such neurons may have been excluded from the results of electrophysiological studies. The majority of neurons (68.3% ± 3.9) are catergorized as NM and neurons in this group spike with an average firing rate

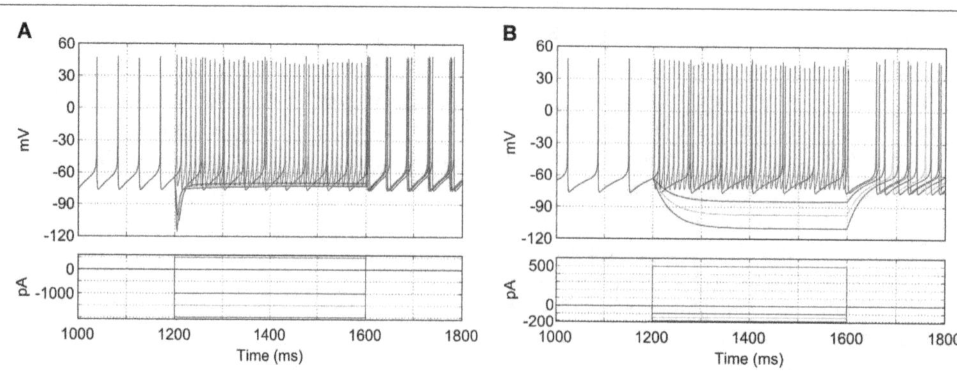

FIGURE 3 | Response of a typical isolated model GP neuron to different current injections. (A) Neuron with normal HCN channel density. Depolarizing current causes fast, regular spiking (green trace), while hyperpolarizing current reveals a sag in membrane potential and rebound firing (red, cyan, and purple traces). With no current injection the neuron fires regularly at approximately 22 Hz (blue trace). **(B)** Neuron with HCN channels removed. Sag in membrane potential is lost and pacemaking is slowed. Note the difference in scale for the injection currents between **(A)** and **(B)**.

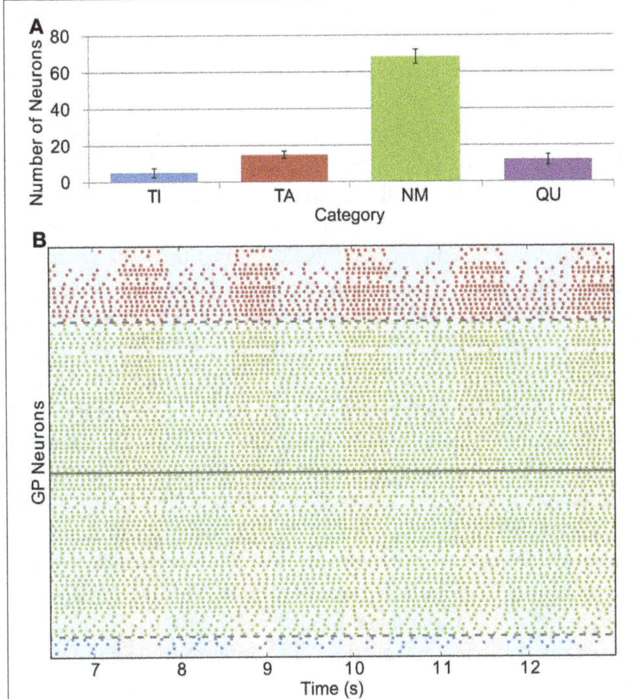

FIGURE 4 | Catergorization and activity of neurons under healthy conditions. (A) The average number of GP neurons in each category across all trials ($n = 12$), showing that most cells do not display prominent modulation by SWA (error bars show standard deviation). **(B)** Raster plot showing the spiking activity of TI, TA and NM neurons in one representative trial. The spike trains above the solid gray line are from neurons whose average spike phase is in the active part of the SWA cycle (light pink shaded background), whilst those below the line have average phases in the inactive part of SWA (light blue shaded background). The spike trains are ordered such that those closer to the solid gray line have lower confidence measures than those further away. The dashed gray lines show the confidence measure boundaries that divide neurons classified as NM from those classified as TI or TA (this boundary is set at 0.1).

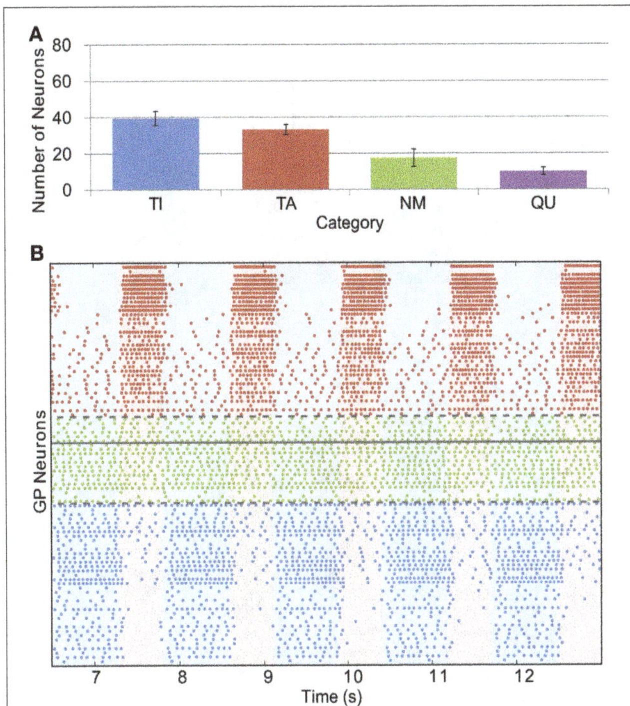

FIGURE 5 | Catergorization and activity of neurons under Parkinsonian conditions. (A) The average number of GP neurons in each category across all trials ($n = 12$), showing that most neurons start to display SWA-modulated firing patterns, either in-phase (TA) or anti-phase (TI). **(B)** Raster plot of Parkinsonian GP neuron activity (description as in **Figure 4B**).

of 12.3 Hz $\pm$ 3.3 and coefficient of variation (CV) of 0.12 $\pm$ 0.04. These statistics are in good agreement with those of neurons recorded from mice GP slices by Chan et al. (2004) (firing rate 12.5, CV 0.18). However, in contrast to these experimental results, which found no effect on firing rate or CV after blocking $GABA_A$ receptors, we would expect the average firing rate of the neurons in our model to increase slightly with inhibition blocked, as the average firing rate in the network is lower than the average pacemaking frequency of isolated model neurons. The average firing frequencies in the (small) TI and TA groups were 3.7 Hz $\pm$1.8 and 10.7 Hz $\pm$ 4.7, respectively.

3.3. PARKINSONIAN NETWORK ACTIVITY

The effects of dopamine lesion were simulated in the model by an increased intensity of STN firing and increased strength of STN-GP excitation and intra-GP inhibition. These changes have a profound effect on activity in the model GP that is similar to what is seen in experiments. As **Figure 5** shows, most neurons begin to preferentially fire during either the active or inactive phase of the SWA. In order to see proportions of TA and TI neurons that were similar to *in vivo* results it was necessary to double the strength of STN-GP and GP-GP synapses ($g_{SG} = 0.2$ nS, $g_{GG} = 1.0$ ns).

The average firing frequency of NM neurons decreased slightly under Parkinsonian conditions while the average firing rates of the TI and TA groups increased to 6.3 Hz $\pm$3.6 and 11.1 Hz $\pm$5.1, respectively (**Figure 6A**). Although the variance of these statistics is fairly large, there does appear to be a trend for different firing rates between the different groups that is not seen *in vivo* (Magill et al., 2001). This difference is perhaps not too surprising given our simplistic and somewhat arbitrary choices for STN-GP and GP-GP connectivity.

In order to investigate the factors that determine whether a neuron becomes TA, TI, NM or QU we examined the following statistics of each neuron: maximum conductance of the NaP persistent sodium channel; initial (before downregulation) maximum conductance of fast and slow HCN channels; total maximum conductance of all excitatory (AMPA) synapses from STN neurons; total maximum conductance of all inhibitory synapses from other GP neurons. In general these statistics were remarkably similar between each of the groups, with two exceptions. Firstly, quiet (QU) neurons have, on average, much lower maximum conductances for their NaP channel (**Figure 6B**). These channels underlie autonomous pacemaking (Mercer et al., 2007) and the intrinsic pacemaking frequency is strongly dependent on the value of the NaP maximum conductance. Since QU neurons have low NaP conductance they are likely to pacemake very slowly

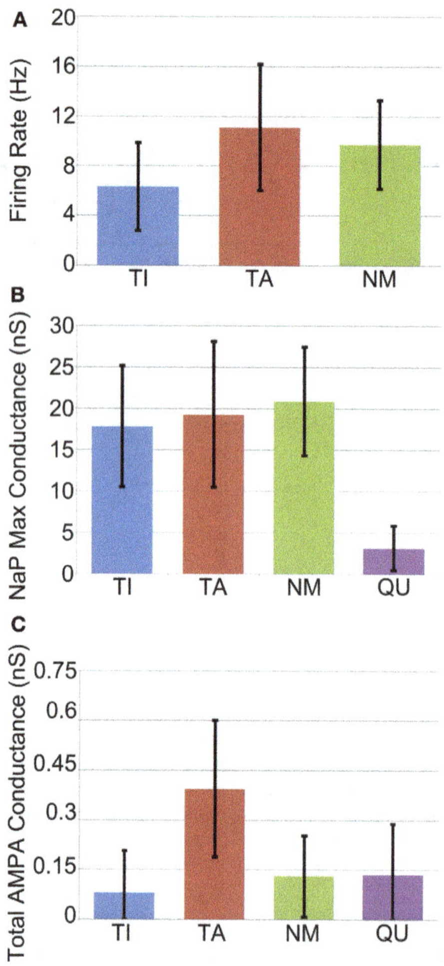

FIGURE 6 | Average cell properties by categorization across all GP neurons from all trials ($n = 1200$). (A) Average firing rate is rather variable but is in general slightly lower for TI neurons. **(B)** Maximum conductance of the persistent sodium channel (NaP) which underlies pacemaking. Quiet neurons can be easily categorized as those with very low NaP conductance. **(C)** Average total maximum conductance due to excitatory synapses. TA neurons receive more excitation on average, but it is highly variable.

or not at all, and it appears (from examination of voltage traces) that the incoming inhibition from other GP neurons is sufficient to prevent them from ever firing. Secondly, TA neurons receive on average more excitatory synaptic input from the STN than the other groups (**Figure 6C**). This result was expected, since STN firing occurs during the active phase of SWA and so it is not surprising that those GP neurons that receive more STN input also fire preferentially during the active phase. In general, however, the simple statistics we examined about membrane properties and synaptic connectivity are not enough to determine which group a particular neuron will fall into. Predicting the classification of a neuron involves knowing the classification of the other GP neurons that it receives inhibition from. This makes the problem complex and extremely difficult to resolve a priori. Instead, when the network is simulated, a dynamic process takes place in which the network self-organizes its activity into the different groups of neurons.

HCN channel downregulation plays a significant, but not essential, role in the emergence of the different groups of neurons in our model. Without this mechanism, many neurons in the TA group continue to fire during the inactive phase due to their intrinsic pacemaker properties. Although this inactive-phase firing is slower than their active-phase firing (due to reduced excitatory input), it is still a source of inhibitory input to other GP neurons and may silence or slow the firing of some which may otherwise be catergorized as TI. With the HCN downregulation mechanism those neurons that receive the most excitatory STN input, and therefore fire at the fastest rate during the active period, will have their maximum HCN conductances reduced. This reduction has the effect of decreasing the intrinsic pacemaking frequency and increasing the hyperpolarization that occurs in response to inhibitory input. To quantify the effect on pacemaking frequency, we ran four simulations using the Parkinsonian parameter values for a period of time long enough for downregulation to take effect (6.5 s) and then removed all synapses and recorded firing rates. The average pacemaker frequency after downregulation was 16.9 Hz ± 2.1, a clear reduction from the normal pacemaker frequency of our model neurons (23.6 Hz $\pm$ 4.0). The proportion of QU neurons after downregulation was 2%, lower than the 4% that we would expect based on the normal pacemaker properties, but we attribute this to statistical noise due to the rather small sample sizes.

These changes to pacemaking affect the competition dynamics during the inactive phase and mean that most TA neurons are no longer able to fire at all during this phase. Although the proportion of neurons classified as either TA or TI is similar with or without HCN downregulation (72.7% $\pm$ 5.4 normally, 68.7% $\pm$ 5.0 without downregulation), TA neuron firing is much more clearly restricted to the active phase with downregulation. This is seen in the average confidence measure (ω) of TA neurons, which is 0.44 ± 0.22 with HCN downregulation and 0.32 ± 0.18 without. The effect is also shown by phase diagrams showing the spiking activity of typical neurons (**Figure 7**). In these plots the background is shaded to show the active (pink) and inactive (blue) parts of the SWA cycle, showing that TI neurons fire preferentially in the inactive part and TA neurons fire preferentially in the active part. The red bars show the average spike phase and their length indicates the confidence measure as a proportion of the total radius.

3.4. LARGER NETWORKS

The results described above were from simulations with 100 GP neurons, each of which made 20 inhibitory synapses onto 20 other (randomly chosen) GP neurons. This level of coupling ($\approx 20\%$) is probably much higher than what is seen in the real GP (Sadek et al., 2007). We ran several simulations, using Parkinsonian parameter settings, where the coupling proportion was decreased by scaling up the number of GP and STN neurons but keeping the number of synapses that each neuron made constant. In the first set of simulations we used 200 GP neurons and 100 STN neurons and in the second set we used 300 GP neurons and 150 STN. These give GP-GP coupling levels of $20/199 \approx 10\%$ and $20/299 \approx 7\%$, respectively. In each case we ran three simulations. For the simulations with 200 GP neurons there were an average

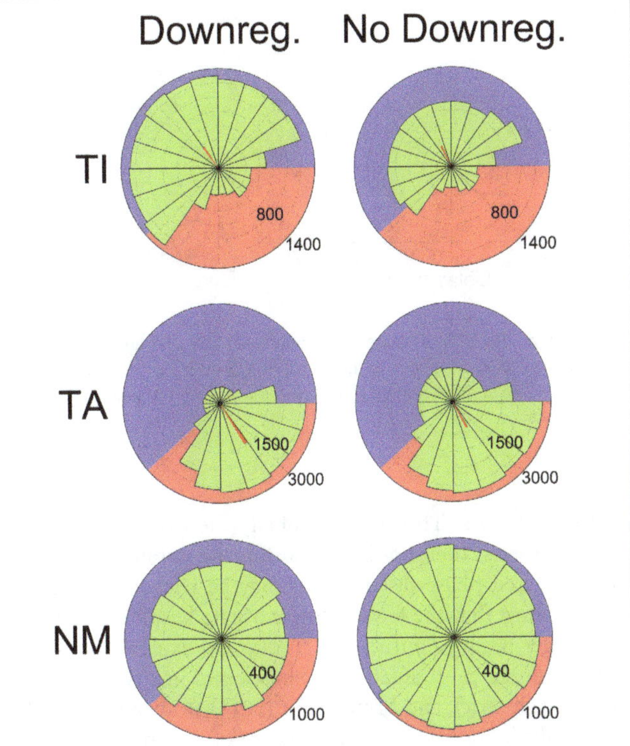

FIGURE 7 | Phase histograms showing the distribution of spikes relative to SWA phase grouped by categorization (Top: TI, Middle: TA, Bottom: NM), demonstrating the effects of HCN downregulation. Numbers indicate the number of spikes in each bin (65 ms bin width). Data are shown from two sets of 12 simulations, one with the HCN downregulation mechanism enabled (left) and one with it disabled (right). The background of each diagram is shaded to illustrate the active (pink, 500 ms) and inactive (blue, 800 ms) parts of the SWA cycle. Downregulation reduces TA neuron firing during the inactive phase **(Middle)**, increases TI firing during the inactive phase **(Top)** and decreases NM firing **(Bottom)**. Spikes from the latter half of simulations (6.5 s out of 13 s) from all neurons (except those categorized as QU) were used to generate the diagrams. The orientation of the red bars shows the average spike phase and their length shows the phase confidence measure (ω) as a proportion of the total radius.

of 71 ± 2.8 TI neurons and 73.7 ± 1.7 TA neurons. For the simulations ($n = 3$) with 300 GP neurons there were an average of 122 ± 4.1 TI neurons and 101.3 ± 2.5 TA neurons. These proportions (particularly in the latter case) are similar to the proportions in the smaller network (see **Figure 5**).

3.5. OTHER FREQUENCY BANDS

We briefly investigated to see if the activity of GP neurons could become entrained to higher frequency cortical rhythms, specifically those in the β band. To do this we generated STN spike trains that were modulated at approximately 14 Hz (70 ms period: 40 ms inactive phase, 30 ms active phase). Although biological experiments on OHDA lesioned rodents find that most neurons fall under the same TI or TA category regardless of whether the cortical rhythm is SWA or β, it was difficult and not effective to use our normal method to categorize neurons because the number of spikes fired by GP neurons in each β cycle was very low. However, examining spike cross-correlations between STN and GP neurons showed that the majority of GP neurons did show oscillatory firing that was in-phase with the STN input (**Figure 8A**). We examined auto-correlations for individual GP neurons and found that the frequency of these neurons' oscillations varied somewhat from neuron to neuron, which suggests that their firing becomes synchronized to some intermediate frequency between the 14 Hz input and their intrinsic pacemaking frequency. We did not see any GP neurons that showed anti-phase oscillations when using our standard Parkinsonian parameters. However, when the degree of intra-GP inhibition is dramatically increased (40% coupling, $g_{GG} = 3.0\,\text{nS}$) then a few neurons do begin to show a preference for anti-phase firing (**Figure 8B**), albeit at a very low rate. It is possible that with different synaptic parameters or connection topology (for example, STN input that preferentially makes contact with a particular group of GP neurons), the synchronized activity of one group could cause a second group to become synchronized in anti-phase.

4. DISCUSSION

4.1. A NEW, BIOLOGICALLY DETAILED, MODEL HELPS US TO STUDY GP DYNAMICS

We have presented what we believe to be a novel model of GP neurons that features much of the biological realism of previous detailed multi-compartmental models but considerably reduced complexity (both computationally and in terms of model construction). This makes our model well-suited to detailed modeling of the dynamics of networks of GP neurons and their connections with other nuclei. We have also introduced a possible computational mechanism for simulating the downregulation of HCN channels and shown that this improves how closely our results fit with biological evidence.

Our results demonstrate a mechanism whereby local inhibitory connections allow two anti-phase oscillatory subpopulations of GP neurons to emerge in response to rhythmic excitatory input from the STN. The two subpopulations appear due to a complex self-organization process and despite the homogenity of the overall population. This effect is only seen when both the STN input and inhibitory GP-GP coupling are sufficiently strong, and there is good experimental evidence that both STN input to the GP and intra-GP coupling increase in rodent models of Parkinson's disease. We therefore claim that our model shows a plausible mechanism for those experimental results which show a prominent increase in the number of TA and TI neurons that occurs in the rodent GP after dopamine lesioning (Magill et al., 2001). In our model, HCN channel downregulation makes oscillatory entrainment of the in-phase group of neurons more prominent but is not essential for the two groups to appear. This may explain the result of Chan et al. (2011) whereby artificial up-regulation of HCN channels via viral transfection restored the cells' ability to autonomously pacemake but did not give any significant improvement to Parkinsonian motor impairment. The fact that we did not see an increase in the number of neurons that were unable to autonomously pacemake following simulations of the Parkinsonian network may indicate that we didn't set the threshold for HCN downregulation low enough.

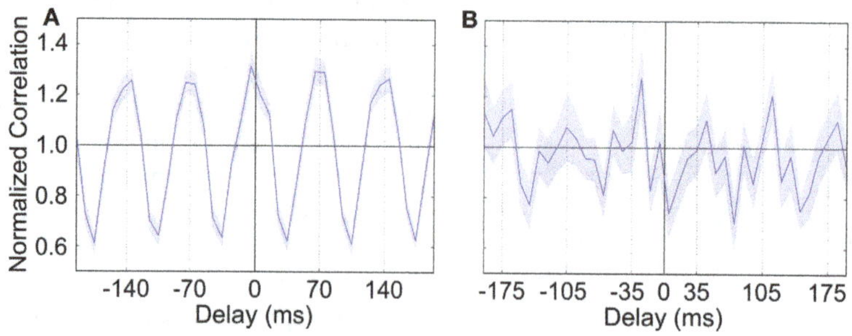

FIGURE 8 | Spike cross-correlation diagrams showing the relationship between STN and GP neuron firing when STN input is modulated at approximately 14 Hz (70 ms period). (A) Typical average cross-correlation between all STN neurons and a single GP neuron showing synchronized in-phase firing. **(B)** STN-GP cross-correlation for a (rare) GP neuron that shows firing that is anti-phase to the β rhythm. Normalization is as in **Figure 2** (Brillinger, 1976) and the shaded area shows the standard deviation across STN neurons.

4.2. RELATIONSHIP TO PREVIOUS STUDIES ON COUPLED OSCILLATORS

Networks of coupled oscillators are found in many areas of science and the dynamics of such networks have therefore been widely studied from a theoretical standpoint. Our model can be thought of as a network of inhibitory coupled oscillators that receive random, sparse excitatory input with a particular global frequency. Although many theoretical studies of similar systems use reduced models, they may still provide insights into the different dynamical behaviors that our model is likely to exhibit.

Most previous theoretical studies do not include common external input to the coupled oscillators, although some may consider the effects of input that is constant in time. Chow (1998) describes the analysis of a neuronal network that consists of a number of oscillators with heterogenous spiking frequencies that are all-to-all coupled by inhibitory connections. Such networks are capable of producing a range of dynamics, including almost-synchronous phase-locking, harmonic locking, and suppression. The stability of these states strongly depends on the details of the neurons' response to synaptic input. This network is similar to our model in the case where STN input is made constant in time, although inhibitory coupling in the GP network is random and relatively sparse rather than all-to-all. Since SWA oscillations are much slower than the GP neurons' intrinsic pacemaking, we can consider the GP network during the active and inactive phases separately, with constant STN input within each phase. Using the terminology of Chow (1998), during the active phase of SWA (high STN input) the TI neurons are in the suppressed state while in the inactive phase the TA neurons are suppressed. We have not observed synchrony between neurons during active or inactive phases, although it's possible that the system would converge to these states after a long period of time with constant input.

As the frequency of the cortical modulation is increased to be closer to the GP neurons' pacemaker frequencies (e.g., into the β band) it no longer makes sense to consider the scenario of constant STN input. In this scenario, theoretical results from oscillator models may be useful for suggesting conditions that support the emergence of in-phase and anti-phase groups. Golomb et al. (1992) describes a network of phase oscillators that all receive common global input that is a function of the phases of the oscillators. This is not explictly the case in our model, but nevertheless their findings regarding the stability of solutions with clustered phase distributions may be relevant. In particular they show that the fewer clusters a state has, the more stable it is (larger basin of attraction). This could explain why the GP network under β modulation organises into just two anti-phase clusters. Kilpatrick and Ermentrout (2011) study a more biologically realistic model for the emergence of gamma rhythms in a network containing a large population of excitatory neurons with a smaller subpopulation of inhibitory interneurons. Interestingly, they show that the number of clusters that emerge in their model depends on the level of spike frequency adaptation in the excitatory neurons, which arises due to a calcium current. Our model contains a calcium channel that activates during fast firing and causes some degree of spike frequency adaptation, which raises the possibility that using different conductances for this channel may result in patterns with more than two clusters. It has also been shown that networks of neurons that have heterogenous synaptic interconnectivity may display clustered dynamics if the connectivity structure satisfies certain conditions (Li et al., 2003)—although this has only been shown for excitatory synapses and so it is not clear whether the same would apply to the GP network.

4.3. STIMULATION OF THE STN MAY REDUCE OSCILLATIONS IN THE HYPERDIRECT PATHWAY

The hypothesis that basal ganglia activity is entrained to cortical rhythms via the hyper-direct pathway in Parkinson's disease offers some explanation of the possible mechanism(s) underlying the clinical effectiveness of STN deep-brain stimulation (DBS), in which an implanted electrode provides constant electrical stimulation of approximately 120 Hz to the STN. The precise effects of this stimulation on neuronal activity in the basal ganglia are not fully understood and are likely to be many and varied (Kringelbach et al., 2010). The computational model of the basal ganglia of Kumar et al. (2011) included the effects of DBS through either a reduction of strength of cortex-STN synapses or inhibitory input onto STN and in both cases DBS was found to reduce oscillatory firing. In this model oscillations appear because the STN and GPe act as a pacemaker circuit due to the excitatory connections between STN neurons. It is clear that if DBS were added to our model in a similar manner then oscillations in the GP would be much reduced, as they are dependent on reasonably strong input from the STN. Another possible mechanism of DBS that has good experimental support is that it antidromically activates the fibers that project from the cortex to the STN (Li et al., 2007). The effect of this antidromic activiation is a reduction of oscillatory activity in the cortical regions that project to the STN. Since our model only includes STN input to the GP, clearly a reduction of oscillatory STN activity would reduce GP oscillations as well. Wilson et al. (2011) found that in a relatively abstract model of the GP consisting of uncoupled phase oscillators synchronized to a common input, chaotic dynamics served to desynchronize the population at frequencies and intensities similar to those that are clinically effecive for DBS. The same may also be true of our model when the GP neurons are entrained to β-frequency STN input but further investigation is required. Our model could also help to test and improve the effectiveness of new forms of DBS, such as that proposed by Popovych and Tass (2012) which involves using multiple electrodes to desynchronize groups of neurons that have become entrained to particular rhythms.

4.4. THE EMERGENCE OF TI/TA GROUPS DEPENDS ON STRONG INHIBITORY COUPLING

One possible weakness of our model is that it relies on intra-GP inhibition being much denser than is currently supported by experimental evidence. It has been estimated that the probability of a given GP neuron synapsing onto any other, randomly-chosen, GP neuron is less than 1% (Sadek et al., 2007) but in most of our simulations this value is 20%. Our preliminary experiments with larger networks have suggested that the level of intra-GP coupling can be reduced while preserving the division into TI and TA groups by increasing the size of the network. Further work will involve investigating even larger (more computationally expensive) networks to see how much further the size of the network can be increased while maintaining the same division.

If further increases in network size cannot generate realistic activity with physiological levels of GP-GP coupling, there are several other possible reasons why the connectivity may be greater than has so far been measured experimentally. It has been suggested that the basal ganglia are organized into a series of partially overlapping "channels" (Alexander and Crutcher, 1990), where neurons preferentially synapse onto other neurons in the same channel. We have previously shown modeling evidence that increased coupling between channels may allow the STN-GP circuit to generate oscillations (Merrison-Hort et al., 2013), but in the present study we suggest that our small population of GP neurons could represent part of a single channel. Under this assumption, the proportion of coupled neurons might be much higher than would be seen from picking pairs of neurons from across the whole GP at random. It is also possible that the projection from GP to STN, which is not included in our model, may contribute to the effect of lateral inhibition since the tri-synaptic GP-STN-GP pathway is a route by which GP neurons inhibit other GP neurons, and there is experimental evidence to suggest the strength of this pathway may be increased under Parkinsonian conditions (Johnson and Napier, 1997). However, it is hard to say whether or not this explanation is plausible without more detailed information about the topology of the STN-GP and GP-STN projections.

Similarly, the increase in GP-GP synaptic conductance that occurs under Parkinsonian conditions in our model may be larger than in reality. Although we have used data from paired-pulse experiments to choose the conductance of GP-GP synapses in the healthy case, it is not clear how much this increases by following loss of dopaminergic input. Miguelez et al. (2012) used an optogentic technique to stimulate a number of GP neurons whilst recording IPSCs and found an increase of approximately 67% after dopamine lesioning. This is considerably smaller than the increase we use under Parkinsonian conditions, where the GP-GP conductance is doubled. However, the increase seen by Miguelez et al. (2012) may be lower than the in conductance at a single GP-GP synapse, since their method simultaneously activates many pre-synaptic GP neurons and the summation of the resulting IPSCs may not be linear.

4.5. FUTURE WORK: STRIATAL INPUT, RECIPROCAL CONNECTIONS AND GP HETEROGENITY MAY IMPROVE OUR RESULTS

The aim of this study was primarily to investigate whether the hyperdirect pathway alone could account for one characteristic of the Parkinsonian GP and we have therefore only included STN-GP and GP-GP synaptic connectivity. However, the main source of synaptic input to the GP is the striatum, and it is clear that adding simulated inhibitory striatal synaptic input could improve our results. Galati et al. (2009) demonstrated that the delivery of a $GABA_A$ antagonist into the GP also causes cortical entrainment of the neurons there and that this effect is dependent on a functioning STN. They suggest that this demonstrates that inhibitory striatal input is also involved in oscillatory entrainment. This result is more difficult to explain in our model, since it is unlikely that decreasing the level of GP-GP inhibition would cause oscillations to appear in the (otherwise) healthy case. However, if the effect of GABA antagonism is to remove *tonic* background inhibition (probably from the striatum) then we could include this in our model as a depolarizing current injection to all GP neurons. This would move their membrane potentials closer to the spike threshold and make them more sensitive to the (weak) rhythmic STN input that is present in the healthy case. Furthermore, Tseng et al. (2001) showed that the activity of striatal projection neurons is modulated by cortical SWA and increases after OHDA lesion. Including the effects of this in our model would probably increase the number of TI neurons and may allow us to reduce the amount of intra-GP inhibition to a more realistic level.

Another possible pathway that could be added to our model is the projection from the GP back to the STN. Computational models of networks that include this connection have shown that the STN and GP can work together to act as a pacemaker circuit (Gillies et al., 2002; Terman et al., 2002; Holgado et al., 2010). Terman et al. (2002) describes the results of simulating a spiking model of the interconnected STN-GPe network in which the tonic activity of both populations can become bursty with a regular bursting rhythm. In fact, the neurons in this model can self-organise into different sized clusters, which allows for the possibility of two anti-phase groups under some conditions. We expect that our model could support similar regimes if the GP-STN connection was added, provided that we also introduced a more realistic STN neuron model.

Although our model has demonstrated that discrete groups of neurons can emerge from a population of GP neurons with homogeneous (unimodally distributed) membrane properties, there is now some evidence that the neurons in the TA and TI groups are distinct in some ways, including the nature of local inhibitory connectivity, the basal ganglia nuclei that they project to, and in their chemistry (Mallet et al., 2012). Similarly, several studies (Nambu and Llinás, 1997; Cooper and Stanford, 2000; Bugaysen et al., 2010) have attempted to categorize GP neurons based on their electrophysiological properties, and their results seem to suggest that several distinct groups may exist (although the boundaries remain fuzzy). It would be very interesting to incorporate these results into our model, perhaps by making the parameter noise for the NaP or HCN channels bi- or tri-modal and by giving one group of neurons a higher degree of local connectivity than another. We expect that this would promote the emergence of the TI, TA and NM groups and would probably reduce the degree of GP-GP connectivity that is required in order to obtain results that are similar to experiments.

ACKNOWLEDGMENTS

We are grateful to A. Korngreen for sharing data regarding IPSPs of GP-GP synapses and P. Magill for friendly and useful feedback about our early experiments. Robert Merrison-Hort would like to acknowledge the generous support for workshop attendance given by the Fields Institute.

FUNDING

Robert Merrison-Hort and Roman Borisyuk are supported by the Faculty of Science and Technology, University of Plymouth.

REFERENCES

Alexander, G. E., and Crutcher, M. D. (1990). Functional architecture of basal ganglia circuits: neural substrates of parallel processing. *Trends Neurosci.* 13, 266–271. doi: 10.1016/0166-2236(90)90107-L

Borisyuk, R. (2002). Oscillatory activity in the neural networks of spiking elements. *Biosystems* 67, 3–16. doi: 10.1016/S0303-2647(02)00058-8

Boyes, J., Bolam, J. P., Shigemoto, R., and Stanford, I. M. (2007). Functional presynaptic hcn channels in the rat globus pallidus. *Eur. J. Neurosci.* 25, 2081–2092. doi: 10.1111/j.1460-9568.2007.05463.x

Brillinger, D. R. (1976). Measuring the association of point processes: a case history. *Am. Math. Mon.* 83, 16–22. doi: 10.2307/2318824

Bugaysen, J., Bronfeld, M., Tischler, H., Bar-Gad, I., and Korngreen, A. (2010). Electrophysiological characteristics of globus pallidus neurons. *PLoS ONE* 5:e12001. doi: 10.1371/journal.pone.0012001

Chan, C. S., Glajch, K. E., Gertler, T. S., Guzman, J. N., Mercer, J. N., Lewis, A. S., et al. (2011). Hcn channelopathy in external globus pallidus neurons in models of parkinson's disease. *Nat. Neurosci.* 14, 85–92. doi: 10.1038/nn.2692

Chan, C. S., Shigemoto, R., Mercer, J. N., and Surmeier, D. J. (2004). Hcn2 and hcn1 channels govern the regularity of autonomous pacemaking and synaptic resetting in globus pallidus neurons. *J. Neurosci.* 24, 9921–9932. doi: 10.1523/JNEUROSCI.2162-04.2004

Chow, C. C. (1998). Phase-locking in weakly heterogeneous neuronal networks. *Physica D* 118, 343–370. doi: 10.1016/S0167-2789(98)00082-7

Cooper, A. J., and Stanford, I. M. (2000). Electrophysiological and morphological characteristics of three subtypes of rat globus pallidus neurone *in vitro*. *J. Physiol.* 527, 291–304. doi: 10.1111/j.1469-7793.2000.t01-1-00291.x

Degos, B., Deniau, J.-M., Chavez, M., and Maurice, N. (2009). Chronic but not acute dopaminergic transmission interruption promotes a progressive increase in cortical beta frequency synchronization: relationships to vigilance state and akinesia. *Cereb. Cortex* 19, 1616–1630. doi: 10.1093/cercor/bhn199

Deister, C. A., Chan, C. S., Surmeier, D. J., and Wilson, C. J. (2009). Calcium-activated sk channels influence voltage-gated ion channels to determine the precision of firing in globus pallidus neurons. *J. Neurosci.* 29, 8452–8461. doi: 10.1523/JNEUROSCI.0576-09.2009

DeLong, M. R. (1990). Primate models of movement disorders of basal ganglia origin. *Trends Neurosci.* 13, 281–285. doi: 10.1016/0166-2236(90)90110-V

Eusebio, A., and Brown, P. (2009). Synchronisation in the beta frequency-band - the bad boy of parkinsonism or an innocent bystander? *Exp. Neurol.* 217, 1–3. doi: 10.1016/j.expneurol.2009.02.003

Galati, S., Stanzione, P., D'Angelo, V., Fedele, E., Marzetti, F., Sancesario, G., et al. (2009). The pharmacological blockade of medial forebrain bundle induces an acute pathological synchronization of the cortico subthalamic nucleus globus pallidus pathway. *J. Physiol.* 587, 4405–4423. doi: 10.1113/jphysiol.2009.172759

Gill, S. S., and Heywood, P. (1997). Bilateral dorsolateral subthalamotomy for advanced parkinson's disease. *Lancet* 350, 1224. doi: 10.1016/S0140-6736(05)63455-1

Gillies, A., Willshaw, D., and Li, Z. (2002). Subthalamic pallidal interactions are critical in determining normal and abnormal functioning of the basal ganglia. *Proc. R. Soc. Lond. B Biol. Sci.* 269, 545–551. doi: 10.1098/rspb.2001.1817

Golomb, D., Hansel, D., Shraiman, B., and Sompolinsky, H. (1992). Clustering in globally coupled phase oscillators. *Phys. Rev. A* 45, 3516–3530. doi: 10.1103/PhysRevA.45.3516

Günay, C., Edgerton, J. R., and Jaeger, D. (2008). Channel density distributions explain spiking variability in the globus pallidus: a combined physiology and computer simulation database approach. *J. Neurosci.* 28, 7476–7491. doi: 10.1523/JNEUROSCI.4198-07.2008

Hassani, O.-K., Mouroux, M., and Féger, J. (1996). Increased subthalamic neuronal activity after nigral dopaminergic lesion independent of disinhibition via the globus pallidus. *Neuroscience* 72, 105–115. doi: 10.1016/0306-4522(95)00535-8

Hernández, A., Ibáñez Sandoval, O., Sierra, A., Valdiosera, R., Tapia, D., Anaya, V., et al. (2006). Control of the subthalamic innervation of the rat globus pallidus by d2/3 and d4 dopamine receptors. *J. Neurophysiol.* 96, 2877–2888. doi: 10.1152/jn.00664.2006

Holgado, A. J. N., Terry, J. R., and Bogacz, R. (2010). Conditions for the generation of beta oscillations in the subthalamic nucleus-globus pallidus network. *J. Neurosci.* 30, 12340–12352. doi: 10.1523/JNEUROSCI.0817-10.2010

Jaeger, D., and Kita, H. (2011). Functional connectivity and integrative properties of globus pallidus neurons. *Neuroscience* 198, 44–53. doi: 10.1016/j.neuroscience.2011.07.050

Jenkinson, N., and Brown, P. (2011). New insights into the relationship between dopamine, beta oscillations and motor function. *Trends Neurosci.* 34, 611–618. doi: 10.1016/j.tins.2011.09.003

Johnson, P. I., and Napier, T. C. (1997). Gaba- and glutamate-evoked responses in the rat ventral pallidum are modulated by dopamine. *Eur. J. Neurosci.* 9, 1397–1406. doi: 10.1111/j.1460-9568.1997.tb01494.x

Kilpatrick, Z. P., and Ermentrout, B. (2011). Sparse gamma rhythms arising through clustering in adapting neuronal networks. *PLoS Comput. Biol.* 7:e1002281. doi: 10.1371/journal.pcbi.1002281

Kringelbach, M. L., Green, A. L., Owen, S. L. F., Schweder, P. M., and Aziz, T. Z. (2010). Sing the mind electric principles of deep brain stimulation. *Eur. J. Neurosci.* 32, 1070–1079. doi: 10.1111/j.1460-9568.2010.07419.x

Kühn, A. A., Kupsch, A., Schneider, G.-H., and Brown, P. (2006). Reduction in subthalamic 35Hz oscillatory activity correlates with clinical improvement in parkinson's disease. *Eur. J. Neurosci.* 23, 1956–1960. doi: 10.1111/j.1460-9568.2006.04717.x

Kumar, A., Cardanobile, S., Rotter, S., and Aertsen, A. (2011). The role of inhibition in generating and controlling parkinson's disease oscillations in the basal ganglia. *Front. Syst. Neurosci.* 5:86. doi: 10.3389/fnsys.2011.00086

Li, S., Arbuthnott, G. W., Jutras, M. J., Goldberg, J. A., and Jaeger, D. (2007). Resonant antidromic cortical circuit activation as a consequence of high-frequency subthalamic deep-brain stimulation. *J. Neurophysiol.* 98, 3525–3537. doi: 10.1152/jn.00808.2007

Litvak, V., Jha, A., Eusebio, A., Oostenveld, R., Foltynie, T., Limousin, P., et al. (2011). Resting oscillatory cortico-subthalamic connectivity in patients with parkinsons disease. *Brain* 134, 359–374. doi: 10.1093/brain/awq332

Li, Y.-X., Wang, Y.-Q., and Miura, R. (2003). Clustering in small networks of excitatory neurons with heterogeneous coupling strengths. *J. Comput. Neurosci.* 14, 139–159.

Loucif, K. C., Wilson, C. L., Baig, R., Lacey, M. G., and Stanford, I. M. (2005). Functional interconnectivity between the globus pallidus and the subthalamic nucleus in the mouse brain slice. *J. Physiol.* 567, 977–987. doi: 10.1113/jphysiol.2005.093807

Lozano, A. M., Lang, A. E., Galvez-Jimenez, N., Miyasaki, J., Duff, J., Hutchison, W. D., et al. (1995). Effect of gpi pallidotomy on motor function in parkinson's disease. *Lancet* 346, 1383–1387. doi: 10.1016/S0140-6736(95)92404-3

Lüthi, A., and McCormick, D. A. (1998). H-current: properties of a neuronal and network pacemaker. *Neuron* 21, 9–12. doi: 10.1016/S0896-6273(00)80509-7

Magill, P. J., Bolam, J. P., and Bevan, M. D. (2001). Dopamine regulates the impact of the cerebral cortex on the subthalamic nucleusglobus pallidus network. *Neuroscience* 106, 313–330. doi: 10.1016/S0306-4522(01)00281-0

Mallet, N., Micklem, B. R., Henny, P., Brown, M. T., Williams, C., et al. (2012). Dichotomous organization of the external globus pallidus. *Neuron* 74, 1075–1086. doi: 10.1016/j.neuron.2012.04.027

Mallet, N., Pogosyan, A., Márton, L. F., Bolam, J. P., Brown, P., and Magill, P. J. (2008a). Parkinsonian beta oscillations in the external globus pallidus and their relationship with subthalamic nucleus activity. *J. Neurosci.* 28, 14245–14258. doi: 10.1523/JNEUROSCI.4199-08.2008

Mallet, N., Pogosyan, A., Sharott, A., Csicsvari, J., Bolam, J. P., Brown, P., et al. (2008b). Disrupted dopamine transmission and the emergence of exaggerated beta oscillations in subthalamic nucleus and cerebral cortex. *J. Neurosci.* 28, 4795–4806. doi: 10.1523/JNEUROSCI.0123-08.2008

Mercer, J. N., Chan, C. S., Tkatch, T., Held, J., and Surmeier, D. J. (2007). Nav1.6 sodium channels are critical to pacemaking and fast spiking in globus pallidus neurons. *J. Neurosci.* 27, 13552–13566. doi: 10.1523/JNEUROSCI.3430-07.2007

Merrison-Hort, R. J., Yousif, N., Njap, F., Hofmann, U. G., Burylko, O., and Borisyuk, R. (2013). An interactive channel model of the basal ganglia: bifurcation analysis under healthy and parkinsonian conditions. *J. Math. Neurosci.* 3, 14–14. doi: 10.1186/2190-8567-3-14

Miguelez, C., Morin, S., Martinez, A., Goillandeau, M., Bezard, E., Bioulac, B., et al. (2012). Altered pallido-pallidal synaptic transmission leads to aberrant firing of globus pallidus neurons in a rat model of parkinson's disease. *J. Physiol.* 590, 5861–5875. doi: 10.1113/jphysiol.2012.241331

Nambu, A., and Llinás, R. (1997). Morphology of globus pallidus neurons: its correlation with electrophysiology in guinea pig brain slices. *J. Comp. Neurol.* 377, 85–94. doi: 10.1002/(SiCi)1096-9861(19970106)377:1<85:AID-CNE8>3.3.CO2-B

Ni, Z., Bouali-Benazzouz, R., Gao, D., Benabid, A.-L., and Benazzouz, A. (2000). Changes in the firing pattern of globus pallidus neurons after the degeneration of nigrostriatal pathway are mediated by the subthalamic nucleus in the rat. *Eur. J. Neurosci.* 12, 4338–4344. doi: 10.1111/j.1460-9568.2000.01346.x

Plenz, D., and Kital, S. T. (1999). A basal ganglia pacemaker formed by the subthalamic nucleus and external globus pallidus. *Nature* 400, 677–682. doi: 10.1038/23281

Popovych, O. V., and Tass, P. A. (2012). Desynchronizing electrical and sensory coordinated reset neuromodulation. *Front. Hum. Neurosci.* 6:58. doi: 10.3389/fnhum.2012.00058

Rubin, J. E., McIntyre, C. C., Turner, R. S., and Wichmann, T. (2012). Basal ganglia activity patterns in parkinsonism and computational modeling of their downstream effects. *Eur. J. Neurosci.* 36, 2213–2228. doi: 10.1111/j.1460-9568.2012.08108.x

Rubin, J. E., and Terman, D. (2004). High frequency stimulation of the subthalamic nucleus eliminates pathological thalamic rhythmicity in a computational model. *J. Comput. Neurosci.* 16, 211–235. doi: 10.1023/B:JCNS.0000025686.47117.67

Sadek, A. R., Magill, P. J., and Bolam, J. P. (2007). A single-cell analysis of intrinsic connectivity in the rat globus pallidus. *J. Neurosci.* 27, 6352–6362. doi: 10.1523/JNEUROSCI.0953-07.2007

Sharott, A., Magill, P. J., Bolam, J. P., and Brown, P. (2005). Directional analysis of coherent oscillatory field potentials in the cerebral cortex and basal ganglia of the rat. *J. Physiol.* 562, 951–963. doi: 10.1113/jphysiol.2004.073189

Terman, D., Rubin, J. E., Yew, A. C., and Wilson, C. J. (2002). Activity patterns in a model for the subthalamopallidal network of the basal ganglia. *J. Neurosci.* 22, 2963–2976.

Tseng, K. Y., Kasanetz, F., Kargieman, L., Riquelme, L. A., and Murer, M. G. (2001). Cortical slow oscillatory activity is reflected in the membrane potential and spike trains of striatal neurons in rats with chronic nigrostriatal lesions. *J. Neurosci.* 21, 6430–6439.

Walters, J., Hu, D., Itoga, C., Parr-Brownlie, L., and Bergstrom, D. (2007). Phase relationships support a role for coordinated activity in the indirect pathway in organizing slow oscillations in basal ganglia output after loss of dopamine. *Neuroscience* 144, 762–776. doi: 10.1016/j.neuroscience.2006.10.006

Wilson, C. J., Beverlin, B., and Netoff, T. I. (2011). Chaotic desynchronization as the therapeutic mechanism of deep brain stimulation. *Front. Syst. Neurosci.* 5:50. doi: 10.3389/fnsys.2011.00050

13

Decomposition of Abnormal Free Locomotor Behavior in a Rat Model of Parkinson's Disease

Benjamin Grieb[1,2]*, Constantin von Nicolai[1,3], Gerhard Engler[1], Andrew Sharott[1,4], Ismini Papageorgiou[5], Wolfgang Hamel[6], Andreas K. Engel[1†] and Christian K. Moll[1†]

[1] Department of Neurophysiology and Pathophysiology, University Medical Center Hamburg-Eppendorf, University of Hamburg, Hamburg, Germany
[2] Department of General Psychiatry, Center for Psychosocial Medicine, University of Heidelberg, Heidelberg, Germany
[3] Centre for Integrative Neuroscience, University of Tübingen, Tübingen, Germany
[4] Medical Research Council, Anatomical Neuropharacology Unit, Department of Pharmacology, University of Oxford, Oxford, UK
[5] Division of General Neurophysiology, Institute of Physiology and Pathophysiology, University of Heidelberg, Heidelberg, Germany
[6] Department of Neurosurgery, University Medical Center Hamburg-Eppendorf, University of Hamburg, Hamburg, Germany

***Correspondence:**
Benjamin Grieb, Department of General Psychiatry, Center for Psychosocial Medicine, University of Heidelberg, Voßstrasse 2, 69115 Heidelberg, Germany
e-mail: benjamin.grieb@med.uni-heidelberg.de

†These authors have contributed equally to this work.

Poverty of spontaneous movement, slowed execution and reduced amplitudes of movement (akinesia, brady- and hypokinesia) are cardinal motor manifestations of Parkinson's disease that can be modeled in experimental animals by brain lesions affecting midbrain dopaminergic neurons. Most behavioral investigations in experimental parkinsonism have employed short-term observation windows to assess motor impairments. We postulated that an analysis of longer-term free exploratory behavior could provide further insights into the complex fine structure of altered locomotor activity in parkinsonian animals. To this end, we video-monitored 23 hours of free locomotor behavior and extracted several behavioral measures before and after the expression of a severe parkinsonian phenotype following bilateral 6-hydroxydopamine (6-OHDA) lesions of the rat dopaminergic substantia nigra. Unbiased stereological cell counting verified the degree of midbrain tyrosine hydroxylase positive cell loss in the substantia nigra and ventral tegmental area. In line with previous reports, overall covered distance and maximal motion speed of lesioned animals were found to be significantly reduced compared to controls. Before lesion surgery, exploratory rat behavior exhibited a bimodal distribution of maximal speed values obtained for single movement episodes, corresponding to a "first" and "second gear" of motion. 6-OHDA injections significantly reduced the incidence of second gear motion episodes and also resulted in an abnormal prolongation of these fast motion events. Likewise, the spatial spread of such episodes was increased in 6-OHDA rats. The increase in curvature of motion tracks was increased in both lesioned and control animals. We conclude that the discrimination of distinct modes of motion by statistical decomposition of longer-term spontaneous locomotion provides useful insights into the fine structure of fluctuating motor functions in a rat analog of Parkinson's disease.

Keywords: 6-OHDA lesions, stereology, spontaneous activity, Parkinson disease, video monitoring

INTRODUCTION

Neurotoxin-induced degeneration of nigral dopamine neurons in experimental animals results in motor abnormalities relevant to motor symptoms of Parkinson's disease (PD; Cenci et al., 2002). One strategy to deplete midbrain dopaminergic neurons in rats is to infuse the neurotoxin 6-hydroxydopamine (6-OHDA) directly into the substantia nigra pars compacta (SNc; Schwarting and Huston, 1996a,b), which can also cause moderate cell death in the neighboring ventral tegmental area (VTA). In the prototypic toxin-induced rat model of PD, unilateral intracerebral 6-OHDA injections lead to the expression of a strictly lateralized hemiparkinsonian phenotype, the behavioral sequelae of which have been described in great detail. A wide variety of different behavioral tests are used to examine motor changes associated with the asymmetrical depletion of the nigrostriatal dopaminergic system, e.g., skilled motor tasks (Mokrý et al., 1995; Truong et al., 2006), footprint-analysis (Metz et al., 2005), treadmill running (Brazhnik et al., 2012), or drug-induced rotation (Ungerstedt, 1971; Kelly, 1975). Compared to the unilateral 6-OHDA model, bilaterally lesioned rats have been used less commonly, although they display a far more severe parkinsonian phenotype. In this respect, the slowness and scarcity of movement observed in the bilateral 6-OHDA rat model resembles more closely the marked expression of PD-like symptoms in monkeys treated systemically with 1-methyl-4-phenyl-1,2,3,6-tetrahydropyridine (Bergman et al., 1990) and cardinal motor manifestations of human PD patients in advanced disease stages. The development of pronounced motor impairment in rats with severe bilateral 6-OHDA lesions is, however, often accompanied by aphagia, adipsia and abulia (Schallert et al., 1978; Sakai and Gash, 1994; Cass et al., 2005; Ferro et al., 2005).

Rat equivalents of akinesia are commonly assessed in an "open-field" environment. Most often, rat motion (including scanning, walking or running, as well as rearing) is detected by consecutively breaking light beams arranged in an array around the arena (Cass et al., 2005; Ferro et al., 2005; Belujon et al., 2007). Other methods to quantify locomotor capacities are wheel (Schallert et al., 1978) or treadmill running (Avila et al., 2010). These standard measurements usually assess a short period of 10–60 min of locomotor activity (Cass et al., 2005; Ferro et al., 2005; Belujon et al., 2007), assuming a stable motor phenotype over time. However, these methods may underestimate the complexity of exploratory behavior, in particular long-term motor fluctuations.

Recently, a novel analytical approach to video-based tracking data utilized the statistical discrimination of rat motor behavior on the basis of speeds (Drai et al., 2000; Drai and Golani, 2001). This form of data analysis showed that naïve rats, but also naïve mice (Drai et al., 2001), use distinctly different modes of motion to explore their environment. The current study aimed to assess the impact of dopamine depletion on these naturally occurring behavioral patterns. We hypothesized that expression of a severe parkinsonian phenotype would not only reduce overall motion speed, as could be assessed with other standard quantification methods, but would also alter the fine spatio-temporal structure of exploratory locomotion modes. To test this, we adapted the analysis approach of Drai and colleagues to video-based tracking data from 23 hours of continuous and spontaneous locomotion of bilaterally 6-OHDA lesioned and control rats.

MATERIALS AND METHODS

ANIMALS

Animal experiments were approved by the local government authorities of Hamburg and carried out in accordance with the European Council Directive 86/609/EEC. All experiments were performed on male Brown Norway rats (Rattus norvegicus; Charles River Laboratories, Sulzfeld, Germany). All efforts were made to minimize suffering. The bilateral 6-OHDA lesion model is known to be associated with high mortality due to aphagia/adipsia and following loss of body weight (Ferro et al., 2005). Careful clinical inspection and weighting of animals was performed on a daily basis. In general, we offered a soft and moist rat chow and 10%-glucose solution in addition to standard chow and water *ad libitum*. To sustain aphagic and adipsic PD rats, we administered a liquid and high caloric nutrition for rodents (Altromin, Lage, Germany) by manual needle feeding. In total, the dropout rate was 5/14 PD rats. Dropouts included perioperative death ($n = 2$ PD) and loss of >20% body weight without stabilization of weight loss within 14 days after surgery ($n = 3$ PD) which led to euthanasia of these animals by decapitation under deep anesthesia (i.p.-injection of ketamine 100 mg/kg, xylazine 6 mg/kg).

EXPERIMENTAL DESIGN

We randomly assigned 14 rats to a PD group receiving bilateral 6-OHDA injections into the SNc and eight rats to a control group receiving bilateral vehicle injections (preoperative weight: 384 ± 32 g, mean ± *SD*). Video tracking of 23 hours of spontaneous locomotor activity was performed prior to surgery. Due to the labor intensity of sustaining PD rats we ran the experiment in two phases. Within the first subset of 10 rats ($n = 8$ PD; $n = 2$ controls) the dropout rate was 4/8 PD rats. The second subset of 12 rats ($n = 6$ PD; $n = 6$ controls) exhibited a dropout rate of 1/6 PD rats. Postoperative locomotor activity was assessed after a recovery period of 12 ± 2 days in the first subset and 28 ± 2 days in the second subset. After postoperative video monitoring, all rats were subsequently used in a separate study. We sacrificed rats after induction of deep anesthesia (ketamine/xylazine) ~14 weeks after lesioning by transcardial perfusion with saline. A midbrain tissue block was immersion-fixed in 4%-PFA-solution (paraformaldehyde in 0.1 M phosphate buffered saline, Sigma-Aldrich) for subsequent histological TH-staining and stereological counting of tyrosine hydroxylase (TH)-positive SNc and VTA neurons.

BILATERAL 6-HYDROXYDOPAMINE LESIONS

Stereotactic injections were performed under general anesthesia introduced with isoflurane (Baxter Germany GmbH, Unterschleißheim, Germany) and maintained with i.p.-injections of ketamine (65 mg/kg, Dr. E. Gräub AG, Bern, Switzerland) and xylazine (3 mg/kg, Bayer Health Care, Leverkusen, Germany). Thirty minutes prior to 6-OHDA or vehicle injections, rats received a bolus i.p.-injection of desipramine (25 mg/kg, Sigma-Aldrich, Munich, Germany) to minimize uptake of 6-OHDA in noradrenergic midbrain neurons (Schwarting and Huston, 1996b). Cardiopulmonary protection was assured by an initial bolus injection of atropine (0.25 mg/kg, B. Braun Melsungen AG, Melsungen, Germany). Body temperature was monitored during surgery with a rectal probe and hypothermia was prevented with an adjustable heating pad (FST, Heidelberg, Germany). In addition, the eyes were covered with dexpanthenol cream to prevent exsiccation. Animals were mounted in a stereotactic frame (David Kopf Instruments, Tujunga, USA). To target the SNc a Hamilton microliter-syringe (FST) was lowered through a burr hole placed at +4 mm AP and ±2.2 mm ML using the interaural line as reference (Paxinos and Watson, 2005). The syringe was slowly lowered to the target depth at −8 mm relative to the dura. Five microliter neurotoxin (3 μg/μl 6-OHDA hydrochloride free base in 0.2% ascorbic acid solution, stored on ice; Sigma-Aldrich) or vehicle (aqua injectabilia, 0.2% ascorbic acid solution; Sigma-Aldrich) was slowly infused at a rate of 0.5 μl/min and the syringe was left in place for 2 min to allow for complete absorption of the toxin. The burr hole was closed with bone wax and the procedure was repeated in the contralateral hemisphere. Rats received s.c.-injections of metamizole (100 mg/kg, Medistar, Holzwickede, Germany) for postoperative analgesia following surgery and on behavioral signs of pain distress.

STEREOLOGY

To count TH-positive dopaminergic cells in PD rats and controls we performed free-floating TH-immunohistochemistry on serial 40 μm coronal sections of the midbrain. **Figure 1A** displays representative examples of photomicrographs depicting TH-stained midbrain sections from a vehicle and 6-OHDA injected rat. Due to technical reasons we could only obtain stereology in a subset of 8/9 PD-rats and 5/8 controls. PFA-fixed tissue blocks containing SNc and VTA were transferred to 30%-sucrose solution and kept at 4°C for 24 hours. Sections were cut with a freezing-microtome

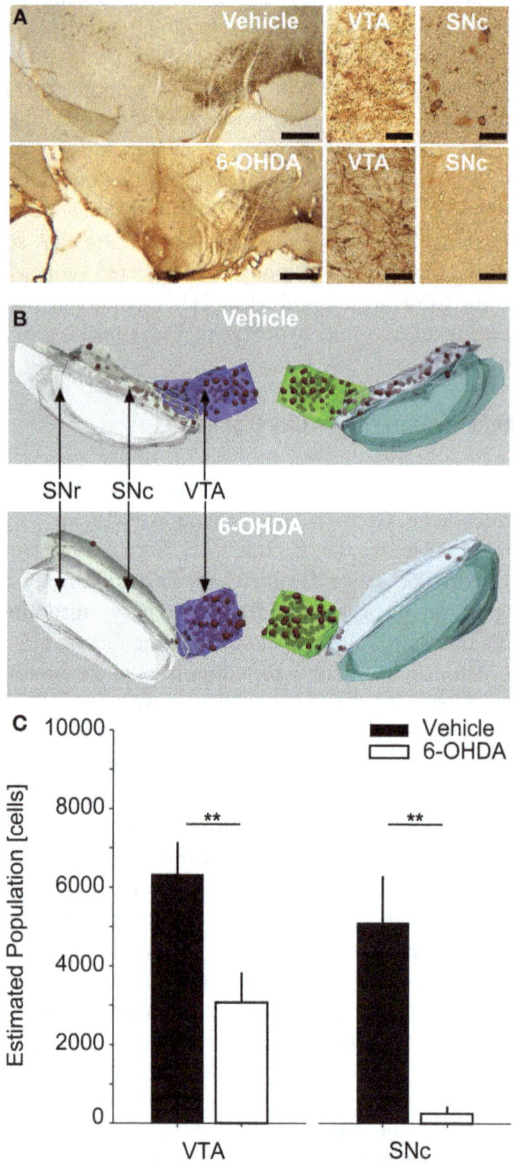

FIGURE 1 | Stereological counting of TH-positive SNc and VTA neurons. (A) Representative photomicrographs of TH-stained midbrain sections of a vehicle and 6-OHDA injected rat (left column, scale bar equals 500 μm) as well as 40× magnifications of VTA and SNc-ROIs (middle and right column, scale bar equals 50 μm). **(B)** 3D-reconstructions of stereological regions of interest for the same vehicle and 6-OHDA injected rats as in **(A)**. Red spheres indicate stereologically counted cells in the SNc and VTA. **(C)** Estimated absolute population of cells in the SNc and VTA for vehicle ($n = 5$) and 6-OHDA ($n = 8$) injected rats. Double asterisks denote $P \leq 0.001$ (uncorrected). TH, tyrosine-hydroxylase; 6-OHDA, 6-hydroxydopamine; VTA, ventral tegmental area; SNc, substantia nigra pars compacta; SNr, substantia nigra pars reticulata.

(Leica Instruments, Wetzlar, Germany) and stained in free-floating fashion for TH-activity. Briefly, sections were washed in phosphate buffer (0.01 M PBS, Sigma-Aldrich), incubated with 3%-H_2O_2-solution for 3 min to block endogenous peroxidase activity and incubated with 2% normal horse serum (added with 0.3% Triton X-100, Sigma-Aldrich) for 30 min. Sections were then incubated over night at 4°C with the primary TH-antibody (1:250, monoclonal mouse antibody, Novocastra reagents, Leica Microsystems, Wetzlar, Germany), followed by the biotinylated secondary antibody (1:400, Novocastra reagents) for 30 min, and afterwards incubated with avidin and biotinylated horseradish peroxidase (ABC kit, Novocastra reagents) for another 30 min. TH was visualized by adding peroxidase substrate (0.02% DAB reagent in 0.003% H_2O_2 in PBS) for 2–10 min duration. Finally, sections were mounted on glass slides, dehydrated in an increasing alcohol row and fixed under a cover slid with Roti Histokitt II (Carl Roth, Karlsruhe, Germany).

Unbiased stereological counting of TH-positive cells in the SNc and VTA was performed using the Stereoinvestigator Software (Version 10.0, MicroBrightField Inc., Williston, Vermont, USA). The hardware consisted of an Olympus Bx61 brightfield microscope (Olympus Deutschland GmbH, Hamburg, Germany) equipped with a Microfire TM A/R camera (Optronics, California, USA) and an x-y-z galvano table (Carl Zeiss AG, Jena, Germany). The optical fractionator probe (West et al., 1991; West, 2002) was applied on series of 40 μm thick coronal sections. To assure sampling of comparable structural parts, the stereological analysis was centered on an independent anatomical hallmark (the rootlets of the oculomotor cranial nerve). Overall we sampled 10 sections (sampling rate of 1.2 ± 0.3 mean ± *SD* sections) spanning ~480 μm in the cranio-caudal dimension. However, due to availability of continuous TH-sections containing SNc and VTA, three rats were investigated using 7, 8, or 9 sections, respectively. Using a 2.5× magnification with numerical aperture of 0.075 we defined three anatomical regions of interest (ROI), i.e., the SNc, the VTA and the substantia nigra pars reticulata (SNr) (Paxinos and Watson, 2005). For examples of anatomical 3-D reconstructions of ROIs and counted cells, see **Figure 1B**. Cell counting was performed using a 40× Plan-Neofluar dry type objective lens with a numerical aperture of 0.75 (Carl Zeiss AG) within the SNc and VTA-ROIs. The counting frame (50 × 50 μm) with dissector height of 20 μm was applied with a uniform random sampling grid of 150 × 150 μm (optical dissector volume of 50,000 μm^3, sampling grid area of 22,500 μm^2, Gundersen, 1986). Schaeffer's estimated coefficient of error ranged between 0.05 and 0.12 for the VTA of both controls and PD animals, as well as the SNc of controls. For SNc-ROIs of PD animals it ranged between 0.3 and 0.9, reflecting the scarceness of TH-positive cells in this area (Gundersen, 1986; West, 2002). The total volume of the sampled SNc and VTA parts was stereologically estimated using the Cavalieri method (Gundersen and Jensen, 1987). Our histological regime resulted in robust sampling >200 neurons per VTA and SNc in vehicle injected controls, enabling us to express TH-positive cell numbers in absolute numbers. Cell counts were calculated separately for each ROI and hemisphere, respectively, and combined across hemispheres ($n = 6$ hemispheres per group).

To assess the symmetry of depletion we calculated the laterality index (*LI*) for each rat (Seghier, 2008), $LI = f \times (E_{LH} - E_{RH})/(E_{LH} + E_{RH})$, where E_{LH} and E_{RH} are the combined VTA and SNc estimates of TH-positive cells for the left and right hemisphere, respectively, and f is a scaling factor set to 1 resulting in the LI to be bound between -1 and 1.

BEHAVIORAL MONITORING

Locomotion of 6-OHDA or vehicle injected rats was investigated via continuous video monitoring of 23 hours of spontaneous behavior in an open field-like environment. We used an infrared video-based tracking system (VideoMot 2.0, TSE Systems, Bad Homburg, Germany) to record movement paths as time series of x-y-positions at a sampling rate of 12.8 Hz. The recording arena was spaced 70 × 100 cm with 40 cm high walls (i.e., 320 × 435 pixel after frame grabbing and offline analysis) and equipped with three food pellet feeders and one water outlet positioned in the corners. The ground was covered with bedding. The arena size was chosen to be ~3 times larger than the size of the rat's home cage to allow for generation of more naturalistic movement patterns including running. The arena was placed in a custom-made recording box lined with foamed plastic to ensure light and acoustic insulation. Recordings took place under constant darkness.

BEHAVIORAL DATA ANALYSIS

To analyze spontaneous long-term behavior we modified a data processing and analysis approach developed for open-field locomotion in rodents (Drai et al., 2000; Drai and Golani, 2001). All routines were written in MATLAB (The Mathworks, Natick, USA). The analytical approach is based on the idea of calculating single speed values (cm/s) from x-y-position time series using a sliding window, separating rest vs. motion episodes and characterizing motion episodes by the maximal speed reached within each episode rather than the average speed of a given episode. Our modified analysis consisted of five separate analysis steps (see **Figure 2**): First, raw x-y-position time series data obtained for 23 hours at a sampling rate of 12.8 Hz (~1,000,000 single data points) contained large amounts of artifacts (see **Figure 2A**). Typically, artifacts resulted from spurious "jumping" within a continuous x-y-position time series to distant places and back. Frequent sources of artifacts lay outside the actual recording arena and could therefore be removed through spatial outlier rejection. However, artifacts also appeared within the arena, generally jumping toward the arena's corners where animals spent most of their resting time (**Figure 2B**). All places on the pixel level that were "visited" twice during the recording time were neglected, eliminating artifacts associated with resting spots (**Figure 2C**). To further de-noise the recordings we applied a low-pass threshold of 80 cm/s (**Figure 2D**), as preliminary data screening showed that no rat reached speed levels >70 cm/s inside the recording arena (data not shown). Single speed values were calculated on position time series with a moving window of 0.3 s (Drai et al., 2000; Drai and Golani, 2001). Separation of resting vs. motion episodes was done by high-pass thresholding speed values at a noise level of 4 cm/s (**Figure 2E**). This threshold was based on previous work of Drai et al. (2000) and adapted to the distribution of single speeds in our data set with a peak at 4 cm/s (data not shown). The remaining motion episodes were used for further analysis (**Figure 2F**). To compensate for erroneous separation of movement episodes resulting from artifact correction we interpolated x-y-coordinates of single missing values.

BEHAVIORAL ENDPOINTS

Smoothed histograms of log transformed maximal speed values, termed "log max-SD," were used to identify different modes of motion in control and PD rats (Drai et al., 2000; Drai and Golani, 2001). A Gaussian mixture model was fitted toward the empirical data to obtain information about the localization of different "gears" of motion within the distribution of speeds. Gears were separated at 10 cm/s, a value consistently derived from preoperative recordings. Descriptive locomotion parameters were calculated for slow (i.e., first gear) and fast (i.e., second gear) episodes. However, as the dissection of second gear episodes allowed a view on full-blown motion, we concentrated our analysis on such episodes.

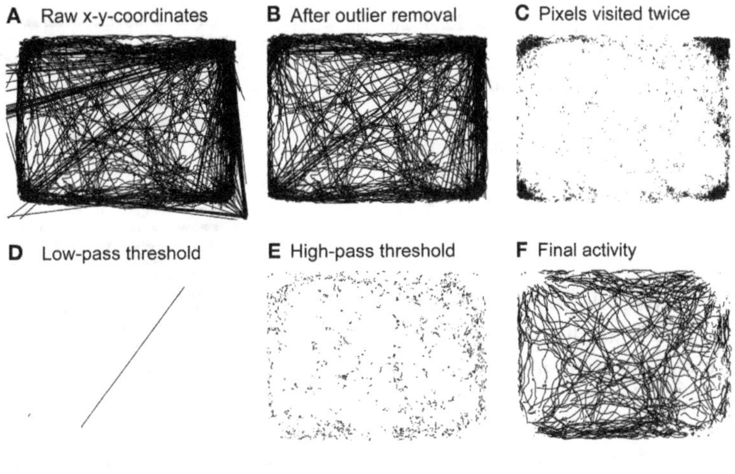

FIGURE 2 | Steps of behavioral analysis. Activity of a representative rat during 23 hours of pre-operative monitoring. **(A)** Raw activity including all artifacts. **(B)** Activity remaining after outlier rejection. **(C)** Spaces on the single pixel level that were "visited" twice during the whole recording time. **(D)** Artifacts excluded through application of a low-pass threshold of 80 cm/s. **(E)** Resting activity excluded through application of a high-pass threshold of 4 cm/s. **(F)** Activity used for subsequent behavioral analyses.

The six different behavioral endpoints were defined as: (1) incidence of fast speed movement episodes, which is the percentage of second gear episodes relative to the number of all motion episodes; (2) absolute distance, calculated as the cumulative sum of the overall covered distance for all motion episodes; (3) average maximal movement speed, corresponding to the mean of all maximal speeds of second gear episodes; (4) dwell time, i.e., the average time it took the rats to execute a motion episode; (5) spatial spread, i.e., the mean distance covered within a motion episode; (6) curvature of movement tracks, i.e., the ratio of the detected real motion track distance and the distance of the virtual line connecting two coordinate pairs directly during temporal windows of 0.5 s. Curvatures were averaged across all windows of a given motion episode.

Our experimental paradigm allowed for *post-hoc* splitting of the experimental groups into rats monitored after 12 ± 2 days and 28 ± 2 days weeks of recovery. We separately analyzed the correlation between the six behavioral endpoints and the estimated absolute population of TH-positive neurons in the SNc and VTA, the corresponding LI of cell depletion and the observed weight reduction for the 6-OHDA and vehicle injected control group. We utilized bootstrap regressions, which do not rely on a normal distribution of data.

STATISTICAL ANALYSIS

All *post-hoc* analyses were performed using the MATLAB Statistics Toolbox and the BRAVO Toolbox for Bootstrap Regression Analysis of Voxelwise Observations. In case of non-normal data distributions, we employed non-parametric statistical testing (Wilcoxon rank sum test). An alpha level of 0.05 was used for all statistical tests. All statistical results are given as mean ± standard deviation (SD). We corrected P-values for multiple comparisons using the false discovery rate (FDR) method (Benjamini and Hochberg, 1995) in case of descriptive behavioral results and multiple bootstrap regression analyses. Bootstrap regressions were performed with 5000 iterations. For descriptive analysis of behavioral endpoints alone, P-values were FDR-corrected for a total of 48 different comparisons (2 experimental groups, 6 behavioral endpoints; 4 different comparisons: preoperative vs. 12 + 28 days postoperative, preoperative vs. 12 days postoperative, preoperative vs. 28 days postoperative and 12 days postoperative vs. 28 days postoperative). For bootstrap regressions, P-values were FDR-corrected for a total of 55 regressions (the estimated neuronal population of the SNc and VTA, the LI, weight reduction and 6 behavioral endpoints).

RESULTS

STEREOLOGICAL COUNTING OF TH-POSITIVE SNc AND VTA NEURONS

Bilateral injections of 15 μg 6-OHDA into the SNc resulted in extensive cell death of dopaminergic neurons in the SNc and intermediate cell death in the VTA (**Figure 1C**). The estimated population of TH-positive neurons for combined SNc-ROIs was reduced by −95% in PD rats compared to controls. The absolute number of cells within combined SNc-ROIs was 253.8 ± 196.9 in PD vs. 5098 ± 1189 in control rats ($P = 0.001$). For combined VTA-ROIs, the estimated population of TH-positive neurons was reduced by −51.4% in PD rats compared to controls. Here, the absolute number of cells within combined VTA-ROIs was 3073 ± 766 in PD vs. 6318 ± 828 in control rats ($P = 0.001$). We also tested whether the cell estimates differed significantly between the two subgroups that were monitored 12 and 28 days after lesioning. No statistically significant difference was found for either VTA or SNc-ROIs of 6-OHDA or vehicle injected rats (P-values > 0.25, data not shown). Furthermore, the estimated populations within single ROIs did not differ significantly between left vs. right hemispheres in PD and control rats, respectively ($P > 0.2$). Likewise, the LI for 6-OHDA treated rats was 0.14 ± 0.2 and 0.08 ± 0.01 for controls ($P = 1$, data not shown).

POSTSURGICAL COURSE

Careful daily inspection of PD and control rats in the home cage environment revealed reduced spontaneous locomotion and movement speed of 6-OHDA-treated rats. Body posture appeared with a hunchback-like shape and hind limb rigidity was detectable upon manual assessment. PD rats displayed aphagia and adipsia leading to a reduction in body weight of $19 \pm 7.7\%$ of the preoperative weight in PD and $1.5 \pm 4.5\%$ in control rats prior to postoperative behavioral monitoring ($P = 0.002$). Three PD rats were euthanized, as they did not exhibit stabilization of weight loss within 12 days after surgery. None of the control rats showed overt movement deficits, aphagia, or adipsia. No additional signs of altered behavior that could indicate persistent pain distress were detected during inspections.

CIRCADIAN ACTIVITY

Free locomotion monitoring took place under constant dark conditions for at least 23 continuous hours. Although no external light cues were given we saw a pattern of locomotor activity reflecting a circadian rhythm in preoperative (data not shown) and postlesion recordings in vehicle injected controls (**Figure 3A**). In most rats we found two activity phases that were separated by a phase of reduced activity lasting ~12 hours each.

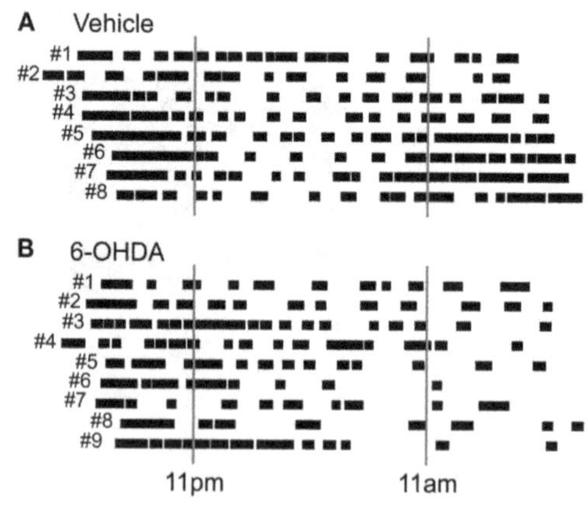

FIGURE 3 | Circadian post-lesion activity. Free locomotor activity of all vehicle **(A)** and all 6-OHDA **(B)** injected rats after lesioning. Animal numbers are given left to the respective vertical bars representing global activity phases. Red solid lines mark light switches at 11 pm (lights on) and 11 am (lights off) that would take place under usual housing conditions. Note that behavioral monitoring was performed under constant dark conditions.

This corresponds to the fact that our rats were accustomed to a 12 hour day/night cycle switching at 11 am (lights off) and 11 pm (lights on). Experiments were usually started between 5 and 6 pm and held under constant dark conditions. In PD rats, however, we found a partially disturbed circadian rhythm (**Figure 3B**) with two major changes. First, PD rats tended to show a prolonged initial global activity period and less distinguishable transition periods. Second, PD rats did not exhibited a clear rebound of activity in the later phase of monitoring.

BIMODAL DISTRIBUTION OF MAXIMAL SPEED VALUES

In prelesion recordings, characterization of movement episodes by the log max-SD resulted in a bimodal distribution (**Figure 4**). In order to distinguish between distinct gears of motion, we fitted a Gaussian mixture model to the empirical distribution of each recording. First gear speeds were centered at a log max-SD of 0.72 ± 0.02 in control and 0.71 ± 0.03 in PD rats, corresponding to a velocity of 5.1 cm/s. Second gear speeds were centered at a log max-SD of 1.24 ± 0.1 in control and 1.24 ± 0.06 in PD rats, i.e., 17.4 cm/s. Notably, 6-OHDA injections resulted in marked changes of the distribution of log max-*SD* values. We observed a partial loss of the bimodal distribution and curve flattening at the center of preoperative second gear episodes. This complicated the fitting of Gaussians and produced spurious results in several animals, e.g., PD rats #1, #2, and #5. Therefore, we separated gears at a log max-SD of 1 (10 cm/s), a value derived from the consistent bimodal distributions of preoperative monitoring.

INCIDENCE OF FAST SPEED MOVEMENT EPISODES

Comparing the number of first gear and second gear episodes per recording, we saw a shift in their incidence after 6-OHDA lesioning (**Figure 5A**). In the PD group, the incidence of second gear episodes decreased from 50.6 ± 4.1% to 36.4 ± 9% (pre- vs. 12 + 28 days postoperatively, $P = 0.01$, corrected). In vehicle injected controls the proportion of first gear and second gear episodes remained the same (51.8 ± 6.1% vs. 47.4 ± 4.7%, pre- vs. 12 + 28 days postoperatively, $P = 0.26$, corrected). Considering the two subpopulations separately, we only saw a significant difference after 12 days of recovery in PD rats ($P = 0.02$ at 12 days vs. $P = 0.08$ at 28 days; $P = 0.35$ for 12 vs. 28 days; corrected).

OVERALL COVERED DISTANCE

6-OHDA injections led to a reduction of the total covered distance within 23 hours of spontaneous locomotion (PD rats: 129.9 ± 25.8 m vs. 94.3 ± 28.7 m, pre- vs. 12 + 28 days postoperatively, $P = 0.05$; control rats: 143.2 ± 38 m vs. 138.9 ± 31.7 m, pre- vs. 12 + 28 days postoperatively, $P = 1$, corrected; **Figure 5B**). Again, this difference was significant for the PD group at 12 days, but not at 28 days of recovery ($P = 0.02$ at 12 days vs. $P = 0.35$ at 28 days; $P = 1$ for 12 vs. 28 days; corrected).

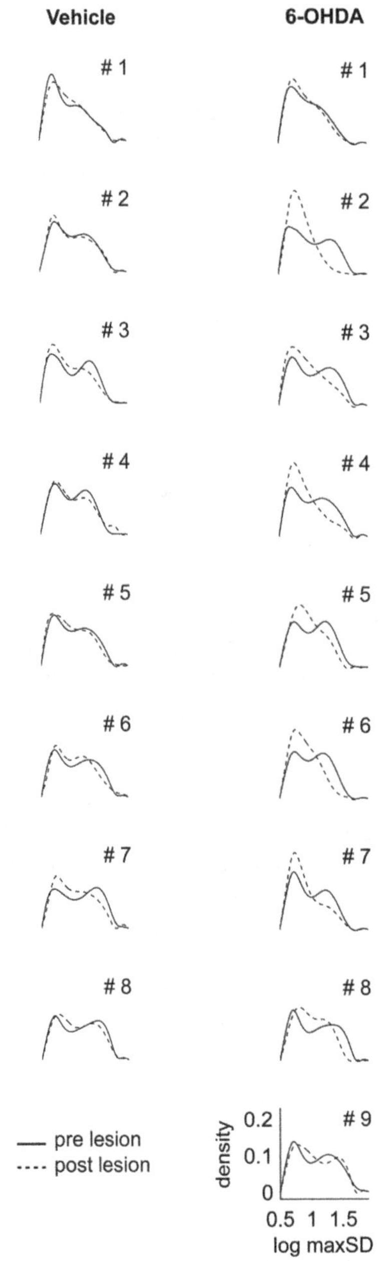

FIGURE 4 | Distribution of maximal speed values. Density functions for logarithmic values of maximal speeds (log max-SD) are shown for all control (left column) and all 6-OHDA lesioned rats (right column). Solid and dashed lines denote log max-SD distributions before and after lesioning, respectively. Animal numbers are given in the right top corner. log max-SD, base 10 logarithm of maximal speed in given movement episode; 6-OHDA, 6-hydroxydopamine.

AVERAGE MAXIMAL MOVEMENT SPEED

The log max-SD across all second gear episodes of full motion was significantly reduced in PD rats (19.9 ± 1.7 cm/s vs. 17 ± 2 cm/s, pre- vs. 12 + 28 days postoperatively, $P = 0.02$; control rats: 20.6 ± 1.8 cm/s vs. 20 ± 1.3 cm/s, pre- vs. 12 + 28 days postoperatively, $P = 1$, corrected; **Figure 5C**). Likewise, the difference was significant also within the PD group at 12 days of recovery ($P = 0.02$ at 12 days vs. $P = 0.18$ at 28 days; $P = 0.92$ for 12 vs. 28 days; corrected). We found no significant difference for first gear episodes ($P = 0.07$ pre- vs. 12 + 28 days postoperatively, $P = 0.25$ at 12 days, $P = 0.09$ at 28 days; $P = 0.26$ for 12 vs. 28 days; corrected).

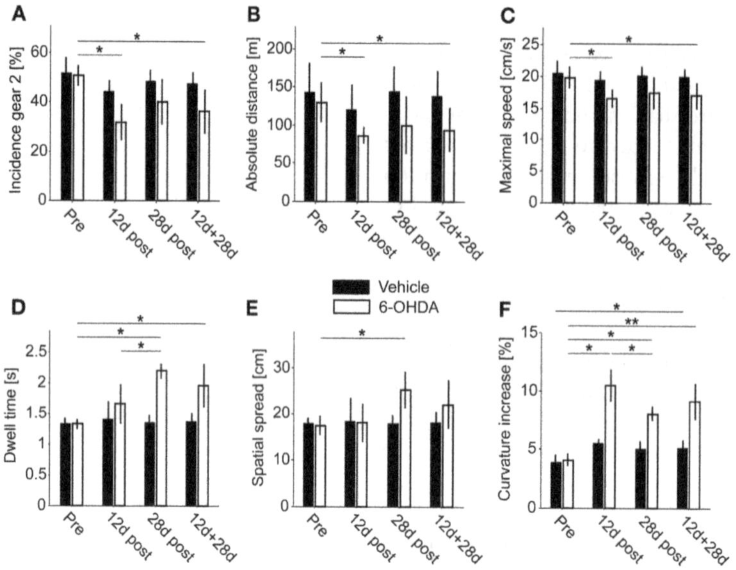

FIGURE 5 | Behavioral endpoints. (A) Incidence of second gear episodes. **(B)** Absolute covered distance. **(C)** Average maximal movement speed of second gear episodes. **(D)** Dwell time of second gear episodes. **(E)** Spatial spread of second gear episodes. **(F)** Increase of curvature in second gear episodes. Single asterisks denote $P \leq 0.05$, double asterisks denote $P \leq 0.001$ (corrected).

DWELL TIME

The average dwell time of second gear episodes was increased in lesioned animals but not in controls (PD rats: 1.32 ± 0.08 s vs. 1.96 ± 0.35 s, pre- vs. 12 + 28 days postoperatively, $P = 0.01$; control rats: 1.33 ± 0.09 s vs. 1.37 ± 0.15 s, pre- vs. 12 + 28 days postoperatively, $P = 0.84$, corrected; **Figure 5D**). Interestingly, the difference in dwell time was also significant in the 28 days subset of PD rats, but not at 12 days post-surgery ($P = 0.17$ at 12 days vs. $P = 0.01$ at 28 days; $P = 0.05$ for 12 vs. 28 days; corrected). Furthermore, the dwell time of first gear episodes was also significantly prolonged ($P = 0.001$ pre- vs. 12 + 28 days postoperatively, $P = 0.01$ at 12 days, $P = 0.008$ at 28 days; $P = 0.98$ for 12 vs. 28 days; corrected).

SPATIAL SPREAD

The spatial spread accomplished within a given episode (averaged across all second gear episodes of full motion) was increased after 6-OHDA lesioning (PD rats: 17.5 ± 2 cm vs. 22.1 ± 5.3 cm, pre- vs. 12 + 28 days postoperatively, $P = 0.08$; control rats: 18 ± 1.2 cm vs. 18 ± 2.6 cm, pre- vs. postoperatively, $P = 0.83$, corrected; **Figure 5E**). Comparable to the dwell time, the difference was significant at 28 days in PD-rats, but not at 12 days or within the combined group ($P = 1$ at 12 days vs. $P = 0.01$ at 28 days; $P = 0.08$ for 12 vs. 28 days; corrected). Similar to the dwell time, the spatial spread was also significantly enlarged for first gear episodes ($P = 0.001$ pre- vs. 12 + 28 days postoperatively, $P = 0.02$ at 12 days, $P = 0.008$ at 28 days; $P = 0.98$ for 12 vs. 28 days; corrected).

CURVATURE

6-OHDA injections led to an increase of the mean curvature of motion tracks (PD-rats: 4.07 ± 0.52% vs. 9.15 ± 1.66%, pre- vs. 12 + 28 days postoperatively, $P = 0.002$). Notably, the curvature was also significantly increased in vehicle injected control rats, but only for the comparison of pre vs. combined postoperative groups (3.850 ± 0.70% vs. 5.15 ± 0.64%, pre- vs. 12 + 28 days postoperatively, $P = 0.02$, corrected; **Figure 5F**). However, in PD rats we saw a stronger increase 12 days after injections ($P = 0.02$ at 12 days) and a significant recovery of curvature ratios 2 weeks later ($P = 0.05$ for 12 vs. 28 days). At the later time point the ratio was still significantly enhanced ($P = 0.01$ at 28 days). The same pattern of statistically significant differences was observed for first gear episodes ($P = 0.001$ pre- vs. 12 + 28 days postoperatively, $P = 0.01$ at 12 days, $P = 0.008$ at 28 days; $P = 0.05$ for 12 vs. 28 days; corrected).

BOOTSTRAP REGRESSIONS

We found a significant correlation for five of 55 independent comparisons (**Figure 6A**) in 6-OHDA treated rats ($n = 8$). The estimated number of VTA, but not of SNc neurons correlated negatively with the magnitude of weight reduction ($R = -0.86$, **Figure 6B1**). Weight loss also correlated with dwell time ($R = 0.8$, **Figure 6B2**) and spatial spread ($R = 0.8$, **Figure 6B3**). Spatial spread also correlated with the incidence of second gear episodes ($R = 0.71$, **Figure 6B4**). Furthermore, the curvature of motion tracks obtained postoperatively correlated negatively with the spatial spread ($R = -0.9$, **Figure 6B5**). Further 9 comparisons were found statistically significant before FDR-correction and yielded P-values < 0.1 after correction (**Figure 6A**). Among them was the only comparison, incidence of second gear episodes vs. maximal speed, that was also found highly correlated in vehicle injected controls ($R = 1$, data not shown).

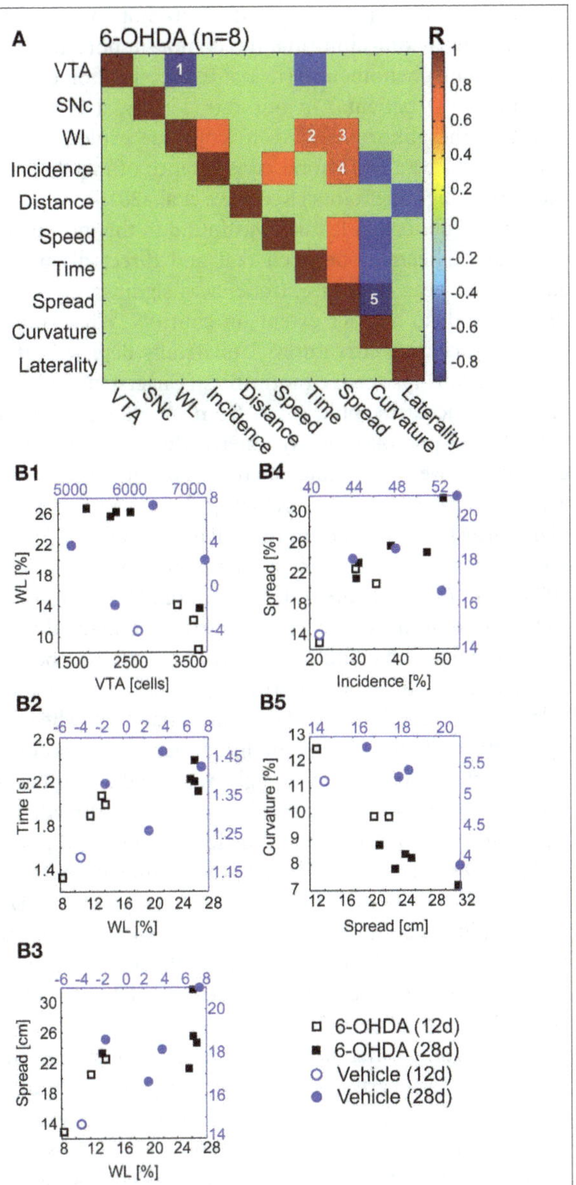

FIGURE 6 | Bootstrap regressions. (A) Independent bootstrap regressions ($n = 55$) of the 6-OHDA group ($n = 8$ animals). The bootstrapping R-value is color-coded and clipped for correlations with $P > 0.1$ after FDR-correction (green fields). **(B1–5)** Correlations with $P < 0.05$ after FDR-correction. Open and filled markers indicate rats from 12 to 28 days subsets, respectively. 6-OHDA, 6-hydroxydopamine.

DISCUSSION

The main findings of our study are that the stereotypical locomotion pattern of rats exhibiting a first and a second gear of motion is partially lost after bilateral dopaminergic denervation. The reduced incidence of second gear episodes points at distinct deficits in the execution of fast motor sequences. However, although generally slowed, bilaterally lesioned rats also displayed bouts of spontaneous locomotion, to some degree similar to kinesia paradoxa observed in PD patients. Contrary to expectation, we observed an abnormally increased spatial spread and increased motion time during episodes of full motion in lesioned rats. Moreover, we noted larger curvature values in movement paths of lesioned rats. Upon acceleration, curvature values showed a reduction toward physiological values. All these changes were accompanied by an alteration of circadian locomotor activity.

The depletion of estimated dopaminergic cell populations in the SNc and VTA in our disease model was comparable to that observed in humans suffering from advanced PD, where the VTA is known to be significantly less depleted than the SNc (Hirsch et al., 1988). However, the mesocorticolimbic dopamine projections are vulnerable in advanced PD as well, and seem to contribute to the complex clinical picture encountered in humans, especially at later disease stages (Thobois et al., 2010). It is worth mentioning that our stereological results were similar to cell-loss estimates of 40–50% in the VTA described in human postmortem studies (Uhl et al., 1985; Hirsch et al., 1988; Dymecki et al., 1996; McRitchie et al., 1997; Thobois et al., 2010). The estimated number of SNc neurons of vehicle injected rats in our study was comparable to the number of TH-positive cells reported by a previous study (Fox et al., 2001) that investigated Fisher 344 × Brown Norway hybrids. Other studies reported significantly higher TH-positive cell counts in different rat strains (Lewis rats, Strackx et al., 2008; Long-Evans rats Healy-Stoffel et al., 2012; Sprague-Dawley rats, Walker et al., 2012) suggesting large differences in the absolute number of midbrain dopaminergic cells in different rat strains.

PD rats in our study displayed a considerable reduction of body weight (~20%). Weight loss and associated metabolic changes might by themselves have an influence on locomotion. We included the reduction of body weight into multiple bootstrap regressions and investigated the interdependence between behavioral endpoints, dopaminergic cell loss and weight reduction. We found a significant negative correlation between the VTA, but not the SNc dopaminergic population, and the magnitude of weight loss. Thus, abnormal feeding behavior and more generally abulia, was related to cell loss within the mesolimbic dopaminergic system in our study (Redgrave et al., 2010).

Our analysis approach allowed the discrimination of naturally occurring motion episodes in severely dopamine depleted and overtly akinetic and bradykinetic rats. The characterization of motion episodes by the maximal rather than the average speed accomplished in a given episode enabled us to analyze rare and, given the pronounced parkinsonian phenotype of our rats, unexpected episodes of qualitatively altered motor activity. These motion episodes were still characterized by a reduced incidence (i.e., poverty of movement or akinesia), reduced overall traveled distance (i.e., hypokinesia) and reduced maximal speed (i.e., bradykinesia) compared to controls. Hence, important hallmark symptoms of PD were clearly detectable in motion episodes of 6-OHDA rats. However, we did not see a significant correlation of these three behavioral endpoints with the estimated populations of the SNc and VTA.

Overall, the quantitative change in traveled distance was rather small. A disruption of the circadian rhythm, a cardinal non-motor symptom in human PD patients (Videnovic and Golombek, 2013) and present in animal models of PD (Kudo et al., 2011; Willison et al., 2013) may introduce a bias. Higher absolute activity values may result from prolongation and fragmentation of activity and reduced sleep phases. Our analysis method could not differentiate between awake resting and true sleep, but conclusions could still be drawn from the overall circadian activity pattern. Here, we observed a more fragmented pattern of activity together with a nearly absent second activity phase. Moreover, PD rats showed a significantly reduced absolute number of motion episodes in comparison to controls (data not shown). Together, this argues against a circadian bias toward higher distance values in our data.

The finding of increased dwell times and spatial spread in first and second gear motion episodes of PD rats was rather unexpected. The spatial spread in the 6-OHDA group was increased to values not seen in any pre-lesion or control recordings. Theoretically, an increased dwell time could be explained as a function of slowed locomotion. To reach the same location, bradykinetic rats may simply need more time. This interdependence should theoretically manifest in a negative correlation between speed and dwell time or spatial spread. To the contrary, our data revealed a positive correlation between speed and spatial spread, albeit not significant after FDR-correction. That is, faster PD rats showed spatially extended second gear episodes. Could a postlesion increase in curvature explain increased dwell times? Arguing against that, curvature values were significantly negatively correlated with spatial spread, and also with dwell time, speed and incidence of second gear episodes (before FDR-correction). Furthermore, a higher incidence of second gear behavior correlated significantly with prolonged spatial spread. Such an increased incidence could be the result of an uneven effect of 6-OHDA lesioning and stronger diminishment of first gear in comparison to second gear activity. This would also be supported by the finding that 6-OHDA induced weight loss correlated positively with the incidence of second gear activity (before FDR-correction). Taken together, increased spatial spread and dwell times constitute an abnormal behavioral characteristic of PD rats.

An abnormal increase of locomotor activity in bilaterally lesioned rats has been described in response to a pharmacological challenge (Schallert et al., 1978). Unexpected bursts of locomotion in otherwise akinetic patients are also well known to occur in selected PD patients or cases with postencephalitic parkinsonism (kinesia paradoxa). The sudden ability of our rats to cover longer distances within a motion episode may thus represent a rat equivalent of this condition. There are, however, important differences to classical kinesia paradoxa, which is often triggered by external sensory cues (Martin, 1967).

One possible explanation for prolonged dwell times and increased spatial spread could be problems with the termination of movement. In PD patients, deficiency in smooth motion termination is known (Dounskaia et al., 2009), along with an inability to promptly change generated force or quickly re-plan current motion. Typically, PD patients show an asymmetric evolution of velocities during the execution of goal-directed behaviors with initial fast accelerations (Flash et al., 1992). In our data we found a symmetric evolution of acceleration between PD and control rats. That is, we saw a linear relationship between the dwell time and the time point where PD or control rats accomplished their maximal speed in a given episode (data not shown). Thus, the observed behavioral abnormalities do not support the presence of the hastening phenomenon (unwanted acceleration of movement in human PD patients) in our rats. Finally, it is also conceivable that the abnormal drive to continue exploration or food search could be a behavioral consequence of metabolic changes accompanying weight loss (Redgrave et al., 2010).

Another abnormal feature was found in the movement path's curvature. The ratio between real and direct distance of first and second gear motion episodes was significantly enlarged in PD rats and, to a lesser extent, in controls. What could be the cause of increased curvatures? Unilaterally depleted rats display a spontaneous ipsiversive motor bias (Ungerstedt, 1971). Hence, curvature increases could result from spontaneous partial turning behavior provoked by asymmetric dopaminergic lesioning in our rats. However, the calculated LI did not correlate with curvature or any other behavioral endpoint except distance (before FDR-correction). Furthermore, unilateral 6-OHDA lesions were shown to shorten steps in spontaneous walking (Metz et al., 2005), thus modeling the shuffling gait of PD patients (Knutsson, 1972). Hind limb rigidity was detected upon manual assessment in our PD rats and could have contributed to disturbed locomotor patterns with reduced step sizes, axial instability and loss of balance during walking. Hemiparkinsonian rats, when tested by e.g., beam-walking, also exhibit difficulties in motor coordination (Truong et al., 2006). Interestingly, we found a significant negative correlation between curvature and spatial spread, as well as maximal speed, dwell time and incidence of second gear activity (before FDR-correction). Thus, faster running or greater spreads were associated with straighter movement paths in PD rats. If limb rigidity was indeed related to the expression of increased curvature values, then the ability of PD rats to generate fast motion with reduced curvature values may reflect an overcoming of rigidity for brief periods.

We saw some differences between lesioned animals that were monitored at an early (12 days) and later stage (28 days) after 6-OHDA lesioning. Most strikingly, the dwell time was significantly longer at 28 days in comparison with 12 days postlesion. Contrary, curvature increases significantly decreased again at the later point of investigation. Importantly, no significant difference in cell counts was observed between the two subsets. It remains difficult to infer which compensatory mechanisms were at work here. The milder but still significant increase of curvature in controls, in conjunction with the significant decrease of curvature values in PD rats with time, could argue for an influence of and recovery from surgery *per se*. The emergence of an abnormally increased behavior such as kinesia paradoxa may have in turn developed over time when the rats recovered fully from surgery. Despite putative effects of recovery from surgery, absolute distance, speed and incidence of second gear activity were comparably decreased at an early and later point of investigation.

We conclude that long-term behavioral observations of spontaneous locomotion offers new perspectives on distinctly different modes of motion in a rat model of advanced PD. The present behavioral analysis, in conjunction with *in-vivo* electrophysiology, may be particularly suited to reveal neural mechanisms underlying motor fluctuations such as kinesia paradoxa, and may provide further insights into the complex pathophysiology of PD.

AUTHOR CONTRIBUTIONS

Benjamin Grieb, Gerhard Engler, Ismini Papageorgiou, Wolfgang Hamel, and Christian K. Moll designed research; Benjamin Grieb, Gerhard Engler, and Ismini Papageorgiou performed experiments; Benjamin Grieb, Constantin von Nicolai, Andrew Sharott, and Ismini Papageorgiou analyzed the data; Benjamin Grieb, Constantin von Nicolai, Andrew Sharott, Andreas K. Engel, and Christian K. Moll wrote the manuscript.

ACKNOWLEDGMENTS

The authors would like to thank Doris Lange for help with the histology. This work was supported by the European Union (MRTN-CT-2005-019247).

REFERENCES

Avila, I., Parr-Brownlie, L. C., Brazhnik, E., Castañeda, E., Bergstrom, D. A., and Walters, J. R. (2010). Beta frequency synchronization in basal ganglia output during rest and walk in a hemiparkinsonian rat. *Exp. Neurol.* 221, 307–319. doi: 10.1016/j.expneurol.2009.11.016

Belujon, P., Bezard, E., Taupignon, A., Bioulac, B., and Benazzouz, A. (2007). Noradrenergic modulation of subthalamic nucleus activity: behavioral and electrophysiological evidence in intact and 6-hydroxydopamine-lesioned rats. *J. Neurosci.* 27, 9595–9606. doi: 10.1523/JNEUROSCI.2583-07.2007

Benjamini, Y., and Hochberg, Y. (1995). Controlling the false discovery rate: a practical and powerful approach to multiple testing. *J. R Stat. Soc. B* 57, 289–300. doi: 10.2307/2346101

Bergman, H., Wichmann, T., and DeLong, M. R. (1990). Reversal of experimental parkinsonism by lesions of the subthalamic nucleus. *Science* 249, 1436–1438. doi: 10.1126/science.2402638

Brazhnik, E., Cruz, A. V., Avila, I., Wahba, M. I., Novikov, N., Ilieva, N. M., et al. (2012). State-dependent spike and local field synchronization between motor cortex and substantia nigra in hemiparkinsonian rats. *J. Neurosci.* 32, 7869–7880. doi: 10.1523/JNEUROSCI.0943-12.2012

Cass, W. A., Peters, L. E., and Smith, M. P. (2005). Reductions in spontaneous locomotor activity in aged male, but not female, rats in a model of early Parkinson's disease. *Brain Res.* 1034, 153–161. doi: 10.1016/j.brainres.2004.12.009

Cenci, M A., Whishaw, I. Q., and Schallert, T. (2002). Animal models of neurological deficits: how relevant is the rat? *Nat. Rev. Neurosci.* 3, 574–579. doi: 10.1038/nrn877

Dounskaia, N., Fradet, L., Lee, G., Leis, B. C., and Adler, C. H. (2009). Submovements during pointing movements in Parkinson's disease. *Exp. Brain Res.* 193, 529–544. doi: 10.1007/s00221-008-1656-6

Drai, D., Benjamini, Y., and Golani, I. (2000). Statistical discrimination of natural modes of motion in rat exploratory behavior. *J. Neurosci. Methods* 96, 119–131. doi: 10.1016/S0165-0270(99)00194-6

Drai, D., and Golani, I. (2001). SEE: a tool for the visualization and analysis of rodent exploratory behavior. *Neurosci. Biobehav. Rev.* 25, 409–426. doi: 10.1016/S0149-7634(01)00022-7

Drai, D., Kafkafi, N., Benjamini, Y., Elmer, G., and Golani, I. (2001). Rats and mice share common ethologically relevant parameters of exploratory behavior. *Behav. Brain Res.* 125, 133–140. doi: 10.1016/S0166-4328(01)00290-X

Dymecki, J., Lechowicz, W., Bertrand, E., and Szpak, G. M. (1996). Changes in dopaminergic neurons of the mesocorticolimbic system in Parkinson's disease. *Folia Neuropathol.* 34, 102–106.

Ferro, M. M., Bellissimo, M. I., Anselmo-Franci, J. A., Angellucci, M. E., Canteras, N. S., and Da Cunha, C. (2005). Comparison of bilaterally 6-OHDA- and MPTP-lesioned rats as models of the early phase of Parkinson's disease: histological, neurochemical, motor and memory alterations. *J. Neurosci. Methods* 148, 78–87. doi: 10.1016/j.jneumeth.2005.04.005

Flash, T., Inzelberg, R., Schechtman, E., and Korczyn, A. D. (1992). Kinematic analysis of upper limb trajectories in Parkinson's disease. *Exp. Neurol.* 118, 215–226. doi: 10.1016/0014-4886(92)90038-R

Fox, C. M., Gash, D. M., Smoot, M. K., and Cass, W. A. (2001). Neuroprotective effects of GDNF against 6-OHDA in young and aged rats. *Brain Res.* 896, 56–63. doi: 10.1016/S0006-8993(00)03270-4

Gundersen, H. J. (1986). Stereology of arbitrary particles. a review of unbiased number and size estimators and the presentation of some new ones, in memory of William R. Thompson. *J. Microsc.* 143(Pt 1), 3–45. doi: 10.1111/j.1365-2818.1986.tb02764.x

Gundersen, H. J., and Jensen, E. B. (1987). The efficiency of systematic sampling in stereology and its prediction. *J. Microsc.* 147(Pt 3), 229–263. doi: 10.1111/j.1365-2818.1987.tb02837.x

Healy-Stoffel, M., Ahmad, S. O., Stanford, J. A., and Levant, B. (2012). A novel use of combined tyrosine hydroxylase and silver nucleolar staining to determine the effects of a unilateral intrastriatal 6-hydroxydopamine lesion in the substantia nigra: a stereological study. *J. Neurosci. Methods* 210, 187–194. doi: 10.1016/j.jneumeth.2012.07.013

Hirsch, E., Graybiel, A. M., and Agid, Y. A. (1988). Melanized dopaminergic neurons are differentially susceptible to degeneration in Parkinson's disease. *Nature* 334, 345–348. doi: 10.1038/334345a0

Kelly, P. H. (1975). Unilateral 6-hydroxydopamine lesions of nigrostriatal or mesolimbic dopamine-containing terminals and the drug-induced rotation of rats. *Brain Res.* 100, 163–169. doi: 10.1016/0006-8993(75)90253-X

Knutsson, E. (1972). An analysis of Parkinsonian gait. *Brain* 95, 475–486. doi: 10.1093/brain/95.3.475

Kudo, T., Loh, D. H., Truong, D., Wu, Y., and Colwell, C. S. (2011). Circadian dysfunction in a mouse model of Parkinson's disease. *Exp. Neurol.* 232, 66–75. doi: 10.1016/j.expneurol.2011.08.003

Martin, J. P. (1967). *The Basal Ganglia and Posture*. Philadelphia, PA: Lippincott.

McRitchie, D. A., Cartwright, H. R., and Halliday, G. M. (1997). Specific A10 dopaminergic nuclei in the midbrain degenerate in Parkinson's disease. *Exp. Neurol.* 144, 202–213. doi: 10.1006/exnr.1997.6418

Metz, G. A., Tse, A., Ballermann, M., Smith, L. K., and Fouad, K. (2005). The unilateral 6-OHDA rat model of Parkinson's disease revisited: an electromyographic and behavioural analysis. *Eur. J. Neurosci.* 22, 735–744. doi: 10.1111/j.1460-9568.2005.04238.x

Mokrý, J. (1995). Experimental models and behavioural tests used in the study of Parkinson's disease. *Physiol. Res.* 44, 143–150.

Paxinos, G., and Watson, C. (2005). *The Rat Brain in Stereotaxic Coordinates*. 5th Edn. Sidney, NSW: Academic Press.

Redgrave, P., Rodriguez, M., Smith, Y., Rodriguez-Oroz, M. C., Lehericy, S., Bergman, H., et al. (2010). Goal-directed and habitual control in the basal ganglia: implications for Parkinson's disease. *Nat. Rev. Neurosci.* 11, 760–772. doi: 10.1038/nrn2915

Sakai, K., and Gash, D. M. (1994). Effect of bilateral 6-OHDA lesions of the substantia nigra on locomotor activity in the rat. *Brain Res.* 633, 144–50. doi: 10.1016/0006-8993(94)91533-4

Schallert, T., Whishaw, I. Q., Ramirez, V. D., and Teitelbaum, P. (1978). Compulsive, abnormal walking caused by anticholinergics in akinetic, 6-hydroxydopamine-treated rats. *Science* 199, 1461–1463. doi: 10.1126/science.564552

Schwarting, R. K., and Huston, J. P. (1996a). Unilateral 6-hydroxydopamine lesions of meso-striatal dopamine neurons and their physiological sequelae. *Prog. Neurobiol.* 49, 215–266. doi: 10.1016/S0301-0082(96)00015-9

Schwarting, R. K., and Huston, J. P.(1996b). The Unilateral 6-hydroxydopamine lesion model in behavioral brain research. Analysis of functional deficits, recovery and treatments. *Prog. Neurobiol.* 50, 275–331. doi: 10.1016/S0301-0082(96)00040-8

Seghier, M. L. (2008). Laterality index in functional MRI: methodological issues. *Magn. Reson. Imaging* 26, 594–601. doi: 10.1016/j.mri.2007.10.010

Strackx, E., Van den Hove, D. L., Steinbusch, H. P., Steinbusch, H. W., Vles, J. S., Blanco, C. E., et al. (2008). A combined behavioral and morphological study on the effects of fetal asphyxia on the nigrostriatal dopaminergic system in adult rats. *Exp. Neurol.* 211, 413–422. doi: 10.1016/j.expneurol.2008.02.006

Thobois, S., Ardouin, C., Lhommée, E., Klinger, H., Lagrange, C., Xie, J., et al. (2010). Non-motor dopamine withdrawal syndrome after surgery for Parkinson's disease: predictors and underlying mesolimbic denervation. *Brain* 133(Pt. 4), 1111–1127. doi: 10.1093/brain/awq032

Truong, L., Allbutt, H., Kassiou, M., and Henderson, J. M. (2006). Developing a preclinical model of Parkinson's disease: a study of behaviour in rats with graded 6-OHDA lesions. *Behav. Brain Res.* 169, 1–9. doi: 10.1016/j.bbr.2005.11.026

Uhl, G. R., Hedreen, J. C., and Price, D. L. (1985). Parkinson's disease: loss of neurons from the ventral tegmental area contralateral to therapeutic surgical lesions. *Neurology* 35, 1215–1218.

Ungerstedt, U. (1971). Postsynaptic supersensitivity after 6-hydroxy-dopamine induced degeneration of the nigro-striatal dopamine system. *Acta Physiol. Scand. Suppl.* 367, 69–93.

Videnovic, A., and Golombek, D. (2013). Circadian and sleep disorders in Parkinson's disease. *Exp. Neurol.* 243, 45–56. doi: 10.1016/j.expneurol.2012.08.018

Walker, Q. D., Johnson, M. L., Van Swearingen, A. E., Arrant, A. E., Caster, J. M., and Kuhn, C. M. (2012). Individual differences in psychostimulant responses of female rats are associated with ovarian hormones and dopamine neuroanatomy. *Neuropharmacology* 62, 2267–2277. doi: 10.1016/j.neuropharm.2012.01.029

West, M. J. (2002). Design-based stereological methods for counting neurons. *Prog. Brain Res.* 135, 43–51. doi: 10.1016/S0079-6123(02)35006-4

West, M. J., Slomianka, L., and Gundersen, H. J. (1991). Unbiased stereological estimation of the total number of neurons in thesubdivisions of the rat hippocampus using the optical fractionator. *Anat. Rec.* 231, 482–497. doi: 10.1002/ar.1092310411

Willison, L. D., Kudo, T., Loh, D. H., Kuljis, D., and Colwell, C. S. (2013). Circadian dysfunction may be a key component of the non-motor symptoms of Parkinson's disease: insights from a transgenic mouse model. *Exp. Neurol.* 243, 57–66. doi: 10.1016/j.expneurol.2013.01.014

14

The Michelin Red Guide of the Brain: Role of Dopamine in Goal-Oriented Navigation

Aude Retailleau[1]* and Thomas Boraud[2,3]

[1] Sagol Department of Neurobiology, University of Haifa, Haifa, Israel
[2] Institut des Maladies Neurodegeneratives UMR 5293, University of Bordeaux, Bordeaux, France
[3] Institut des Maladies Neurodegeneratives UMR 5293, CNRS, Bordeaux, France

Correspondence:
Aude Retailleau, Neural Representations Lab, Sagol Department of Neurobiology, University of Haifa, 99 Aba Khoushy Ave, Mount Carmel, Haifa 3498838, Israel
e-mail: retailleau@campus.haifa.ac.il

Spatial learning has been recognized over the years to be under the control of the hippocampus and related temporal lobe structures. Hippocampal damage often causes severe impairments in the ability to learn and remember a location in space defined by distal visual cues. Such cognitive disabilities are found in Parkinsonian patients. We recently investigated the role of dopamine in navigation in the 6-Hydroxy-dopamine (6-OHDA) rat, a model of Parkinson's disease (PD) commonly used to investigate the pathophysiology of dopamine depletion (Retailleau et al., 2013). We demonstrated that dopamine (DA) is essential to spatial learning as its depletion results in spatial impairments. Our results showed that the behavioral effect of DA depletion is correlated with modification of the neural encoding of spatial features and decision making processes in hippocampus. However, the origin of these alterations in the neural processing of the spatial information needs to be clarified. It could result from a local effect: dopamine depletion disturbs directly the processing of relevant spatial information at hippocampal level. Alternatively, it could result from a more distributed network effect: dopamine depletion elsewhere in the brain (entorhinal cortex, striatum, etc.) modifies the way hippocampus processes spatial information. Recent experimental evidence in rodents, demonstrated indeed, that other brain areas are involved in the acquisition of spatial information. Amongst these, the cortex—basal ganglia (BG) loop is known to be involved in reinforcement learning and has been identified as an important contributor to spatial learning. In particular, it has been shown that altered activity of the BG striatal complex can impair the ability to perform spatial learning tasks. The present review provides a glimpse of the findings obtained over the past decade that support a dialog between these two structures during spatial learning under DA control.

Keywords: dopamine, hippocampus, basal ganglia, spatial navigation, striatum

INTRODUCTION: OF PARKINSON'S DISEASE, DISORIENTATION, DOPAMINE AND HIPPOCAMPUS

Parkinson disease (PD) has long been characterized as a motor disease (Agid, 1991). Emphasis has been stressed for long on the so-called triad of akinesia, rigidity and tremor. However classic drug and surgical therapies are now able to control more or less these symptoms, often at the cost of disabling side effects such as drug-induced dyskinesia (Boraud et al., 2001). Nevertheless, the increased autonomy acquired by the Parkinsonian patients unmasked cognitive symptoms previously underestimated (Sawamoto et al., 2002). It was previously thought that cognitive alteration was a late feature of the disease but, in fact, it occurs early in about 15–20% of the patients (Weintraub et al., 2011; Svenningsson et al., 2012). Amongst cognitive symptoms we can identify spatial disorientation, which has been described as an early landmark 25 years ago but left unexplored for a long time (Hovestadt et al., 1987; Taylor et al., 1989) despite its impact on life quality and public health problem (Crizzle et al., 2012).

Spatial cognition includes all the processes that allow animals to acquire process, memorize and use spatial information to perform goal-directed movements. Animals perceive space and extract pertinent information relevant to their spatial behavior using two types of sensory information: external cues supplied by the environment and internal cues supplied by their own movements. Navigation strategies are based on internal cues (path integration), external cues (taxon navigation) or on both (local navigation; O'Keefe and Conway, 1978; Gallistel, 1990; Trullier et al., 1997) Navigation could be represented in space by two systems of coordinates: an external coordinate system (allocentric representation) or an internal frame (egocentric representation; Berthoz, 1991; Poucet and Benhamou, 1997; Benhamou and Poucet, 1998). Several structures are considered to be important for building the neural representation of these spatial coordinates often called cognitive maps: amongst them the hippocampus is considered as the corner stone (O'Keefe and Dostrovsky, 1971; O'Keefe, 1979). Dopaminergic afferents to the hippocampal formation arise from both the ventral tegmental area (VTA, A10) and *substantia nigra pars compacta* (SNc, A8–A9) dopaminergic cell groups (Scatton et al., 1980). In addition, intra-hippocampal injections of D1 agonists and D2 antagonists improve memory (Packard and White, 1991; Wilkerson and Levin, 1999), while 6-Hydroxy-dopamine (6-OHDA) lesions of dopaminergic inputs to hippocampus induce spatial working memory deficits (Gasbarri et al., 1996). The dorsal part of Cornu Ammonis areas 3 (CA3), considered to be involved in the rapid acquisition of new memory (Kesner, 2007), is the target of dopamine (DA) projections from VTA and SNc (Scatton et al., 1980; Luo et al., 2011). DA innervation together with a higher liability of place fields as compared to those of CA1 (Barnes et al., 1990; Mizumori, 2006), makes CA3 a good candidate for the detection of the contextual significance of spatial features (Penner and Mizumori, 2012).

These facts raise the question of what happens in this brain structure when dopamine is depleted in Parkinsonian patient. We recently addressed this issue in the 6-OHDA rat, a model of PD commonly used to investigate the pathophysiology of dopamine depletion (Retailleau et al., 2013). We demonstrated that hippocampus played not only a role in the identification of locations in an environment and in the planning of the trajectories to goals and path selection as previously showed (Morris et al., 1990; Bannerman et al., 1995; Whishaw and Jarrard, 1995; Whishaw and Tomie, 1996; Hollup et al., 2001; Johnson and Redish, 2007; Rolls, 2007), but also in goal encoding. Behavioral analysis showed that sham rats are able to maximize their behavior in a baited Y-maze in order to increase the total amount of reward income over the course of the session. This behavior is correlated to an increase in the mean firing rate of neurons in CA3 at both decision point and reward location. Moreover, the lesion of the dopaminergic neurons of Substantia Nigra disrupted this ability and uncorrelated firing rate of CA3 neurons from decision and reward location (**Figure 1**).

However, the origin of these alterations in the neural processing of the spatial features needs to be clarified. It could result from a local effect: dopamine depletion disturbs directly the processing of relevant spatial information at hippocampal level. Alternatively, it could result from a more distributed network effect: dopamine depletion elsewhere in the brain (entorhinal cortex, striatum, etc.) modifies the way hippocampus processes spatial information. In this mini-review we address as survey of arguments in the literature that can support eachtheory.

INFLUENCE OF DA IN THE HIPPOCAMPUS

Dopamine from SNc and VTA provides a reward prediction error signal to the dorsal and ventral striatum (Schultz, 2006). It is tempting to assume that similar mechanisms are involved in the hippocampus itself. There are strong elements to support this assumption. Hippocampus is one of the rare brain areas where the 5 subtypes of DA receptors are found, D2-like (Brouwer et al., 1992) and D1-like families (Gingrich et al., 1992; Laurier et al., 1994; Sokoloff and Schwartz, 1995). In addition, intra-hippocampal injections of D1 agonists and D2 antagonists improves memory (Packard and White, 1991; Wilkerson and Levin, 1999), while 6-OHDA lesions of dopamine input to hippocampus result in spatial working memory deficits (Gasbarri et al., 1996). Exposure to a novel context increases hippocampal dopamine release (Ihalainen et al., 1999), which in turn facilitates long term potentiation (LTP) induction (Li et al., 2003; Lemon and Manahan-Vaughan, 2006). Detection of a context change by hippocampus can be used to update memory systems, which in turn may signal dopamine neurons to increase dopamine release. The subsequent increase in dopamine release in hippocampus seems to excite hippocampal neurons and so increase the duration of neural responses to glutamatergic input (Smialowski, 1987; Smialowski and Bijak, 1987) contributing as such to the increased stabilization of place fields typically observed as rats become familiar with new environmental conditions (Frank et al., 2004).

All of these data strengthened the hypothesis of a local effect of DA in the hippocampus, but there is a major drawback, which is that dopaminergic direct input to hippocampus, is very sparse and poorly described despite intensive search. As far as we know, we found only one study which described that a few fibers arise from both the VTA, A10 and SNc, A8–A9 dopaminergic cell groups (Scatton et al., 1980). But sparseness doesn't mean inefficiency and the contrast with the reasonably high density of DA receptors in the hippocampus pleads for an actual functional effect.

BASAL GANGLIA AND SPATIAL NAVIGATION

Experimental approaches in rodents have provided behavioral evidence that pharmacological manipulations of the nucleus accumbens (NAc—part of the ventral striatum) impair acquisition and/or performance in spatial learning tasks (Annett et al., 1989; Wiener, 1993; Ploeger et al., 1994; Gal et al., 1997; Smith-Roe et al., 1999; Atallah et al., 2007; Ferretti et al., 2007). Packard and McGaugh's seminal experiments (Packard and McGaugh, 1996) introduced the hypothesis that the striatum contributed to egocentric learning. However, recent data have generated controversy and show that the striatum is also involved in other aspects of spatial learning. Various studies examined the involvement of different sub-regions of the striatum in allocentric and egocentric learning (Voorn et al., 2004). Their results suggest that the Dorso Lateral Striatum (DLS) plays a role in egocentric spatial learning (Yin and Knowlton, 2004) based on cue-action association (van der Meer et al., 2010) and both the NAc and the Dorso Medial Striatum (DMS) plays a role in allocentric learning (Lavoie and Mizumori, 1994; Mizumori et al., 2004; Ferretti et al., 2007). The central role of the ventral striatum in spatial decision making has been confirmed by electrophysiological approach (Lansink et al., 2009; van der Meer et al., 2010; van der Meer and Redish, 2011).

These findings pave the way for integration between allocentric and egocentric process in the striatum. Striatum is a highly convergent structure where huge overlaps exist between the different functional territories (Parent and Hazrati, 1995). Thorn et al. (2010) recently demonstrated that DMS and DLS display contrasting patterns of activity during task performance that developed concurrently with sharply different dynamics. It suggests that this integration can be a cooperative (additive) process or a competition process that would contribute to multimodal

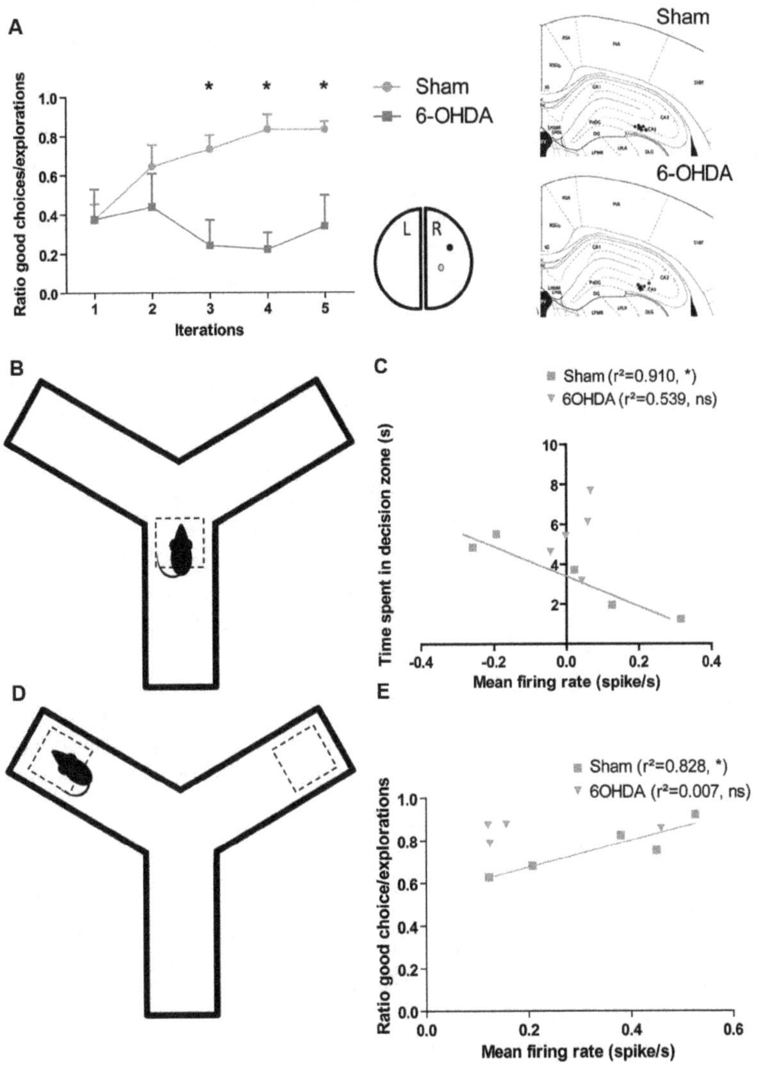

FIGURE 1 | Dopamine depletion modifies the encoding of decision process and reward location in CA3 (adapted form Retailleau et al., 2013). (A) In a baited Y-maze, the rat has to choose one of the arms where the reward is located. Rat with a 6-OHDA lesion in the right medial forebrain bundle had difficulties to find the reward when it is in the right arm as it is shown by its low ratio of good choice (i.e., the baited arm)/the number of exploration. We correlated the behavior in the maze with population responses in the right CA3 (A, right). The time spent by the animal in the decision zone **(B)** is correlated with the population firing rate of CA3 neurons of Sham, but not 6-OHDA rats **(C)**. The ratio of good choice/total number of exploration is correlated with the population firing rate of CA3 neurons of Sham, but not 6-OHDA rats **(E)** when the animal is in the reward location **(D)**.

decision making using mechanisms similar to those that have been modeled for action selection (Leblois et al., 2006; Guthrie et al., 2013).

INFLUENCE OF DA IN THE BASAL GANGLIA

The regulation of striatal input by tonic and phasic dopamine release is so well known and described that there is not enough space in this mini-review to detail and we report the reader to more comprehensive review (Goto et al., 2007; Schultz, 2007; Humphries et al., 2012). Briefly, dopamine presysnaptic button connect the base of dendritic spines of the Medium Spiny Neurons of the striatum. From this key position they control the effect of the other inputs connecting the head of the spine (Parent and Hazrati, 1993) and play a key role in synaptic plasticity.

The role of DA at striatal level in the control of spatial navigation has been evidenced both in its ventral and dorsal part. In the ventral part, evidences are accumulated since the late 1980s. Mogenson was the first to highlight that the hippocampal signal transmission to the pedunculopontine tegmental nucleus is regulated by dopamine receptors of the NAc (Mogenson et al., 1987). The integrative role of the NAc and subpallidal area in relaying hippocampal signals to the mesencephalic locomotor region in the brainstem was investigated electrophysiologically in urethane-anaesthetized rats. A behavioral study of the functional connections was also performed in freely moving rats. In the electrophysiological experiments, subpallidal output neurons to the pedunculopontine nucleus were first identified by their antidromic responses to electrical stimulation of the pedunculopontine nucleus. Hippocampal stimulation was then shown to inhibit orthodromically some of these subpallidal neurons. The inhibitory response was attenuated following microinjection of a dopamine D2 agonist, but not a D1 agonist, into the NAc. This suggests that signal transmission from the hippocampus to the subpallidal output neurons to the pedunculopontine nucleus is modulated by a D2 receptor-mediated mechanism in the NAc. Injections of N-methyl-D-aspartate into the ventral subiculum of the hippocampus resulted in a threefold increase in locomotor responses. Injection of a D2 agonist into the accumbens reduced the hyperkinetic response dose-dependently and suggests that D2 receptors regulate locomotor responses initiated by the hippocampal-accumbens pathway. These results provide evidence of limbic (e.g., hippocampus) influences on locomotor activity by way of NAc-subpallidal-pedunculopontine nucleus connections that may contribute to adaptive behavior.

Concerning the dorsal part (DMS and DLS), the role of DA in controlling spatial navigation has been partially demonstrated only much more recently (for review: Penner and Mizumori, 2012). What is known so far is that, DA depletion in the DLS interfere with strategy shifting, but no experiments has been conducted yet in order to assess if it induced disruption of the egocentric learning.

Thus despite it is highly probable that DA depletion in the striatum could explain the effect on spatial behavior, there is no definitive evidences yet.

TOWARDS AN INTEGRATIVE REPRESENTATION

This quick review of the literature highlighted the multilevel implication of DA in the process of spatial information by the nervous system, however, it remains to determine at which level(s) the disruption of the dopaminergic function impacts spatial navigation in order to unravel the origin of spatial disorientation in PD patients (Hovestadt et al., 1987; Taylor et al., 1989).

The classical segregation between allocentric and egocentric learning seems too schematic and does not take into account the different modalities of perception of the environment. Hippocampus and striatum both contribute to encoding the spatial representation and seem to be involved in various modalities of perception. The hippocampus is related to the building of a spatial map (where am I?) but recent study evidenced that many place cells recorded from rats performing place or cue navigation tasks also discharged when they are at the goal location (Hok et al., 2007). The striatum provides reinforcing values to several aspects of the environment (where is my reward?), the ventral part to the pure localization aspects while the medial part encodes external cues. Meanwhile the dorsal striatum encodes the procedure (from here, which sequence of actions do I have to take in order to get my reward? (Retailleau et al., 2012). This taxonomy overlaps with the one recently proposed by Khamassi and Humphries (2012), which proposed that allocentric framework encompassed a model-based learning process while egocentric is more related to model free associative learning. It seems obvious that DA plays a key role in the striatum and that striatal DA depletion partly disrupts these processes. It is also highly probable that the rich density of DA receptors together with the response to reward location and decision processes we evidenced in CA3 (Retailleau et al., 2013) argue for also a local effect. So both mechanisms should be involved in the spatial disorientation observed in PD patients, but what remains to be established is in which proportion.

HOW EMERGES A SPATIAL STRATEGY?

It has been shown that different spatial strategies can be used and that lesion of the hippocampus or one of the striatal territories may shift the dominant strategy used by the subject (Packard and McGaugh, 1996; Mizumori et al., 2004; Penner and Mizumori, 2012) It strongly suggests that the neural mechanism of the specific selection of one of these modalities is based on competition mechanisms.

We demonstrated that action selection and decision making are emerging properties of the architecture of the frontal and dorsal part of the cortex-basal ganglia (BG) loop (Leblois et al., 2006; Guthrie et al., 2013). It makes it a perfect analogous of the actor in the actor-critic model of Sutton and Barto (1998), working under the supervision of a critic. Actor and critic are interfaced by DA at striatal level. The exact role of DA is still discussed and may be different in different structures (Khamassi and Humphries, 2012). While it is almost evident that it acts as error prediction signal in dorsal territories it may be simple reward signal elsewhere. In fact the neural substrate underlying

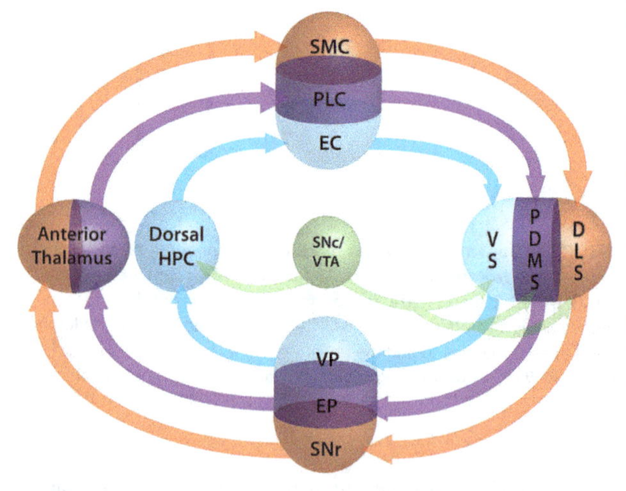

FIGURE 2 | Schematic representation of the three loops involved in spatial Inavigation. The loops are embedded in the fronto-cortical structures (SMC: sensorimotor cortex, PLC: prelimbic cortex, EC: entorhinal cortex), the basal ganglia (BG) segregated roughly into ventral (VS: ventral striatum, VP: ventral pallidum), dorsomedial (DMS: dorsomedial striatum, EP: entopeduncular nucleus) and dorsolateral (DLS: dorsolat- eral striatum, SNr: substantia nigra pars reticulata) parts, the anterior thalamus and the dorsal part of the hippocampus (Dorsal HPC). Dopamine projections from the SNc and ventral tegmantal area (VTA) are shown in green. The three functional loops are shown in blue for allocentric navigation by localization, in purple for allocentric navigation by external cues and in red for egocentric navigation. Convergence at BG level allows the system to perform selection of one of the modalities through a competition mechanism similar to those of the action selection loop (adapted form Retailleau et al., 2012).

the critic is still unknown and different sub-population of the actor structures can be involved (Lansink et al., 2009; Gläscher et al., 2010). For a comprehensive review of the involvement of the structures in different modalities of critic processing, we report the reader to Khamassi and Humphries (2012). We propose here to extend our model of the actor to the modalities of spatial navigation. The three modalities (external coordinates, external cues and internal coordinates) are supported by three different loops. The first loop passing through the ventral BG and the hippocampus, the second supported by the medial BG and thalamus respectively, and the third loop passing through the dorsal BG (**Figure 2**). The competition mechanism would allow the activation of one of the three modalities. During learning, dopamine would induce plasticity at various levels (ventral/medial or dorsal striatum, hippocampus) and modify the respective weight of each loop. According to the phase of learning and the reinforcing value of one of the aspects, one of the three networks would win the competition and therefore take over the control of the spatial navigation. This theory has the advantage of taking into account both the competitive and the collaborative aspects of their interactions and explains why, when all loops are functional, one can take over from another during the course of learning while, when one is disrupted, a different loop is able to take over the spatial navigation function. At the beginning of learning the system switches from one modality to another randomly due to the system noise level. Meanwhile, each system learns in parallel from the outcomes. From Packard and McGaugh (1996) work, we can infer that the more ventral system learns first and drives animal behavior after a moderate period of learning. After longer practice, the dorsal system is strengthened, takes over from the ventral system and drives the animal behavior. Inhibition of the stronger partner of the system (the ventral in the early phase, the dorsal in the later phase) allows the weaker system to take control of the behavior. According to the topography of the lesion, dopamine depletion as in PD may disrupt one or several of these systems. Where this disruption occurs and can it be compensated for by another system is still an open question to be investigated.

REFERENCES

Agid, Y. (1991). Parkinson's disease: pathophysiology. *Lancet* 337, 1321–1324. doi: 10.1016/0140-6736(91)92989-F

Annett, L. E., McGregor, A., and Robbins, T. W. (1989). The effects of ibotenic acid lesions of the nucleus accumbens on spatial learning and extinction in the rat. *Behav. Brain Res.* 31, 231–242. doi: 10.1016/0166-4328(89)90005-3

Atallah, H. E., Lopez-Paniagua, D., Rudy, J. W., and O'Reilly, R. C. (2007). Separate neural substrates for skill learning and performance in the ventral and dorsal striatum. *Nat. Neurosci.* 10, 126–131. doi: 10.1038/nn1817

Bannerman, D. M., Good, M. A., Butcher, S. P., Ramsay, M., and Morris, R. G. (1995). Distinct components of spatial learning revealed by prior training and NMDA receptor blockade. *Nature* 378, 182–186. doi: 10.1038/378182a0

Barnes, C. A., McNaughton, B. L., Mizumori, S. J., Leonard, B. W., and Lin, L. H. (1990). Comparison of spatial and temporal characteristics of neuronal activity in sequential stages of hippocampal processing. *Prog. Brain Res.* 83, 287–300. doi: 10.1016/s0079-6123(08)61257-1

Benhamou, S., and Poucet, B. (1998). Landmark use by navigating rats: contrasting geometrical and featural information. *J. Comp. Psychol.* 112, 317–322. doi: 10.1037/0735-7036.112.3.317

Berthoz, A. (1991). "Reference frames for the perception and control of movement," in *Brain and Space*, ed J. Paillard (Oxford, UK: Oxford University Press), 81–111.

Boraud, T., Bezard, E., Bioulac, B., and Gross, C. E. (2001). Dopamine agonist-induced dyskinesias are correlated to both firing pattern and frequency alterations of pallidal neurones in the MPTP-treated monkey. *Brain* 124, 546–557. doi: 10.1093/brain/124.3.546

Brouwer, N., Van Dijken, H., Ruiters, M. H., Van Willigen, J. D., and Ter Horst, G. J. (1992). Localization of dopamine D2 receptor mRNA with non-radioactive in situ hybridization histochemistry. *Neurosci. Lett.* 142, 223–227. doi: 10.1016/0304-3940(92)90378-k

Crizzle, A. M., Classen, S., and Uc, E. Y. (2012). Parkinson disease and driving: an evidence-based review. *Neurology* 79, 2067–2074. doi: 10.1212/WNL.0b013e3182749e95

Ferretti, V., Sargolini, F., Oliverio, A., Mele, A., and Roullet, P. (2007). Effects of intra-accumbens NMDA and AMPA receptor antagonists on short-term spatial learning in the Morris water maze task. *Behav. Brain Res.* 179, 43–49. doi: 10.1016/j.bbr.2007.01.009

Frank, M. J., Seeberger, L. C., and O'Reilly, R. C. (2004). By carrot or by stick: cognitive reinforcement learning in parkinsonism. *Science* 306, 1940–1943. doi: 10.1126/science.1102941

Gal, G., Joel, D., Gusak, O., Feldon, J., and Weiner, I. (1997). The effects of electrolytic lesion to the shell subterritory of the nucleus accumbens on delayed non-matching-to-sample and four-arm baited eight-arm radial-maze tasks. *Behav. Neurosci.* 111, 92–103. doi: 10.1037/0735-7044.111.1.92

Gallistel, C. R. (1990). Representations in animal cognition: an introduction. *Cognition* 37, 1–22. doi: 10.1016/0010-0277(90)90016-d

Gasbarri, A., Sulli, A., Innocenzi, R., Pacitti, C., and Brioni, J. D. (1996). Spatial memory impairment induced by lesion of the mesohippocampal dopaminergic system in the rat. *Neuroscience* 74, 1037–1044. doi: 10.1016/s0306-4522(96)00202-3

Gingrich, J. A., Dearry, A., Falardeau, P., Bates, M. D., Fremeau, R. T. Jr., and Caron, M. G. (1992). Location and molecular cloning of D1 dopamine receptor. *Neurochem. Int.* 20, 9S–15S. doi: 10.1016/0197-0186(92)90204-5

Gläscher, J., Daw, N., Dayan, P., and O'Doherty, J. P. (2010). States versus rewards: dissociable neural prediction error signals underlying model-based and model-free reinforcement learning. *Neuron* 66, 585–595. doi: 10.1016/j.neuron.2010.04.016

Goto, Y., Otani, S., and Grace, A. A. (2007). The Yin and Yang of dopamine release: a new perspective. *Neuropharmacology* 53, 583–587. doi: 10.1016/j.neuropharm.2007.07.007

Guthrie, M., Leblois, A., Garenne, A., and Boraud, T. (2013). Interaction between cognitive and motor cortico-basal ganglia loops during decision making: a computational study. *J. Neurophysiol.* 109, 3025–3040. doi: 10.1152/jn.00026.2013

Hok, V., Lenck-Santini, P. P., Roux, S., Save, E., Muller, R. U., and Poucet, B. (2007). Goal-related activity in hippocampal place cells. *J. Neurosci.* 27, 472–482. doi: 10.1523/jneurosci.2864-06.2007

Hollup, S. A., Kjelstrup, K. G., Hoff, J., Moser, M. B., and Moser, E. I. (2001). Impaired recognition of the goal location during spatial navigation in rats with hippocampal lesions. *J. Neurosci.* 21, 4505–4513.

Hovestadt, A., de Jong, G. J., and Meerwaldt, J. D. (1987). Spatial disorientation as an early symptom of Parkinson's disease. *Neurology* 37, 485–487. doi: 10.1212/WNL.37.3.485

Humphries, M. D., Khamassi, M., and Gurney, K. (2012). Dopaminergic control of the exploration-exploitation trade-off via the basal ganglia. *Front. Neurosci.* 6:9. doi: 10.3389/fnins.2012.00009

Ihalainen, J. A., Riekkinen, P. Jr., and Feenstra, M. G. (1999). Comparison of dopamine and noradrenaline release in mouse prefrontal cortex, striatum and hippocampus using microdialysis. *Neurosci. Lett.* 277, 71–74. doi: 10.1016/s0304-3940(99)00840-x

Johnson, A., and Redish, A. D. (2007). Neural ensembles in CA3 transiently encode paths forward of the animal at a decision point. *J. Neurosci.* 27, 12176–12189. doi: 10.1523/jneurosci.3761-07.2007

Kesner, R. P. (2007). Behavioral functions of the CA3 subregion of the hippocampus. *Learn. Mem.* 14, 771–781. doi: 10.1101/lm.688207

Khamassi, M., and Humphries, M. D. (2012). Integrating cortico-limbic-basal ganglia architectures for learning model-based and model-free navigation strategies. *Front. Behav. Neurosci.* 6:79. doi: 10.3389/fnbeh.2012.00079

Lansink, C. S., Goltstein, P. M., Lankelma, J. V., McNaughton, B. L., and Pennartz, C. M. (2009). Hippocampus leads ventral striatum in replay of place-reward information. *PLoS Biol.* 7:e1000173. doi: 10.1371/journal.pbio.1000173

Laurier, L. G., O'Dowd, B. F., and George, S. R. (1994). Heterogeneous tissue-specific transcription of dopamine receptor subtype messenger RNA in rat brain. *Brain Res. Mol. Brain Res.* 25, 344–350. doi: 10.1016/0169-328x(94)90170-8

Lavoie, A. M., and Mizumori, S. J. (1994). Spatial, movement- and reward-sensitive discharge by medial ventral striatum neurons of rats. *Brain Res.* 638, 157–168. doi: 10.1016/0006-8993(94)90645-9

Leblois, A., Boraud, T., Meissner, W., Bergman, H., and Hansel, D. (2006). Competition between feedback loops underlies normal and pathological dynamics in the basal ganglia. *J. Neurosci.* 26, 3567–3583. doi: 10.1523/jneurosci.5050-05.2006

Lemon, N., and Manahan-Vaughan, D. (2006). Dopamine D1/D5 receptors gate the acquisition of novel information through hippocampal long-term potentiation and long-term depression. *J. Neurosci.* 26, 7723–7729. doi: 10.1523/jneurosci.1454-06.2006

Li, S., Cullen, W. K., Anwyl, R., and Rowan, M. J. (2003). Dopamine-dependent facilitation of LTP induction in hippocampal CA1 by exposure to spatial novelty. *Nat. Neurosci.* 6, 526–531. doi: 10.1038/nn1049

Luo, A. H., Tahsili-Fahadan, P., Wise, R. A., Lupica, C. R., and Aston-Jones, G. (2011). Linking context with reward: a functional circuit from hippocampal CA3 to ventral tegmental area. *Science* 333, 353–357. doi: 10.1126/science.1204622

Mizumori, S. J. (2006). Hippocampal place fields: a neural code for episodic memory? *Hippocampus* 16, 685–690. doi: 10.1002/hipo.20209

Mizumori, S. J., Yeshenko, O., Gill, K. M., and Davis, D. M. (2004). Parallel processing across neural systems: implications for a multiple memory system hypothesis. *Neurobiol. Learn. Mem.* 82, 278–298. doi: 10.1016/j.nlm.2004.07.007

Mogenson, G. J., Ciriello, J., Garland, J., and Wu, M. (1987). Ventral pallidum projections to mediodorsal nucleus of the thalamus: an anatomical and electrophysiological investigation in the rat. *Brain Res.* 404, 221–230. doi: 10.1016/0006-8993(87)91373-4

Morris, R. G., Schenk, F., Tweedie, F., and Jarrard, L. E. (1990). Ibotenate lesions of hippocampus and/or subiculum: dissociating components of allocentric spatial learning. *Eur. J. Neurosci.* 2, 1016–1028. doi: 10.1111/j.1460-9568.1990.tb00014.x

O'Keefe, J. (1979). A review of the hippocampal place cells. *Prog. Neurobiol.* 13, 419–439. doi: 10.1016/0301-0082(79)90005-4

O'Keefe, J., and Conway, D. H. (1978). Hippocampal place units in the freely moving rat: why they fire where they fire. *Exp. Brain Res.* 31, 573–590. doi: 10.1007/bf00239813

O'Keefe, J., and Dostrovsky, J. (1971). The hippocampus as a spatial map. Preliminary evidence from unit activity in the freely-moving rat. *Brain Res.* 34, 171–175. doi: 10.1016/0006-8993(71)90358-1

Packard, M. G., and McGaugh, J. L. (1996). Inactivation of hippocampus or caudate nucleus with lidocaine differentially affects expression of place and response learning. *Neurobiol. Learn. Mem.* 65, 65–72. doi: 10.1006/nlme.1996.0007

Packard, M. G., and White, N. M. (1991). Dissociation of hippocampus and caudate nucleus memory systems by posttraining intracerebral injection of dopamine agonists. *Behav. Neurosci.* 105, 295–306. doi: 10.1037//0735-7044.105.2.295

Parent, A., and Hazrati, L. N. (1993). Anatomical aspects of information processing in primate basal ganglia. *Trends Neurosci.* 16, 111–116. doi: 10.1016/0166-2236(93)90135-9

Parent, A., and Hazrati, L. N. (1995). Functional anatomy of the basal ganglia. I. The cortico-basal ganglia-thalamo-cortical loop. *Brain Res. Brain Res. Rev.* 20, 91–127. doi: 10.1016/0165-0173(94)00007-C

Penner, M. R., and Mizumori, S. J. (2012). Neural systems analysis of decision making during goal-directed navigation. *Prog. Neurobiol.* 96, 96–135. doi: 10.1016/j.pneurobio.2011.08.010

Ploeger, G. E., Spruijt, B. M., and Cools, A. R. (1994). Spatial localization in the Morris water maze in rats: acquisition is affected by intra-accumbens injections of the dopaminergic antagonist haloperidol. *Behav. Neurosci.* 108, 927–934. doi: 10.1037/0735-7044.108.5.927

Poucet, B., and Benhamou, S. (1997). The neuropsychology of spatial cognition in the rat. *Crit. Rev. Neurobiol.* 11, 101–120. doi: 10.1615/critrevneurobiol.v11.i2-3.10

Retailleau, A., Etienne, S., Guthrie, M., and Boraud, T. (2012). Where is my reward and how do I get it? Interaction between the hippocampus and the basal ganglia during spatial learning. *J. Physiol. Paris* 106, 72–80. doi: 10.1016/j.jphysparis.2011.10.002

Retailleau, A., Dejean, C., Fourneaux, B., Leinekugel, X., and Boraud, T. (2013). Why am I lost without dopamine? Effects of 6-OHDA lesion on the encoding of reward and decision process in CA3. *Neurobiol. Dis.* 59, 151–164. doi: 10.1016/j.nbd.2013.07.014

Rolls, E. T. (2007). An attractor network in the hippocampus: theory and neurophysiology. *Learn. Mem.* 14, 714–731. doi: 10.1101/lm.631207

Sawamoto, N., Honda, M., Hanakawa, T., Fukuyama, H., and Shibasaki, H. (2002). Cognitive slowing in Parkinson's disease: a behavioral evaluation independent of motor slowing. *J. Neurosci.* 22, 5198–5203.

Scatton, B., Simon, H., Le Moal, M., and Bischoff, S. (1980). Origin of dopaminergic innervation of the rat hippocampal formation. *Neurosci. Lett.* 18, 125–131. doi: 10.1016/0304-3940(80)90314-6

Schultz, W. (2006). Behavioral theories and the neurophysiology of reward. *Annu. Rev. Psychol.* 57, 87–115. doi: 10.1146/annurev.psych.56.091103.070229

Schultz, W. (2007). Behavioral dopamine signals. *Trends Neurosci.* 30, 203–210. doi: 10.1016/j.tins.2007.03.007

Smialowski, A. (1987). Repeated imipramine enhances sensitivity of the brain dopaminergic system related to exploratory behavior. *J. Neural. Transm.* 69, 201–209. doi: 10.1007/bf01244341

Smialowski, A., and Bijak, M. (1987). Excitatory and inhibitory action of dopamine on hippocampal neurons in vitro. Involvement of D2 and D1 receptors. *Neuroscience* 23, 95–101. doi: 10.1016/0306-4522(87)90274-0

Smith-Roe, S. L., Sadeghian, K., and Kelley, A. E. (1999). Spatial learning and performance in the radial arm maze is impaired after N-methyl-D-aspartate (NMDA) receptor blockade in striatal subregions. *Behav. Neurosci.* 113, 703–717. doi: 10.1037/0735-7044.113.4.703

Sokoloff, P., and Schwartz, J. C. (1995). Novel dopamine receptors half a decade later. *Trends Pharmacol. Sci.* 16, 270–275. doi: 10.1016/s0165-6147(00)89044-6

Sutton, R. S., and Barto, A. G. (1998). *Reinforcement Learning: An Introduction.* Cambridge, MA: MIT Press.

Svenningsson, P., Westman, E., Ballard, C., and Aarsland, D. (2012). Cognitive impairment in patients with Parkinson's disease: diagnosis, biomarkers, and treatment. *Lancet Neurol.* 11, 697–707. doi: 10.1016/S1474-4422(12)70152-7

Taylor, A., Lang, A. E., and Saint-Cyr, J. A. (1989). Spatial disorientation in PD. *Neurology* 39, 879–880. doi: 10.1212/WNL.39.6.879-a

Thorn, C. A., Atallah, H., Howe, M., and Graybiel, A. M. (2010). Differential dynamics of activity changes in dorsolateral and dorsomedial striatal loops during learning. *Neuron* 66, 781–795. doi: 10.1016/j.neuron.2010.04.036

Trullier, O., Wiener, S. I., Berthoz, A., and Meyer, J. A. (1997). Biologically based artificial navigation systems: review and prospects. *Prog. Neurobiol.* 51, 483–544. doi: 10.1016/s0301-0082(96)00060-3

van der Meer, M. A., Kalenscher, T., Lansink, C. S., Pennartz, C. M., Berke, J. D., and Redish, A. D. (2010). Integrating early results on ventral striatal gamma oscillations in the rat. *Front. Neurosci.* 4:300. doi: 10.3389/fnins.2010.00300

van der Meer, M. A., and Redish, A. D. (2011). Theta phase precession in rat ventral striatum links place and reward information. *J. Neurosci.* 31, 2843–2854. doi: 10.1523/JNEUROSCI.4869-10.2011

Voorn, P., Vanderschuren, L. J., Groenewegen, H. J., Robbins, T. W., and Pennartz, C. M. (2004). Putting a spin on the dorsal-ventral divide of the striatum. *Trends Neurosci.* 27, 468–474. doi: 10.1016/j.tins.2004.06.006

Weintraub, D., Doshi, J., Koka, D., Davatzikos, C., Siderowf, A. D., Duda, J. E., et al. (2011). Neurodegeneration across stages of cognitive decline in Parkinson disease. *Arch. Neurol.* 68, 1562–1568. doi: 10.1001/archneurol.2011.725

Whishaw, I. Q., and Jarrard, L. E. (1995). Similarities vs. differences in place learning and circadian activity in rats after fimbria-fornix section or ibotenate removal of hippocampal cells. *Hippocampus* 5, 595–604. doi: 10.1002/hipo.450050610

Whishaw, I. Q., and Tomie, J. (1996). Of mice and mazes: similarities between mice and rats on dry land but not water mazes. *Physiol. Behav.* 60, 1191–1197. doi: 10.1016/s0031-9384(96)00176-x

Wiener, S. I. (1993). Spatial and behavioral correlates of striatal neurons in rats performing a self-initiated navigation task. *J. Neurosci.* 13, 3802–3817.

Wilkerson, A., and Levin, E. D. (1999). Ventral hippocampal dopamine D1 and D2 systems and spatial working memory in rats. *Neuroscience* 89, 743–749. doi: 10.1016/s0306-4522(98)00346-7

Yin, H. H., and Knowlton, B. J. (2004). Contributions of striatal subregions to place and response learning. *Learn. Mem.* 11, 459–463. doi: 10.1101/lm.81004

15

Linking Reward Processing to Behavioral Output: Motor and Motivational Integration in the Primate Subthalamic Nucleus

Juan-Francisco Espinosa-Parrilla, Christelle Baunez and Paul Apicella*

Institut de Neurosciences de la Timone, CNRS-Aix-Marseille Université, Marseille, France

***Correspondence:**
Paul Apicella, Institut de Neurosciences de la Timone, CNRS-Aix-Marseille Université, 27 boulevard Jean Moulin, 13005 Marseille, cedex 05, France
e-mail: paul.apicella@univ-amu.fr

The expectation and detection of motivationally relevant events is a major determinant of goal-directed behavior and there is a strong interest in the contribution of basal ganglia in the integration of motivational processes into behavioral output. Recent research has focused on the role of the subthalamic nucleus (STN) in the motivational control of action, but it remains to be determined how information about reward is encoded in this nucleus. We recorded the activity of single neurons in the STN of two behaving monkeys to examine whether activity was influenced by the delivery of reward in an instrumental task, a Pavlovian stimulus-reward association, or outside of a task context. We confirmed preliminary findings indicating that STN neurons were sensitive not only to rewards obtained during task performance, but also to the expectation of reward when its delivery was delayed in time. Most of the modulations at the onset of reaching movement were combined with modulations following reward delivery, suggesting the convergence of signals related to the animal's movement and its outcome in the same neurons. Some neurons were also influenced by the visuomotor contingencies of the task, i.e., target location and/or movement direction. In addition, modulations were observed under conditions where reward delivery was not contingent on an instrumental response, even in the absence of a reward predictive cue. Taken as a whole, these results demonstrate a potential contribution of the STN to motivational control of behavior in the non-human primate, although problems in distinguishing neuronal signals related to reward from those related to motor behavior should be considered. Characterizing the specificity of reward processing in the STN remains challenging and could have important implications for understanding the influence of this key component of basal ganglia circuitry on emotional and motivated behaviors under normal and pathological conditions.

Keywords: basal ganglia, reinforcement, reward expectation, context processing, single-neuron activity, monkey

INTRODUCTION

Although it is traditionally considered that the subthalamic nucleus (STN) is important in motor control, an increasing number of studies has been conducted to investigate the role of this nucleus in the processing of reward-related information. Evidence in favor of the STN involvement in motivational processes comes primarily from lesions studies in behaving rats showing that STN dysfunction leads to increased responding for a food reward (Baunez et al., 2002). In addition, STN lesions could have a differential impact on the incentive motivational properties of natural reinforcers and drugs of abuse, the STN-lesioned rats becoming more motivated as they work to obtain food reward and less motivated when cocaine was used as the reward (Baunez et al., 2005), suggesting that processing of different types of rewards can be dissociated at the STN level.

Clinical studies also support the notion that the STN is a component of reward circuitry. In particular, deep brain stimulation (DBS) of this nucleus, which is effective at alleviating motor symptoms in patients with Parkinson's disease, can also interfere with brain circuits that mediate mood and reward signals leading to enhanced motivation and decreased apathy in some of these patients (Funkiewiez et al., 2003; Takeshita et al., 2005), although an interference with decreased dopaminergic medication cannot be excluded. It has been also reported that DBS of the STN can either increase (Houeto et al., 2002; Schüpbach et al., 2005) or decrease (Witjas et al., 2005; Lhommée et al., 2012; Eusebio et al., 2013) the addiction of parkinsonian patients for their levodopa treatment. Since abnormal repetitive behaviors (i.e., compulsions) include an emotional component, the observation that obsessive–compulsive disorders can be improved by DBS of the STN is also an argument in favor of the contribution of this nucleus in emotional and motivational processes (Mallet et al., 2002; Baunez et al., 2011). Taking into account those elements, it has been suggested that the STN may represent a promising target for the treatment of addiction (Pelloux and Baunez, 2013).

Although, functional neuroimaging research in humans poses challenges to the interpretation of changes in activity of small subcortical brain structures (Keuken et al., 2013; reviewed in Péron et al., 2013), studies in this field have recently confirmed the role of the STN in behavioral inhibition highlighted by animal studies, such as the ability to cancel planned or already initiated actions (Aron and Poldrack, 2006; Li et al., 2008). While the role of this nucleus in motivation has received much less attention, the contribution of other parts of the basal ganglia, particularly the ventral striatum, in emotion and reward processes has been studied in many experiments using monetary or taste rewards under a variety of behavioral paradigms (Delgado, 2007). So far, hemodynamic changes restricted to the STN area which may be linked to anticipation and experience of reward have not been reported. However, as mentioned above, such an approach is still limited by the relatively poor spatial resolution of brain imaging techniques. On the other hand, neuronal recordings from the STN in patients with Parkinson's disease or obsessive–compulsive disorders during DBS surgery or after electrode implantation (local field potentials, LFPs) have provided evidence that the STN region is active during the processing of information related to emotional aspects of behavior (Kühn et al., 2005; Brücke et al., 2007; Burbaud et al., 2013). A potential disturbance of emotional information processing at the STN level could account for the mood changes reported in parkinsonian patients subjected to STN stimulation (Krack et al., 2001; Schneider et al., 2003).

More direct evidence for the involvement of STN in motivational processes is obtained from single-neuron recording experiments in animals performing controlled behavioral tasks. Several components of the basal ganglia circuitry, including the striatum, globus pallidus and substantia nigra pars reticulata, have been implicated in the processing of reward-related information and in linking motivation to action (reviewed in Schultz et al., 2000 and Hikosaka et al., 2006). In contrast, there are few data in direct support of reward processing at the STN level. Previous studies in behaving rats have reported that STN neurons can be modulated after the presentation of stimuli associated with reward and at the time of the reward delivery (Teagarden and Rebec, 2007; Lardeux et al., 2009, 2013). Moreover, STN neurons show differential responses to reward-related cues according to the quality of the expected reward, i.e., the degree of sweetness of a sucrose solution (Lardeux et al., 2009), and they can also discriminate between food and drug reinforcement, showing a specialization according to the relative preference for the reward (Lardeux et al., 2013). These findings are consistent with the existing literature on the impact of STN inactivation in rodents, supporting a role for this nucleus in reward processing. Conversely, much less information about the role of the STN in motivation is available in the primate. In a preliminary report, we have examined the relation of STN neuronal activity to movement and reward in one monkey performing an arm reaching task (Darbaky et al., 2005). In that study, we showed that the discharge of STN neurons was often modulated during the movement period of the task and at the time of the reward delivery, suggesting that STN neurons carrying signals related to motor activity could also be informed about the reception of the reinforcer. However, the details as to how the association of reward information with motor processes occurs in this nucleus remain unclear.

The purpose of our study was to further examine in monkeys the activity of STN neurons which could be related to reward delivered in distinct behavioral situations. The activity was analyzed during performance of visually-triggered movements leading to reward and in conditions with no contingency between movement and reward. Our objective was to determine whether the information contained in the discharge of individual STN neurons could be related to reward and by the behavioral context in which rewards were experienced.

MATERIALS AND METHODS

ANIMALS

Two adult macaque monkeys (G and P, *Macaca fascicularis)*, weighing 5–6 kg, were used as subjects. Experimental setup, surgical procedures and recording procedures were the same as described previously (Deffains et al., 2010). Both animals were fully trained to perform visually triggered arm-reaching movements for liquid rewards before being surgically prepared for neuronal recordings. During the training and recording periods, the monkeys were deprived of water in their home cage and received apple juice during the experiments. Unlimited water access was allowed for at least one day each week. All experiments were in accordance with the guidelines of the National Institutes of Health Guide for the Care and Use of Laboratory Animals and the French laws on animal experimentation.

BEHAVIORAL TESTING CONDITIONS

The monkeys were seated in a specially designed restraining box, facing a panel 30 cm from its head. The panel contained two metal knobs (10 × 10 mm) separated by 20 cm horizontally, and two light-emitting diodes (two-colored LEDs red/green), one above each knob, at eye level of the animal (**Figure 1A**). An unmovable metal bar mounted at the center of the panel served as a starting point for the reaching movement. Each trial began by keeping the hand on the bar. There was no fixation point signaling the trial initiation or constraining the monkey's eye movements. After a period of at least 1 s, a visual cue (green light) was presented randomly, either to the right or left, for 0.5 s. Cue presentation was followed by a 1-s delay period at the end of which the trigger stimulus (red light) appeared in the same location, indicating that the monkey should release the bar and touch the corresponding target. The delivery of reward (0.3 ml of apple juice) occurred immediately after target contact, under the control of a solenoid valve placed outside the experimental room. After target contact, the monkey moved back to the bar and waited for the total duration of the current trial (5 s) to elapse before a new trial began. An error trial was recorded when monkeys took longer than 1 s to initiate or execute the movement (omission trials). The two monkeys received training until they achieved a consistent correct performance rate of > 90% in the reaching task before the neuronal recording started.

In the basic task condition, reward was delivered immediately after the correct hand reaching for a target ("immediate reward") (**Figure 1A**, left). We also employed another condition in which a constant delay of 0.5 s was introduced between target contact

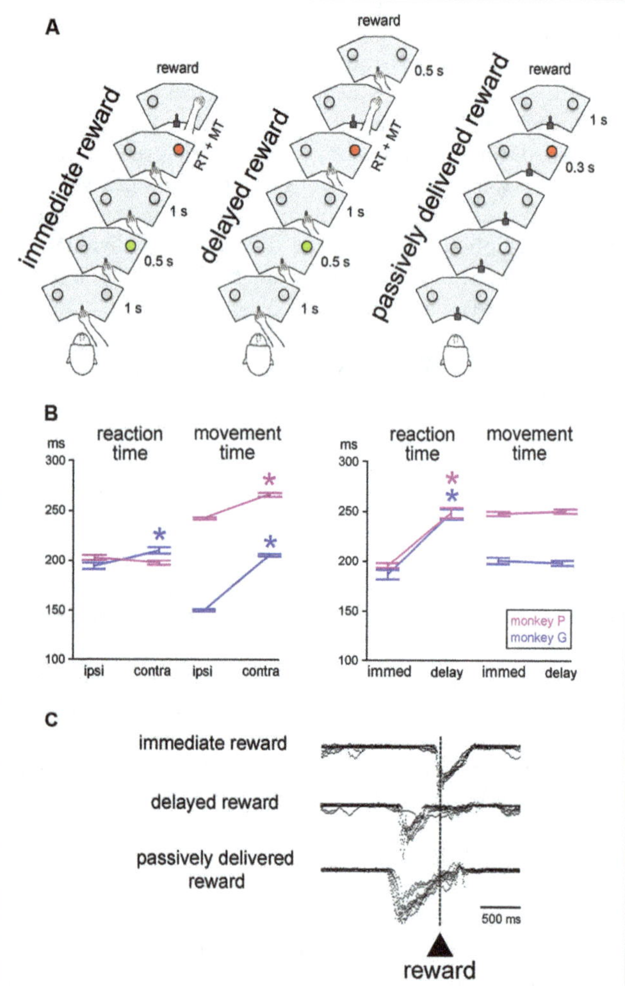

FIGURE 1 | Sequences of events and behavior in the testing conditions. (A) In the reaching task, monkey started a trial by keeping the hand on a bar. A first visual stimulus (green light) was presented for 0.5 s at one of the two locations. A second visual stimulus (red light) was presented 1 s later at the same location. The animal was then required to release the bar and reach for the target located below the light, which it had to touch to receive a liquid reward. In the *immediate reward* condition, the reward was given immediately after correct target contact. In the *delayed reward* condition, the reward was delivered at the end of a 0.5-s interval after target contact. In the *passively delivered reward* condition, the monkey remained motionless without any access to the bar. This is a Pavlovian protocol in which a visual stimulus signaled the delivery of reward 1 s later, independently of a motor action. The three conditions were tested in separate blocks of trials. RT, MT. **(B)** Reaching task performance for the two monkeys. Each value of RT and MT was obtained by calculating the mean for all correct trials (± SEM) for the different locations of the target stimulus (*ipsi* and *contra* refer to the location of the stimulus ipsilateral and controlateral to the moving arm, respectively) and timing of reward delivery (*immed* and *delay* refer to immediate and delayed delivery of reward after target contact, respectively). An asterisk indicates that the value was significantly different between the two target locations or reward timing conditions (paired *t*-test, $P < 0.05$). **(C)** Licking behavior in the three conditions. Superimposed traces of mouth movement records are aligned on reward valve activation occurring with target contact in the immediate reward condition, 0.5 s after target contact in the delayed reward condition, and 1 s after the onset of the visual stimulus in the Pavlovian protocol, i.e., when reward was passively delivered.

and reward delivery ("delayed reward") (**Figure 1A**, middle), trials being similar to the immediate condition in all other aspects of appearance and timing. In particular, the trigger light remained illuminated until target contact, regardless of the moment of reward delivery. In a few cases, the 0.5-s delay was replaced by a 1.0-s delay when single neuron isolation was maintained long enough to complete an additional test. Because this happened infrequently, it was not possible for the monkey to predict the further lengthening of the target-reward interval. In all conditions, trials lasted 5 s so that a temporally less well-defined period began with reward delivery and ended with the cue of the subsequent trial (i.e., intervals between reward and the next cue varied from ~2 s to 3 s in the 1.0-s delay and immediate reward conditions, respectively). The immediate and delayed reward conditions were conducted in separate blocks of 40–60 trials, the change in condition not being indicated by any explicit cues. However, because of the block design, it did not take monkeys many trials to adjust their expectation after a switch in testing condition. Before the recording experiments started, both monkeys were well-trained in the immediate reward condition, whereas the delayed reward condition was used only occasionally during recording sessions.

We also employed a condition in which the liquid reward was delivered in a passive manner after a period of 1 s after one LED was illuminated with a red light (**Figure 1A**, right). This was a Pavlovian conditioning procedure in which reward was not contingent on behavior (Apicella et al., 1997). In this testing condition, the sliding door located at the front of the restraining box was closed to prevent manual access to the panel. In addition to the testing of the monkeys in the Pavlovian protocol, we also delivered the liquid at unpredictable times, in the absence of any cue to precisely time when the reward would be delivered. The change from instrumentally to passively delivered reward was indicated by the experimenter entering the experimental room to open or close the sliding door of the box. Conversely, there was no signal indicating that the Pavlovian protocol was about to be changed to a block of trials in which reward was delivered alone. Passively delivered reward conditions were presented using the same trial duration as used in the reaching task, thus preserving the overall temporal structure of the testing condition.

NEURONAL RECORDINGS

On completion of training, each monkey underwent sterile surgery under sodium pentobarbital anesthesia. An opening was made in the skull over the left hemisphere and a stainless steel recording chamber (25 mm OD) was implanted over the hole, its center being aimed at the anterior commissure (AC), approximately 5 mm anterior to the rostral pole of the STN. The chamber was held in place by dental acrylic anchored with stainless steel screws drilled into the skull. Two stainless steel cylinders were also embedded in dental acrylic for subsequent head fixation during recording sessions. Antibiotics and analgesics were administered after surgery. Extracellular activity of single neurons was recorded with tungsten microelectrodes, as described previously (Deffains et al., 2010). In both monkeys, with their heads restrained while performing the behavioral tasks, neuronal recordings were carried out first from striatum. After several months of recording mainly targeted at the putamen, finding the accurate location of the STN was relatively easy using the striatal tracks, particularly at the level of the posterior putamen. Parallel electrode tracks were then made vertically, through the thalamus, zona incerta, STN and substantia nigra pars reticulata, in that order, the transition between these structures being obvious because of grossly different spontaneous neuronal activity. The electrode was driven by a hydraulic microdrive (MO-95; Narishige, Tokyo, Japan) through a stainless steel guide tube, which was used to penetrate the dura. After penetration of the dura, the electrode was advanced until the dorsal border of the STN was identified by an increase of background noise and typical large-amplitude irregular spike activity after passing the white matter area below the thalamus (i. e., fields of Forel) and zona incerta (Matsumura et al., 1992; Wichmann et al., 1994; Isoda and Hikosaka, 2008). Signals from neuronal activity were conventionally amplified, filtered (bandpass, 0.3–1.5 kHz), and converted to digital pulses through a window discriminator. During the recording of any neuron, activity in the immediate reward version of the reaching task was generally studied first, and, if the isolation could be sustained for a sufficient period of time, the tests were continued in the other conditions. It needs to be pointed out that the relative lack of stability of recording in the primate STN did not always ensure the isolation of individual neurons over successive trial blocks for different conditions (Wichmann et al., 1994). We have succeeded in helding stable neurons for two or more blocks in only a few cases. Presentation of visual stimuli, delivery of reward, collection of movement parameters, mouth movements and single-neuron activity were controlled by a computer, using custom software written by E. Legallet.

DATA ANALYSIS

Performance in the reaching task was assessed by measuring the reaction time (RT), i.e., the time between the onset of the trigger stimulus and release of the bar, and the movement time (MT), i.e., the time taken to contact a target after releasing the bar. The analysis included data from all correctly performed trials and all recording sessions, excluding error trials (omissions of the trigger stimulus) and premature responses (RTs < 100 ms). The tube conducting reward liquid to the spout positioned directly in front of the monkey's mouth was equipped with a strain gauge circuit with which we monitored the licking movements as analog signals (sampling rate: 100 Hz). The timing characteristics of the mouth movements that monkeys performed in the different conditions were assessed off-line by single-trial analysis.

To analyze neuronal correlates of the initiation of movement, we calculated the mean firing rate in a 300-ms time window extending from 200 ms before movement onset until 100 ms after movement onset, called the "perimovement period", and in another 300-ms time window extending from 400 to 700 ms after target contact, called the "postreward period". The mean discharge rate in each task period was compared with that in the control period (the 1 s duration before the cue onset) to examine whether the neuron showed significant task-related activities. If the mean discharge rate in a given period was significantly different from that in the control period (two-tailed Student t-test, $P < 0.05$), the neuron was considered to show task-related activity in that period. We tested for changes in activity during these two period for each recorded neuron.

The selectivity of the task-related activity for a particular location of the target stimulus was judged to be present if the magnitudes of the perimovement activity were significantly different between the two locations (two-way ANOVA, period (control, perimovement) × location (left, right), $p < 0.05$).

To determine the response latency of a neuron to a particular task event, onset and offset times of statistically significant changes in activity were assessed using a previously established procedure based on a sliding time window analysis (Deffains et al., 2010). Briefly, baseline activity was determined in the 1-s period that preceded the onset of the cue (control period). A test window of 100 ms was moved in steps of 10 ms, starting at the onset of the cue. We then compared activity from the baseline period to activity in the sliding window. Neurons showing a statistically significant difference in activity during ≥ 20 consecutive steps (Wilcoxon signed-rank test, $P < 0.05$) were considered as modulated. The latency of a significant change in neuronal activity was defined as the beginning of the first of 20 consecutive steps showing a significant difference as against the baseline activity during the control period.

In addition to the assessment of activity changes of the individual STN neurons, we also summed activity of all neurons tested in a given condition or for a particular location of the target stimulus and made population histograms. For each neuron, a normalized perievent time histogram was obtained by dividing the content of each bin by the number of trials. The population histogram was obtained by averaging all normalized histograms referenced to a particular event. These histograms were constructed from neurons recorded in monkeys P and G in each testing condition.

HISTOLOGY

We confirmed our recording sites by histological verification in one monkey, whereas the location of recorded neurons was determined solely on the basis of the electrophysiological information concerning the boundaries of the STN and surrounding structures in the other monkey. After the experiments had been completed, monkey P was sacrificed with an intravenous overdose of pentobarbital and perfused transcardially with 0.9% saline followed by a fixative (4% paraformaldehyde, pH 7.4 phosphate buffer). The brain was cut in 50-μm coronal sections, mounted on slides, and stained with cresyl violet. We identified the recording sites that had been marked with small electrolytic lesions in and around the STN at the end of neuronal data collection. Electrode penetrations were then reconstructed in serial sections through the STN by referring to the marking lesions.

RESULTS

TASK PERFORMANCE DATA

The mean RT and MT for different target locations and reward timing for each monkey are presented in **Figure 1B**. Consistent with previous reports from our lab (Ravel et al., 2006; Deffains et al., 2010), RTs to target stimuli presented contralaterally to the moving arm were slightly but significantly longer than RTs to ipsilateral target stimuli in monkey G (Student's t-test, $P < 0.01$), whereas the effect of spatial location on RT was no significant in monkey P ($P > 0.05$). On the other hand, MTs for contralateral movements were longer than MTs for ipsilateral ones in both monkeys ($P < 0.01$). It is possible that monkey P used prior information about the target location efficiently to prepare the movement and then improve speed during initiation, thus explaining the lack of spatial response bias in the initiation phase of movement in this animal.

As also shown in **Figure 1B**, comparing the RTs obtained during blocks where the reward was delivered immediately after target contact with those where the reward was delayed by 0.5 s after target contact, yielded significant longer RTs in the latter condition in both monkeys (two-way ANOVA) with the factors target location and reward timing, effect of reward timing: monkey G: (F (1, 401) = 73.82, $P < 0.01$; monkey P: (F (1, 364) = 96.16, $P < 0.01$). In contrast, for MT, there was no significant difference between the two conditions (monkey G: F (1, 401) = 0.47, $P > 0.05$; monkey P: F (1, 364) = 0.65, $P > 0.05$). There was no interaction between target location and reward timing regarding RT and MT in monkey G ($P > 0.05$), whereas such interactions were detected for RT ($P < 0.05$) and MT ($P < 0.01$) in monkey P. These findings indicate that monkeys took longer to initiate reaching movements when the timing of the reward outcome was delayed. These results differ from what was found in a previous study, using a similar reaching task, in which we reported that neither RT and MT were influenced by the delayed delivery of reward after target contact (Ravel et al., 2001). This lack of concordance could be attributed to differences in training levels, the small sample of neurons tested in the delayed reward condition in the present study did not allow enough training. In a few cases (1 and 4 trial blocks in monkeys G and P, respectively), a 1-s delay was employed in order to further lengthen the period of expectation of reward after target contact. This test was only used when stable recordings were obtained on neurons that were modulated during the target-reward interval of 0.5 s. In monkey P, two-way ANOVA performed with target location and reward timing (immediate, delay 0.5-s, delay 1.0-s) as factors revealed a significant main effect of reward timing on RT (F (2, 266) = 31.01, $P < 0.01$), so that RT was longer in the delay 1.0-s than the delay 0.5-s conditions. In contrast, the MTs varied insignificantly by reward timing (F (2, 266) = 1.97, $P > 0.05$). When monkeys were tested with delayed reward conditions, whether a 0.5-s or a 1.0-s delay, they moved immediately their hand back to the bar after having touched the target and then waited for the delay before reward. In this regard, there were no noticeable differences in gross behavior between immediate and delayed reward conditions while the animal was resting the hand on the bar in order to initiate the next trial.

Representative mouth movement recordings are illustrated in **Figure 1C**. They were essentially the same as those described in earlier studies using similar behavioral situations (Ravel et al., 2001; Apicella et al., 2009). The monkey started to lick the spout on or slightly before target contact in the instrumental task, regardless of the timing of reward, and these movements were prolonged until the receipt of liquid when a 0.5-s delay was introduced between target contact and reward delivery. Licking movements occurred during the 1-s interval separating the presentation of the visual stimulus from the delivery of reward, indicating that the stimulus served as a trigger for mouth movements in anticipation of the upcoming reward. This served as a well-established behavioral marker of the Pavlovian stimulus-reward association.

GENERAL

While the monkeys performed the reaching task, we recorded from 74 neurons in the STN (51 and 23 from monkey G and P, respectively) with a background firing rate of 23.5 ± 16.4 spikes/s (mean ± SEM). Most neurons ($n = 59$) had medium to high firing rates (mean 28.6, range 10.3–71.3), a small number ($n = 15$) had firing below 10 spikes/s (mean 3.4). The firing characteristics of STN neurons were similar to what has been reported previously in behaving monkeys in terms of spiking irregularity and baseline firing rate (Matsumura et al., 1992; Wichmann et al., 1994; Isoda and Hikosaka, 2008).

Based on the location of recording sites identified histologically in monkey P, these neurons were recorded between 5 and 7 mm posterior to the AC, over the mediolateral extent of the STN, except its most medial part. A summary plot of all neurons recorded is shown in **Figure 2**, including those that could not be recorded for enough number of trials. On the basis of histological analysis of electrode tracks in this monkey, it appears that we failed to adequately sample the most medial portion of the nucleus in its more anterior parts. As regards the recording sites of well isolated neurons, the two major groups of task-related changes in activity (i.e., those occurring during the perimovement period and/or the postreward period) did not show clear regional differences in the STN explored.

In general, STN neurons exhibited a variety of changes in activity during various periods of the reaching task, with some neurons being modulated before the onset of the movement and others being modulated later, after the monkey's hand contacted the target and was immediately followed by the delivery of reward. These modulations could consist in either excitation or inhibition. As we point out below, the same neurons often displayed changes in activity during two distinct task periods, namely around the initiation of movement and after target contact.

ACTIVITY AFTER TARGET CONTACT

The activity of 70% (52/74) of neurons (13 of 23 in monkey P, 39 of 51 in monkey G) was significantly modulated after reaching toward the correct target. **Figure 3A** shows an example of neuron with increased activity after target contact (right part). This neuron also showed increased activity, although to a weaker degree, before the initiation of movement (left part). As is demonstrated by this case, the temporal linkage to movement onset was clearly apparent by aligning neuronal activity on bar release. The activity was rapidly decreased immediately after the onset of movement and increased again after movement termination, lasting more than 1 s after target contact. About three quarters of the detected changes occurring after target contact consisted of increases and one quarter of decreases.

As illustrated in **Figure 3A**, the majority of neurons (35/52) significantly modulated after target contact also showed a significant change in activity around the initiation of movement. Thirty three neurons changed their activity in the same direction for both movement initiation and after target contact (28 increases,

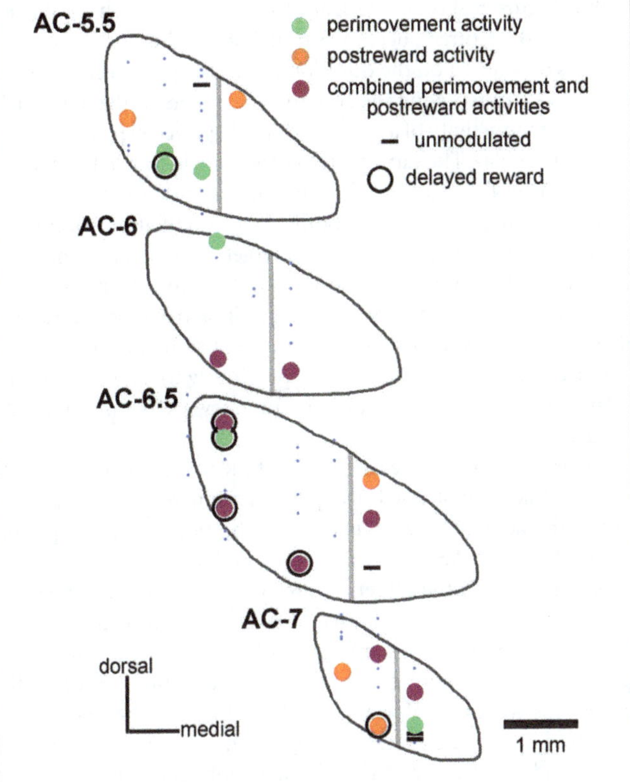

FIGURE 2 | Histological verification of recording sites in the STN of one monkey. Data from monkey P are plotted on coronal sections of the STN referenced to the AC. Neurons studied during the performance of the reaching task were classified as being modulated around the initiation of movement (*perimovement activity*), after the delivery of reward (*postreward activity*), at both periods of the task (*combined perimovement and postreward activities*), or without any change in their firing in these two periods (*unmodulated*). Neurons whose recordings were not sufficiently stable to permit adequate testing are represented by small blue dots. Neurons displaying a sustained change in activity when a delay between target contact and reward delivery was introduced are surrounded by a black circle (*delayed reward*). Gray lines indicate the approximate boundary of the "sensorimotor" and "cognitive-limbic" parts of the STN.

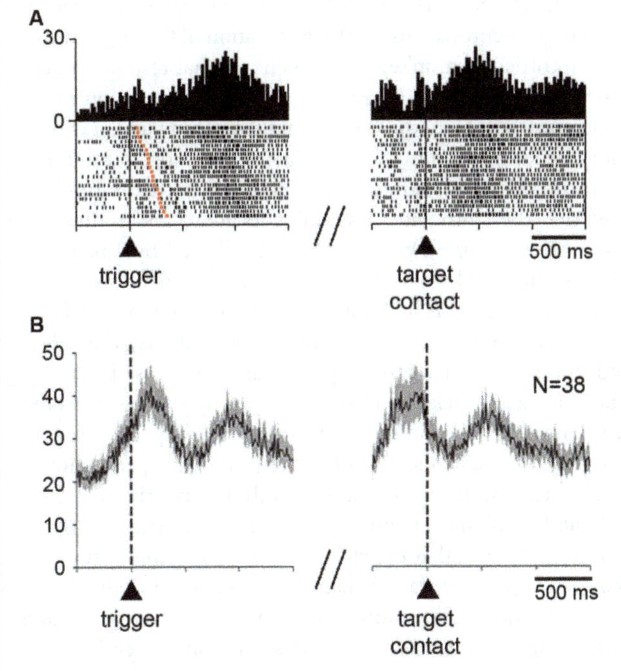

FIGURE 3 | Neuronal activity in the STN during the performance of the reaching task. (A) An example of neuron showing an increase in firing rate before the initiation of movement and after target contact immediately followed by reward delivery. Each dot in the raster displays represents one neuronal impulse, and each line of dots represents the neuronal activity during a single trial. Dot displays and perievent time histograms are aligned on the onset of the movement triggering stimulus (left) or the contact with the target (right), which are marked by vertical lines. The raster was sorted in order of increasing RT, i.e., increasing interval from trigger onset to the onset of movement (red squares in each row). Histogram scale: impulses/bin. Binwidth for histograms: 20 ms. **(B)** Modulation of population activity in the reaching task. Only neurons showing increases in firing rate after target contact, pooled from both monkeys, are included in this analysis. Average activity is aligned on the trigger stimulus (left) or target contact (right), which are marked by vertical dashed lines. Vertical scale: impulses/s. N: number of neurons included for the population histogram.

5 decreases), whereas only 2 neurons had opposite changes in activity (an increase for movement initiation and a decrease after target contact). Changes in activity occurring specifically after target contact were observed in 17 neurons (10 increases, 7 decreases) and 15 neurons showed an exclusive change in activity around the initiation of movement (10 increases, 5 decreases).

We examined the time course of activity changes at the level of the whole sample of neurons modulated during the postreward period (**Figure 3B**). Only neurons showing increases in their firing rate were included in this population average. The average activity reached a first peak of increased activity slightly after the presentation of the trigger stimulus that elicited movements. A second peak of increased activity occurred later after target contact. It is noticeable that this latter peak was well located in the 300-ms time window we have chosen for analysis (i.e., 400–700 ms after target contact), indicating that the majority of activations following target contact were relatively late increases.

The relative late onset of peak firing after target contact suggests that changes in STN neuronal activity did not occur directly in response to target contact. Also, peak firing did not appear to be associated with the monkey's movement back to the resting bar. Although a possible relationship to the consumption of liquid must be taken into account, it seems that the motor aspects of orofacial activity were not the only explanation, particularly for those neurons which began to be modulated with a relatively long latency after target contact. This explanation, however, does not hold for other neurons that became active earlier, during the reaching movement, a task period in which preparation and initiation of mouth movements took place.

We next examined whether the magnitude of the change in activity during the perimovement period was affected by the location of the target stimulus and/or the direction of the associated movement. Target location had a significant effect ($P < 0.05$; two-way ANOVA) on perimovement activity in 22 of the 74 neurons tested (19 and 3 neurons in monkeys G and P, respectively). Among them, 19 showed increases in activity around the initiation of movement and 3 showed decreases. The fact that most of the neurons sensitive to the location of the target stimulus were recorded in monkey G in which a spatial response bias was observed behaviorally (**Figure 1B**), suggests that a contralateral preference in STN modulations could emerge in parallel with slow movement initiation in the contralateral direction. We found that 14 of the 22 neurons displaying spatially selective modulations preferred the contralateral stimulus location, and 8 the ipsilateral one ($P < 0.05$; two-way ANOVA followed by Tukey's test). This is illustrated by data from two example neurons classified as spatially selective in **Figure 4A**. The first neuron (left part) is an example of directional preparatory activity, the selective activation being manifested by a sustained increase in discharge rate during the delay period prior to contralateral movement, whereas a corresponding reduction in activity occurred with ipsilateral movements. The other neuron (right part) showed a contralateral-selective activation in advance of trigger presentation and until movement onset. It is noteworthy, in the two example neurons, that the change in activity terminated with the onset of movement, rather than the presentation of the stimulus triggering movement. Moreover, a phasic component occurring just before the movement onset was still visible even in the case of ipsilateral movements, suggesting the presence of a neuronal signal related to movement initiation that did not depend on the spatial features of the task.

Separate population histograms were constructed from all neurons showing target location selectivity (**Figure 4B**). This analysis was confined to data from neurons recorded in monkey G showing increased activity during the perimovement period and in which a significant effect of spatial location was detected. Despite the small number of neurons, the spatial preference in terms of magnitude of change in the average activity was obvious when the stimulus was presented contralaterally to the reaching arm. As shown in **Figure 4B**, the selectivity for ipsilateral target location appeared less evident at the level of the population average, compared to contralateral location.

INFLUENCE OF DELAYING THE REWARD AFTER TARGET CONTACT

Additional tests were performed for characterizing changes in activity following target contact. In particular, we wanted to separate in time movement termination from the receipt of liquid by delaying the reward for 0.5 s, occasionally 1 s, after the contact of the monkey's hand with the target. In 21 neurons (8 and 13 from monkeys P and G, respectively), single neuron isolation could be successfully maintained during recording in both the immediate and delayed reward conditions. Of these, 16 neurons showed a sustained change in activity through the delay between target contact and reward delivery, consisting of increases and decreases in activity in 10 and 6 neurons, respectively. For 5 of the 16 neurons showing a sustained change in their activity during the 0.5-s delay (2 increases, 3 decreases), data were also collected when the target–reward interval was further lengthened to 1 s and we verified that the change in activity was prolonged accordingly. This is consistent with previous studies demonstrating that STN neurons recorded in behaving monkeys can display sustained changes in activity as a possible reflection of a state of expectation of the delivery of reward (Matsumura et al., 1992; Darbaky et al., 2005). **Figure 5** shows data from two neurons which have been fully tested in three successive trial blocks, illustrating activity profiles dependent on the duration of the delay between reaching the target and receiving the reward. The rasters in the left panels represent the activity of a neuron which displayed elevated activity during the delay. The same pattern of activity is seen in the neuron illustrated in the right panels, but consisting in a suppression of activity during the delay. In both cases, modulations occurring during the delay began just before target contact and continued until reward delivery. Despite the limited size of our data set, it is noticeable that sustained changes in activity before reward delivery were frequently found in the ventral half of the nucleus (**Figure 2**) which has been shown previously to contain neurons related to reward expectation in monkey (Matsumura et al., 1992).

In order to investigate whether the task-related changes in STN neuronal activity showed a dependency on reward timing, we tested the activity of each neuron in the perimovement period with a three-way ANOVA with factors: period × target location × reward timing. Of the 21 neurons recorded in both the immediate and delayed reward conditions, 16 were modulated in a similar manner and 5 showed a significant difference in the magnitude of perimovement activity between the two conditions. Specifically, 3 neurons were modulated more strongly when the reward was delivered immediately after the target contact, whereas 2 neurons were modulated more strongly when monkeys received reward 0.5 s after the target contact. It therefore appears that there was no systematic relationship between the level of modulation and reward timing, suggesting that changes in movement speed were not linked to perimovement changes in STN firing as a function of reward timing. On the other hand, a significant difference in the magnitude of postreward activity between the two conditions was detected in 15 of the 21 neurons, with 10 of them being modulated more strongly when the reward was delivered immediately after the target contact and 5 neurons being modulated more strongly when reward was delayed by 0.5 s. This suggests that modulations of postreward activity can be explained, at least for some STN neurons, by the subjective value of reward which decayed as the time to its delivery was delayed. The small number of neurons tested with the 0.5-s and 1.0-s delays prevented a similar analysis.

INFLUENCE OF DELIVERING REWARDS NOT CONTINGENT UPON INSTRUMENTAL REACTIONS

The relationship of changes in neuronal activity to the expectation and detection of reward was further examined when the liquid was delivered outside of the reaching task. Twenty neurons (16 and 4 neurons in monkeys G and P, respectively) were studied in the Pavlovian protocol. **Figure 6A** (left panel) shows a neuron that displayed two consecutive components of neuronal modulation, i.e., a brief increase in firing after the presentation of the visual stimulus and another increase after the subsequent delivery of reward. The same neuron was also recorded when the reward was delivered alone, in the absence of the preceding stimulus (right panel), and an increase in firing was still detected after this single event.

A notable feature of STN neurons recorded in the Pavlovian protocol is the substantial variability in the temporal profile of

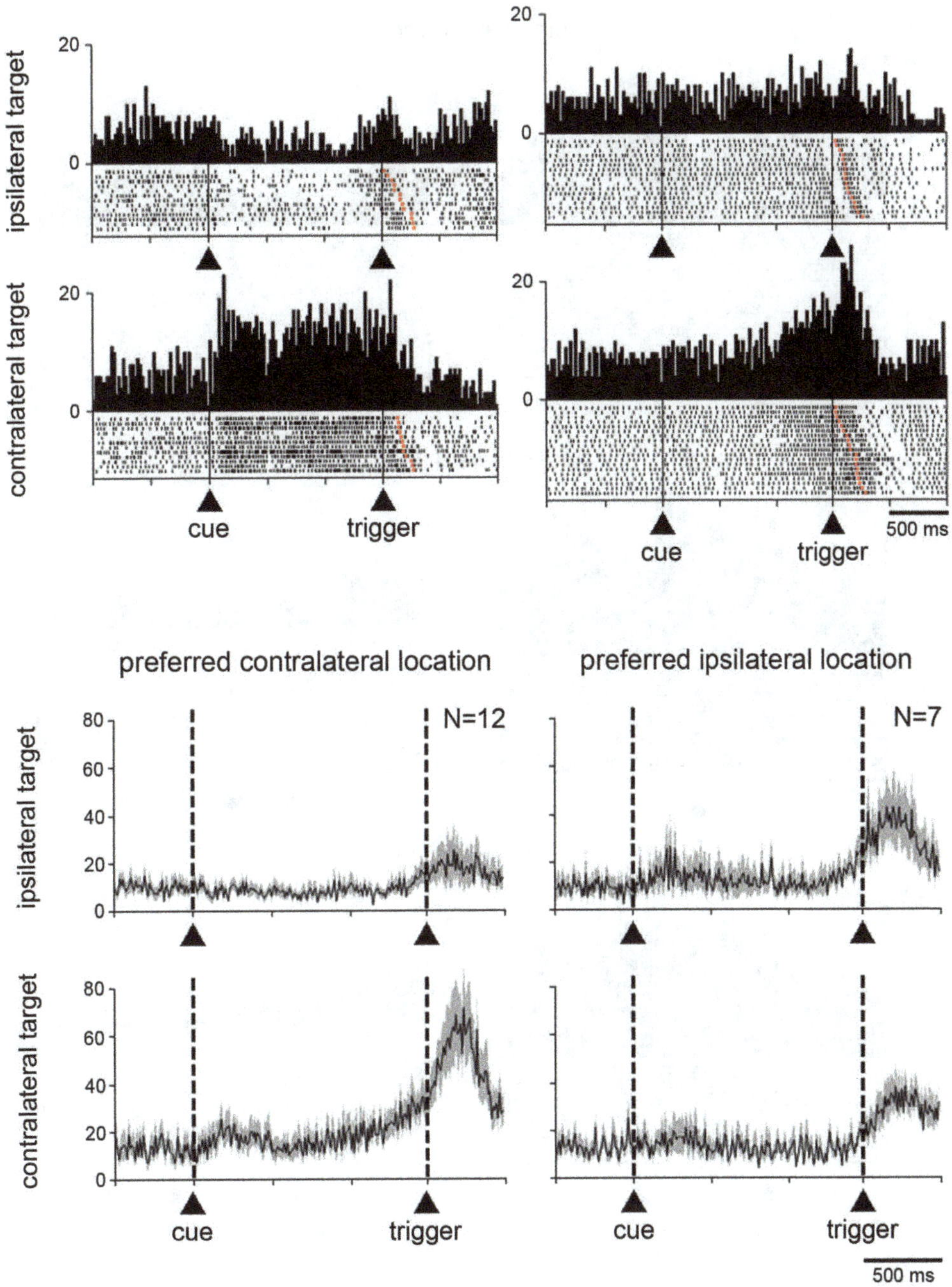

FIGURE 4 | Neuronal activity in the STN related to the spatial location of the target stimulus. (A) Two examples neurons showing a spatial preference for target stimuli presented on the side contralateral to the moving arm. Data were separated off-line according to the location of the target stimulus. Same conventions as in **Figure 3A**. **(B)** Modulation of population activity dependent on the location of the target stimulus. Populations included all neurons with a spatial selectivity in the magnitude of their modulation, separately for each preferred location. The data were taken from monkey G. Same conventions as in **Figure 3B**.

their changes in activity. To quantitatively assess this, the times of onset and offset of modulation were determined for each neuron with the use of the sliding window procedure (see Section Materials and Methods). The distribution of temporal profiles of activity relative to stimulus onset for every recorded neuron is presented in **Figure 6B** (left). We found that 17 neurons were significantly modulated after the presentation of the visual stimulus (10 increases, 7 decreases), the remaining 3 neurons being modulated only after the delivery of reward (2 increases, 1 decrease). As can be seen in this figure, the change in activity after stimulus onset was maintained in the time period immediately following stimulus onset for 16 neurons and even extended beyond reward delivery for 15 neurons. Two neurons were modulated only after the presentation of the stimulus (2 increases). Some

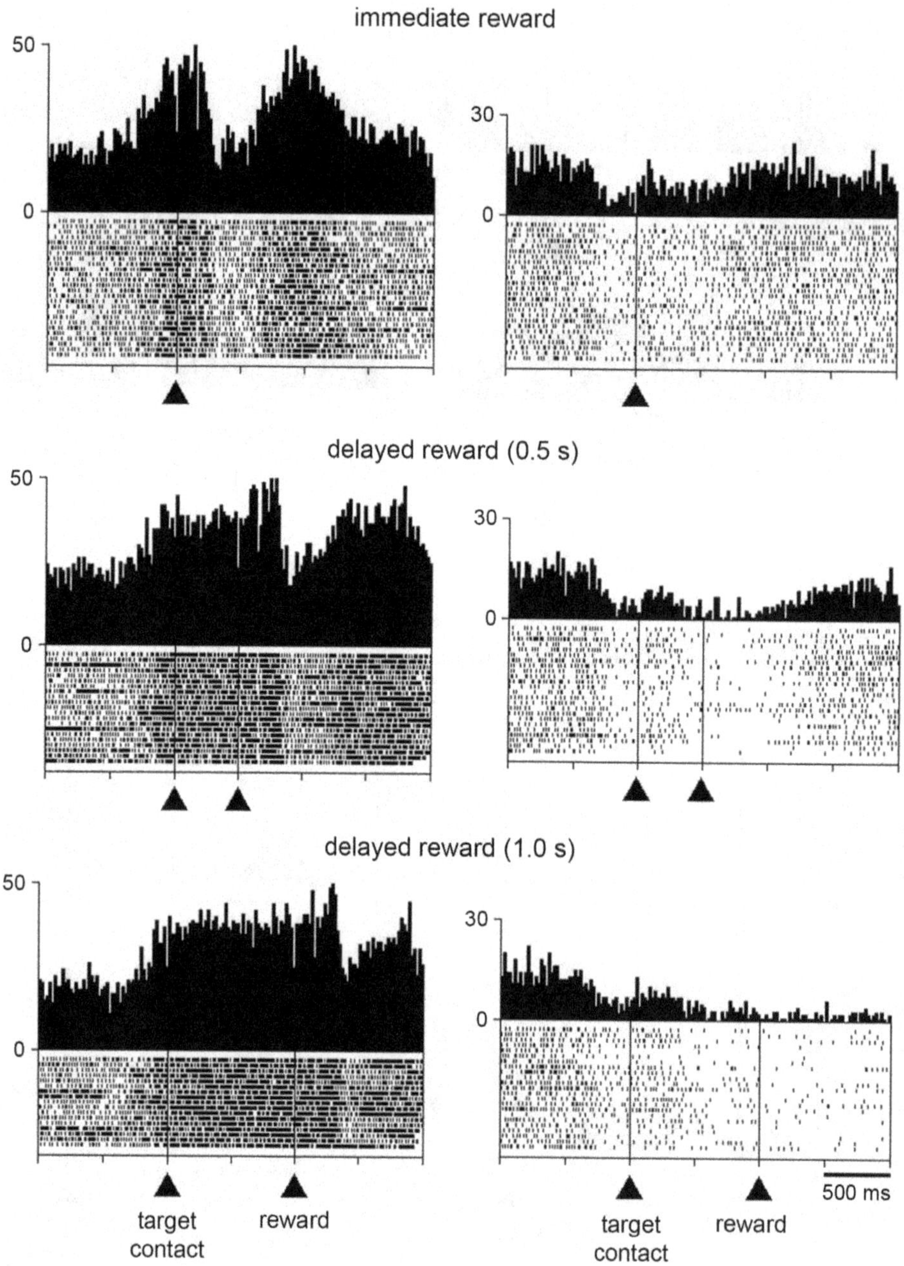

FIGURE 5 | Influence of delaying the time of reward delivery in the reaching task in two STN neurons. For each recorded neuron, the change of condition occurred over three successive blocks of trials in which reward was delivered immediately, 0.5 s, or 1 s after target contact. Same conventions as in **Figure 3A**.

activity changes began after stimulus onset, lasted before reward delivery and then restarted later after the delivery of reward, whereas others persisted through the delay until the delivery of reward. Overall, it appears that the distributions of onset of modulation overlapped substantially among neurons with task-related increases and decreases in activity. In 10 neurons, the receipt of reward produced a change in activity of the same sign as the change following stimulus onset, whereas 5 neurons had bidirectional changes in activity. These observations are consistent with the idea that STN neurons were not exclusively sensitive to the reinforcement of an instrumental response. We examined the population activity for the sample of 20 neurons recorded in the Pavlovian protocol (**Figure 6C**). Considering the complex pattern of changes in activity described above, we combined all neurons, regardless of their increase and/or decrease in firing rate. Two phases of increased activity were visible after each task event in the population average. The first phase appeared relatively homogeneous, whereas the second phase included multiple components.

Finally, it was of special interest to examine STN neuronal activity when the monkey received reward without any predictive

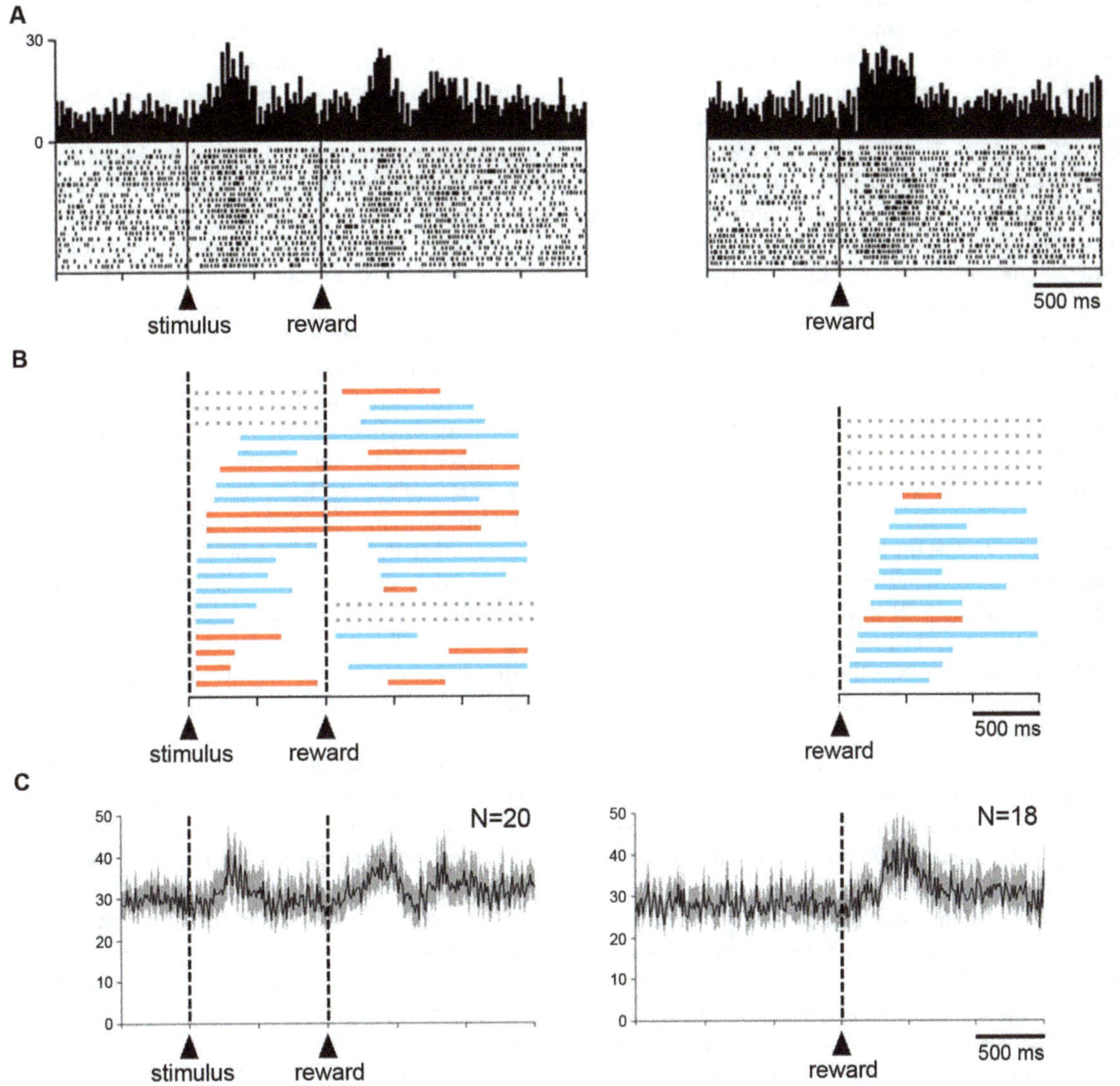

FIGURE 6 | Influence of reward delivery that is not contingent on behavior on the STN neuronal activity. **(A)** An example of neuron showing an increased in firing rate after the visual stimulus that signals the delivery of reward and after the reward itself under the Pavlovian condition (left). The same neuron also displayed an increased in firing rate after the delivery of reward not signaled by a predictive cue (right). Same conventions as in **Figure 3A**. **(B)** Time course of changes in activity of all neurons tested in the Pavlovian protocol (left) and during the delivery of reward alone (right). Each colored horizontal line represents the period with a statistically significant increase (blue) or decrease (red) in activity for a single neuron. Lines are ordered according to onsets of activity change after the presentation of the visual stimulus or the delivery of reward. Gray horizontal dashed lines indicate a lack of significant change in discharge rate after a given event. **(C)** Modulation of population activity. Population included all neurons (i.e., both increases and decreases) recorded in the two testing situations. Same conventions as in **Figure 3A**.

cues. Among a sample of 18 neurons (3 and 15 neurons from monkey P and G, respectively), 13 displayed changes in activity after the delivery of reward (11 increases, 2 decreases). The remaining 5 neurons showed no detectable change in activity during the test. As mentioned above, the example neuron shown in **Figure 6A** (right) increased its activity in response to reward given alone. The temporal parameters of the changes in activity were also analyzed for each neuron tested in this condition and the results of this analysis are illustrated in **Figure 6B** (right). It can be seen that the increases in firing occurred more frequently than the decreases. We then performed a population analysis for these 18 neurons and by comparing it with the average activity obtained in the Pavlovian protocol, it appears that the modulation in response to the delivery of reward was more homogeneous in the former condition.

DISCUSSION

Although clinical and neurophysiological evidence has long pointed to the role of STN in regulating motor function, recent studies have also implicated this nucleus in the processing of reward-related information. Consistent with this idea, we found that STN neurons displayed changes in activity after the delivery of reward, regardless of the need to make a movement to obtain reward. When monkeys were actively engaged in target reaching, the reward signals carried by STN neurons were often combined with modulations around the time of movement onset, demonstrating that STN neurons are sensitive to the movement and its reward outcome. These observations confirmed earlier findings from only a single monkey performing a reaching task to obtain reward (Darbaky et al., 2005). In the present study, we have provided further details of reward-related changes in STN activity under varying contextual conditions, i.e., during instrumental and Pavlovian conditioning tasks and even in the absence of any reward predictive cue. In addition, our findings have emphasized the presence of STN neurons exhibiting sustained changes in activity in advance of reward whose delivery was delayed in the reaching task, indicating that STN neuronal activity is influenced by the state of expectation of future rewards. Altogether, these results obtained in non-human primates are consistent with the idea that the STN is a component of basal ganglia circuitry that mediates motivational processes.

REWARD-RELATED ACTIVITY IN THE STN

Even if increasingly more clinical and animal lesion studies are highlighting the role of the STN in reward circuitry, only a few studies of neuronal activity in the STN have documented the sensitivity of individual neurons to the delivery of reward during the performance of motor tasks in both rodents (Teagarden and Rebec, 2007; Lardeux et al., 2009, 2013) and monkeys (Matsumura et al., 1992; Darbaky et al., 2005). Previously, we have shown in a preliminary study that STN neuronal activity was modulated by reward delivered after an instrumental response, and preliminary work done at that time indicated that reward-related modulations were still detected when reward was passively delivered in a Pavlovian manner (Darbaky et al., 2005). The activity changes reported here confirm these preliminary findings and further indicate that STN neurons were responsive to unpredicted deliveries of reward. It therefore appears that STN neurons have firing rates that are sensitive to appetitive events themselves, whether or not a motor response was required to obtain reward and even outside of Pavlovian or instrumental response control. However, as we discuss below, circumstances in which rewards are passively experienced by animals do not exclude a possible influence of motor constraints to consume the liquid.

Earlier reported changes in STN neuronal activity after reward delivered have been reported in rats performing instrumental tasks (Teagarden and Rebec, 2007; Lardeux et al., 2009, 2013) and are comparable to those reported here in monkeys. In addition, Lardeux et al. (2009) have further demonstrated that STN activity may be related to reward quality (i.e., different sweetness of a liquid sucrose reward). These same authors have recently reported that different populations of STN neurons were modulated by the delivery of an appetitive liquid or administration of a psychoactive drug (Lardeux et al., 2013), suggesting that distinct neuronal circuits within the STN mediate the positive value of stimuli.

Several basal ganglia structures with neuronal activity linked to the rewarding significance of conditioned stimuli as well as to reward itself have been extensively investigated in both rodents and monkeys (Schultz et al., 2000; Hikosaka et al., 2006). It appears that the STN also contributes to the processing of motivational information. How reward sensitivity is encoded in the STN compared with that found in other components of the basal ganglia circuitry, particularly the striatum, remains to be clarified.

Although our results showed, at the single-neuron level, the contribution of the STN in the detection of rewarding events, they did not allow to firmly establish whether the observed changes in activity were related to the hedonic nature of the reward. In particular, the possibility that the reward-related activity encoded some aspects of orofacial behavior was not totally eliminated. In an attempt to dissociate mouth movements from the delivery of reward *per se*, we have examined the timing characteristics of licks at the spout during neuronal recordings. As already pointed out in our previous study (Darbaky et al., 2005), the reward-related activity was not directly related to the licking patterns in terms of onset and duration. For example, in the reaching task, the majority of modulations of STN neuron firing which occurred after target contact were relatively late changes, suggesting that they were unlikely to be coupled to preparation or initiation of mouth movements which began earlier. We cannot exclude, however, that they could be involved in later phases of liquid consumption, such as swallowing. Moreover, the variability in the time course of the observed changes in neuronal activity during Pavlovian conditioned behavior challenges the notion that STN neurons may encode the highly stereotyped pattern of licking movements elicited in this condition.

HETEROGENEITY OF REWARD-RELATED ACTIVITIES IN THE STN

Consistent with previous electrophysiological studies, we have found that STN neurons were either excited or inhibited by rewarding events, increases being more common than decreases. Interestingly, the prevalence of increases in STN neuronal activity became particularly evident when switching from a Pavlovian association between stimulus and reward to a situation in which reward was not signaled by a cue, thus suggesting a change in the way that the reward itself is processed by STN neurons. For comparison with our earlier study (Darbaky et al., 2005), it was also noticed that increases in STN neuronal activity were more frequent when reward was given outside of a learning context. In the rat experiments, modulations of STN firing following reward delivery also consisted of either an increase or a decrease in firing (Teagarden and Rebec, 2007; Lardeux et al., 2009, 2013), although the respective proportions of changes in opposite direction could be different from one study to another, and an influence of context on reward-related activities was also highlighted in the case of changes in reward values (Lardeux et al., 2009, 2013). Because behavior-related increases and decreases in the activity of STN neurons are assumed to have opposing effects on behavioral output, it is important to understand the significance of these opposing changes in activity. Indeed, increases in STN activity are thought to suppress movement execution by increasing inhibition of thalamic and brainstem targets via basal ganglia output structures and the reverse may occur in the case of decreases in STN activity.

CHANGES IN STN NEURONAL ACTIVITY RELATED TO SPECIFIC ASPECTS OF TARGET REACHING

Our findings have shown two main and temporally distinct patterns of task-related activity in the STN during performance in the reaching task, one occurring around the initiation of movement and the other after target contact, immediately followed by reward delivery. Previous studies in behaving rats have also shown that most neurons in the STN carry signals related to both motor behavior and reward outcomes (Teagarden and Rebec, 2007; Lardeux et al., 2009, 2013). These observations point to an influence of motor and motivational aspects of task performance at the single-neuron level, possibly reflecting the fact that reward signals generated by STN neurons are linked to the performance of specific actions.

In the present study, we have examined the involvement of the STN in motor aspects of performance specifically regarding the visuospatial features of the reaching task. We found that a number of STN neurons displayed preferences for one location of the triggering stimulus and/or direction of its associated motor response, most of them preferring the location and/or direction opposite to the moving arm. In at least one monkey, this spatial preference was accompanied by a variation in the speed of the motor response to the stimulus. A link between STN neuronal activity and spatial information provided by stimuli eliciting movements in various directions has been reported in previous monkey studies (Georgopoulos et al., 1983; DeLong et al., 1985; Isoda and Hikosaka, 2008). However, it is unknown whether this spatial selectivity was related to the location of the trigger stimulus and/or the direction of the movement associated with that stimulus. Indeed, in these studies (including our own), the motor response was directed toward the spatial location of the trigger stimulus, so that it cannot be established whether the observed changes in activity were dependent on the "sensory" or "motor" constraints. Only a few studies have attempted to dissociate these two aspects while studying task-related neuronal activity in basal ganglia (Alexander and Crutcher, 1990; Ravel et al., 2006). However, in rats trained to make a constant motor reaction (i.e., cessation of lever pressing) to different spatial locations of a movement-triggering stimulus, no influence of location was reported on the activity of STN neurons (Lardeux et al., 2009).

CHANGES IN STN NEURONAL ACTIVITY RELATED TO REWARD EXPECTATION DURING TASK PERFORMANCE

We have found that STN neurons may exhibit persistent changes in firing throughout a time interval introduced between correct target contact and reward delivery in the reaching task. These findings are consistent with previous observations in monkeys that showed the influence of variations in reward timing on STN activity (Matsumura et al., 1992; Darbaky et al., 2005). In addition, we showed that monkeys were sensitive to the presence of a reward delay after target reaching, suggesting that they discounted the value of a reward when it is delayed in time. We found that few neurons exhibited non-systematic differences in firing around the initiation of movement which leads to an immediate or delayed reward. On the other hand, a relatively large number of neurons showed stronger changes in activity following reward delivered immediately after completion of movement, compared with delayed reward, suggesting that they may participate in the time-discounted encoding of reward value. In the present study, sustained changes in activity were extended when the target-reward interval was prolonged to 0.5 to 1 s, suggesting that this activity may be interpreted as reflecting a representation of outcomes which is crucial for the control of reward-guided behavior. Again, we cannot exclude completely the alternative explanation that the observed changes in neuronal activity may reflect preparation to consume the liquid (Roesch and Olson, 2003). The observed modulations in STN neuronal activity did not appear to be related to the simultaneously occurring mouth movements, suggesting that these modulations might be related more to reward expectation than to motor preparation, but this needs to be further clarified. In addition, our task manipulation did not allow a clear-cut dissociation between motivation and attention (Maunsell, 2004). Since STN has been shown to be involved in attention (Baunez and Robbins, 1997, 1999), we cannot rule out a contribution of attentional processes in the neuronal changes reported here. Additional work is needed to clarify this issue.

IS REWARD-RELATED ACTIVITY CONFINED TO SPECIFIC REGIONS OF THE STN?

Based on anatomical studies of corticosubthalamic circuitry, it is thought that regions of the STN can be functionally delineated along distinct territories. Although neuroimaging data do not provide the spatial resolution required to examine these distinctions, recording studies at a single-neuron resolution level may be helpful to analyze the fine distribution of neurons displaying specific response properties. Previous studies have reported that neurons related to limb movements are located primarily in the dorsolateral STN region (Georgopoulos et al., 1983; DeLong et al., 1985; Wichmann et al., 1994), whereas neurons related to visuomotor functions were generally located more ventrally (Matsumura et al., 1992; Isoda and Hikosaka, 2008). Although anatomical connectivity defines an organization in subterritories (Groenewegen and Berendse, 1990), the functional evidence is less clear for the rodent STN for which researchers refer to task-related activities without attempting to parcel out the subdivisions (Teagarden and Rebec, 2007; Lardeux et al., 2009, 2013). Despite some limitations on the extent of the area over which we recorded STN neurons, our results based on histological examination in one monkey did not show regional differences that were particularly obvious in the pattern of distribution of task-related neurons. In particular, neurons sensitive to reward were scattered throughout the parts of the STN explored, without preferential location in the ventromedial part, which receives inputs from the orbitofrontal cortex and anterior cingulate cortex and is considered the « limbic » part of the STN in primates (Takada et al., 2001; Karachi et al., 2005; Haynes and Haber, 2013). This observation confirms what had been previously noted in our preliminary study (Darbaky et al., 2005). Also, neurons sensitive to movement did not appear to be clustered in the dorsolateral part of the STN, which is connected to motor and premotor cortical areas, and corresponds to the « motor »part of the STN. Although the small number of neurons sampled did not allow us to state whether the present findings are representative of STN recordings in general, the presence of neurons sensitive to expectation of reward in the ventral part of the STN is consistent with the findings of Matsumura et al. (1992).

FUNCTIONAL SIGNIFICANCE OF REWARD-RELATED ACTIVITY IN STN

Although our findings add to the growing body of literature highlighting the role of the STN in motivation, it is not yet clear how reward signals found in the STN are used to influence behavioral output. One could speculate that changes in STN neuronal activity related to reward expectation or to the detection of the reward itself contribute to behaviors directed at obtaining the reward by maintaining the representation of an expected outcome and by monitoring the positive feedback which may serve to shape future behavior. An important feature of the reward signals generated by STN neurons in an instrumental task was their frequent combination with signals related to the movement. These combined changes in STN firing may reflect a mechanism linking the generation of motor behavior with the rewarding outcome. The specific function of STN in reward-guided behavior thus appears to be complex and further investigations of changes in STN neuronal activity employing appropriately designed tasks are needed to understand how this nucleus contribute to motor and reward processing in the basal ganglia circuitry.

Recently, the STN has been considered to be a key component of the brain network which mediates behavioral inhibition, particularly under circumstances requiring the active suppression of inadequate movements when several conflicting actions compete (Frank et al., 2007). At the moment, it is unclear how this conception can be matched with reward signals generated by STN neurons such as those described here. However, even seemingly simple motor behaviors consist of a spatiotemporal organization of distinct motor components, and STN neurons may intervene to facilitate or suppress these components to complete the whole behavior. In this regard, combined increases and decreases in STN activity may reflect a mechanism that releases from inhibition actions and maintains inhibitory control over others which is crucial for reward-oriented behavior.

CONCLUSION

In summary, the data gathered in the present study provide further evidence for a contribution of the STN to motivational control of behavior in the non-human primate. Detailed understanding of the specificity of reward processing within single STN neurons could lead to a better appreciation of the influence of this nucleus on motivated behaviors under normal and pathological conditions in humans. This is particularly relevant in view of the current interest for surgical therapy aimed at treating psychiatric disorders associated with impaired reward and motivational processes, including drug addiction.

AUTHOR CONTRIBUTIONS

Juan-Francisco Espinosa-Parrilla and Paul Apicella designed the study, collected the data, and performed the analyses. Paul Apicella wrote the manuscript with the help of Christelle Baunez.

ACKNOWLEDGMENTS

We thank E. Legallet for designing the computer programs, I. Balansard for assistance with surgery, and M. Deffains and S. Ravel for help with data collection. This work was supported by Centre National de la Recherche Scientifique. Juan-Francisco Espinosa-Parrilla was funded by a French ANR grant to Christelle Baunez.

REFERENCES

Alexander, G. E., and Crutcher, M. D. (1990). Preparation for movement: neural representations of intended direction in three motor areas of the monkey. *J. Neurophysiol.* 64, 133–150.

Apicella, P., Deffains, M., Ravel, S., and Legallet, E. (2009). Tonically active neurons in the striatum differentiate between delivery and omission of expected reward in a probabilistic task context. *Eur. J. Neurosci.* 30, 515–526. doi: 10.1111/j.1460-9568.2009.06872.x

Apicella, P., Legallet, E., and Trouche, E. (1997). Responses of tonically discharging neurons in the monkey striatum to primary rewards delivered during different behavioral states. *Exp. Brain Res.* 116, 456–466. doi: 10.1007/pl00005773

Aron, A. R., and Poldrack, R. A. (2006). Cortical and subcortical contributions to stop signal response inhibition: role of the subthalamic nucleus. *J. Neurosci.* 26, 2424–2433. doi: 10.1523/jneurosci.4682-05.2006

Baunez, C., Amalric, M., and Robbins, T. W. (2002). Enhanced food-related motivation after bilateral lesions of the subthalamic nucleus. *J. Neurosci.* 22, 562–568.

Baunez, C., Dias, C., Cador, M., and Amalric, M. (2005). The subthalamic nucleus exerts opposite control on cocaine and 'natural' rewards. *Nat. Neurosci.* 8, 484–489. doi: 10.1038/nn1429

Baunez, C., and Robbins, T. W. (1997). Bilateral lesions of the subthalamic nucleus induce multiple deficits in an attentional task in rats. *Eur. J. Neurosci.* 9, 2086–2099. doi: 10.1111/j.1460-9568.1997.tb01376.x

Baunez, C., and Robbins, T. W. (1999). Effects of dopamine depletion of the dorsal striatum and further interaction with subthalamic nucleus lesions in an attentional task in the rat. *Neuroscience* 92, 1343–1356. doi: 10.1016/s0306-4522(99)00065-2

Baunez, C., Yelnik, J., and Mallet, L. (2011). Six questions on the subthalamic nucleus: lessons from animal models and from stimulated patients. *Neuroscience* 198, 193–204. doi: 10.1016/j.neuroscience.2011.09.059

Brücke, C., Kupsch, A., Schneider, G.-H., Hariz, M. I., Nuttin, B., Kopp, U., et al. (2007). The subthalamic region is activated during valence-related emotional processing in patients with Parkinson's disease. *Eur. J. Neurosci.* 26, 767–774. doi: 10.1111/j.1460-9568.2007.05683.x

Burbaud, P., Clair, A. H., Langbour, N., Fernandez-Vidal, S., Goillandeau, M., Michelet, T., et al. (2013). Neuronal activity correlated with checking behaviour in the subthalamic nucleus of patients with obsessive-compulsive disorder. *Brain* 136, 304–317. doi: 10.1093/brain/aws306

Darbaky, Y., Baunez, C., Arecchi, P., Legallet, E., and Apicella, P. (2005). Reward-related neuronal activity in the subthalamic nucleus of the monkey. *Neuroreport* 16, 1241–1244. doi: 10.1097/00001756-200508010-00022

Deffains, M., Legallet, E., and Apicella, P. (2010). Modulation of neuronal activity in the monkey putamen associated with changes in the habitual order of sequential movements. *J. Neurophysiol.* 104, 1355–1369. doi: 10.1152/jn.00355.2010

Delgado, M. R. (2007). Reward-related responses in the human striatum. *Ann. N Y Acad. Sci.* 1104, 70–88. doi: 10.1196/annals.1390.002

DeLong, M. R., Crutcher, M. D., and Georgopoulos, A. P. (1985). Primate globus pallidus and subthalamic nucleus: functional organization. *J. Neurophysiol.* 53, 530–543.

Eusebio, A., Witjas, T., Cohen, J., Fluchère, F., Jouve, E., Régis, J., et al. (2013). Subthalamic nucleus stimulation and compulsive use of dopaminergic medication in Parkinson's disease. *J. Neurol. Neurosurg. Psychiatry* 84, 868–874. doi: 10.1136/jnnp-2012-302387

Frank, M. J., Samanta, J., Moustafa, A. A., and Sherman, S. J. (2007). Hold your horses: impulsivity, deep brain stimulation and medication in parkinsonism. *Science* 318, 1309–1312. doi: 10.1126/science.1146157

Funkiewiez, A., Ardouin, C., Krack, P., Fraix, V., Van Blercom, N., Xie, J., et al. (2003). Acute psychotropic effects of bilateral subthalamic nucleus stimulation and levodopa in Parkinson's disease. *Mov. Disord.* 18, 524–530. doi: 10.1002/mds.10441

Georgopoulos, A. P., DeLong, M. R., and Crutcher, M. D. (1983). Relations between parameters of step-tracking movements and single cell discharge in the globus pallidus and subthalamic nucleus of the behaving monkey. *J. Neurosci.* 3, 1586–1598.

Groenewegen, H. J., and Berendse, H. W. (1990). Connections of the subthalamic nucleus with ventral striatopallidal parts of the basal ganglia in the rat. *J. Comp. Neurol.* 294, 607–622. doi: 10.1002/cne.902940408

Haynes, W. I., and Haber, S. N. (2013). The organization of prefrontal-subthalamic inputs in primates provides an anatomical substrate for both functional specificity and integration: implications for Basal Ganglia models and deep brain stimulation. *J. Neurosci.* 33, 4804–4814. doi: 10.1523/JNEUROSCI.4674-12.2013

Hikosaka, O., Nakamura, K., and Nakahara, H. (2006). Basal ganglia orient eyes to reward. *J. Neurophysiol.* 95, 567–584. doi: 10.1152/jn.00458.2005

Houeto, J. L., Mesnage, V., Mallet, L., Pillon, B., Gargiulo, M., du Moncel, S. T., et al. (2002). Behavioural disorders, Parkinson's disease and subthalamic stimulation. *J. Neurol. Neurosurg. Psychiatry* 72, 701–707. doi: 10.1136/jnnp.72.6.701

Isoda, M., and Hikosaka, O. (2008). Role for subthalamic nucleus neurons in switching from automatic to controlled eye movement. *J. Neurosci.* 28, 7209–7218. doi: 10.1523/JNEUROSCI.0487-08.2008

Karachi, C., Yelnik, J., Tandé, D., Tremblay, L., Hirsch, E. C., François, C., et al. (2005). The pallidosubthalamic projection: an anatomical substrate for nonmotor functions of the subthalamic nucleus in primates. *Mov. Disord.* 20, 172–180. doi: 10.1002/mds.20302

Keuken, M. C., Bazin, P.-L., Schafer, A., Neumann, J., Turner, R., and Forstmann, B. U. (2013). Ultra-high 7T MRI of structural age-related changes of the subthalamic nucleus. *J. Neurosci.* 33, 4896–4900. doi: 10.1523/JNEUROSCI.3241-12.2013

Krack, P., Kumar, R., Ardouin, C., Limousin Dowsey, P., McVicker, J. M., Benabid, A. L., et al. (2001). Mirthful laughter induced by subthalamic nucleus stimulation. *Mov. Disord.* 16, 867–875. doi: 10.1002/mds.1174

Kühn, A. A., Hariz, M. I., Silberstein, P., Tisch, S., Kupsch, A., Schneider, G.-H., et al. (2005). Activation of the subthalamic region during emotional processing in Parkinson disease. *Neurology* 65, 707–713. doi: 10.1212/01.wnl.0000174438.78399.bc

Lardeux, S., Paleressompoulle, D., Pernaud, R., Cador, M., and Baunez, C. (2013). Different populations of subthalamic neurons encode cocaine versus sucrose reward and predict future error. *J. Neurophysiol.* 110, 1497–1510. doi: 10.1152/jn.00160.2013

Lardeux, S., Pernaud, R., Paleressompoulle, D., and Baunez, C. (2009). Beyond the reward pathway: coding reward magnitude and error in the rat subthalamic nucleus. *J. Neurophysiol.* 102, 2526–2537. doi: 10.1152/jn.91009.2008

Lhommée, E., Klinger, H., Thobois, S., Schmitt, E., Ardouin, C., Bichon, A., et al. (2012). Subthalamic stimulation in Parkinson's disease: restoring the balance of motivated behaviours. *Brain* 135, 1463–1477. doi: 10.1093/brain/aws078

Li, C. S., Yan, P., Sinha, R., and Lee, T. W. (2008). Subcortical processes of motor response inhibition during a stop signal task. *Neuroimage* 41, 1352–1363. doi: 10.1016/j.neuroimage.2008.04.023

Mallet, L., Mesnage, V., Houeto, J. L., Pelissolo, A., Yelnik, J., Behar, C., et al. (2002). Compulsions, Parkinson's disease and stimulation. *Lancet* 360, 1302–1304. doi: 10.1016/s0140-6736(02)11339-0

Matsumura, M., Kojima, J., Gardiner, T. W., and Hikosaka, O. (1992). Visual and oculomotor functions of monkey subthalamic nucleus. *J. Neurophysiol.* 67, 1615–1632.

Maunsell, J. H. (2004). Neuronal representations of cognitive state: reward or attention? *Trends Cogn. Sci.* 8, 261–265. doi: 10.1016/j.tics.2004.04.003

Pelloux, Y., and Baunez, C. (2013). Deep brain stimulation for addiction: why the subthalamic nucleus should be favored. *Curr. Opin. Neurobiol.* 23, 713–720. doi: 10.1016/j.conb.2013.02.016

Péron, J., Frühholz, S., Vérin, M., Grandjean, D. (2013). Subthalamic nucleus: a key structure for emotional component synchronization in humans. *Neurosci. Biobehav. Rev.* 37, 358–373. doi: 10.1016/j.neubiorev.2013.01.001

Ravel, S., Sardo, P., Legallet, E., and Apicella, P. (2001). Reward unpredictability inside and outside of a task context as a determinant of the responses of tonically active neurons in the monkey striatum. *J. Neurosci.* 21, 5730–5739.

Ravel, S., Sardo, P., Legallet, E., and Apicella, P. (2006). Influence of spatial information on responses of tonically active neurons in the monkey striatum. *J. Neurophysiol.* 95, 2975–2986. doi: 10.1152/jn.01113.2005

Roesch, M. R., and Olson, C. R. (2003). Impact of expected reward on neuronal activity in prefrontal cortex, frontal and supplementary eye fields and premotor cortex. *J. Neurophysiol.* 90, 1766–1789. doi: 10.1152/jn.00019.2003

Schneider, F., Habel, U., Volkmann, J., Regel, S., Kornischka, Sturm, V., et al. (2003). Deep brain stimulation of the subthalamic nucleus enhances emotional processing in Parkinson disease. *Arch. Gen. Psychiatry* 60, 296–302. doi: 10.1001/archpsyc.60.3.296

Schultz, W., Tremblay, L., and Hollerman, J. R. (2000). Reward processing in primate orbitofrontal cortex and basal ganglia. *Cereb. Cortex* 10, 272–283. doi: 10.1093/cercor/10.3.272

Schüpbach, W. M., Chastan, N., Welter, M. L., Houeto, J. L., Mesnage, V., Bonnet, A. M., et al. (2005). Stimulation of the subthalamic nucleus in Parkinson's disease: a 5 year follow up. *J. Neurol. Neurosurg. Psychiatry* 76, 1640–1644. doi: 10.1136/jnnp.2005.063206

Takada, M., Tokuno, H., Hamada, I., Inase, M., Ito, Y., Imanishi, M., et al. (2001). Organization of inputs from cingulate motor areas to basal ganglia in macaque monkey. *Eur. J. Neurosci.* 14, 1633–1650. doi: 10.1046/j.0953-816x.2001.01789.x

Takeshita, S., Kurisu, K., Trop, L., Arita, K., Akimitsu, T., Verhoeff, N. P., et al. (2005). Effect of subthalamic stimulation on mood state in Parkinson's disease: evaluation of previous facts and problems. *Neurosurg. Rev.* 28, 179–186. doi: 10.1007/s10143-005-0387-4

Teagarden, M. A., and Rebec, G. V. (2007). Subthalamic and striatal neurons concurrently process motor, limbic and associative information in rats performing an operant task. *J. Neurophysiol.* 97, 2042–2058. doi: 10.1152/jn.00368.2006

Wichmann, T., Bergman, H., and DeLong, M. R. (1994). The primate subthalamic nucleus. I. Functional properties in intact animals. *J. Neurophysiol.* 72, 494–506.

Witjas, T., Baunez, C., Henry, J. M., Delfini, M., Regis, J., Cherif, A. A., et al. (2005). Addiction in Parkinson's disease: impact of subthalamic nucleus deep brain stimulation. *Mov. Disord.* 20, 1052–1055. doi: 10.1002/mds.20501

16

Primary Motor Cortex of the Parkinsonian Monkey: Altered Neuronal Responses to Muscle Stretch

Benjamin Pasquereau and Robert S. Turner*

Department of Neurobiology, Center for Neuroscience and The Center for the Neural Basis of Cognition, University of Pittsburgh, Pittsburgh, PA, USA

Correspondence:
Robert S. Turner, Department of Neurobiology, Center for Neuroscience and The Center for the Neural Basis of Cognition, University of Pittsburgh, 4047 BST-3, 3501 Fifth Avenue, Pittsburgh, PA 15261, USA
e-mail: rturner@pitt.edu

Exaggeration of the long-latency stretch reflex (LLSR) is a characteristic neurophysiologic feature of Parkinson's disease (PD) that contributes to parkinsonian rigidity. To explore one frequently-hypothesized mechanism, we studied the effects of fast muscle stretches on neuronal activity in the macaque primary motor cortex (M1) before and after the induction of parkinsonism by unilateral administration of 1-methyl-4-phenyl-1,2,3,6-tetrahydropyridine (MPTP). We compared results from the general population of M1 neurons and two antidromically-identified subpopulations: distant-projecting pyramidal-tract type neurons (PTNs) and intra-telecenphalic-type corticostriatal neurons (CSNs). Rapid rotations of elbow or wrist joints evoked short-latency responses in 62% of arm-related M1 neurons. As in PD, the late electromyographic responses that constitute the LLSR were enhanced following MPTP. This was accompanied by a shortening of M1 neuronal response latencies and a degradation of directional selectivity, but surprisingly, no increase in single unit response magnitudes. The results suggest that parkinsonism alters the timing and specificity of M1 responses to muscle stretch. Observation of an exaggerated LLSR with no change in the magnitude of proprioceptive responses in M1 is consistent with the idea that the increase in LLSR gain that contributes to parkinsonian rigidity is localized to the spinal cord.

Keywords: stretch reflex, primary motor cortex, MPTP, Parkinson's disease, rigidity

INTRODUCTION

Rigidity, one of the cardinal signs of Parkinson's disease (PD), is defined clinically as a sustained increase in resistance to passive movement of a joint throughout its range (Stebbins and Goetz, 1998). Although various possible contributing factors have been studied for decades at the central (Cantello et al., 1991; Aminoff et al., 1997; Strafella et al., 1997; Young et al., 1997), spinal (Angel and Hofmann, 1963; Dietrichson, 1971; Andersson and Sjolund, 1978; Delwaide et al., 1991; Lelli et al., 1991; Marchand-Pauvert et al., 2011) and muscle (Dietz et al., 1981; Lee and Tatton, 1982; Noth et al., 1988) levels, the exact pathophysiologic mechanisms of parkinsonian rigidity remain elusive. Many observations have suggested that the stretch reflex plays a key role in the generation of rigidity, but controversies persist regarding the precise relationship (Lee and Tatton, 1975; Berardelli et al., 1983; Rothwell et al., 1983; Meara and Cody, 1992; Xia et al., 2009).

In neurologically-intact animals, the stretch reflex appears to regulate limb stiffness to maintain precise control of multi-joint posture during interactions with an unstable environment (Rothwell, 1990; Shemmell et al., 2010; Pruszynski et al., 2011a). The stretch reflex involves at least two components: a short-latency response mediated by fast-conducting segmental pathways (Magladery et al., 1951; Burke et al., 1984), and a long-latency component mediated, at least in part, by a transcortical pathway (Hammond, 1955; Marsden et al., 1972; Capaday et al., 1991; Day et al., 1991; Matthews, 1991; Palmer and Ashby, 1992; Pruszynski et al., 2011b). The idea that cortex contributes to the long-latency component (i.e., the long latency stretch reflex, LLSR) is supported by observations that neurons in primary motor cortex (M1) respond to proprioceptive perturbations at delays (20–60 ms prior to the late muscle reaction) appropriate for them to participate in this long-latency component (Evarts, 1973; Conrad et al., 1975; Evarts and Tanji, 1976; Cheney and Fetz, 1984; Abbruzzese et al., 1985; Aminoff et al., 1997; Mackinnon et al., 2000). The ability of unilateral muscle stretches to evoke bilateral LLSRs in cases of congenital corticospinal tract malformation (Matthews et al., 1990; Capaday et al., 1991) provides strong support for the view that a component of the LLSR is mediated via a transcortical route. It is important to note, however, that slow-conducting spinal reflex pathways also contribute to the LLSR (Berardelli et al., 1983; Cody et al., 1986).

In PD, the short-latency component of the stretch reflex appears essentially normal (Berardelli et al., 1983; Rothwell et al., 1983; Cody et al., 1986; Meara and Cody, 1993; Hayashi et al., 2001), but the LLSR is markedly exaggerated (Tatton and Lee, 1975; Mortimer and Webster, 1979; Berardelli et al., 1983; Rothwell et al., 1983; Cody et al., 1986; Meara and Cody, 1993; Hayashi et al., 2001; Xia et al., 2009). By increasing the activation of muscles that oppose passive stretch, an abnormally-increased LLSR may be a key factor in the genesis of parkinsonian rigidity. Indeed, several studies have documented a correlation between the magnitude of the LLSR and the severity of parkinsonian rigidity (Lee and Tatton, 1975; Mortimer and Webster, 1979; Tatton et al., 1984; Xia et al., 2009). Other studies failed to confirm such a clear relationship (Berardelli et al., 1983; Rothwell et al., 1983; Cody et al., 1986), most likely because additional reflex abnormalities, such as the aberrant activation of the shortening muscle, also contribute (Andrews et al., 1972; Xia et al., 2006, 2009). Further support for the LLSR's role in parkinsonian rigidity comes from observations that treatments for PD (i.e., dopaminergic medication, pallidotomy and subthalamic stimulation) clearly reduce stretch-related muscled activation, and ameliorate muscle stiffness proportionately (Teravainen et al., 1989; Limousin et al., 1999; Fung et al., 2000; Hayashi et al., 2001; Lee et al., 2002; Xia et al., 2006; Levin et al., 2009; Marchand-Pauvert et al., 2011; Raoul et al., 2012).

Two straightforward possibilities may account for the exaggerated LLSR of PD. The trans-cortical hypothesis states that abnormal neuronal activity transmitted from the parkinsonian basal ganglia (BG) (Delong and Wichmann, 2007) causes increased somatosensory responsiveness in the M1 neurons that participate in the LLSR. Indeed, neurons in the BG and thalamus of parkinsonian subjects have larger-than-normal responses to proprioceptive stimulation and reduced response selectivity with respect to the joint and limb stimulated (Filion et al., 1988; Bergman et al., 1994; Pessiglione et al., 2005). According to this model, increased proprioceptive responsiveness might be transmitted to M1 where it would appear as (1) a greater incidence of neuronal responses to proprioceptive stimulation in the population of M1 neurons, (2) an increase in the balance of torque-evoked increases over decreases, or (3) an increase in the magnitude of torque-evoked responses in individual M1 neurons. It is unclear, however, how this simple model can be reconciled with the abundant evidence that the M1 of parkinsonian subjects has reduced responsiveness to somatosensory inputs as measured by electroencephalography (Rossini et al., 1989; Aminoff et al., 1997; Rickards and Cody, 1997; Lewis and Byblow, 2002; Schrader et al., 2008; Degardin et al., 2009), transcranial magnetic stimulation (Lewis and Byblow, 2002), and functional imaging (Boecker et al., 1999). The alternative model hypothesizes that the exaggerated LLSR of PD is mediated by abnormal function of slow-conducting spinal reflex pathways (Berardelli et al., 1983; Cody et al., 1986; Simonetta Moreau et al., 2002; Marchand-Pauvert et al., 2011; Raoul et al., 2012).

Primary motor cortex is composed of a complex collection of distinct cell types that differ with respect to intrinsic physiology (McCormick et al., 1985; Connors and Gutnick, 1990; Stewart and Foehring, 2000; Hattox and Nelson, 2007; Kiritani et al., 2012) and afferent innervation (Swadlow, 1994). These subtypes may perform dissimilar functions in the LLSR and may be affected differently in the parkinsonian state (Pasquereau and Turner, 2011). For example, distant-projecting lamina 5b pyramidal tract-type neurons (PTNs) and intratelencephalic-projecting corticostriatal neurons (CSNs) in the M1 have markedly different somatosensory responsiveness (Bauswein et al., 1989; Turner and Delong, 2000). PTNs are positioned to play a relatively direct role in the expression of the abnormal LLSR in PD due to their direct projections to segmental motor nuclei (Landgren et al., 1962; Brodal, 1978; Kuypers, 1981). The CSNs of M1, in contrast, provide an important glutamatergic input to motor regions of the striatum, and thus, are in a position to influence, for better or worse, the disordered physiology of the dopamine-depleted striatum (Mallet et al., 2006).

Despite clear implication of the motor cortex in the LLSR, only a few studies have compared cerebral responses to proprioceptive inputs and abnormalities in the LLSR in parkinsonian subjects (Rossini et al., 1989, 1991; Aminoff et al., 1997), and these used a non-invasive electrocerebral approach. These studies reported the seemingly paradoxical finding that an exaggerated LLSR was correlated with *attenuation* of a sensory evoked potential that is thought to emanate from precentral cortical areas. To elucidate the changes in cortical function associated with the exaggerated LLSR of PD, we performed single unit recording in the M1 of parkinsonian macaques and studied the short latency neuronal responses to rapid muscle stretch. Based on previous observations that the spontaneous activity of PTN and CSN populations are affected differently in parkinsonism (Mallet et al., 2006; Pasquereau and Turner, 2011), we hypothesized that the responses of PTNs and CSNs to muscle stretch would be affected differently in parkinsonism. To address this issue, antidromically-identified neurons (PTNs and CSNs) were studied in the arm area of M1 in two rhesus monkeys. The stretch reflex was evoked by sudden rotations of the animal's elbow or wrist and recordings were obtained before and after induction of parkinsonism by unilateral intra-carotid administration of 1-methyl-4-phenyl-1,2,3,6-tetrahydropyridine (MPTP).

METHODS

ANIMALS, APPARATUS, TASKS

Two female monkeys (*Macaca mulatta*) were used for these experiments (monkeys V and L). All aspects of animal care were in accord with the *Guide for the Care and Use of Laboratory Animals* (National Research Council, 1996), and all procedures were approved by the institutional animal care and use committee.

Data from these animals were part of a recent publication describing changes in resting cortical activity associated with parkinsonism (Pasquereau and Turner, 2011). Many aspects of the experimental approach were described in detail in that report. In brief, the animals performed a visuomotor step-tracking task similar to one used in previous studies of cortical and BG neuronal activity (Alexander, 1987; Mitchell et al., 1987; Alexander and Crutcher, 1990; Turner and Delong, 2000). The animal sat in a primate chair and faced a computer monitor. The right arm was secured into a close-fitting padded cradle attached to a one-dimensional torquable manipulandum. The wrist (monkey L) or elbow (monkey V) joint was aligned with the manipulandum's axis of rotation. Flexion and extension movements rotated the manipulandum in the horizontal plane and thereby controlled the horizontal position of an onscreen cursor. A trial began when a center target appeared and the monkey made the appropriate joint movement to align the cursor with the target. The monkey maintained this position for the duration of a start-position hold period (random duration, 2–5 s), during which the animal could not predict the location of the upcoming lateral target. The target then shifted to the left or right (chosen at random), and the animal moved the cursor to capture the lateral target. The animal received a drop of juice for successful completion of the task.

On two-thirds of the trials (selected at random), single flexing or extending torque impulses (0.1 Nm–50 ms duration) were applied to the manipulandum by a DC brushless torque motor (TQ40W, Aerotech Inc., Pittsburgh PA) at an unpredictable time beginning 1–2 s (uniform randomized distribution) after initial capture of the center target. Each square-wave torque impulse induced an angular displacement of the joint (mean = 10-deg) causing a sudden stretch of arm extensor or flexor muscles. The animals were not trained to produce a specific response to these unpredictable perturbations, but the animals naturally adopted a strategy that returned the joint to its initial pre-impulse position.

Later aspects of the behavioral trial, which evaluated instruction-related neuronal activity, are irrelevant to the current study.

SURGERY

The animals were prepared surgically using aseptic techniques under Isoflurane inhalation anesthesia (Pasquereau and Turner, 2011). A cylindrical stainless steel chamber was implanted at an angle of 35° in the coronal plane to allow access to the arm-related regions of the left M1 and the posterior putamen. The chamber and hardware for head fixation were fixed to the skull with bone screws and methyl methacrylate polymer.

Pairs of fine Teflon-insulated multistranded stainless steel wires were implanted into multiple arm muscles: flexor carpi ulnaris, flexor carpi radialis, biceps longus, brachioradialis, and triceps lateralis in monkey L; and posterior deltoid, trapezius, triceps longus, triceps lateralis and brachioradialis in monkey V. The wires were led subcutaneously to a connector fixed to the skull implant. Accurate placement of electromyographic (EMG) electrodes was verified post-surgically. Following surgery, animals were given prophylactic antibiotics and analgesic medication.

PLACEMENT OF ELECTRODES FOR ANTIDROMIC IDENTIFICATION

PTNs and CSNs were identified by antidromic activation from electrodes implanted in the cerebral peduncles and posterolateral striatum. Sites for implantation were identified using standard electrophysiological mapping techniques (Turner and Delong, 2000). Arm-related areas of the putamen were identified by sensorimotor examination of striatal activity and microstimulation effects. The arm-related fiber tract in the pre-pontine cerebral peduncle (ventral to the substantia nigra) was located using similar techniques.

Custom-built PtIr microwire electrodes were implanted at arm-related sites in putamen and the peduncle (Turner and Delong, 2000). After implantation, stimulation through the electrodes evoked arm movements similar to those observed at the target sites during microelectrode mapping. In both animals, three such electrodes were implanted in the posterior putamen between the planes of HC anterior 8 and 14, and one electrode was implanted in the arm-responsive portion of the pre-pontine peduncle (for details, see Turner and Delong, 2000). Histologic reconstruction confirmed that the striatal and peduncle electrodes were at sites known from anatomical studies to receive the bulk of M1 CSN and PTN projections, respectively (Brodal, 1978; Flaherty and Graybiel, 1991; Takada et al., 1998; Turner and Delong, 2000).

DATA ACQUISITION

Areas of M1 related to the primary joint used in the task were identified using microstimulation and sensorimotor mapping. We preformed trans-dural extracellular recording using single glass-coated PtIr microelectrodes mounted in a hydraulic microdrive (MO-95, Narishige Intl., Tokyo). A cortical region was targeted for data collection if neurons responded to active and/or passive movement of the arm and microstimulation at low currents evoked contraction of forelimb muscles (<40-μA, 10 biphasic pulses at 300-Hz). Microelectrode penetrations were performed throughout the targeted cortical area using sequential stimulation of each putamen and peduncle stimulating site as search stimuli (biphasic current pulses of 700-μA, 0.2-ms duration separated by 0.1-ms, >1.5-s between successive biphasic shocks). Neurons were selected for data collection if they were activated antidromically or if they were located in close proximity (<0.5-mm) to an antidromically-activated neuron. Standard tests for antidromic identification were used: constant antidromic latency (<0.2-ms jitter), reliable following of a high-frequency train of stimuli (three or four shocks at 200-Hz), and collision of antidromic spikes with spontaneously occurring spikes (Fuller and Schlag, 1976; Turner and Delong, 2000).

Neuronal activity was collected while the animal performed the step-tracking task. The microelectrode signal was amplified $\times 10^4$ and bandpass filtered (0.3–10 KHz, DAM-80, WPI Inc.). The action potentials of single neurons (sampled at 60-kHz) were discriminated on-line using template-based spike sorting (MultiSpike Detector, Alpha Omega Engineering, Nazareth, Israel). The timing of detected spikes and of relevant task events was sampled digitally at 1 kHz and saved to disk for offline analysis. EMG signals were differentially amplified (gain = 10-K), band-pass filtered (20-Hz to 5-kHz), rectified and then low-pass filtered (100-Hz). EMG data were collected during only a subset of data recording sessions. (No usable EMG signal was available in monkey L after MPTP administration.) Analog data reflecting angular position of the manipulandum (i.e., joint angle), the torque produced by the motor, and EMG were digitized at either 200-Hz (monkey L) or 500-Hz (monkey V).

ADMINISTRATION OF MPTP

After an adequate number of neurons were sampled from the neurologically-normal state, a hemiparkinsonian syndrome was induced by injection of MPTP into the left internal carotid artery [0.5-mg/kg, (Bankiewicz et al., 1986; Wu et al., 2007)]. This model of parkinsonism was chosen to facilitate care of the animals during the months-long period of post-intoxication recording and to increase the likelihood that animals would continue performing the operant task following intoxication (Bankiewicz et al., 2001). The MPTP administration procedure was performed under general anesthesia (1–3% Isoflurane) and prophylactic antibiotics and analgesics were administered post-surgically. Both animals developed stable signs of parkinsonism contralateral to the infusion (i.e., on the right side of the body). Quantitative measures of the severity of parkinsonism, of its impact on task performance, and histologic evidence of dopamine depletion are documented in a previous report (Pasquereau and Turner, 2011). Post-MPTP recording sessions started >30-days after MPTP administration.

HISTOLOGY

After the last recording session, each monkey was given a lethal dose of sodium pentobarbital and was perfused transcardially with saline followed by 10% formalin in phosphate buffer and then sucrose. The brains were processed histologically to localize microelectrode tracks (using cresyl violet staining) and to document the loss of dopaminergic cells in the substantia nigra *pars compacta* (SNc) using tyrosine hydroxylase (TH) immunochemistry (See Pasquereau and Turner (2011) for details concerning histologic results).

DATA ANALYSIS

The present report addresses only the short-latency joint movements and changes in neuronal activity evoked by torque perturbation during the start-position hold period. The general features of task performance before and after MPTP have been reported previously (Pasquereau and Turner, 2011).

The digitized signal reflecting manipulandum angle was filtered and differentiated [low-pass 25-Hz (Hamming, 1983)]. The onset of torque-evoked movement, peak velocity, and movement termination were detected automatically using angle, velocity, and duration criteria. A velocity threshold of 5-deg/s was used to detect movement. Session-by-session means of kinematic measures were entered into Three-Way ANOVAs to test for effects of MPTP administration, movement direction and animal.

EMG data were analyzed using methods similar to those described previously (Turner et al., 1995). For each muscle, peri-torque means of the digitized EMG signals were constructed for all valid torque perturbations in each direction (flexion and extension). The signal was normalized by subtracting the background activity recorded 200-ms prior to the onset of the torque perturbation.

Neuronal data were screened based on the location, quality, and duration of the recording. Data were included in the analysis database if they met the following criteria: (1) The recording was obtained from a location within 3-mm of the anterior bank of the central sulcus from which movements of the arm could be evoked by microstimulation (i.e., <40-μA, 10 pulses at 300-Hz). (2) Adequate single unit isolation was maintained throughout the recording. Isolation was controlled during acquisition by adjusting electrode position and spike sorting. Adequate isolation was verified off-line by testing whether a neuron's inter-spike intervals (ISIs) obeyed a refractory period (>2-ms). (3) Neurons were studied if they were either responsive to antidromic stimulation or were encountered within 0.5-mm of an antidromically activated neuron.

The analyses presented here were performed on data extracted from completely different task time periods than those used in our previous publication (Pasquereau and Turner, 2011). In addition, not all neurons were recorded from under all task conditions, so the neuronal populations studied here overlap only partially with those used in (Pasquereau and Turner, 2011).

For each torque perturbation, continuous neuronal activation functions [spike density functions (SDFs)] were generated by convolving a spike train's delta function (1-ms resolution) with an asymmetric Gamma function kernel ($k = 1.5$ and $\theta = 20$). SDFs are traditionally constructed as a sum of Gaussian functions centered on the times of each discriminated action potential (Szucs, 1998). Gaussian functions, however, exert influence backward in time (Thompson et al., 1996; Isoda and Hikosaka, 2008; Heitz et al., 2010) such that SDFs constructed using a Gaussian kernel occasionally gave spurious results, indicating that torque-evoked responses began prior to torque onset. The Gamma function, which approximates the timecourse of a postsynaptic potential, avoided this problem by exerting influence only forward in time. Mean peri-torque SDFs (averaged across trials) were constructed separately for the two torque directions for neurons studied during at least 5 repetitions of each torque direction. A neuron's baseline firing rate was calculated as the mean of the SDFs across the 500-ms epoch immediately preceding torque pulse onset. Phasic responses to a torque perturbation were detected by comparing SDF values (millisecond-by-millisecond) during a post-torque epoch (200-ms) relative to a cell's baseline firing rate (2-tailed t-test). The threshold for significance was adjusted to account for multiple comparisons [$p < 0.01/(200\text{-ms epoch}/40\text{-ms gamma filter half-width} = 5 \text{ independent comparisons}) = 0.002$]. A neuron was judged to be torque-related if it generated a significant post-torque response for at least one movement direction. Response onset times, defined as the time at which the SDF first crossed the $p = 0.002$ threshold, were determined separately for each torque direction. For comparisons between neuronal populations, a cell's earliest response onset across directions was used as that cell's latency. We only analyzed cortical responses that began at relatively short latencies (between 20–60-ms), so as to exclude responses related to volitional compensatory movements (Evarts, 1973; Pruszynski et al., 2011b). The time of offset of a neuronal response was calculated using a similar method, searching for the time point at which the SDF first returned within the $p = 0.002$ threshold relative to baseline firing rate.

The magnitude of a torque-evoked response was measured using three separate measures. First, the mean firing rate during the response was calculated (i.e., mean of the SDF between times of response onset and offset). Second, we calculated the maximum change of firing rate away from baseline between times of response onset and offset. And third, we calculated the area under the curve in the SDF between times of response onset and offset. The temporal dispersion of a response was measured as its full-width half-maximum (FWHM).

The directional selectivity of torque-evoked responses was parameterized using a directional selectivity index (DSI) (Suarez et al., 1995): $DSI = |1 - (NP/P)|$, where NP equals the maximum change infiring rate from baseline in the non-preferred direction and P equals the maximum change in firing rate in the preferred direction during the post-torque period (200-ms).The preferred direction is defined as the direction that elicits the largest change from baseline firing rate (either positive or negative).By this convention, $DSI = 0$ meant that the response to torque perturbation was equal for both directions and therefore was not directionally selective (classified as *non-directional)*. DSI ≈1 meant that the cell response (either increase or decrease in firing) was present for only one movement direction (classified as *unidirectional activity*). A cell's torque response was considered directionally selective if the DSI was >0.50 (i.e., P/2>NP). Responses with DSIs between 0.5 and 1 were defined as *bidirectional* whereas those with DSIs >1 were considered *reciprocal* (changes of opposite sign for opposing directions of movement).

To study MPTP-related changes for different subsets of cells, we corrected for multiple comparisons using the Bonferroni–Holm method (Holm, 1979). Then, two separate analyses were performed to determine if MPTP-induced alterations in neuronal responses correlated with behavioral measures of rigidity. The first analysis tested for relationships across recording sessions. We tested for correlations between mean measures of neuronal responses (magnitudes and latencies) and mean measures of reflex movements for those sessions (behavioral indexes: peak velocity of movements and magnitude of EMG responses). Spearman's rank correlations were performed and the threshold for significance was adjusted to account for multiple comparisons [$p < 0.05/(4 \text{ comparisons}) = 0.0125$]. The second analysis tested for relationships within individual recording sessions. We tested for correlations between a single neuron's trial-to-trial response latency and an animal's trial-to-trial response to torque perturbations (peak velocity and EMG). Spearman's rank correlations were performed for individual cells and results were compared between populations recorded pre- and post-MPTP.

RESULTS

DATABASE

Single unit recordings were obtained from the arm-related areas of the left M1 of two monkeys. A total of 227 neurons were studied in the neurologically normal state. Of these, 66 were activated antidromically from peduncle stimulation (PTNs: 49 in monkey V and 17 in monkey L; **Table 1**) and 56 were activated from the putamen (CSNs: 31 in monkey V and 25 in monkey L). Of the 232 neurons collected during the post-MPTP period, 65 were PTNs (54 in monkey V and 11 in monkey L) and 58 were CSNs (48 in monkey V and 10 in monkey L). Only 3 cells were activated antidromically from both the putamen and the peduncle (0.5% of neurons studied). These three cells were included in the general "M1" category (i.e., all cells studied including PTNs, CSNs and non-activated cells), but they were excluded from "PTN" and "CSN" categories. The remainder of the neurons (105 pre-MPTP and 109 post-MPTP) were not activated antidromically (NA), but were recorded either at the same time as PT or CS recordings or were sampled within 0.5-mm of an antidromically activated neuron along the same microelectrode track.

Paralleling our previous report (Pasquereau and Turner, 2011), in neurologically-normal animals, resting neuronal firing rates measured immediately prior to torque onset were markedly higher for PTNs (mean rate: 16.3-spikes/s, range: 0.2–45; **Table 1**) than for CSNs (mean rate: 3.6-spikes/s, range: 0–22; Mann–Whitney U-test, $p < 0.001$). This result is consistent with previous descriptions of the marked differences in resting firing rates between intra-telencephalic-like CSNs and PTNs (Bauswein et al., 1989; Turner and Delong, 2000).

Table 1 | Effects of MPTP on two distinct subpopulations of M1 cells.

		M1	PTN	CSN
Number of cells	Pre-MPTP	227	66	56
	Post-MPTP	232	65	58
Baseline firing rate (Sp/s)	Pre-MPTP	11.8 ± 10.3	18.3 ± 8.6	3.2 ± 4.0
	Post-MPTP	9.5 ± 9.2*	13.9 ± 9.6***	4.2 ± 4.8
Antidromic latency (ms)	Pre-MPTP	3.3 ± 2.3	1.9 ± 0.9	5.1 ± 2.3
	Post-MPTP	3.6 ± 3.1	1.9 ± 0.8	6.1 ± 3.4**
Torque-related cells	Pre-MPTP	141/227 (62%)	43/66 (65%)	19/56 (34%)
	Post-MPTP	143/232 (62%)	46/65 (71%)	16/58 (28%)
Ratio of excitatory responses (Flexion and Extension)	Pre-MPTP	91/111 and 95/106 (86%)	19/34 and 28/33 (70%)	13/13 and 10/11 (96%)
	Post-MPTP	105/119 and 95/108 (88%)	26/35 and 24/32 (75%)	11/13 and 8/9 (86%)##

*Mean values ± SD before and after MPTP treatment are calculated for all M1 cells (left), for PTNs (middle), and for CSNs (right). *p < 0.05, **p < 0.01, ***p < 0.001 (Mann–Whitney U-test); and ##p < 0.01 (χ^2 test). All statistical results in this table compare results within the indicated category for pre- vs. post-MPTP periods.*

Also consistent with previous reports (Pasquereau and Turner, 2011) the spontaneous activity of the general population of M1 cells decreased by 17% after MPTP treatment (Mann–Whitney U-test, $p < 0.05/2$). MPTP had markedly different effects on the two identified neuronal populations. The pre-torque firing rate of PTNs was reduced by 27% following MPTP treatment (Mann–Whitney U-test, $p < 0.001$; **Table 1**) whereas the mean activity of CSNs remained unchanged (Mann–Whitney U-test, $p = 0.5$). The antidromic latencies of PTNs remained unchanged between pre- and post-MPTP periods (mean = 1.9-ms; Mann–Whitney U-test, $p = 0.9$; **Table 1**) whereas those of CSNs were significantly longer following MPTP administration (means = 5.1 and 6.1-ms, pre- and post-MPTP, respectively; Mann–Whitney U-test, $p < 0.05/3$).

BEHAVIORAL EFFECTS OF MPTP

Intracarotid administration of MPTP rendered the animals moderately parkinsonian as evidenced by increased reaction times, decreased movement velocities and reduced movement extents in the behavioral task [for details, see Pasquereau and Turner (2011)]. Monkeys showed limited variation in the severity of these impairments throughout the post-MPTP recording period (maximum 117-days).

Induction of parkinsonism also led to a slowing of torque-induced displacements of the arm (ANOVA; $F > 515, p < 0.001$; **Figure 1**) and a reduction in movement amplitude ($F > 49, p < 0.01$). More specifically, the mean peak velocity and the amplitude of torque-induced displacements averaged across recording sessions were reduced by 16.2% and 6.6%, respectively, following MPTP administration, consistent with an increase of rigidity in the parkinsonian condition. The latencies of torque-induced displacements remained unmodified post-MPTP ($F < 0.2$ and

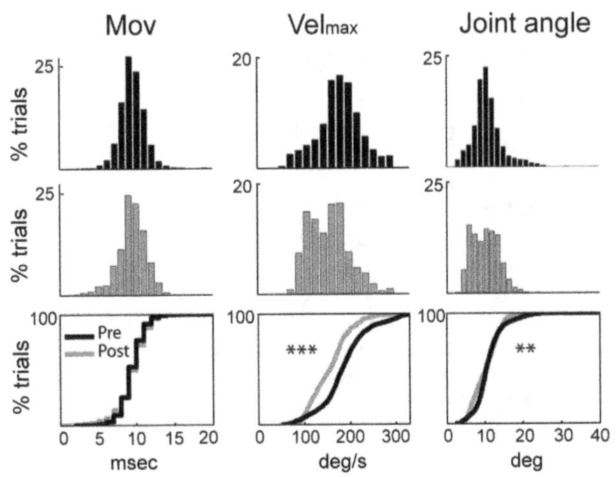

FIGURE 1 | Rigidity was increased following MPTP administration. Kinematic measures (cross-session means) from pre-MPTP (black) and post-MPTP (gray) periods for flexion movements following torque perturbations. Cumulative distributions are shown at the bottom. Movement onsets (*Mov*), peak velocities (Vel_{max}), and movement amplitudes (*Joint angle*) were compared between MPTP states (ANOVA; $^{**}p < 0.01$, $^{***}p < 0.001$).

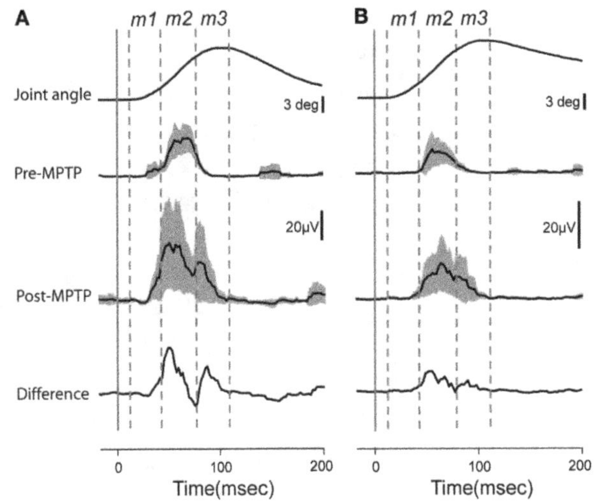

FIGURE 2 | Averaged and rectified grand-average EMG responses (±95% confidence intervals) to elbow flexion from triceps longus (A) and triceps lateralis (B). Lower traces reflect the differences between EMG responses recorded before or after MPTP administration. Time zero indicates the time at which the torque impulse was turned on to initiate the arm displacement. Vertical lines show the putative onset of each muscle component (*m1*, *m2*, and *m3*).

$p > 0.05$; **Figure 1**), but we found significant differences in the effects of MPTP for the two torque directions ($F > 94$ and $p < 0.001$). Because of this, data were analyzed separately for flexion and extension torque directions.

EMG responses to sudden, unpredictable muscle stretches were analyzed in their separate latency components (**Figure 2**). The short-latency response defined as the *m1* component (muscle activity occurring between 15 ± 3 and 40 ± 4-ms post-torque) was poorly formed and generally much smaller than the long-latency response (*m2*; 41 ± 4 and 80 ± 7-ms post-torque). Following the administration of MPTP, the *m2* component was markedly larger (Kolmogorov two-sample test, $p < 0.05$; **Figure 2**). The total duration of EMG responses to torque perturbations also increased (from 57 ± 6 to 79 ± 3-ms; Kolmogorov two-sample test, $p < 0.001$), primarily due to the appearance of an *m3* component. The *m1* short-latency response remained weak in all the case, and latencies of the earliest EMG responses showed no significant change ($p > 0.05$).

TORQUE-EVOKED NEURONAL RESPONSES – PREVALENCE

A large fraction of the general population of M1 cells (62%, 284/459, of all CSNs, PTNs, and NA cells) responded to torque perturbations with a phasic response at short latency (<60-ms, **Figure 3A**). Half of these torque-related cells (124/284, 44%) responded for only one direction of rotation (flexion or extension). **Figures 3B,C** illustrate examples of neuronal responses to torques in which a CSN responded to flexion torques only **(3B)**, and a PTN that responded to both flexion and extension torques **(3C)**. Monophasic increases in firing constituted a large fraction of the torque response in M1 (87%) whereas torque-evoked decreases in firing were observed infrequently (13% of all M1 neurons; **Table 1**). Consistent with previous observations (Turner and Delong, 2000), PTNs were more responsive to proprioceptive stimulation than CSNs. Torque responses were observed in 68% (89/131) of PTNs but only 31% (35/114) of CSNs ($\chi^2 = 32.3$, $p < 0.001$; **Table 1** and **Figure 3A**).

TORQUE-EVOKED NEURONAL RESPONSES – PRE- vs. POST-MPTP

Contrary to predictions from a simple model for exaggerated LLSRs in PD (see Introduction), induction of parkinsonism did not increase the prevalence of torque responses in the general population of M1 cells (62% for both states), in CSNs (26%), or in PTNs (68%; $\chi^2 < 6.4$ $p > 0.05/3$; **Figure 3A**, **Table 1**). These results are broken down in a more fine-grained manner for the two monkeys in the Supplementary Table. The small number of proprioceptive-responsive CSNs studied post-MPTP prevented more in-depth analysis of response timing in this neuronal type.

Induction of parkinsonism also did not alter the balance of torque-elicited increases and decreases in firing. For PTNs, most torque-evoked changes in activity consisted of an increase in firing (72% of responses; 97 of 134 responses counting responses to flexions and extensions separately; **Figure 4A** and **Table 1**). That high prevalence of torque-evoked increases in firing did not differ between pre- and post-MPTP periods ($\chi^2 = 0.1$, $p = 0.7$; **Table 1**). The magnitudes of torque-evoked responses also did not differ between pre- and post-MPTP periods. Response magnitudes were compared for M1 cells, and again for PTNs separately, using three different measures of magnitude: (1) the mean change of firing rate relative to pre-torque baseline, (2) the maximum change of firing rate, and (3) the area under the curve in the SDF. None of these comparisons yielded a significant difference between pre- and post-MPTP periods (Kolmogorov two-sample test and Mann–Whitney *U*-test, all *p*'s > 0.15; **Figure 4A**). To

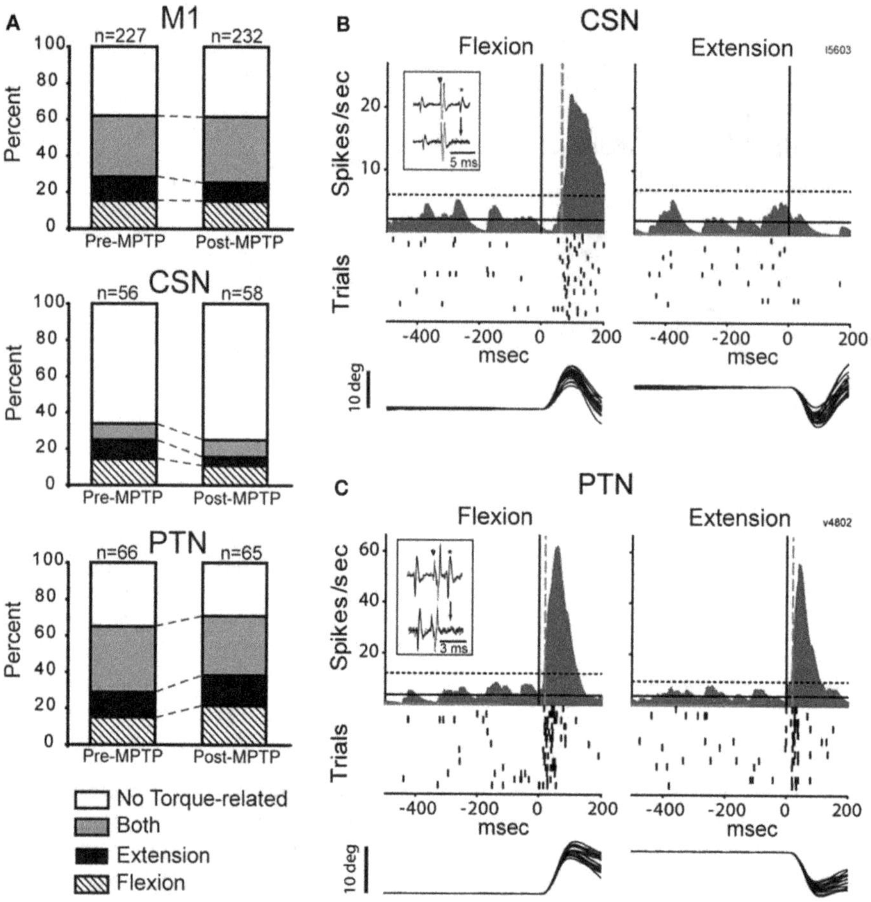

FIGURE 3 | MPTP did not alter torque responsiveness. (A) The fractions of neurons that were torque-related to one or both stretch directions (flexion and extension) did not change following MPTP administration for the general population of M1 cells (top), for CSNs (middle), or for PTNs (bottom) (χ^2 test, $p > 0.05/3$). **(B,C)** Representative short latency responses to torque perturbations for CSNs **(B)** and PTNs **(C)**. The torque responses of CSNs tended to be small in magnitude and in one direction only, whereas the responses of PTNs were most commonly sensitive to both directions. Mean SDFs, rasters, and overlaid traces of single trial joint are aligned on the onset of flexing or extending torques (*vertical black lines*). The *vertical gray dotted lines* show neuronal response latencies detected using significant threshold computed from the pre-torque period (*horizontal dotted lines*, $p < 0.01/(5$ comparisons$) = 0.002$). *Inset figures* in each panel illustrate antidromic activation and collision tests for the neuron that has its torque response shown.

control for the possibility that these results were biased by the MPTP-induced global slowing of torque-induced displacements of the arm (see *Behavioral effects of MPTP*, above), we selected subsets of recording sessions from pre- and post-MPTP sessions in which velocities were equivalent (range: 130–200 deg/s, Mann–Whitney U-test, $p > 0.05$; Supplementary Figure 1). We confirmed our main result in this subset by observing that MPTP did not change the magnitude of torque-evoked responses in M1 (Mann–Whitney U-test, all p's > 0.19).

The latencies of torque-evoked responses, however, were significantly shorter following MPTP administration. This observation held true for the general population of M1 neurons and specifically for PTNs, and for responses to flexions and extensions, all considered separately (Kolmogorov two-sample test, all p's < 0.05; **Figure 4B**). For PTNs, the mean latency of responses was reduced by 17% from a pre-MPTP value of 46-ms (45-ms for flexions, and 46-ms for extensions) to a post-MPTP value of 38-ms (37-ms for flexions, and 39-ms for extensions). Similarly, for the general population of M1 neurons, mean response latencies were reduced by 15% from 41-ms pre-MPTP (40-ms for flexions, and 42-ms for extensions) to 35-ms post-MPTP (36-ms for flexions, and 35-ms for extensions; Kolmogorov two-sample test, $p < 0.01$). M1 response latencies were reduced by similar degrees for flexion and extension directions (Kolmogorov two-sample test, $p = 0.52$; **Figure 4B**). This latency shortening effect could not be attributed to history effects (e.g., increasing experience by the animal or cumulative recording tracks) because we found no correlation between the latencies of torque-evoked responses and the days of training an animal experienced (monkey V: Spearman $|\text{rho}| = 0.02$ $p = 0.85$; monkey L: Spearman $|\text{rho}| = 0.08$ $p = 0.68$).

In addition to the shift in latencies, torque-evoked increases in PTN activity were more tightly synchronized or time-locked to the torque perturbation following MPTP (**Figure 4A**). For these responses, the response FWHM was reduced by 31% from a mean of 73-ms (80-ms for flexion, and 66-ms for extension) pre-MPTP to 50-ms (54-ms for flexion, and 46-ms for extension) post-MPTP (Mann–Whitney U-test, p's < 0.05).

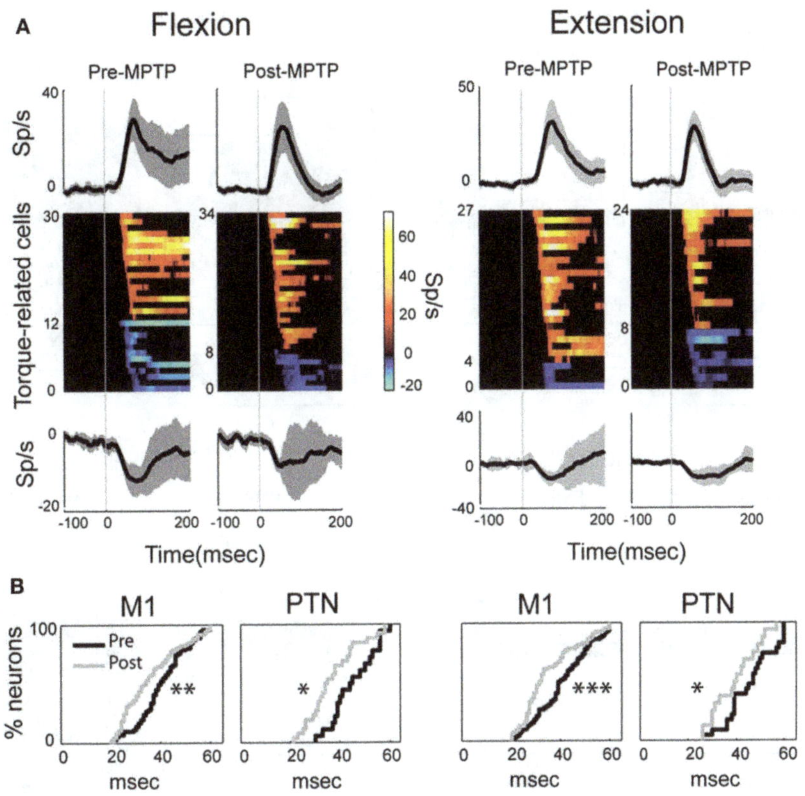

FIGURE 4 | MPTP altered the M1 response latencies to torque perturbations. The latency of response shifted significantly in PTNs or in the general population of M1 cells, although its magnitude remained unchanged between MPTP periods. **(A)** Population mean spike density functions (SDFs) averaged across all positive (top) or negative (bottom) phasic responses in PTNs for flexion or extension movements (left and right panels, respectively). Gray shadings and vertical gray lines indicate ± *SE* and the time of torque onset (time 0), respectively. Color plot of all SDFs (one row per PTN) classified neurons according to latency and polarity of responses. Colors along each horizontal band indicate the significant changes in firing rate of one PTN induced by torque perturbation (red-yellow = increases; blue-cyan = decreases; firing rate scale in the bar). Black = no significant change in a SDF. **(B)** Following MPTP, the cumulative distributions for M1 (left) or for PTNs (right) showed a reduction of response latency to torque perturbation (Kolmogorov two-sample test; ****p* < 0.001, ***p* < 0.01, **p* < 0.05).

RESPONSE DIRECTIONALITY – PRE- vs. POST-MPTP

In the general population of M1 cells, the directional selectivity of torque responses was reduced following MPTP. Prior to MPTP, a large proportion of the torque-responsive cells in M1 responded differently for the two directions of torque perturbation (**Figure 5**; 143/231, 62% of all torque-responsive cells). By classifying the torque-evoked responses of M1 neurons according to their directional selectivity indices (DSI, *Methods*), it became clear that highly directional (reciprocal and unidirectional) response types became less common following MPTP administration (10% reduction in incidence), and bi-directional or non-directional response types became more common (10% increase in incidence; $\chi^2 = 22.2$, $p < 0.001$; ### in **Figure 6**). Non-significant reductions ($p > 0.05/2$, likely due to small N) in the incidence of highly directional response patterns were observed in CSN and PTN sub-populations. This general decrease in directional selectivity could not be attributed directly to MPTP-induced changes in resting firing rates because pre-torque mean firing rates did not differ between the different directional categories (One-Way ANOVA, $F = 0.77$ and $p = 0.46$). In addition, EMG responses to torque perturbations did not show alterations in directional selectivity or sign of co-contraction between antagonist muscles (Supplementary Figure 2).

ANALYSIS OF NEURAL-BEHAVIORAL CORRELATIONS

Although torque-evoked cortical responses, movement velocity, and the *m2* component of EMG reflex activity were all affected by MPTP administration, we found no correlation between the modifications in M1 responses and variations in the LLSR. That question was addressed first by testing for correlations between session-by-session measures of the mean PTN response latency and mean measures of the LLSR (i.e., peak velocity of movements, and magnitude of the *m2* muscle component). This analysis was restricted to the relatively homogenous population of PTNs because their activity was known to be affected by MPTP administration. No significant correlation was found for either analysis (Vel_{max}, Spearman $|rho| < 0.18$ $p > 0.05$; or $m2_{max}$, $|rho| < 0.26$ $p > 0.05$). A second approach searched for correlations trial-by-trial between torque-evoked neuronal responses and measures of the LLSR (Vel_{max} or $m2_{max}$). Measures of PTN response latencies did not correlate with any of the measures of LLSR (Spearman $|rho| < 0.34$; $p > 0.05$). Similar negative results were obtained

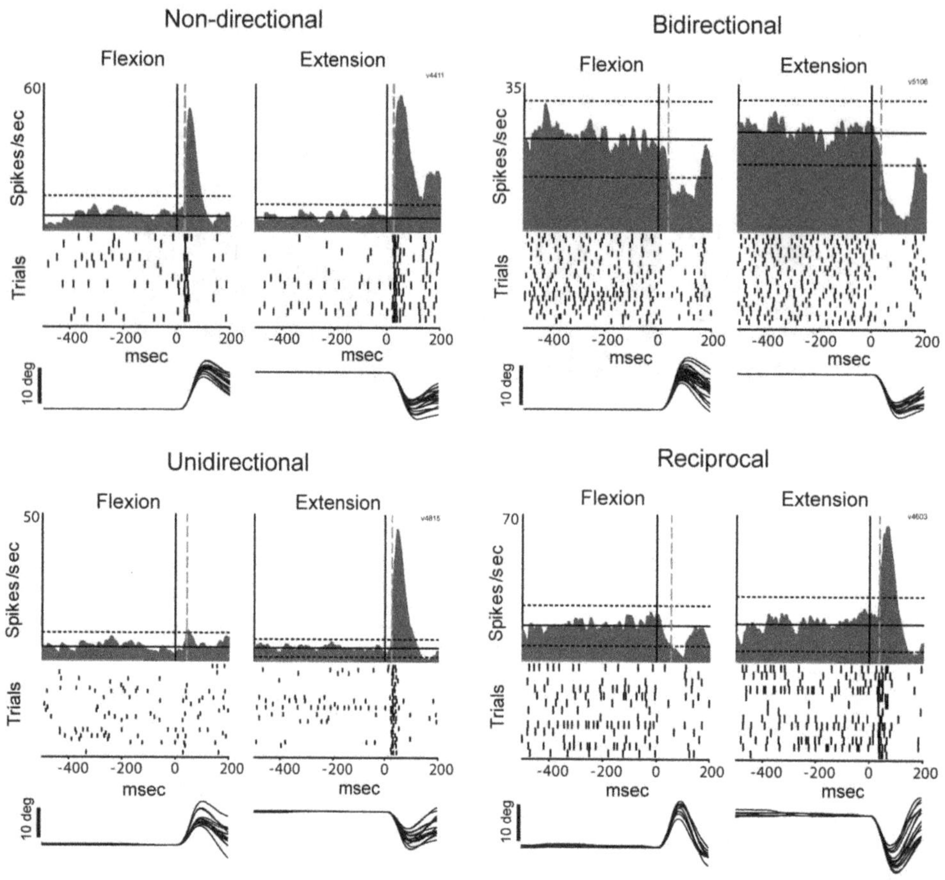

FIGURE 5 | Representative examples of directional peri-torque activity in PTNs. *Non-directional* neuron similarly responded to torque perturbation for both directions (flexion and extension; DSI = 0). *Unidirectional* activity indicates that torque response only occurred for the preferred direction (the direction associated with a maximal change in firing; DSI = 1). *Bidirectional* neuron was considered directionally selective with a change in firing for the preferred direction ≥2 times the magnitude of that for the opposing direction (0.5 < DSI < 1). *Reciprocal* responses indicate that changes in firing were opposite sign (increase and decrease in firing for preferred and non-preferred directions,respectively) for opposing directions of movement (DSI >1). These figures follow the conventions of **Figure 3** to illustrate mean SDFs, rasters, and arm positions.

from correlation analyses of the general population of M1 cells (results not shown).

DISCUSSION

The present study addresses a long-standing but untested hypothesis for why the long-latency component of the stretch reflex is exaggerated in Parkinson's disease. Despite the fact that exaggeration of the LLSR is a significant contributor to parkinsonian rigidity (Lee and Tatton, 1975; Mortimer and Webster, 1979; Tatton et al., 1984; Xia et al., 2009), the CNS correlates of the parkinsonian stretch reflex have seldom been examined (Rossini et al., 1989; Aminoff et al., 1997) and never, to our knowledge, using single unit recording. One straightforward hypothesis states that the LLSR is exaggerated in PD because of increased corticospinal sensitivity to muscle stretch (Rothwell et al., 1983). Alternative hypotheses implicate increased gain in slow-conducting spinal reflex pathways (Berardelli et al., 1983). We tested the trans-cortical hypothesis by measuring the stretch-evoked responses of identified sub-populations of M1 neurons prior to and following the induction of parkinsonism. Contrary to the predictions of the trans-cortical model, we did not observe an increase in M1 responsiveness to proprioceptive stimuli. Rather, the MPTP-induced increase in rigidity and LLSR was associated with shortened M1 response latency and a reduction in directional selectivity. The sections below address each of these findings in turn.

ABSENCE OF INCREASED RESPONSE PREVALENCE OR MAGNITUDE

We found no evidence that the induction of parkinsonism lead to a greater incidence of neuronal responses to proprioceptive stimuli in the population of M1 neurons, an increase in the balance of torque-evoked increases over decreases, or an increase in the magnitude of torque-evoked responses in individual M1 neurons. These observations run contrary to predictions of the simple trans-cortical model for the exaggerated LLSR of PD. In their key study of the LLSR in PD patients, Rothwell et al. stated that "if the stretch reflex excitability is indeed enhanced in PD, the gain must be increased at some central site"(Rothwell et al., 1983, p. 35). The M1, and its population of PTNs in particular, is one of the few central nodes in the circuit that mediates the LLSR.

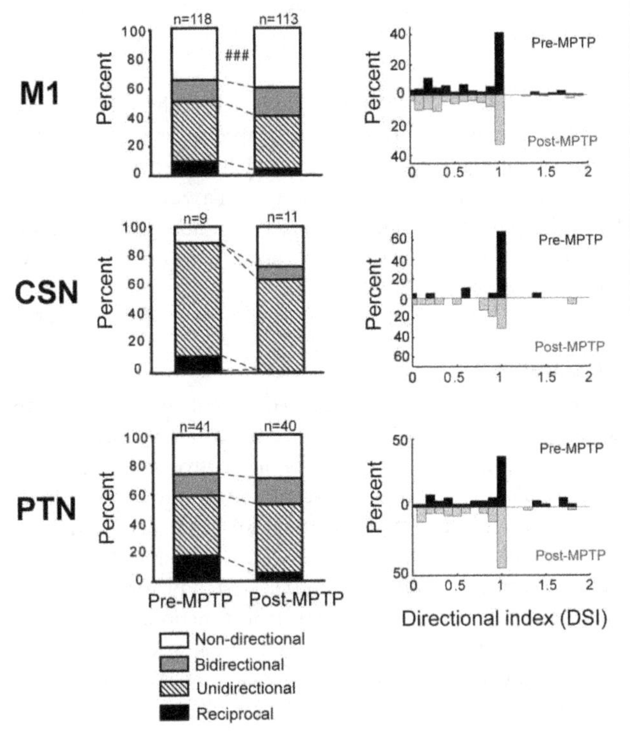

FIGURE 6 | MPTP altered the directionally selective responses. Compared to the pre-MPTP period, the short latency torque responses of M1 were directionally selective less frequently following the MPTP treatment: a smaller proportion of neurons had reciprocal or unidirectional activities, whereas the responses were most commonly non-directional or bidirectional. These modifications were partly attributable to PTNs, for instance, whose reciprocal responses were less frequent in post-MPTP. The small number of CSNs showing directionally selective responses further limited the statistical analysis. χ^2 test; $^{###}p < 0.001$.

A straightforward interpretation of Rothwell et al.'s statement predicts that neurons in this circuit will show an increased prevalence of stretch-evoked neuronal responses or increased neuronal response magnitudes. We found no evidence of either in the activity of single units in M1.

Although inconsistent with the simple trans-cortical hypothesis, this result agrees with the abundant evidence that somatosensory-evoked responses are not enhanced in the sensorimotor cortex of parkinsonian subjects (Rossini et al., 1989; Aminoff et al., 1997; Rickards and Cody, 1997; Boecker et al., 1999; Lewis and Byblow, 2002; Schrader et al., 2008). The classical rate model of PD pathophysiology also proposes that excessive inhibitory outflow from the parkinsonian BG attenuates thalamocortical responses (Delong and Wichmann, 2007). Despite the limitations of the rate model (Montgomery, 2007), evidence continues to support the model's prediction that parkinsonism is associated with a reduction in M1 excitability (Lefaucheur, 2005; Brown et al., 2009; Pasquereau and Turner, 2011; Viaro et al., 2011; Leon-Sarmiento et al., 2013). From this perspective, it might be seen as surprising that we did not observe more profound *decreases* in the prevalence or magnitude of M1 responses to proprioceptive stimulation. Our failure to observe an attenuation of proprioceptive responsiveness, as predicted by indirect measures of brain activity (Rossini et al., 1989; Aminoff et al., 1997; Rickards and Cody, 1997; Boecker et al., 1999; Lewis and Byblow, 2002; Schrader et al., 2008), may be explained by the idea that M1 is organized into dissociable sub-circuits that are affected differently with the induction of parkinsonism (Shepherd, 2013).

Numerous studies have reported that neurons in BG structures and in the motor thalamus of parkinsonian animals show marked increases in the prevalence and magnitude of proprioceptive responses (Filion et al., 1988; Bergman et al., 1994; Pessiglione et al., 2005; Bronfeld and Bar-Gad, 2011). Our results suggest that this exaggerated proprioceptive responsiveness in subcortical structures is not relayed to cortex in any simple way. This result is congruent with other lines of evidence that indicate that the BG-thalamo-cortical pathway does not operate as a simple driver of cortical activity (Inase et al., 1996; Rubin and Terman, 2004; Kuramoto et al., 2009; Goldberg and Fee, 2012).

Our observation of an elevated LLSR (**Figure 2**) combined with no change in prevalence or magnitude of stretch-evoked neuronal responses in PTNs is consistent with the view that the alteration in reflex function that mediates the exaggerated LLSR of PD is localized to the spinal cord (Simonetta Moreau et al., 2002; Marchand-Pauvert et al., 2011; Raoul et al., 2012). Several abnormalities in segmental function have been observed in PD and there is no consensus as to which of them contribute most significantly to the LLSR or rigidity. Some studies implicate slow-conducting group II spindle afferents (Cody et al., 1986; Marchand-Pauvert et al., 2011). Others suggest impairments in inhibition (Tsai et al., 1997; Meunier et al., 2000), perhaps via underactivation of the IB interneuron (Delwaide et al., 1991), or, alternatively, an abnormality in homosynaptic depression (Raoul et al., 2012). For all of these, dysfunction within the BG may affect segmental motor function via descending BG projections to the pedunculopontine nucleus and from there to spinal cord projecting brainstem nuclei (Delwaide et al., 2000). Degeneration of the noradrenergic projection to the spinal cord may also play an important role (Simonetta Moreau et al., 2002).

ALTERED RESPONSE LATENCIES AND DIRECTIONALITY

The stretch-evoked neuronal responses in M1 began at shorter latencies following MPTP administration (**Figure 4B**). The fact that very similar latency shifts were observed for responses to torque perturbations in the flexion and extension directions suggests that the latency shift was a primary effect of parkinsonism and not a by-product of altered postural bias or background muscle activity. The mechanisms that might mediate such a shift in response latency remain unclear as do its functional implications.

We also found that the directional specificity of neuronal responses was reduced following MPTP administration (**Figure 6**). Similar reductions in somatosensory specificity have been reported for neuronal activity in BG structures and in the thalamus of parkinsonian subjects (Filion et al., 1988; Bergman et al., 1994; Pessiglione et al., 2005). Our observation of reduced encoding of movement direction in M1 is consistent with the general concept that a reduction in functional specificity may be an important component of the pathophysiology of PD (Bronfeld and Bar-Gad, 2011). More specifically, the increased prevalence of non-directional and bidirectional responses may contribute to the genesis of EMG "shortening reactions," which are abnormal muscle reflex responses to passive joint rotation that appear in the muscles that are shortened by the rotation (Andrews et al., 1972; Berardelli and Hallett, 1984). Recent evidence implicates the shortening reaction in the lead-pipe nature of parkinsonian rigidity (Xia et al., 2009, 2011). The deficient directional specificity observed in M1 may contribute to the genesis of shortening reactions by producing corticospinal excitation of segmental circuit elements that should, under normal conditions, be suppressed (e.g., in the motor neuron pool of the shortened muscle). A similar mechanism may account for the more transient responses observed following MPTP administration (**Figure 4**).

METHODOLOGIC CONSIDERATIONS

This is the first study to our knowledge to examine single unit activity in M1 related to the exaggerated LLSR of parkinsonism. We examined the torque-evoked responses of M1 neurons while our research subjects were engaged in a behavioral task that required postural stabilization. This approach allowed us to maintain relative control over the behavioral state of our animal subjects across the induction of moderate parkinsonism. We used the well-established non-human primate MPTP model of PD (Bankiewicz et al., 1986, 2001) and we studied the activity of two distinct sub-populations of cortical neurons, PTNs and CSNs, as identified by antidromic activation. The divergent effects of MPTP intoxication on the two neuronal populations is consistent with the view that the two play different roles in the pathophysiology of PD (Shepherd, 2013).

It is important to recognize several limitation to the methodology used. First, we did not pre-load the muscle to be stretched or control for the level of muscle activity prior to delivery of torque perturbations, as is often done in studies of the stretch reflex (Rothwell et al., 1983). It is unlikely that this represents a serious confound for the principal results, however, because the trans-cortical component of the LLSR appears to be insensitive to the pre-perturbation level of muscle activity (Pruszynski et al., 2011b).

Second, the contribution of the trans-cortical pathway to the LLSR appears to vary between effectors, being maximal for finger muscles (Marsden et al., 1983; Noth et al., 1991) and of less importance for muscles around more proximal joints such as the wrist and elbow (Berardelli et al., 1983; Cody et al., 1986). We might have obtained different results if we had studied, for example, the effects in M1 of proprioceptive perturbations delivered to intrinsic muscles of the hand.

Third, the peak velocity and amplitude of torque-evoked joint movements were significantly smaller following MPTP administration (**Figure 1**). The magnitude of the LLSR is known to be modulated in proportion to the velocity of muscle stretches (Rothwell et al., 1983; Powell et al., 2012). The stretch-evoked neuronal responses in M1 might have been more numerous or larger in magnitude if the perturbation kinematics had been identical pre- and post-MPTP. However, the difference in kinematics is unlikely to invalidate the significance of our main results. Even when data were selected from subsets of recording sessions that had equivalent velocities, we found that response magnitudes were very similar in the pre-and post-MPTP periods (Supplementary Figure 1).

Fourth, different results might have been observed if we had induced more severe parkinsonian symptoms or bilateral parkinsonism. Although our animals showed clear behavioral and histologic signs of moderate parkinsonism (Pasquereau and Turner, 2011), the symptoms of our animals were not as severe as those rendered by other MPTP intoxication protocols (Bankiewicz et al., 2001; Emborg, 2007).

CONCLUSIONS

In summary, our results are not consistent with the idea that the exaggerated LLSR of PD is mediated by an increase in transcortical reflex gain. The most likely alternative is that reflex gain is abnormally increased in slow-conducting segmental pathways, such as those driven by group II spindle afferents (Cody et al., 1986; Marchand-Pauvert et al., 2011). The reduced directional specificity of M1 responses to muscle stretch provides additional evidence for the general breakdown in functional specificity in parkinsonism. This breakdown in directional specificity may contribute to the abnormal shortening reactions that contribute to parkinsonian rigidity.

FUNDING

This work was supported by National Institute of Neurological Disorders and Stroke at the National Institutes of Health (grant numbers NS044551 and NS055197 to Robert S. Turner and the Center for Neuroscience Research in Non-human Primates, 1P30NS076405).

REFERENCES

Abbruzzese, G., Berardelli, A., Rothwell, J. C., Day, B. L., and Marsden, C. D. (1985). Cerebral potentials and electromyographic responses evoked by stretch of wrist muscles in man. *Exp. Brain Res.* 58, 544–551. doi: 10.1007/BF00235870

Alexander, G. E. (1987). Selective neuronal discharge in monkey putamen reflects intended direction of planned limb movements. *Exp. Brain Res.* 67, 623–634. doi: 10.1007/BF00247293

Alexander, G. E., and Crutcher, M. D. (1990). Preparation for movement: neural representations of intended direction in three motor areas of the monkey. *J. Neurophysiol.* 64, 133–150.

Aminoff, M. J., Siedenberg, R., and Goodin, D. S. (1997). Changes of forearm EMG and cerebral evoked potentials following sudden muscle stretch during isometric contractions in patients with Parkinson's disease. *Brain Res.* 757, 254–259. doi: 10.1016/S0006-8993(97)00226-6

Andersson, G., and Sjolund, B. (1978). The ventral spino-olivocerebellar system in the cat. IV. Spinal transmission after administration of clonidine and L-dopa. *Exp. Brain Res.* 33, 227–240. doi: 10.1007/BF00238062

Andrews, C. J., Burke, D., and Lance, J. W. (1972). The response to muscle stretch and shortening in Parkinsonian rigidity. *Brain* 95, 795–812. doi: 10.1093/brain/95.4.795

Angel, R. W., and Hofmann, W. W. (1963). The H Reflex in Normal, Spastic, and Rigid Subjects. *Arch. Neurol.* 9, 591–596. doi: 10.1001/archneur.1963.00460060021002

Bankiewicz, K. S., Oldfield, E. H., Chiueh, C. C., Doppman, J. L., Jacobowitz, D. M., and Kopin, I. J. (1986). Hemiparkinsonism in monkeys after unilateral internal carotid artery infusion of 1-methyl-4-phenyl-1,2,3,6-tetrahydropyridine (MPTP). *Life Sci.* 39, 7–16. doi: 10.1016/0024-3205(86)90431-5

Bankiewicz, K. S., Sanchez-Pernaute, R., Oiwa, Y., Kohutnicka, M., Cummins, A., and Eberling, J. (2001). Preclinical models of Parkinson's Disease. *Curr. Protoc. Neurosci.* 9.4, 1–32. doi: 10.1002/0471142301.ns0904s09

Bauswein, E., Fromm, C., and Preuss, A. (1989). Corticostriatal cells in comparison with pyramidal tract neurons: contrasting properties in the behaving monkey. *Brain Res.* 493, 198–203. doi: 10.1016/0006-8993(89)91018-4

Berardelli, A., and Hallett, M. (1984). Shortening reaction of human tibialis anterior. *Neurology* 34, 242–245. doi: 10.1212/WNL.34.2.242

Berardelli, A., Sabra, A. F., and Hallett, M. (1983). Physiological mechanisms of rigidity in Parkinson's disease. *J. Neurol. Neurosurg. Psychiatry* 46, 45–53. doi: 10.1136/jnnp.46.1.45

Bergman, H., Wichmann, T., Karmon, B., and Delong, M. R. (1994). The primate subthalamic nucleus. II. Neuronal activity in the MPTP model of parkinsonism. *J. Neurophysiol.* 72, 507–520.

Boecker, H., Ceballos-Baumann, A., Bartenstein, P., Weindl, A., Siebner, H. R., Fassbender, T., et al. (1999). Sensory processing in Parkinson's and Huntington's disease: investigations with 3D H(2)(15)O-PET. *Brain* 122, 1651–1665. doi: 10.1093/brain/122.9.1651

Brodal, P. (1978). The corticopontine projection in the rhesus monkey. Origin and principles of organization. *Brain* 101(part 2), 251–283. doi: 10.1093/brain/101.2.251

Bronfeld, M., and Bar-Gad, I. (2011). Loss of specificity in Basal Ganglia related movement disorders. *Front. Syst. Neurosci.* 5:38. doi: 10.3389/fnsys.2011.00038

Brown, A. R., Hu, B., Antle, M. C., and Teskey, G. C. (2009). Neocortical movement representations are reduced and reorganized following bilateral intrastriatal 6-hydroxydopamine infusion and dopamine type-2 receptor antagonism. *Exp. Neurol.* 220, 162–170. doi: 10.1016/j.expneurol.2009.08.015

Burke, D., Gandevia, S. C., and McKeon, B. (1984). Monosynaptic and oligosynaptic contributions to human ankle jerk and H-reflex. *J. Neurophysiol.* 52, 435–448.

Cantello, R., Gianelli, M., Bettucci, D., Civardi, C., De Angelis, M. S., and Mutani, R. (1991). Parkinson's disease rigidity: magnetic motor evoked potentials in a small hand muscle. *Neurology* 41, 1449–1456. doi: 10.1212/WNL.41.9.1449

Capaday, C., Forget, R., Fraser, R., and Lamarre, Y. (1991). Evidence for a contribution of the motor cortex to the long-latency stretch reflex of the human thumb. *J. Physiol.* 440, 243–255.

Cheney, P. D., and Fetz, E. E. (1984). Corticomotoneuronal cells contribute to long-latency stretch reflexes in the rhesus monkey. *J. Physiol.* 349, 249–272.

Cody, F. W., Macdermott, N., Matthews, P. B., and Richardson, H. C. (1986). Observations on the genesis of the stretch reflex in Parkinson's disease. *Brain* 109(Pt 2), 229–249. doi: 10.1093/brain/109.2.229

Connors, B. W., and Gutnick, M. J. (1990). Intrinsic firing patterns of diverse neocortical neurons. *Trends Neurosci.* 13, 99–103. doi: 10.1016/0166-2236(90)90185-D

Conrad, B., Meyer-Lohmann, J., Matsunami, K., and Brooks, V. B. (1975). Precentral unit activity following torque pulse injections into elbow movements. *Brain Res.* 94, 219–236. doi: 10.1016/0006-8993(75)90058-X

Day, B. L., Riescher, H., Struppler, A., Rothwell, J. C., and Marsden, C. D. (1991). Changes in the response to magnetic and electrical stimulation of the motor cortex following muscle stretch in man. *J. Physiol.* 433, 41–57.

Degardin, A., Houdayer, E., Bourriez, J. L., Destee, A., Defebvre, L., Derambure, P., et al. (2009). Deficient "sensory" beta synchronization in Parkinson's disease. *Clin. Neurophysiol.* 120, 636–642. doi: 10.1016/j.clinph.2009.01.001

Delong, M. R., and Wichmann, T. (2007). Circuits and circuit disorders of the basal ganglia. *Arch. Neurol.* 64, 20–24. doi: 10.1001/archneur.64.1.20

Delwaide, P. J., Pepin, J. L., De Pasqua, V., and De Noordhout, A. M. (2000). Projections from basal ganglia to tegmentum: a subcortical route for explaining the pathophysiology of Parkinson's disease signs? *J. Neurol.* 247(Suppl. 2), II75–II81. doi: 10.1007/PL00007765

Delwaide, P. J., Pepin, J. L., and Maertens De Noordhout, A. (1991). Short-latency autogenic inhibition in patients with Parkinsonian rigidity. *Ann. Neurol.* 30, 83–89. doi: 10.1002/ana.410300115

Dietrichson, P. (1971). Phasic ankle reflex in spasticity and Parkinsonian rigidity. The role of the fusimotor system. *Acta Neurol. Scand.* 47, 22–51. doi: 10.1111/j.1600-0404.1971.tb07462.x

Dietz, V., Quintern, J., and Berger, W. (1981). Electrophysiological studies of gait in spasticity and rigidity. Evidence that altered mechanical properties of muscle contribute to hypertonia. *Brain* 104, 431–449. doi: 10.1093/brain/104.3.431

Emborg, M. E. (2007). Nonhuman primate models of Parkinson's disease. *ILAR J.* 48, 339–355. doi: 10.1093/ilar.48.4.339

Evarts, E. V. (1973). Motor cortex reflexes associated with learned movement. *Science* 179, 501–503. doi: 10.1126/science.179.4072.501

Evarts, E. V., and Tanji, J. (1976). Reflex and intended responses in motor cortex pyramidal tract neurons of monkey. *J. Neurophysiol.* 39, 1069–1080.

Filion, M., Tremblay, L., and Bedard, P. J. (1988). Abnormal influences of passive limb movement on the activity of globus pallidus neurons in parkinsonian monkeys. *Brain Res.* 444, 165–176. doi: 10.1016/0006-8993(88)90924-9

Flaherty, A. W., and Graybiel, A. M. (1991). Corticostriatal transformations in the primate somatosensory sstem. Projections from physiologically mapped body-part representations. *J. Neurophysiol.* 66, 1249–1263.

Fuller, J. H., and Schlag, J. D. (1976). Determination of antidromic excitation by the collision test: problems of interpretation. *Brain Res.* 112, 283–298. doi: 10.1016/0006-8993(76)90284-5

Fung, V. S., Burne, J. A., and Morris, J. G. (2000). Objective quantification of resting and activated parkinsonian rigidity: a comparison of angular impulse and work scores. *Mov. Disord.* 15, 48–55. doi: 10.1002/1531-8257(200001)15:1<48::AID-MDS1009>3.0.CO;2-E

Goldberg, J. H., and Fee, M. S. (2012). A cortical motor nucleus drives the basal ganglia-recipient thalamus in singing birds. *Nat. Neurosci.* 15, 620–627. doi: 10.1038/nn.3047

Hamming, R. W. (1983). *Digital Filters.* Englewood Cliffs NJ: Prentice Hall.

Hammond, P. H. (1955). Involuntary activity in biceps following the sudden application of velocity to the abducted forearm. *J. Physiol.* 127, 23P–25P.

Hattox, A. M., and Nelson, S. B. (2007). Layer V neurons in mouse cortex projecting to different targets have distinct physiological properties. *J. Neurophysiol.* 98, 3330–3340. doi: 10.1152/jn.00397.2007

Hayashi, R., Hashimoto, T., Tada, T., and Ikeda, S. (2001). Relation between changes in long-latency stretch reflexes and muscle stiffness in Parkinson's disease–comparison before and after unilateral pallidotomy. *Clin. Neurophysiol.* 112, 1814–1821. doi: 10.1016/S1388-2457(01)00642-3

Heitz, R. P., Cohen, J. Y., Woodman, G. F., and Schall, J. D. (2010). Neural correlates of correct and errant attentional selection revealed through N2pc and frontal eye field activity. *J. Neurophysiol.* 104, 2433–2441. doi: 10.1152/jn.00604.2010

Holm, S. (1979). A Simple Sequentially Rejective Multiple Test Procedure. *Scand. J. Stat.* 6, 65–70.

Inase, M., Buford, J. A., and Anderson, M. E. (1996). Changes in the control of arm position, movement, and thalamic discharge during local inactivation in the globus pallidus of the monkey. *J. Neurophysiol.* 75, 1087–1104.

Isoda, M., and Hikosaka, O. (2008). Role for subthalamic nucleus neurons in switching from automatic to controlled eye movement. *J. Neurosci.* 28, 7209–7218. doi: 10.1523/JNEUROSCI.0487-08.2008

Kiritani, T., Wickersham, I. R., Seung, H. S., and Shepherd, G. M. (2012). Hierarchical connectivity and connection-specific dynamics in the corticospinal-corticostriatal microcircuit in mouse motor cortex. *J. Neurosci.* 32, 4992–5001. doi: 10.1523/JNEUROSCI.4759-11.2012

Kuramoto, E., Furuta, T., Nakamura, K. C., Unzai, T., Hioki, H., and Kaneko, T. (2009). Two types of thalamocortical projections from the motor thalamic nuclei of the rat: a single neuron-tracing study using viral vectors. *Cereb. Cortex* 19, 2065–2077. doi: 10.1093/cercor/bhn231

Kuypers, H. G. (1981). "Anatomy of the descending pathways," in *Handbook of Physiology. The Nervous System. Motor Control. Section 1, Part 1.*, Vol. 2, eds J. M. Brookhart, V. B. Mountcastle, V. B. Brooks and S. R. Geiger (Bethesda, ML: American Physiological Society), 597–666.

Landgren, S., Phillips, C. G., and Porter, R. (1962). Minimal synaptic actions of pyramidal impulses on some alpha motoneurones of the baboon's hand and forearm. *J. Physiol.* 161, 91–111.

Lee, H. M., Huang, Y. Z., Chen, J. J., and Hwang, I. S. (2002). Quantitative analysis of the velocity related pathophysiology of spasticity and rigidity in the elbow flexors. *J. Neurol. Neurosurg. Psychiatry* 72, 621–629. doi: 10.1136/jnnp.72.5.621

Lee, R. G., and Tatton, W. G. (1975). Motor responses to sudden limb displacements in primates with specific CNS lesions and in human patients with motor system disorders. *Can. J. Neurol. Sci.* 2, 285–293.

Lee, R. G., and Tatton, W. G. (1982). Long latency reflexes to imposed displacements of the human wrist: dependence on duration of movement. *Exp. Brain. Res.* 45, 207–216.

Lefaucheur, J. P. (2005). Motor cortex dysfunction revealed by cortical excitability studies in Parkinson's disease: influence of antiparkinsonian treatment and cortical stimulation. *Clin. Neurophysiol.* 116, 244–253. doi: 10.1016/j.clinph.2004.11.017

Lelli, S., Panizza, M., and Hallett, M. (1991). Spinal cord inhibitory mechanisms in Parkinson's disease. *Neurology* 41, 553–556. doi: 10.1212/WNL.41.4.553

Leon-Sarmiento, F. E., Rizzo-Sierra, C. V., Bayona, E. A., Bayona-Prieto, J., Doty, R. L., and Bara-Jimenez, W. (2013). Novel mechanisms underlying inhibitory and facilitatory transcranial magnetic stimulation abnormalities in Parkinson's disease. *Arch. Med. Res.* 44, 221–228. doi: 10.1016/j.arcmed.2013.03.003

Levin, J., Krafczyk, S., Valkovic, P., Eggert, T., Claassen, J., and Botzel, K. (2009). Objective measurement of muscle rigidity in Parkinsonian patients treated with subthalamic stimulation. *Mov. Disord.* 24, 57–63. doi: 10.1002/mds.22291

Lewis, G. N., and Byblow, W. D. (2002). Altered sensorimotor integration in Parkinson's disease. *Brain* 125, 2089–2099. doi: 10.1093/brain/awf200

Limousin, P., Brown, R. G., Jahanshahi, M., Asselman, P., Quinn, N. P., Thomas, D., et al. (1999). The effects of posteroventral pallidotomy on the preparation and execution of voluntary hand and arm movements in Parkinson's disease. *Brain* 122(Pt 2), 315–327. doi: 10.1093/brain/122.2.315

Mackinnon, C. D., Verrier, M. C., and Tatton, W. G. (2000). Motor cortical potentials precede long-latency EMG activity evoked by imposed displacements of the human wrist. *Exp. Brain Res.* 131, 477–490. doi: 10.1007/s002219900317

Magladery, J. W., Porter, W. E., Park, A. M., and Teasdall, R. D. (1951). Electrophysiological studies of nerve and reflex activity in normal man. IV. The two-neurone reflex and identification of certain action potentials from spinal roots and cord. *Bull. Johns Hopkins Hosp.* 88, 499–519.

Mallet, N., Ballion, B., Le Moine, C., and Gonon, F. (2006). Cortical inputs and GABA interneurons imbalance projection neurons in the striatum of parkinsonian rats. *J. Neurosci.* 26, 3875–3884. doi: 10.1523/JNEUROSCI.4439-05.2006

Marchand-Pauvert, V., Gerdelat-Mas, A., Ory-Magne, F., Calvas, F., Mazevet, D., Meunier, S., et al. (2011). Both L-DOPA and HFS-STN restore the enhanced group II spinal reflex excitation to a normal level in patients with Parkinson's disease. *Clin. Neurophysiol.* 122, 1019–1026. doi: 10.1016/j.clinph.2010.08.015

Marsden, C. D., Merton, P. A., and Morton, H. B. (1972). Servo action in human voluntary movement. *Nature* 238, 140–143. doi: 10.1038/238140a0

Marsden, C. D., Rothwell, J. C., and Day, B. L. (1983). Long-latency automatic responses to muscle stretch in man: origin and function. *Adv. Neurol.* 39, 509–539.

Matthews, P. B. (1991). The human stretch reflex and the motor cortex. *Trends Neurosci.* 14, 87–91. doi: 10.1016/0166-2236(91)90064-2

Matthews, P. B., Farmer, S. F., and Ingram, D. A. (1990). On the localization of the stretch reflex of intrinsic hand muscles in a patient with mirror movements. *J. Physiol.* 428, 561–577.

McCormick, D. A., Connors, B. W., Lighthall, J. W., and Prince, D. A. (1985). Comparative electrophysiology of pyramidal and sparsely spiny stellate neurons of the neocortex. *J. Neurophysiol.* 54, 782–806.

Meara, R. J., and Cody, F. W. (1992). Relationship between electromyographic activity and clinically assessed rigidity studied at the wrist joint in Parkinson's disease. *Brain* 115(Pt 4), 1167–1180. doi: 10.1093/brain/115.4.1167

Meara, R. J., and Cody, F. W. (1993). Stretch reflexes of individual parkinsonian patients studied during changes in clinical rigidity following medication. *Electroencephalogr. Clin. Neurophysiol.* 89, 261–268. doi: 10.1016/0168-5597(93)90105-X

Meunier, S., Pol, S., Houeto, J. L., and Vidailhet, M. (2000). Abnormal reciprocal inhibition between antagonist muscles in Parkinson's disease. *Brain* 123(Pt 5), 1017–1026. doi: 10.1093/brain/123.5.1017

Mitchell, S. J., Richardson, R. T., Baker, F. H., and Delong, M. R. (1987). The primate globus pallidus: Neuronal activity related to direction of movement. *Exp. Brain Res.* 68, 491–505. doi: 10.1007/BF00249793

Montgomery, E. B. Jr. (2007). Basal ganglia physiology and pathophysiology: a reappraisal. *Parkinsonism Relat. Disord.* 13, 455–465. doi: 10.1016/j.parkreldis.2007.07.020

Mortimer, J. A., and Webster, D. D. (1979). Evidence for a quantitative association between EMG stretch responses and Parkinsonian rigidity. *Brain Res.* 162, 169–173. doi: 10.1016/0006-8993(79)90768-6

Noth, J., Schurmann, M., Podoll, K., and Schwarz, M. (1988). Reconsideration of the concept of enhanced static fusimotor drive in rigidity in patients with Parkinson's disease. *Neurosci. Lett.* 84, 239–243. doi: 10.1016/0304-3940(88)90415-6

Noth, J., Schwarz, M., Podoll, K., and Motamedi, F. (1991). Evidence that low-threshold muscle afferents evoke long-latency stretch reflexes in human hand muscles. *J. Neurophysiol.* 65, 1089–1097.

Palmer, E., and Ashby, P. (1992). Evidence that a long latency stretch reflex in humans is transcortical. *J. Physiol.* 449, 429–440.

Pasquereau, B., and Turner, R. S. (2011). Primary motor cortex of the parkinsonian monkey: differential effects on the spontaneous activity of pyramidal tract-type neurons. *Cereb. Cortex* 21, 1362–1378. doi: 10.1093/cercor/bhq217

Pessiglione, M., Guehl, D., Rolland, A. S., Francois, C., Hirsch, E. C., Feger, J., et al. (2005). Thalamic neuronal activity in dopamine-depleted primates: evidence for a loss of functional segregation within basal ganglia circuits. *J. Neurosci.* 25, 1523–1531. doi: 10.1523/JNEUROSCI.4056-04.2005

Powell, D., Threlkeld, A. J., Fang, X., Muthumani, A., and Xia, R. (2012). Amplitude- and velocity-dependency of rigidity measured at the wrist in Parkinson's disease. *Clin. Neurophysiol.* 123, 764–773. doi: 10.1016/j.clinph.2011.08.004

Pruszynski, J. A., Kurtzer, I., Nashed, J. Y., Omrani, M., Brouwer, B., and Scott, S. H. (2011a). Primary motor cortex underlies multi-joint integration for fast feedback control. *Nature* 478, 387–390. doi: 10.1038/nature10436

Pruszynski, J. A., Kurtzer, I., and Scott, S. H. (2011b). The long-latency reflex is composed of at least two functionally independent processes. *J. Neurophysiol.* 106, 449–459. doi: 10.1152/jn.01052.2010

Raoul, S., Roualdes, V., Deligny, C., Leduc, D., Lamy, J. C., Lackmy-Vallee, A., et al. (2012). Subthalamic nucleus stimulation reverses spinal motoneuron activity in parkinsonian patients. *Brain* 135, 139–147. doi: 10.1093/brain/awr267

Rickards, C., and Cody, F. W. (1997). Proprioceptive control of wrist movements in Parkinson's disease. Reduced muscle vibration-induced errors. *Brain* 120(Pt 6), 977–990. doi: 10.1093/brain/120.6.977

Rossini, P. M., Babiloni, F., Bernardi, G., Cecchi, L., Johnson, P. B., Malentacca, A., et al. (1989). Abnormalities of short-latency somatosensory evoked potentials in parkinsonian patients. *Electroencephalogr. Clin. Neurophysiol.* 74, 277–289. doi: 10.1016/0168-5597(89)90058-0

Rossini, P. M., Paradiso, C., Zarola, F., Bernardi, G., Caramia, M. D., Margari, L., et al. (1991). Brain excitability and long latency muscular arm responses: non-invasive evaluation in healthy and parkinsonian subjects. *Electroencephalogr. Clin. Neurophysiol.* 81, 454–465. doi: 10.1016/0168-5597(91)90055-3

Rothwell, J. C. (1990). Long latency reflexes of human arm muscles in health and disease. *Electroencephalogr. Clin. Neurophysiol. Suppl.* 41, 251–263.

Rothwell, J. C., Obeso, J. A., Traub, M. M., and Marsden, C. D. (1983). The behaviour of the long-latency stretch reflex in patients with Parkinson's disease. *J. Neurol. Neurosurg. Psychiatry* 46, 35–44. doi: 10.1136/jnnp.46.1.35

Rubin, J. E., and Terman, D. (2004). High frequency stimulation of the subthalamic nucleus eliminates pathological thalamic rhythmicity in a computational model. *J. Comput. Neurosci.* 16, 211–235. doi: 10.1023/B:JCNS.0000025686.47117.67

Schrader, C., Peschel, T., Dauper, J., Rollnik, J. D., Dengler, R., and Kossev, A. R. (2008). Changes in processing of proprioceptive information in Parkinson's disease and multiple system atrophy. *Clin. Neurophysiol.* 119, 1139–1146. doi: 10.1016/j.clinph.2008.01.005

Shemmell, J., Krutky, M. A., and Perreault, E. J. (2010). Stretch sensitive reflexes as an adaptive mechanism for maintaining limb stability. *Clin. Neurophysiol.* 121, 1680–1689. doi: 10.1016/j.clinph.2010.02.166

Shepherd, G. M. (2013). Corticostriatal connectivity and its role in disease. *Nat. Rev. Neurosci.* 14, 278–291. doi: 10.1038/nrn3469

Simonetta Moreau, M., Meunier, S., Vidailhet, M., Pol, S., Galitzky, M., and Rascol, O. (2002). Transmission of group II heteronymous pathways is enhanced in rigid lower limb of *de novo* patients with Parkinson's disease. *Brain* 125, 2125–2133. doi: 10.1093/brain/awf201

Stebbins, G. T., and Goetz, C. G. (1998). Factor structure of the unified Parkinson's disease rating scale: motor examination section. *Mov. Disord.* 13, 633–636. doi: 10.1002/mds.870130404

Stewart, A., and Foehring, R. C. (2000). Calcium currents in retrogradely labeled pyramidal cells from rat sensorimotor cortex. *J. Neurophysiol.* 83, 2349–2354.

Strafella, A., Ashby, P., Lozano, A., and Lang, A. E. (1997). Pallidotomy increases cortical inhibition in Parkinson's disease. *Can. J. Neurol. Sci.* 24, 133–136.

Suarez, H., Koch, C., and Douglas, R. (1995). Modeling direction selectivity of simple cells in striate visual cortex within the framework of the canonical microcircuit. *J. Neurosci.* 15, 6700–6719.

Swadlow, H. A. (1994). Efferent neurons and suspected interneurons in motor cortex of the awake rabbit: axonal properties, sensory receptive fields, and subthreshold synaptic inputs. *J. Neurophysiol.* 71, 437–453.

Szucs, A. (1998). Applications of the spike density function in analysis of neuronal firing patterns. *J. Neurosci. Methods* 81, 159–167. doi: 10.1016/S0165-0270(98)00033-8

Takada, M., Tokuno, H., Nambu, A., and Inase, M. (1998). Corticostriatal projections from the somatic motor areas of the frontal cortex in the macaque monkey: segregation versus overlap of input zones from the primary motor cortex, the supplementary motor area, and the premotor cortex. *Exp. Brain Res.* 120, 114–128. doi: 10.1007/s002210050384

Tatton, W. G., Eastman, M. J., Bedingham, W., Verrier, M. C., and Bruce, I. C. (1984). Defective utilization of sensory input as the basis for bradykinesia, rigidity and decreased movement repertoire in Parkinson's disease: a hypothesis. *Can. J. Neurol. Sci.* 11, 136–143.

Tatton, W. G., and Lee, R. G. (1975). Evidence for abnormal long-loop reflexes in rigid parkinsonian patients. *Brain Res.* 100, 671–676. doi: 10.1016/0006-8993(75)90167-5

Teravainen, H., Tsui, J. K., Mak, E., and Calne, D. B. (1989). Optimal indices for testing parkinsonian rigidity. *Can. J. Neurol. Sci.* 16, 180–183.

Thompson, K. G., Hanes, D. P., Bichot, N. P., and Schall, J. D. (1996). Perceptual and motor processing stages identified in the activity of macaque frontal eye field neurons during visual search. *J. Neurophysiol.* 76, 4040–4055.

Tsai, C. H., Chen, R. S., and Lu, C. S. (1997). Reciprocal inhibition in Parkinson's disease. *Acta Neurol. Scand.* 95, 13–18. doi: 10.1111/j.1600-0404.1997.tb00061.x

Turner, R., and Delong, M. (2000). Corticostriatal activity in primary motor cortex of the macaque. *J. Neurosci.* 20, 7096–7108.

Turner, R. S., Owens, J. W. Jr., and Anderson, M. E. (1995). Directional variation of spatial and temporal characteristics of limb movements made by monkeys in a two-dimensional work space. *J. Neurophysiol.* 74, 684–697.

Viaro, R., Morari, M., and Franchi, G. (2011). Progressive motor cortex functional reorganization following 6-hydroxydopamine lesioning in rats. *J. Neurosci.* 31, 4544–4554. doi: 10.1523/JNEUROSCI.5394-10.2011

Wu, A. K., McCairn, K. W., Zada, G., Wu, T., and Turner, R. S. (2007). Motor cortex stimulation: mild transient benefit in a primate model of Parkinson disease. *J. Neurosurg.* 106, 695–700. doi: 10.3171/jns.2007.106.4.695

Xia, R., Markopoulou, K., Puumala, S. E., and Rymer, W. Z. (2006). A comparison of the effects of imposed extension and flexion movements on Parkinsonian rigidity. *Clin. Neurophysiol.* 117, 2302–2307. doi: 10.1016/j.clinph.2006.06.176

Xia, R., Powell, D., Rymer, W. Z., Hanson, N., Fang, X., and Threlkeld, A. J. (2011). Differentiation between the contributions of shortening reaction and stretch-induced inhibition to rigidity in Parkinson's disease. *Exp. Brain Res.* 209, 609–618. doi: 10.1007/s00221-011-2594-2

Xia, R., Sun, J., and Threlkeld, A. J. (2009). Analysis of interactive effect of stretch reflex and shortening reaction on rigidity in Parkinson's disease. *Clin. Neurophysiol.* 120, 1400–1407. doi: 10.1016/j.clinph.2009.05.001

Young, M. S., Triggs, W. J., Bowers, D., Greer, M., and Friedman, W. A. (1997). Stereotactic pallidotomy lengthens the transcranial magnetic cortical stimulation silent period in Parkinson's disease. *Neurology* 49, 1278–1283. doi: 10.1212/WNL.49.5.1278

17

A Neurocomputational Theory of How Explicit Learning Bootstraps Early Procedural Learning

Erick J. Paul*[1] *and F. Gregory Ashby*[2]

[1] *Beckman Institute for Advanced Science and Technology, University of Illinois at Urbana, Champaign, IL, USA*
[2] *Department of Psychological and Brain Sciences, University of California, Santa Barbara, Santa Barbara, CA, USA*

Correspondence:
F. Gregory Ashby, Department of Psychological and Brain Sciences, University of California, 552 University Road, Santa Barbara, Santa Barbara, CA 93106, USA
e-mail: ashby@psych.ucsb.edu

It is widely accepted that human learning and memory is mediated by multiple memory systems that are each best suited to different requirements and demands. Within the domain of categorization, at least two systems are thought to facilitate learning: an explicit (declarative) system depending largely on the prefrontal cortex, and a procedural (non-declarative) system depending on the basal ganglia. Substantial evidence suggests that each system is optimally suited to learn particular categorization tasks. However, it remains unknown precisely how these systems interact to produce optimal learning and behavior. In order to investigate this issue, the present research evaluated the progression of learning through simulation of categorization tasks using COVIS, a well-known model of human category learning that includes both explicit and procedural learning systems. Specifically, the model's parameter space was thoroughly explored in procedurally learned categorization tasks across a variety of conditions and architectures to identify plausible interaction architectures. The simulation results support the hypothesis that one-way interaction between the systems occurs such that the explicit system "bootstraps" learning early on in the procedural system. Thus, the procedural system initially learns a suboptimal strategy employed by the explicit system and later refines its strategy. This bootstrapping could be from cortical-striatal projections that originate in premotor or motor regions of cortex, or possibly by the explicit system's control of motor responses through basal ganglia-mediated loops

Keywords: basal ganglia, categorization, computational model, COVIS, declarative, non-declarative, procedural learning

INTRODUCTION

The existence of multiple memory systems was theorized as early as the 1970s (Tulving, 1972), and the idea was more formally stated in the mid-1980s (Tulving, 1985). The distinction between declarative (i.e., explicit, conscious memory for specific events or facts) and non-declarative (i.e., implicit) memory systems is now well established (e.g., Poldrack and Packard, 2003).

The fundamental ideas driving multiple memory system theories have been applied more recently to the domain of category learning. Perhaps the most successful multiple system model of category learning is COVIS (Ashby et al., 1998). COVIS assumes two interacting systems that each map onto previously hypothesized human memory systems (Ashby and O'Brien, 2005). The COVIS explicit system uses declarative memory and mediates learning in tasks that require hypothesis testing, logical reasoning, and the application of verbalizable rules. In contrast, the procedural system uses non-declarative memory and learns to gradually associate motor programs with regions of perceptual space through reinforcement learning (Ashby and Waldron, 1999; Ashby et al., 2007).

Computational and mathematical models based on other theories of human category learning have been described, tested, and compared (e.g., Homa et al., 1979; Hintzman, 1984; Nosofsky, 1986; Kruschke, 1992; Ashby and Maddox, 1993; Smith and Minda, 2000; Love et al., 2004), and even other multiple-systems accounts have been proposed (Erickson and Kruschke, 1998; Anderson and Betz, 2001), though no other model has been formulated with such deep ties to known neurobiology as COVIS. It is precisely because of these neurobiological constraints that COVIS has been such a successful model of human category learning.

The neurobiology underlying its two distinct systems has been well described (Ashby et al., 1998; Ashby and Valentin, 2005; Ashby and Ennis, 2006). Furthermore, the neurobiological motivation of COVIS serves to constrain the model by utilizing the known neural basis of the constituent memory systems responsible for category learning to define the function and implementation of each system. Following is a brief description of the two systems of COVIS.

COVIS

As mentioned above, the explicit system of COVIS learns in tasks that require logical reasoning and explicit rules. This system tests simple hypotheses about category membership by allocating executive attention to single stimulus dimensions and then formulating explicit rules using Boolean algebra (e.g., logical conjunctions). Working memory is used to store candidate rules during testing. The COVIS explicit system is assumed to be mediated by a broad neural network that includes the prefrontal cortex (PFC), the anterior cingulate cortex (ACC), the head of the caudate nucleus, and medial temporal lobe (MTL) structures.

The procedural system of COVIS learns to associate motor programs with multidimensional stimuli via reinforcement learning (Ashby and Waldron, 1999). The neuroanatomical basis is the direct pathway through the basal ganglia. More specifically, for visual stimuli the relevant structures are early visual cortex (excluding V1) and parietal visual areas, posterior putamen, the internal segment of the globus pallidus (GPi), the ventral-anterior and ventral-lateral thalamic nuclei, and premotor cortex [i.e., supplementary motor area (SMA) and/or dorsal premotor cortex (PMd)]. The key site of learning is at cortical-striatal synapses, and plasticity there follows reinforcement learning rules, with dopamine from the substantia nigra pars compacta (SNpc) serving as the training signal.

COVIS assumes that the explicit system dominates in rule-based (RB) category-learning tasks. In RB tasks, the categories can be separated by a rule that is easy to describe verbally. In many cases, only a single stimulus dimension is relevant, although tasks where the optimal strategy is a logical conjunction are also RB. An example is shown in the bottom panel of **Figure 1**. Here, stimuli are discs with alternating black/white bars that vary in their orientation and thickness (or spatial frequency). A simple rule on the thickness dimension successfully accounts for the separation of the categories.

The top panel of **Figure 1** shows an example of an information-integration (II) category–learning task. Here, information about both stimulus dimensions (i.e., orientation and spatial frequency) must be (pre-decisionally) integrated to respond optimally. Note that there is no way to verbalize the optimal strategy in this task (i.e., denoted by the diagonal boundary). RB strategies could be (and frequently are) adopted in II tasks, but such strategies lead to suboptimal performance. COVIS assumes that when the explicit system fails to learn a task of this kind, it passes control to the procedural system.

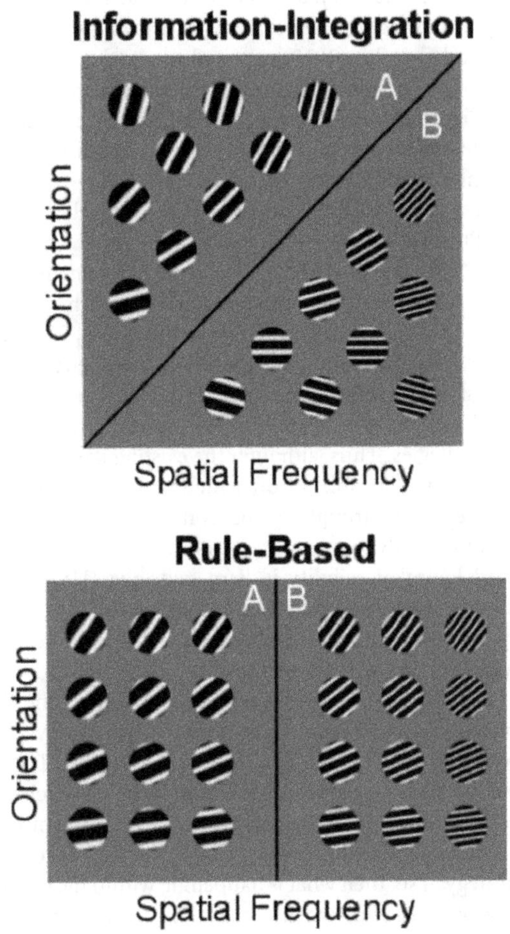

FIGURE 1 | Examples of information-integration and rule-based category-learning tasks. The optimal boundary separating categories is shown as a solid black line.

Many dissociations in learning RB and II categories have been observed across a variety of methodologies and in numerous human and non-human populations (see Ashby and Maddox, 2005, 2011 for reviews). These dissociations strongly support the hypothesis that multiple memory systems contribute to category learning.

INTERACTIONS BETWEEN DECLARATIVE AND PROCEDURAL MEMORY

Although overwhelming evidence now supports the existence of functionally separate declarative and procedural memory systems, much less is known about how these systems interact. The first important question to answer is how a single response is selected, given that either system can presumably control behavior?

Logically, there are at least three possible ways to select a single response when two learning and memory systems are simultaneously active. One possibility is that the outputs of the constituent systems are mixed or blended to produce the final output. This assumption is made by several currently popular categorization models (Erickson and Kruschke, 1998; Anderson and Betz, 2001). Mixture models assume that all categorization responses reflect a mixture of declarative and procedural processes, so that the difference between RB and II tasks is quantitative rather than qualitative—that is, the mixture might weight the declarative output more heavily in an RB task than in an II task, but some weight is always given to both systems. The problem for mixture models is to account for the many behavioral dissociations that have been reported between performance in RB and II tasks. For example, a simultaneous dual task greatly interferes with RB category learning, but not with II learning (Waldron and Ashby, 2001; Zeithamova and Maddox, 2006). If the dual task interferes with the use of declarative memory and responding is always a mixture of declarative and procedural memory processes then it seems that a dual task should interfere with both RB and II learning.

A second logical possibility, which we call *soft switching*, is that only one system controls each response, but that control is passed back and forth between the systems on a trial-by-trial basis. This is the assumption made by the original version of COVIS. More specifically, COVIS assumes that the response on each trial is generated by whichever system is most confident in the accuracy of its response (weighted by a system bias parameter).

Ashby and Crossley (2010) reported results that argue against soft switching. These experiments used hybrid categories (illustrated in **Figure 2**) that were constructed so that perfect performance is possible if participants use a 1D rule on disks with steep orientations and an II strategy on disks with shallow orientations. Nevertheless, fewer than 5% of participants were able to adopt a strategy of the optimal type (solid black line). On the other hand, Erickson (2008) reported the results of an experiment in which about 40% of his participants appeared to switch successfully between declarative (i.e., RB) and procedural (i.e., II) strategies on a trial-by-trial basis. But this experiment provided participants with several explicit cues that signaled which memory system to use on each trial. Despite all of these cues, most participants failed to switch strategies. Thus, although the existing data suggest that some participants are able to soft switch under some conditions, the evidence argues strongly against soft switching as the default mechanism to resolve system interactions.

A third logical possibility is *hard switching* (HS), in which one system is used exclusively and a single switch is made to the other system (when the task demands it). This hypothesis seems most consistent with the available data—in that it accounts for all the RB vs. II behavioral dissociations, as well as the data of Erickson (2008) and Ashby and Crossley (2010). Nevertheless, hard switching faces numerous theoretical challenges. For example, consider an II category-learning task. A hard-switch version of COVIS assumes that participants begin experimenting with explicit strategies, and then when these all fail, switch to a procedural strategy. If so, then what is happening within the procedural system early in learning when declarative memory systems control behavior? One possibility is that no procedural learning occurs until the procedural system controls behavior. This model makes a strong prediction. A suboptimal explicit strategy will

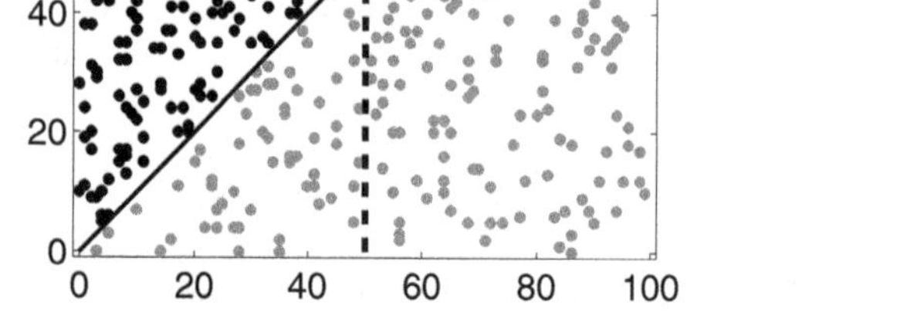

FIGURE 2 | Hybrid categories used by Ashby and Crossley (2010). Each black and gray dot marks the 2D coordinates of a stimulus (e.g., disks varying in spatial frequency and orientation as in **Figure 1**). The solid black line represents the optimal boundary; the dashed black line represents a suboptimal rule-based boundary. Note that the axes are in arbitrary units.

almost always yield performance that is significantly above chance in an II task. Thus, if the procedural system cannot learn while the explicit system controls behavior, then a hard-switch model must predict that accuracy will rise to well above chance and then suddenly fall back to chance when control is passed to the procedural system. To our knowledge, none of the many published II studies has ever reported this strange data pattern.

The second possibility is that the procedural system learns on trials when the explicit system is controlling behavior. COVIS actually predicts such learning because it assumes that each system receives its own separate feedback signal that rewards or punishes the system for recommending either the correct or incorrect response, respectively, regardless of whether that recommendation was used to select the single response made on that trial. These separate feedback signals allow both systems to learn independently of the other, and regardless of whether or not they control responding.

The assumption that the explicit and procedural category-learning systems each receive their own independent feedback signal on every trial is very strong. In most category learning experiments, only a single feedback signal is given that is based entirely on the emitted (observable) response; independent feedback would require sophisticated self-monitoring that might for example, send a reward signal to the procedural system on trials when the emitted response was incorrect. The explicit system might have such flexibility: evidence suggests that the PFC can handle abstract forms of feedback and generate second-order feedback (Ashby et al., 2002; Maddox et al., 2003; Cools et al., 2006; Maddox et al., 2008; Wallis and Kennerley, 2010). On the other hand, the available evidence does not support the hypothesis that the procedural system can self-monitor and generate its own feedback. Learning in the procedural system depends on dopamine signals in the striatum. Dopamine neurons in SNpc respond to rewards and reward-predicting stimuli, and also encode reward prediction error (Schultz et al., 1997, 2000; Tobler et al., 2003), which depends in part on the valence of the feedback. This suggests that the basal ganglia are unable to flexibly manipulate feedback signals, and instead respond to the valence (and expectation) of feedback (and reward). As such, the possibility of independent feedback seems unlikely.

A more plausible solution is to assume that each system receives the feedback elicited by the observable response and that each system must use this common feedback to guide learning. The theoretical challenge for this hypothesis is to show how one system can learn from feedback that is based on the response of the other system. Because the evidence is good that the explicit system dominates during early responding, this question is moot for any tasks that are learned by the explicit system (e.g., RB tasks), because in such cases, evidence suggests that the procedural system is never used. In II tasks however, we expect the explicit system to control early learning and the procedural system to control late learning. The key question addressed by this article is how the procedural system can learn during trials when the explicit system controls responding and there is only a single source of feedback.

To begin, we need to identify a candidate neural mechanism that mediates the competition between the two systems. The hypothesis that the procedural system is able to learn while the explicit system is in control suggests that when in control, the explicit system prevents the procedural system from accessing motor output systems, but does not interfere with learning. Some independent evidence supports this hypothesis (e.g., Packard and McGaugh, 1996; Foerde et al., 2006, 2007).

Given these considerations, Ashby and Crossley (2010) proposed that frontal cortex and the subthalamic nucleus (STN) control system interactions via the hyperdirect pathway through the basal ganglia. The hyperdirect pathway begins with direct excitatory glutamate projections from frontal cortex (via presupplementary cortex, preSMA) to the STN, which sends excitatory glutamate projections directly to the internal segment of the globus pallidus (GPi; Parent and Hazrati, 1995; Joel and Weiner, 1997), making it more difficult for striatal activity to affect cortex. The evidence that the preSMA is in this circuit comes from several sources. First, Hikosaka and Isoda (2010) reviewed evidence that the preSMA is crucial for switching between controlled and automatic responding. Second, Waldschmidt and Ashby (2011) reported that after 20 sessions of practice, the only brain areas in which neural activation correlated with accuracy in an II task were the preSMA and SMA.

Evidence for a role of the STN in this model comes largely from studies using the stop-signal task where participants initiate a motor response as quickly as possible when a cue is presented. On some trials, a second cue is presented soon after the first signaling participants to inhibit their response. A variety of evidence implicates the STN in this task (Aron and Poldrack, 2006; Aron et al., 2007; Mostofsky and Simmonds, 2008). A popular model is that the second cue generates a "stop signal" in cortex that is rapidly transmitted through the hyperdirect pathway to the GPi, where it cancels out the "go signal" being sent through the striatum.

Ashby and Crossley (2010) hypothesized that when the explicit system is controlling behavior a stop signal may inhibit a potentially competing response generated by the procedural system: the PFC could increase STN output via the hyperdirect pathway, preventing the procedural system from influencing cortical motor systems, thereby allowing the explicit system to control the overall response. Note that because the inhibition occurs downstream from the striatum, this hypothesis theoretically allows procedural learning to occur within the striatum. The next section describes several different model architectures that will be used to explore the conditions under which procedural learning can occur with a single source of feedback.

SIMULATION SET 1—COVIS ARCHITECTURES

The basic model that we will use in all investigations is COVIS (Ashby et al., 1998, 2011). The original version of COVIS assumed soft switching and independent feedback. However, to gain more insight into system interactions, we will explore a number of alternative model architectures. For the reasons described above, our focus will be on two model features: the nature of the feedback signal (separate signals to each system vs. a single feedback signal); and the switching mechanism (soft vs. hard). Following are descriptions of three alternative versions of COVIS that explore the effects of varying these two features.

MODEL 0: INDEPENDENT FEEDBACK, SOFT SWITCHING

Our first goal is to implement COVIS computationally as described in Ashby et al. (2011). Only components critical to the simulations will be described; interested readers are encouraged to review the complete description elsewhere (e.g., Ashby et al., 1998, 2011; Hélie et al., 2012a,b). Model 0 is simply the independent feedback model previously described with some simplifications made to each system to improve the likelihood of learning in the procedural system, and to maximize computational efficiency.

First, because our goal is not to elucidate the nature of learning in the explicit system, it was heavily simplified to respond with the most accurate possible one-dimensional rule from the outset of the simulated experiment (in normal applications, the explicit system selects and tests a variety of rules). Thus, in current applications, the explicit system has no free parameters and reduces to the equation below. The response rule is: respond A on trial n if $h_E(x) < 0$; respond B if $h_E(x) > 0$; and the discriminant function is defined as:

$$h_E(x) = x_d - C_d - \varepsilon_E, \tag{1}$$

where x_d is the value of stimulus x on dimension d, C_d is a constant that plays the role of a decision criterion (typically learned; hard-coded here) and ε_E is a normally distributed random variable with mean 0 and variance σ_E^2 that models the variability in both stimulus perception and memory of the decision criterion. When σ_E^2 is large, the discriminant value becomes less deterministic, so σ_E^2 was set to zero in the present application.

The COVIS procedural system is a two-layer connectionist network. The input layer includes 625 input units arranged in a 25 × 25 grid (i.e., because the simulations will use stimuli that vary on two stimulus dimensions). Each input unit is tuned to a particular stimulus, in the sense that it is maximally activated when its preferred stimulus is presented, and it is less activated when similar stimuli are presented. The activation in sensory cortical unit K on trial n is given by

$$I_K(n) = e^{\frac{-d(K,\,\text{stimulus})^2}{\sigma_R}} \tag{2}$$

where $d(K, \text{stimulus})$ is the Euclidean distance (in stimulus space) between the stimulus preferred by unit K and the presented stimulus (i.e., in units of 25 × 25 space). Equation 2 is a radial basis function (e.g., Kruschke, 1992; Riesenhuber and Poggio, 1999). The constant σ_R has the effect of expanding or narrowing the width of the radial basis function, much like a variance.

The output layer in the COVIS procedural system is assumed to represent the striatum. The model includes the same number of output units as there are alternative responses. All simulations described here used two categories (A and B), so all models included two output units. Activation of striatal unit J in the output layer is determined by the weighted sum of activations from the input layer projecting to it:

$$S_J(n) = \sum_{K=1}^{625} w_{K,J}(n) I_K(n) \tag{3}$$

where $w_{K,J}(n)$ is the strength of the synapse between cortical unit K and striatal cell J on trial n. The decision rule in the procedural system is similar to that of the explicit system. The decision rule is: respond A on trial n if $S_A(n) > S_B(n)$; otherwise respond B. The relative activity between striatal units changes as the model learns, and learning is accomplished by adjusting the synaptic weights, $w_{K,J}$ (n), up or down from trial-to-trial via reinforcement learning.

The weights in the procedural system are updated based on the three factors: (1) pre-synaptic activation, (2) post-synaptic activation, and (3) dopamine levels (e.g., Arbuthnott et al., 2000; Ashby and Hélie, 2011). Specifically, $w_{K,J}(n)$ is updated after each trial using the following learning rule:

$$\begin{aligned} w_{K,J}(n+1) = w_{K,J}(n) + \alpha I_K(n)\left[S_J(n) - \theta_{\text{NMDA}}\right]^+ \\ \left[D(n) - D_{\text{base}}\right]^+ \left[w_{\max} - w_{K,J}(n)\right] \\ -\beta I_K(n)\left[S_J(n) - \theta_{\text{NMDA}}\right]^+ \left[D_{\text{base}} - D(n)\right]^+ w_{K,J}(n) \\ -\gamma I_K(n)\left[\theta_{\text{NMDA}} - S_J(n)\right]^+ \left[S_J(n) - \theta_{\text{AMPA}}\right]^+ w_{K,J}(n) \end{aligned} \quad (4)$$

The function $[g(n)]^+ = g(n)$ if $g(n) > 0$, and otherwise $g(n) = 0$. The constant D_{base} is the baseline dopamine level, $D(n)$ is the amount of dopamine released on trial n following feedback, and α, β, γ, θ_{NMDA}, and θ_{AMPA} are all constants. The first three of these (i.e., α, β, and γ) operate like standard learning rates because they determine the magnitudes of increases and decreases in synaptic strength. The constants θ_{NMDA} and θ_{AMPA} represent the activation thresholds for post-synaptic NMDA and AMPA (more precisely, non-NMDA) glutamate receptors, respectively. The numerical value of $\theta_{\text{NMDA}} > \theta_{\text{AMPA}}$ because NMDA receptors have a higher threshold for activation than AMPA receptors. This is critical because NMDA receptor activation is required to strengthen cortical-striatal synapses (Calabresi et al., 1996).

The positive term in Equation (4) describes the conditions under which synapses are strengthened (i.e., striatal activation above the threshold for NMDA receptor activation and dopamine above baseline) and the two negative terms describe conditions that cause the synapse to be weakened. The first possibility (line 3) is that post-synaptic activation is above the NMDA threshold but dopamine is below baseline (as on an error trial), and the second possibility is that striatal activation is between the AMPA and NMDA thresholds. Note that synaptic strength does not change if post-synaptic activation is below the AMPA threshold.

The Equation (4) model of reinforcement learning requires that the amount of dopamine released in response to the feedback signal [that is, the $D(n)$ term] is specified on every trial. COVIS adopts the popular model that, over a wide range, dopamine firing is proportional to the reward prediction error (RPE) (e.g., Schultz et al., 1997; Tobler et al., 2003):

$$\text{RPE} = \text{Obtained Reward} - \text{Predicted Reward} \quad (5)$$

The procedural system of COVIS uses a simple model of dopamine release by first computing both obtained and predicted reward, and then by estimating the amount of dopamine released as a function of RPE.

In applications that do not vary the valence of the rewards, the obtained reward R_n on trial n is defined as

$$R_n = \begin{cases} +1 & \text{if correct feedback} \\ 0 & \text{if no feedback is given} \\ -1 & \text{if error feedback} \end{cases} \quad (6)$$

In models that assume separate, independent feedback signals, the reward signal is based on the response suggested by the procedural system regardless of which system initiated the response. In models that assume a single feedback signal, the reward is based on the observable response. The single-operator learning model (Bush and Mosteller, 1955) is used to compute predicted reward, P_n:

$$P_n = P_{n-1} + \alpha_{\text{pr}}\left(R_{n-1} - P_{n-1}\right) \quad (7)$$

It is well known that when computed in this fashion, P_n converges exponentially to the mean reward value and then fluctuates around this value (until reward contingencies change). The parameter α_{pr} governs how quickly P_n converges.

Finally, to compute the dopamine release to the feedback, a simple model matching empirical results reported by Bayer and Glimcher (2005) is used:

$$D(n) = \begin{cases} 1 & \text{if RPE} > 1 \\ 0.8\text{RPE} + 0.2 & \text{if } -0.25 \leq \text{RPE} \leq 1 \\ 0 & \text{if RPE} < -0.25 \end{cases} \quad (8)$$

Note that the baseline dopamine level is 0.2 (i.e., when RPE = 0) and that dopamine levels increase linearly with RPE between a floor of 0 and a ceiling of 1.

For the final simplification, a strong form of lateral inhibition at the level of the striatum was assumed. Computationally, this amounts to updating only the weights associated with the striatal unit matching the response suggested by the procedural system. For example, if the procedural system suggests an "A" response, only the weights associated with the "A" striatal unit are modified. This simplification effectively serves a dual-purpose: it accelerates learning in the procedural system because only the weights relevant to that trial are updated and improves computational efficiency.

In order to resolve the competition between the systems and to select an overall model response, confidence is measured on every trial by calculating a discriminant value for each system. For the explicit system, the discriminant value equals the distance from the stimulus to the decision bound used by the explicit system. The confidence of the explicit system, which equals $|h_E(n)|$, will be large on any trial where the stimulus is far (in stimulus space) from the response criterion. In the procedural system, confidence is measured by the difference in striatal unit activity and is defined by:

$$|h_P(n)| = |S_A(n) - S_B(n)| \quad (9)$$

Note that as with the explicit system, the procedural system will be highly confident when it strongly favors one response over another. Hence, the explicit system is more confident when the stimulus is far from the bound and the procedural is more confident when the stimulus is strongly associated with one motor response but not the other.

The trust placed in each system is determined by overall system weights, $\theta_E(n)$ and $\theta_P(n)$, where $\theta_E(n) + \theta_P(n) = 1$. Because humans are naturally rule preferring and there is no procedural learning at the beginning of an experiment, COVIS assumes that trust in the explicit system is initially much higher than in the procedural system, hence $\theta_E(1) = 0.99$. Throughout each experiment, the system weights are adjusted based on the success of the explicit system. When the explicit system suggests a correct response,

$$\theta_E(n+1) = \theta_E(n) + \Delta_{OC}\left[1 - \theta_E(n)\right], \tag{10}$$

where Δ_{OC} is a learning rate constant. If instead the explicit system suggests an incorrect response then

$$\theta_E(n+1) = \theta_E(n) - \Delta_{OE}\theta_E(n), \tag{11}$$

where Δ_{OE} is another rate constant. The two regulatory terms on the ends of Eqs. 10 and 11 restrict $\theta_E(n)$ to the range $0 \leq \theta_E(n) \leq 1$. Finally, on every trial, $\theta_P(n) = 1 - \theta_E(n)$. Thus, Equations 10 and 11 also guarantee that $\theta_P(n)$ falls in the range $0 < \theta_P(n) < 1$. The parameters Δ_{OC} and Δ_{OE} control how fast $\theta_E(n)$ changes in response to correct and incorrect feedback, respectively; thus, they also control how quickly $\theta_P(n)$ changes, which is related to how frequently the procedural system will be allowed to generate the overall system response.

The overall system decision rule is to emit the response suggested by the explicit system if $\theta_E(n) \times \mid h_E(n) \mid > \theta_P(n) \times |h_P(n)|$; otherwise emit the response suggested by the procedural system. Notice that this is done on a trial-by-trial basis and that either system may be responsible for the overall response generated depending on the confidence and trust; hence, this a soft-switching model.

All exploratory analyses will be conducted with this model, so that Model 0 will serve as a baseline to compare the effects of modifications to this standard implementation. The simplifications made to the model serve only to optimize learning performance and computational efficiency. It is important to emphasize that the simplifications will only help the procedural system learn faster, so all results should be interpreted as a best-case learning scenario.

MODEL 1: SINGLE SOURCE OF FEEDBACK, HARD SWITCH

The first modified COVIS model follows the revisions suggested by the evidence reviewed above. Specifically, this model only receives a single source of feedback based on the response of the controlling system and assumes that the switch from the explicit to the procedural system is a one-time, hard switch.

The goal of the present research is not to specify exactly how this hard switch is implemented computationally, but instead to evaluate learning in the procedural system under explicit-system controlled responding. For this reason, Model 1 never switches from the explicit to the procedural system. The hyperdirect pathway model places the switching gate downstream from learning in the procedural system (i.e., downstream from the striatum), so the procedural system weights are still modified on every trial. The absence of any switching is a worst-case scenario for a hard-switch model in a procedurally learned task, but it is also the best way to evaluate the ability of the procedural system to learn while the explicit system controls responding (by design, the procedural system will necessarily learn after a switch).

With a single feedback source, and because the model never switches, RPE (Equations 5 and 7) and therefore dopamine Equation (8) will always be driven by the responses of the explicit system. Concretely, reward, R_n is determined only by the explicit system's response to the stimulus (affecting RPE and dopamine calculations). The procedural system will suggest its response normally, but the weights will be updated based on the feedback elicited by the explicit system response. All other features of this model are identical to the implementation of Model 0.

MODEL 2: SINGLE SOURCE OF FEEDBACK, SOFT SWITCH

The second modified COVIS model is a simple modification of Model 0 in which a single source of feedback is used in conjunction with soft switching. Models 1 and 2 together allow procedural-system learning with a single source of feedback to be evaluated both under hard- and soft-switching architectures.

As with Model 0, the switching algorithm described above was used to select between procedural and explicit system responses on every trial. The difference from Model 0 is that, while the explicit system controls the overall response, the procedural system (specifically, RPE and dopamine) is updated using the feedback signal generated by the explicit system's response. On the other hand, whenever the procedural system controls the overall response, the feedback signal is guaranteed to be congruent with the response suggested by the procedural system. All other features of this model are identical to the implementation of Model 0.

A summary of these models and their differences appears in **Table 1**.

METHOD—SIMULATION SET 1

CATEGORIZATION SIMULATIONS

Information-integration categories

Each model was evaluated through simulation to determine whether the procedural system could learn II categories (e.g., as in **Figure 1**, top panel). Human participants reliably learn categories like these, so any multiple systems model of category learning must pass this basic performance benchmark. These simulations served as a first-pass elimination round—any model performing poorly on this category structure should be considered unviable while all successful models will move on to a second simulation experiment. A total of 300 sample stimuli were drawn from each of two bivariate normal distributions (with the category means and variances in **Table 2**). The sample category distributions used are shown in **Figure 3**. Maximum performance by the explicit system on these categories is 78.5%, and the explicit one-dimensional bound (the dashed line) was set to guarantee that the explicit system reached this level of performance.

Model 0 should have no trouble learning these categories as each subsystem receives independent feedback. Models 1 and 2

Table 1 | Summary of each model and brief description of differences.

Name	Feedback type	Switching type	Description
Model 0 (2FB-SS)	Independent (2FB)	Soft (SS)	Original formulation of COVIS where each system receives independent feedback and either system controls responding on a trial-by-trial basis.
Model 1 (1FB-HS)	Single (1FB)	Hard (HS)	Each system is only updated with a single feedback signal from the responding system; switching from explicit to procedural responding occurs once.
Model 2 (1FB-SS)	Single (1FB)	Soft (SS)	Each system is only updated with a single feedback signal from the responding system; system switching is on a trial-by-trial basis.

Table 2 | Mean, variance, and covariance parameters for each category in Figure 3.

Category	μ_x	μ_y	σ_x^2, σ_y^2	$Cov_{x,y}$
A	40	60	167.59	151.26
B	60	40	167.59	151.26

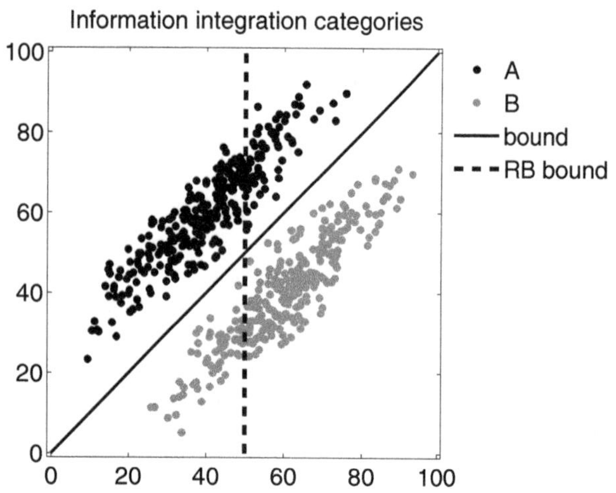

FIGURE 3 | Information integration (II) categories used in the simulation experiments. Each black and gray dot marks the 2D coordinates of a stimulus (e.g., disks varying in spatial frequency and orientation as in **Figure 1**). The solid black line represents the optimal boundary; the dashed black line represents a suboptimal rule-based boundary. Note that the axes are in arbitrary units.

are particularly interesting because, currently, it is unknown if any COVIS model will successfully learn II categories without independent feedback.

Hybrid categories (Ashby and Crossley, 2010)

All models that successfully learned the benchmark II category structures were tested on the hybrid categories shown in **Figure 2** (Ashby and Crossley, 2010). These categories require a 1D rule on disks with steep orientations and an II strategy on disks with shallow orientations, so optimal responding requires trial-by-trial system switching. As mentioned earlier, Ashby and Crossley (2010) reported that only 4% of participants showed any evidence of trial-by-trial switching. An obvious prediction is that soft-switching models will perform well on these categories (i.e., better than human participants), but it is not clear how well hard-switching models will perform.

The hybrid categories shown in **Figure 2** were used in this simulation. A total of 300 stimuli were uniformly sampled from each of two categories separated by the hybrid bound. Maximum performance by the explicit system on these categories is 88.33%, and the one-dimensional bound of the explicit system (the dashed line) was set to this optimal position.

ASSESSMENT OF MODEL PERFORMANCE—PARAMETER SPACE PARTITIONING

The goal of our simulation analyses is not to ask how well each particular model can fit some data set, but rather to ask whether each model is or is not capable of learning. Before concluding that a model cannot learn, it is vital to examine its performance under a wide range of parameter settings. Similarly, when a model does learn, it is important to know whether the learning is representative of the model, or restricted to a small set of parameter settings. Because of these unique modeling goals, we chose to evaluate the performance of each model using a parameter space partitioning (PSP) analysis (Pitt et al., 2006, 2008). PSP is a technique used to investigate the global performance of cognitive models. The basic idea is to exhaustively explore the parameter space (defined by the free parameters of the model) and to map out regions that lead to qualitatively different behaviors (called data patterns).

The end result is a disjoint partitioning of the parameter space into regions that each produces a qualitatively unique behavior (data pattern). The finite set of data patterns must be defined by the experimenter. In order to map out the space, discrete "steps" in the parameter space are each assigned a data pattern. A step is defined as a particular set of numerical values for every parameter that defines the space. Because the computational demands of searching the parameter space increase dramatically with the number of parameters, PSP uses an efficient Markov chain Monte Carlo search algorithm (Pitt et al., 2006). Recall that the implementation of COVIS used here was optimized for computational efficiency so that the parameter space search would be computationally tractable. Once the entire parameter space has been mapped, volumes (i.e., contiguous regions) of the space are computed to quantify the range of parameters that produce a particular data pattern. These volumes describe how likely a behavior is to be produced by the model.

Figure 4 offers a schematic representation of this analysis and related concepts. In this hypothetical example, a simple model is defined by two parameters (θ_1, θ_2). By simultaneously varying these parameters, the model can account for three qualitatively different behaviors or data patterns. These could be almost anything. For example, pattern 1 might be that performance is significantly better in an experimental condition than in a control condition (e.g., at least 5% better), pattern 2 could be the reverse ordering, and pattern 3 might be that performance in the two conditions is not significantly different. The PSP analysis measures the area (or volume when there are 3 or more parameters) of the parameter space that predicts each of the three patterns. In this case, the analysis reveals that for most pairs of parameters, data pattern 1 is produced, but for more restricted sets of parameters, patterns 2 or 3 occur.

IMPLEMENTATION OF PSP

In the following analyses, a MATLAB implementation of the PSP algorithm was obtained from the website of J. I. Myung (http://faculty.psy.ohio-state.edu/myung/personal/psp.html). For the PSP search algorithm to proceed, the model must produce deterministic output (i.e., produce the same behavior) for a given set of parameters. In order to accomplish this, all randomized features of the model must be fixed. All models used here omit the noise (e.g., perceptual and criterial) terms typically included. Thus, the only probabilistic features are the random initial weights for each striatal unit and the randomized stimulus ordering.

In normal applications of the model the stimulus ordering is completely randomized in every simulation. Because of this, the performance of the model averaged across many (i.e., 100 or more) simulations will be robust to stimulus ordering. This is important because Pitt et al. (2006) observed that other models of category learning (e.g., ALCOVE; Kruschke, 1992) are sensitive to stimulus ordering. In addition, the effect of stimulus ordering interacts with the particular initial randomization of weights in the procedural system. To handle these random ordering and initialization effects, it is necessary to choose a fixed random sample on which to run all PSP analyses. For these reasons a random set of 19 random stimulus orderings and weight initializations were generated. Each simulation (each step in the parameter space) was tested on this set, and the model performance was averaged across them. This allowed for deterministic output and relatively stable estimates of the model behavior.

It is necessary to select the parameters defining the parameter space. Including every parameter of the model would be inefficient because the parameter space would be very high dimensional and many parameters interact in predictable ways. For example, in COVIS, if the AMPA and NMDA thresholds (Equation 4) are set too high, then the procedural system will be unable to learn regardless of the values of any other parameters.

Our goal is only to evaluate the ability of learning to proceed in the procedural system, so the parameter space was constrained to parameters that directly affect procedural learning: the learning rates, α and β (Equation 4), and α_{pr} (Equation 7), which determines how fast predicted reward converges to the expected reward value, and therefore affects the trial-by-trial dopamine fluctuations and weight adjustment.

Additionally, for Model 2 only, the system switching rate parameters Δ_{OC} and Δ_{OE} (Equations 10, 11) were also included in the PSP analysis. These parameters directly affect system-switching behavior and learning in the procedural system (note that this is not true for model 0 because the procedural system always receives independent feedback). **Table 3** summarizes the function and search range for each manipulated parameter. Every other parameter was fixed to the specific value shown in **Table 4.** The learning rate parameter γ (Equation 4) was irrelevant because the AMPA and NMDA thresholds were set low enough that the model would never be above AMPA but below NMDA (e.g., line 3 of Equation 4).

The next choice in a PSP analysis is to define the qualitative behaviors (data patterns) that determine the partitioning of the parameter space. We chose to partition based on the accuracy of the procedural system separated into deciles from 0 to 100%; hence, a total of 10 data patterns were possible. For example, data pattern 1 occurs if the procedural system accuracy falls between

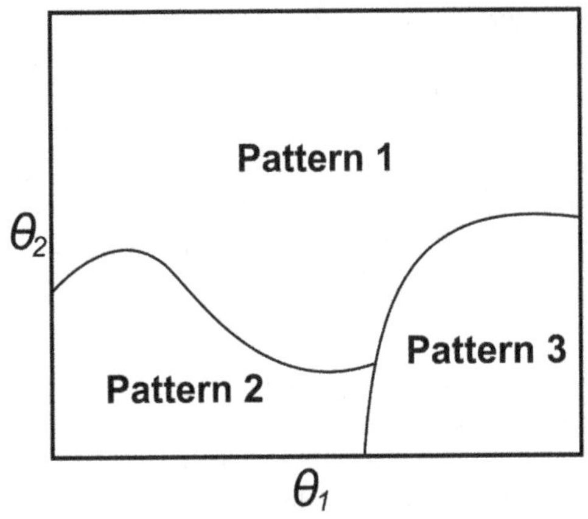

FIGURE 4 | A hypothetical example of parameter space partitioning (PSP) for a model with two parameters, (θ_1 and θ_2). In this example, varying these two parameters allows the model to produce three qualitatively different data patterns. The PSP algorithm efficiently steps through the space to determine which data pattern is produced by each combination of parameters. The curves separate regions where different patterns are predicted. The PSP algorithm returns the area (or volume) of each of these three regions. In this example, pattern 1 accounts for more than 50% of the total area.

Table 3 | Function and search range for each parameter in the PSP analysis.

Parameter	Function	Range
α_{pr}	Controls how fast predicted reward converges, affecting dopamine.	[0.005, 1]
α	Learning rate for strengthening weights.	[0.001, 1]
β	Learning rate for weakening weights.	[0.001, 1]
Δ_{OC}	Controls how explicit system bias grows for correct responses	[0.001, 0.2]
Δ_{OE}	Controls how explicit system bias decays for incorrect responses	[0.001, 0.2]

Table 4 | Values of all parameters that remained fixed across all simulations.

Parameter	Function	Value (for each model)
σ_R	Width of the RBF	4.5
θ_{AMPA}	AMPA threshold	0.01
θ_{NMDA}	NMDA threshold	0.1

0 and 10%, pattern 2 occurs if accuracy falls between 10 and 20%, and so forth. This simple definition of data patterns easily allows for a rough quantification of how well the procedural system performs on the category structure after the weights have been trained.

The PSP analysis proceeded in two stages: the initial partitioning stage, and an evaluation of robustness stage. For the initial stage, each step in the parameter space was tested on all 19 initializations. Each initialization included a training phase, where the model was trained with feedback on the sample stimuli, and a testing phase where end-of-simulation (learned) procedural system weights were run forward through the stimuli again simply to estimate the asymptotic procedural system accuracy. The test performance of the model was averaged over all 19 initializations to determine the final data pattern for each step in the parameter space. The PSP algorithm proceeded for six search cycles to obtain a reliable partitioning of the parameter space.

The complete PSP search returned the volume of parameter space that was associated with each of the 10 data patterns, and a specific set of parameter values that generated each discovered pattern. The robustness stage further tested each model in 200 random stimulus orderings and weight initializations using the parameters returned for each discovered data pattern. This two-stage approach was used because the initial PSP analysis is computationally demanding, so running hundreds of simulations per step in parameter space would be prohibitively time consuming. The second stage is important, though, because it essentially establishes the reliability of the parameters to produce a particular behavior (pattern).

RESULTS—SIMULATION SET 1

MODEL 0: INDEPENDENT FEEDBACK, SOFT SWITCH

Recall that Model 0 is simply the COVIS model as previously described. It is an independent feedback model (i.e., both systems learn independently and receive a separate feedback signal), and uses soft switching (either system can potentially control the overall system response on every trial). This version of Model 0 will be referred to as Model 0 (2FB-SS) because it receives two independent feedback (2FB) signals and uses soft switching (SS).

Information integration categories

Figure 5 shows the percentage of the volume of parameter space that produced each data pattern that was discovered. Note that Model 0 (2FB-SS) showed robust learning of the II categories in the majority of the parameter space (**Figure 5**, first column). A total of three data patterns were found. Over 99.99% of the volume of the parameter space learned the categories at or above

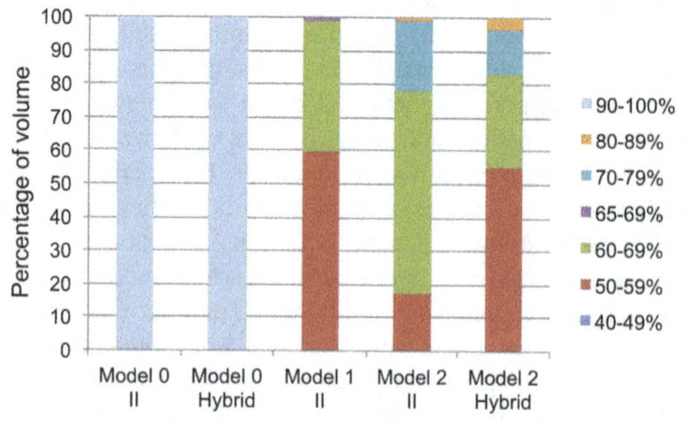

FIGURE 5 | Percentage of volume of the parameter space for each data pattern discovered for every model and category structure. The legend corresponds to test phase accuracy of the procedural system (i.e., possible data patterns). Each color represents a unique data pattern discovered by the PSP for that combination of model/category structure, and the height of the color in the bar corresponds to the volume of parameter space producing that data pattern. The range from 65 to 69% is a special pattern only searched for in model 1 (see text for details).

90% accuracy (Pattern 10). The remaining two data patterns accounted for less than 0.01% of the parameter space volume and corresponded to accuracy in the 70–79% and the 80–89% deciles (Patterns 8 and 9).

Recall that in the Stage 2 analysis, representative parameter values were chosen that produced each of the three observed data patterns and then the model was tested on 200 random stimulus orderings and weight initializations for each of these three parameter settings. In all cases, the performance of the model on these new tests was virtually identical to the performance on the 19 stimulus orderings and weight initializations used in the PSP analysis. Thus, learning in Model 0 (2FB-SS) is highly robust.

Finally, **Figure 6** shows the learned procedural system weights for each striatal unit at the end of training (again, averaged across 200 simulations). It is clear from the figure that a progression of weight strength follows the data patterns: parameters producing the worst model performance led to noisier, smaller weights than parameters producing the best model performance. Still, the success of Model 0 (2FB-SS) in the II categories suggests that it will learn equally well in the hybrid category structures.

Hybrid categories

As with the II categories, Model 0 (2FB-SS) showed very good learning throughout the parameter space with the hybrid categories (**Figure 5**, second column). A total of five data patterns were found. Over 99.94% of the parameter space learned the hybrid categories at or above 90% accuracy. Less than 0.06% of the parameter space was accounted for by data patterns corresponding to the four accuracy deciles between 50 and 90%.

As with the II categories, Model 0 (2FB-SS) showed very robust learning in each region of the parameter space. In all cases, performance on the 200 random initializations was virtually identical to performance on the 19 training initializations. The behavior of the model appears to be very similar for both hybrid and II categories. An examination of the weights showed that they closely mimicked the structure of the hybrid categories (e.g., as the **Figure 6** weights mimic the structure of the II categories).

MODEL 1: SINGLE SOURCE OF FEEDBACK, HARD SWITCH

Recall that Model 1 receives only one feedback signal, and uses hard switching (the explicit system controls responding until it yields control to the procedural system, at which point the procedural system controls responding), so we refer to this model as Model 1 (1FB-HS). Also recall that in these simulations the procedural system is never allowed to respond—in other words, the hard switch never occurs. This way, the ability of the procedural system to learn during explicit system responding can be fully evaluated.

Information integration categories

The partitioning for Model 1 (1FB-HS) required a slight modification to acquire a higher resolution partitioning of the space. In the first partitioning, approximately 62% of the parameter space volume was between 40 and 59% test performance accuracy, and about 38% of the volume was associated with test performance accuracy between 60 and 69%. To create a finer-grained partitioning, for Model 1 (1FB-HS) only the 60–69% decile was subdivided into 60–64 and 65–69% ranges.

Figure 5 shows that the model performed poorly on the II categories. Approximately 60% of the parameter space performed at between 40 and 59% in the test phase, suggesting that, for more than half of the volume, the model produced no measurable learning. About 39% of the parameter space volume showed between 60 and 64% test accuracy and slightly more than 1% of the volume was above 65% test accuracy. The robustness analysis, described in **Figure 7**, shows that **Figure 5** actually overestimates the performance of Model 1 (1FB-HS). While the test performance of the model clearly produces the expected output when averaged across the 19 fixed initializations (dark gray bars), every set of parameters (i.e., for each discovered data pattern) performs no better than 52% in the test phase when averaged across 200 random initializations (light gray bars). Because of the model's II categorization learning failure, the hybrid categories were not explored.

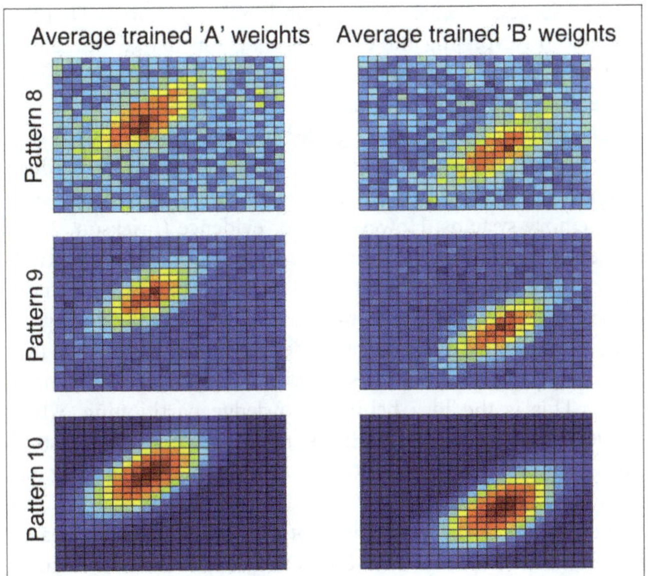

FIGURE 6 | "A" and "B" striatal weights in the procedural system of model 0 (2FB-SS) after training in information integration categories, averaged across 200 simulations. Blue (cool colors) represent small weights whereas red (warm colors) represent large weights. Patterns 8, 9, and 10 refer to the 70–79, 80–89, and 90–100% performance deciles, respectively. Note the good correspondence between the high-performing bottom row weights (Pattern 3) and the stimuli plotted in **Figure 3**, and also the weaker correspondence in the lower-performing weights.

MODEL 2: SINGLE SOURCE OF FEEDBACK, SOFT-SWITCH

Model 2 (1FB-SS) receives only one source of feedback [as in Model 1 (1FB-HS)], and uses soft switching [either system can potentially control the overall system response on every trial [as in Model 0 (2FB-SS)].

Information integration categories

The partitioning for Model 2 (1FB-SS) was comparatively diverse, suggesting that this model is capable of a wider range of behaviors. A total of 6 data patterns were discovered for the II categories (**Figure 6**, fourth column). The percentage of volume associated with each data region is also shown in **Table 5**. Although the model is capable of responding with accuracy above 90%, this behavior occurs only for a very small proportion of the parameter space. In fact, accuracy in the test phase was below 70% for approximately 80% of the parameter space. Overall, each data pattern appeared relatively robust across the 200 simulations. Only data patterns 3 and 4 performed worse (10 and 6%, respectively) on the 200 simulations than on the 19 fixed initializations. Hence, the performance of this model seems to be reliable.

Although only a small proportion (approximately 1%) of the overall parameter space was associated with test performance at or above 80% after training, the results suggest that for a restricted range of parameters, this model can successfully learn II categories with only a single source of feedback.

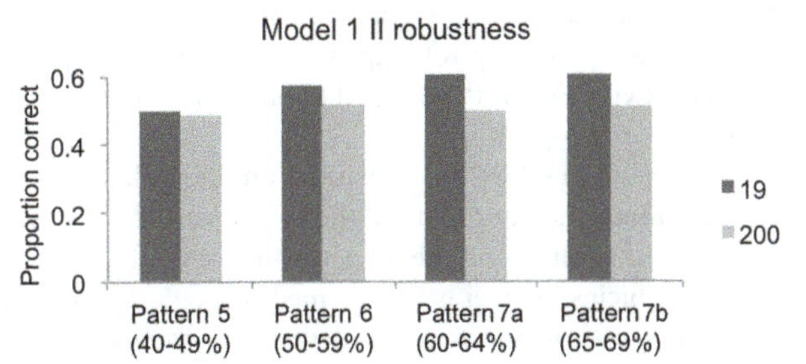

FIGURE 7 | Robustness of Model 1 (1FB-HS) in II categories for each of four discovered data patterns. Dark gray bars represent the performance of the model (proportion correct in the test phase) for the 19 fixed initializations used in the PSP analysis; light gray bars represent the performance of the model across 200 random initializations. In every case, the stage 2 analysis using 200 simulations failed to reproduce the patterns observed in the PSP across the 19 fixed initializations suggesting that the observed PSP performance was not robust. Note that the 60–69% performance decile was separated into two patterns (7a and 7b) for a more fine-grained evaluation.

Table 5 | Percentage of parameter space volume for each observed data pattern (or test phase accuracy ranges) for Model 2 (1FB-SS).

Category	Test phase accuracy range (data patterns)					
	40–49%	50–59%	60–69%	70–79%	80–89%	≥90%
II	0.002	17.075	61.113	20.718	0.949	0.143
Hybrid	0.032	54.875	28.374	13.036	3.556	0.127

Hybrid categories

The performance of Model 2 (1FB-SS) on the hybrid categories was similar to its performance on the II categories. The same data patterns were observed, and the parameter space volumes associated with each of these patterns were similar (compare the 4th and 5th columns of **Figure 5**). When tested across the 200 random initializations, the model's performance was robust.

Soft switching drives learning in the procedural system

The ability of Model 2 (1FB-SS) to learn at all is in stark contrast to Model 1. The only difference between those models is the switching mechanism—Model 1 uses hard switching, whereas Model 2 uses soft switching. These results suggest that the switching mechanism is allowing the procedural system to learn in Model 2 (1FB-SS). For example, when the model switches to the procedural system, the procedural system receives veridical feedback, which should facilitate procedural learning. Note that this hypothesis predicts that model accuracy should increase with the proportion of trials controlled by the procedural system. To test this prediction, we computed the correlations between accuracy and the number of procedural system responses for Model 2 (1FB-SS) separately on the II and hybrid categories, both for the 19 training initializations and the 200 random initializations. All four of these correlations were $r \geq 0.97$ (all $p < 0.001$).

Given that the procedural system only learns when it is parameterized so that it generates the majority (nearly 90%) of responses, a follow-up test was conducted to evaluate whether the procedural system would take over control of responding with simple RB categories (**Figure 1**, bottom panel). The RB categories were created by rotating the II categories (**Figure 3**) counter-clockwise so that the optimal bound (solid black line) is vertical.

The model was run for 200 simulations on these RB categories using the parameters that produced the best II learning (i.e., pattern 6). In these simulations, the RB performance was hard-coded so that the explicit system either performed at 90, 95, 99, or 100% accuracy. These simulations revealed that the average proportion of trials where the procedural system controlled responding was 0.84, 0.76, 0.41, and 0.00, respectively. This is fundamentally problematic because the explicit system should overwhelmingly control responding in RB tasks, especially when it is performing at such high accuracy levels.

DISCUSSION—SIMULATION SET 1

The results of the PSP analyses reveal the strength and limitations imposed by the feedback signal. First, when each system receives independent feedback (Model 0, 2FB-SS), the procedural system of COVIS readily learns to respond accurately in both II and hybrid categories. This is problematic because the model performs substantially better than humans in the hybrid task. Soft switching allows the model to pass control to the procedural system, which easily learns the hybrid categories. It is important to recall that Model 0 (2FB-SS) was designed deliberately to maximize learning. For this reason, our results represent a best-case scenario for this model.

In contrast, procedural learning was seriously compromised when both systems received the same feedback signal. Although the PSP for Model 1 hinted at a small amount of learning in the procedural system, that learning depended critically on the exact ordering of the stimuli during training, because during test the apparent learning disappeared. Note that Model 1 failed to learn even though the explicit system received correct feedback more than 75% of the time. This was because the feedback was independent of any activation within the procedural system, and thus it had the same effect as if the feedback was random.

Of course, the procedural system of Model 1 would learn *after* the hard switch occurs. But our results show clearly that the procedural system learns nothing until it controls responding in the task. Thus, in the II task simulated here, Model 1 predicts that accuracy should drop from around 75% correct to chance on the trial of the hard switch. As noted earlier, we know of no II studies that have reported such a mid-session drop in accuracy.

Finally, the results from Model 2 (1FB-SS) show that with soft switching, the procedural system of COVIS can learn provided that it controls responding for the majority of trials in the experiment. In other words, when the procedural system is allowed to generate the overall response for a large proportion of the training trials, it successfully learns to respond to the categories. That this occurs is unsurprising and essentially suggests that, within a narrow range of parameterizations, the model learns with one source of feedback in a serial fashion.

The empirical evidence (e.g., Ashby and Crossley, 2010) suggests that soft switching is not the dominant method via which humans resolve competition between declarative and procedural memory systems. However, other evidence (Erickson, 2008) suggests that a minority of humans seem to be able to switch trial-by-trial if given enough cues, so it may be the case that under some conditions, soft switching could occur naturally during the course of learning. When the task demands are clear, people may successfully adopt different strategies and flexibly shift among them. This is the idea behind knowledge partitioning, where participants learn to apply different strategies to different stimuli within one task (Lewandowsky and Kirsner, 2000; Yang and Lewandowsky, 2004).

Regardless of the plausibility of soft switching, the greatest problem with Model 2 (1FB-SS) is that it only predicts learning in the procedural system when the procedural system dominates responding in the task, regardless of whether that task is RB or II. This is problematic because the model predicts that even one-dimensional RB tasks will frequently be learned procedurally—a prediction that is strongly contradicted by the literature (e.g., Waldron and Ashby, 2001).

The results of these simulations largely suggest that with a single feedback source, simply modifying the system switching mechanism is not sufficient to account for human learning data. Regardless of the switching mechanism, the results show that learning in the procedural system is possible only if the procedural system controls responding throughout the majority of training.

ADDITIONAL COVIS MODIFICATIONS—THE BOOTSTRAPPING HYPOTHESIS

All of the models so far investigated predict no procedural learning while the explicit system controls responding. If we take for granted that the procedural system learns even while it does not control responding, then it appears that another modification to the architecture of COVIS may be necessary. One possibility is that the explicit system somehow trains or bootstraps the procedural system while it controls responding.

Although speculative, this could occur if the procedural system is somehow informed of the response the explicit system generates. As discussed above, the problem with the single feedback models so far investigated is that when the explicit system controls responding, the feedback it elicits is independent of activity within the procedural system. In other words, any change in cortical-striatal weights is as likely to be rewarded as any other change. If the procedural system is somehow fed information about the explicit system response, however, then this independence could disappear, which might allow the procedural system to learn from the explicit system.

IMPLEMENTING BOOTSTRAPPING IN COVIS

In order to implement bootstrapping in COVIS, a simple modification was made. Recall from earlier that, on every trial, the explicit system generates a discriminant value, $h_E(n)$, that quantifies the overall output of the explicit system's response. Also recall that, on every trial, each striatal unit produces an overall activation value that is driven by the stimulus. For example, activation in striatal unit J on trial n is denoted by $S_J(n)$ (i.e., see Equation 3). Using these values, the following modification was made to reflect the hypothesis that the procedural system is privy to the response generated by the explicit system whenever the explicit system controls responding. If the explicit system controls the overall response and emits a response corresponding to category J on trial n, set

$$S_J(n) = S_J(n) + \mid h_E(n) \mid \tag{12}$$

and make no changes to $S_K(n)$, for all $K \neq J$.

This modification makes no changes to the parameters of the model; it only makes a new assumption about the flow of information when the explicit system is generating the overall system response. Specifically, it assumes that information about the explicit system's response is fed back into the procedural system at the level of the striatum and only to the striatal unit matching the response of the explicit system. Ramping up the activity of the striatal unit corresponding to the response generated by the explicit system translates into larger changes in the weights associated with that striatal unit (see the reinforcement learning equation, Equation 4). The timing of this ramping-up of activity only needs to occur before feedback is given to the model, and because the explicit system discriminant value $h_E(n)$ is related to the explicit system decision, one can further assume that this information transfer occurs in tandem with the explicit system decision.

One attractive property of this modification is that it does not necessarily override the output of the procedural system. For example, suppose that the procedural system has been partially trained in an II categorization task, so its weights have been modified to respond accurately. The explicit system may make an incorrect "A" response to a stimulus, but because the procedural system has been trained, it is suggesting a correct "B" response with high confidence. The explicit system discriminant value $h_E(n)$ would be added to the striatal unit response $S_A(n)$, but $S_B(n)$ could still be larger and thus, the procedural system's output would not be washed out by the explicit system.

Early in training when the procedural system has not yet learned anything, both $S_A(n)$ and $S_B(n)$ will be approximately equal, so the explicit system's output will nudge learning in the procedural system in the direction of the explicit system's response when the weights are updated. The end result should be procedural system weights that are updated to reflect the response strategy of the explicit system as long as the explicit system controls responding.

SIMULATION SET 2—BOOTSTRAPPED COVIS ARCHITECTURES

This section explores two COVIS architectures (Models 1 and 2) with bootstrapping implemented. The general methodology and presentation of results will follow those already described and presented. Bootstrapping Model 0 (2FB-SS) is unnecessary as it receives independent feedback in each system.

MODEL 1: SINGLE SOURCE OF FEEDBACK, HARD SWITCH, BOOTSTRAPPED

This model is exactly as described above with the additional bootstrapping modification. It will be referred to as Model 1 (1FB-HS-B) because it receives only a single source of feedback (1FB), assumes hard switching, and is bootstrapped (B) by the explicit system.

MODEL 2: SINGLE SOURCE OF FEEDBACK, SOFT SWITCH, BOOTSTRAPPED

Model 2 (1FB-SS-B) is exactly as described above with the additional bootstrapping modification.

METHOD—SIMULATION SET 2

The methods of assessment for both models were identical to those described for simulation set 1.

RESULTS—SIMULATION SET 2

MODEL 1 (1FB-HS-B)

Information integration categories

The PSP on Model 1 (1FB-HS-B) was definitive: only one data pattern was discovered, corresponding to test phase accuracies greater than 90%. This suggests that across all parameter values (at least for the parameters defining the parameter space) the model learns II categories handily. The robustness analysis showed that the performance of the model across the 200 random simulations were essentially identical as across the 19 training simulations. Thus, the model is highly robust. Recall, however, that the suboptimal explicit strategy only performs at about 78% correct in II categories. How, then can the procedural system outperform the suboptimal strategy it was trained on?

A careful evaluation of the procedural system weights provides insight. The average trained procedural system weights across 200 simulations appear different than in previous models; the weights now show a residual trace of the vertical bound used by the explicit system (**Figure 8**, top). The effects of the explicit system training are most easily seen in the bottom of **Figure 8**, which shows a ratio of the A and B weights (i.e., A/B and B/A). Here, the solid red vertical line approximately corresponds to the boundary used by the explicit system. Note the small regions to the right and left of the bound in the A/B and B/A ratios, respectively. These are the regions where the procedural system weights are driven to zero due to the incorrect responses being made by the explicit system (top row, yellow arrows).

In other words, the procedural system not only learns to make the responses that the explicit system gets correct, but it also learns to avoid responses made by the explicit system that were incorrect. This analysis resolves the apparent paradox of how the procedural system was able to outperform the system that trained it.

Hybrid categories

The partitioning for Model 1 (1FB-HS-B) on the hybrid categories was similar to the II partitioning. The PSP algorithm discovered two data patterns corresponding to 80–89% test phase accuracy and greater than 90% test phase accuracy. The volume estimate was nearly 100% for the pattern corresponding to >90% test accuracy. The model's performance was also very robust across 200 simulations.

As with the II categories, the weights learned by the procedural system show a residual trace of the explicit system training. This is most easily seen in **Figure 9**, which shows a ratio of the A and B weights. Note that, as with the II categories, the procedural system weights for the striatal unit where incorrect responses are made appear to be driven toward zero in the region where the explicit system responds incorrectly. Specifically, notice in the bottom right panel that there are some large positive values to the left of the explicit system's approximated bound. These large positive values in the ratio are due to the A-weights being very close to zero in those regions. Again, the procedural system learns what response not to make in this region.

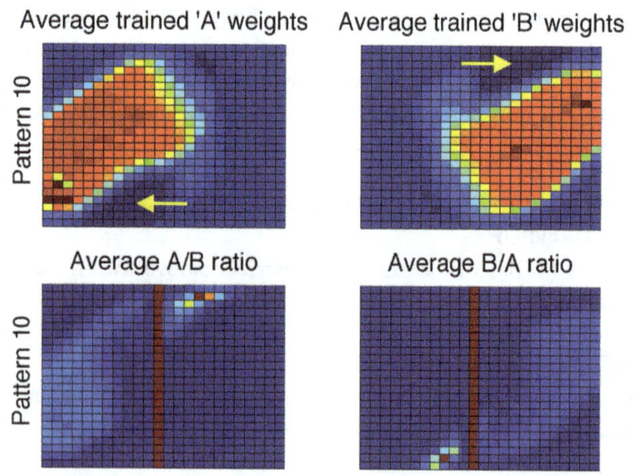

FIGURE 8 | Top: Striatal weights in the procedural system of Model 1 (1FB-HS-B) trained on II categories, averaged across 200 simulations. Blue (cool colors) represent small weights whereas red (warm colors) represent large weights. Note the qualitative difference between these weights and those in **Figure 6**. **Bottom:** Ratio of procedural system weights. Solid vertical line approximately corresponds to the explicit system rule-based bound. Note that large values in the ratio correspond to regions where the weights in the denominator are driven toward zero (darkest blue regions in the top row indicated by yellow arrows).

MODEL 2 (1FB-SS-B)

Information integration categories

The PSP analysis found only two data patterns corresponding to 80–89% and >90% test phase accuracy. Again, the volume of parameter space was nearly 100% for the >90% data pattern, and again, the model's performance was very stable across 200 simulations using random stimulus orderings and weight initializations. The pattern of weights learned by Model 2 (1FB-SS-B) were functionally identical to the weights learned by Model 1 (1FB-HS-B).

The only noteworthy difference between the models is that in Model 2 (1FB-SS-B), the procedural system is sometimes allowed to generate the overall system response. Recall that, in Model 2 (1FB-SS), the procedural system could learn, but only when the procedural system dominated responding (nearly 90% of all responses). This, however, was not a learning requirement in Model 2 (1FB-SS-B). Across 200 simulations, for pattern 9 (80–89% accuracy in the test phase), the procedural system only generated 7% of the overall responses on average; for pattern 2 (>90% test phase accuracy), the procedural system generated about 40% of the overall responses.

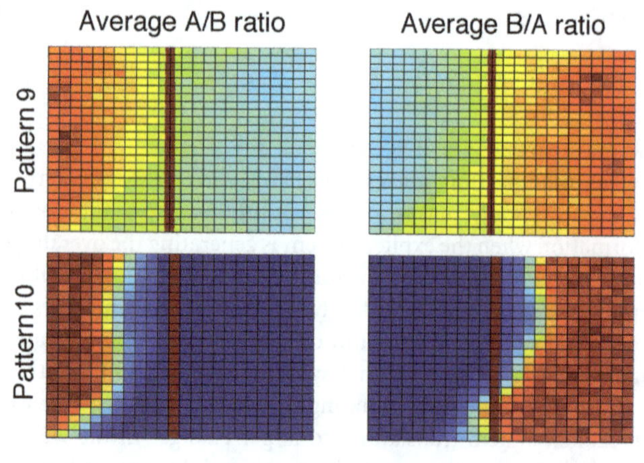

FIGURE 9 | Ratio of procedural system weights in Model 1 (1FB-HS-B) trained with hybrid categories. Solid vertical line approximately corresponds to the explicit system rule-based bound.

Thus, procedural system learning in Model 2 (1FB-SS-B) is not critically dependent on the procedural system taking over the task.

Hybrid categories

Again, the PSP analysis only found two data patterns for Model 2 (1FB-SS-B) in the hybrid categories and nearly 100% of the volume of the parameter space was assigned to the pattern corresponding to >90% test phase accuracy. The performance of the model was also very robust across 200 simulations. The learned weights to those learned by Model 1 (1FB-HS-B).

Finally, as with the II categories, the success of Model 2 (1FB-SS-B) no longer hinged critically on the procedural system dominating the training phase. Across 200 simulations, the procedural system of Model 2 (1FB-SS-B) never accounted for more than 7% of the overall responses, on average (i.e., no parameterization caused the procedural system to dominate responding as before).

DISCUSSION—SIMULATION SET 2

With the addition of bootstrapping, there was a striking difference in the model's performance using only a single source of feedback. Basically, the bootstrapping modification allowed the feedback elicited by the responses of the explicit system to become useful to the procedural system. Model 1 failed to learn without bootstrapping whereas, with bootstrapping, it learned the categories well, even without ever generating a response. Model 2's performance previously depended on soft switching, which allowed the procedural system to dominate responding, but with the bootstrapping mechanism implemented, the model no longer required control.

Notably, the bootstrapping models learn both to respond and to not respond in certain regions of stimulus space, effectively allowing the procedural system to learn the categories better than the explicit system even though the procedural system only gets feedback based on the suboptimal explicit system strategy. This is a unique and strong prediction, which should be interpreted with some caution—recall that the models were biased toward learning very well, so it may be that, with a full explicit system and noise, the procedural system might not show such a dramatic performance improvement. This would be more in line with observed learning in human studies (i.e., learning curves generally have no large discontinuities from sudden drops or jumps in accuracy). However, even with noise, the weights in the procedural system should change in the same general fashion, so it seems that, with bootstrapping, the procedural system is capable of learning a little better than the explicit system, and once it is allowed to take over, refine its strategy.

Finally, it is interesting that in the soft switching Model 2 (1FB-SS-B), the procedural system was able to make as many as 40% of the overall responses with II categories, but not more than 7% with hybrid categories. This result is in line with the observation in Ashby and Crossley (2010) that humans tend to persist with suboptimal RB strategies with hybrid categories. Overall, learning in both models presented here is nearly identical. The current simulations, therefore, do not support a hard switching mechanism over a soft switching mechanism. With the assumption of bootstrapping, these simulations only confirm that the procedural system can learn with one source of feedback, regardless of the switching mechanism.

GENERAL DISCUSSION

The simulations show clearly that the procedural system can learn with one source of feedback as long as the response generated by the explicit system is communicated back to the procedural system (i.e., via bootstrapping). Specifically, the model assumes that this information is passed back to the procedural system at the level of the striatum. COVIS is a model constrained by neurobiology, so although the simulations reported above verify that bootstrapping is a plausible computational mechanism that allows the procedural system to learn during explicit system control, an ideal model would identify a neurobiologically plausible explanation for how bootstrapping could work in a human brain.

There are a number of possible specific pathways via which the procedural system could receive an efferent copy of the explicit system motor response. In general, the challenge for all these accounts is that this efferent motor signal must project to the same striatal targets in the procedural system that receive the relevant visual input. Unfortunately, current neuroanatomy is not precise enough to draw any strong conclusions. Thus, the possibilities considered in this section must all be considered speculative. Hopefully, future research will clarify this issue.

The organizing scheme of the basal ganglia is characterized by parallel cortical-striatal-cortical projection loops (Alexander et al., 1986; Parent and Hazrati, 1995; DeLong and Wichmann, 2007). For this reason, one obvious hypothesis is that an efferent copy of the explicit system response is passed back to the striatum via direct cortical-striatal projections from premotor or motor areas of cortex to the striatal regions responsible for procedural learning. Within premotor areas, one intriguing possibility is that the signal originates in ventral premotor cortex (PMv), which is a likely candidate for the first motor-target of the explicit system.

Tracing and direct stimulation studies have found that premotor and motor regions project to distinct regions of the striatum (Takada et al., 1998; Nambu et al., 2002). Specifically, neurons from primary motor cortex (M1) send projections to medial aspects of the putamen, and neurons in premotor cortex project to dorsolateral regions of the putamen. Further evidence suggests connectivity patterns are both segregated and overlapping (Draganski et al., 2008), and also in accordance to the same somatotopic organization in cortex (Jones et al., 1977; Flaherty and Graybiel, 1993; Takada et al., 1998), which together suggest that the projections may indeed terminate in the general regions of the striatum responsible for executing the motor responses of the procedural system.

Recent studies have found different kinds of projections from M1 cortical layer V into the striatum. For example, Parent and Parent (2006) found not only direct projections from M1 into the striatum, but also indirect projections via long-range pyramidal tract neurons that form en passant synapses across wide regions. It is believed that these different projections actually stem from two different classes of layer V pyramidal neurons (Molnár and Cheung, 2006): those that send projections within the cortex and basal ganglia (IT-type) and those that send projections to deeper structures, brain stem, and spinal cord (PT-type; Reiner et al., 2003, 2010).

Another well-known organizing principle within the basal ganglia is the direct- and indirect-pathways (Albin et al., 1989; Gerfen, 1992; Pollack, 2001). Both pathways receive excitatory cortical input, but the direct pathway has the effect of increasing striatal output whereas the indirect pathway has the opposite effect. Some evidence now suggests that direct pathway striatal neurons receive input predominantly from IT-type neurons, whereas the indirect pathway neurons receive input largely from PT-type neurons (Reiner et al., 2003, 2010; Lei et al., 2004), and that short projecting IT-type neurons convey a different motor signal to the striatum than the motor signal conveyed to the spinal cord via long projecting neurons (Bauswein et al., 1989; Turner and DeLong, 2000). In contrast, the long projecting PT-type neurons may communicate to the striatum an efferent copy of the motor signals being sent to the spinal cord (Parent and Parent, 2006). Reiner et al. (2010) thus proposed a theory that these inputs ultimately lead to different kinds of motor modulation within the striatum. Specifically, they suggested that IT-type neuronal projections to the striatum facilitate planned motor actions along the direct pathway and that PT-type projections stymie conflicting motor actions along the indirect pathway.

This hypothesis suggests that projections to the indirect pathway might teach the procedural system what responses not to make early on during explicit system control by driving weights toward zero in regions where the suboptimal explicit strategy yields incorrect responses. Similarly, projections to the direct pathway could teach the procedural system when there is agreement between the explicit system's strategy and the categories by increasing weights. Broadly speaking, the differential effects of these cortical-striatal projections would translate to increasing one striatal response and decreasing another, which has the overall effect of increasing the output of the elicited motor response relative to the not-elicited response. Although there is no indirect pathway in COVIS, this is computationally the effect achieved by adding the output of the explicit system to the procedural system. Furthermore, it would be straightforward to implement COVIS with the addition of the indirect pathway. Even if this dichotomy between projections to the striatum is incorrect, the existence of projections from cortical motor regions to the striatal nuclei hypothesized to mediate procedural learning is well-established, and thus a plausible pipeline through which explicit system responses are communicated to the procedural system.

A very different alternative possibility is that the explicit system executes its motor response by activating the striatum, in which case the information about its response might automatically be communicated to the striatum. In other words, this hypothesis predicts that the striatum is involved in explicitly produced, volitional movements, either at the level of generation or execution of motor movements. Striatal involvement in volitional movement is corroborated by PET (Roland et al., 1982; Jueptner and Weiller, 1998), and fMRI (Cunnington et al., 2002) experiments. Neurophysiological studies in non-human primates provide more direct evidence (e.g., Romo et al., 1992; Schultz and Romo, 1992). In those experiments, striatal neurons responded to self-initiated movement, either leading up to the movement (suggesting involvement in generating the motor action), or with the movement (suggesting involvement in executing the motor action).

Although the exact computational mechanism is currently unknown, the available neurobiological evidence supports the possibility that the procedural system of COVIS can be bootstrapped by the explicit system before it takes over responding in a perceptual category-learning task. This bootstrapping could be from cortical-striatal projections from premotor or motor regions into the striatum, or possibly by the explicit system's control of motor responses through basal ganglia-mediated loops.

ACKNOWLEDGMENTS

This research was supported in part by AFOSR grant FA9550-12-1-0355, NIH (NINDS) Grant No. P01NS044393, and by Grant No. W911NF-07-1-0072 from the U.S. Army Research Office through the Institute for Collaborative Biotechnologies.

REFERENCES

Albin, R. L., Young, A. B., and Penney, J. B. (1989). The functional anatomy of basal ganglia disorders. *Trends Neurosci.* 12, 366–375. doi: 10.1016/0166-2236(89)90074-X

Alexander, G., DeLong, M. R., and Strick, P. L. (1986). Parallel organization of functionally segregated circuits linking basal ganglia and cortex. *Annu. Rev. Neurosci.* 9, 357–381. doi: 10.1146/annurev.neuro.9.1.357

Anderson, J. R., and Betz, J. (2001). A hybrid model of categorization. *Psychon. Bull. Rev.* 8, 629–647. doi: 10.3758/BF03196200

Arbuthnott, G. W., Ingham, C. A., and Wickens, J. R. (2000). Dopamine and synaptic plasticity in the neostriatum. *J. Anat.* 196, 587–596. doi: 10.1046/j.1469-7580.2000.19640587.x

Aron, A. R., Behrens, T. E., Smith, S., Frank, M. J., and Poldrack, R. A. (2007). Triangulating a cognitive control network using diffusion-weighted magnetic resonance imaging (MRI) and functional MRI. *J. Neurosci.* 27, 3743–3752. doi: 10.1523/JNEUROSCI.0519-07.2007

Aron, A. R., and Poldrack, R. A. (2006). Cortical and subcortical contributions to stop signal response inhibition: role of the subthalamic nucleus. *J. Neurosci.* 26, 2424–2433. doi: 10.1523/JNEUROSCI.4682-05.2006

Ashby, F. G., Alfonso-Reese, L. A., Turken, A. U., and Waldron, E. M. (1998). A neuropsychological theory of multiple systems in category learning. *Psychol. Rev.* 105, 442–481. doi: 10.1037/0033-295X.105.3.442

Ashby, F. G., and Crossley, M. J. (2010). Interactions between declarative and procedural-learning categorization systems. *Neurobiol. Learn. Mem.* 94, 1–12. doi: 10.1016/j.nlm.2010.03.001

Ashby, F. G., and Ennis, J. M. (2006). The role of the basal ganglia in category learning. *Psychol. Learn. Motiv.* 46, 1–36. doi: 10.1016/S0079-7421(06)46001-1

Ashby, F. G., Ennis, J. M., and Spiering, B. J. (2007). A neurobiological theory of automaticity in perceptual categorization. *Psychol. Rev.* 114, 632–656. doi: 10.1037/0033-295X.114.3.632

Ashby, F. G., and Hélie, S. (2011). A tutorial on computational cognitive neuroscience: modeling the neurodynamics of cognition. *J. Math. Psychol.* 55, 273–289. doi: 10.1016/j.jmp.2011.04.003

Ashby, F. G., and Maddox, W. T. (1993). Relations between prototype, exemplar, and decision bound models of categorization. *J. Math. Psychol.* 37, 372–400. doi: 10.1006/jmps.1993.1023

Ashby, F. G., and Maddox, W. T. (2005). Human category learning. *Annu. Rev. Psychol.* 56, 149–178. doi: 10.1146/annurev.psych.56.091103.070217

Ashby, F. G., Maddox, W. T., and Bohil, C. J. (2002). Observational versus feedback training in rule-based and information-integration category learning. *Mem. Cogn.* 30, 666–677. *doi: 10.3758/BF03196423*

Ashby, F. G., and O'Brien, J. B. (2005). Category learning and multiple memory systems. *Trends Cogn. Sci.* 2, 83–89. doi: 10.1016/j.tics.2004.12.003

Ashby, F. G., Paul, E. J., and Maddox, W. T. (2011). "COVIS," in *Formal Approaches in Categorization*, eds E. M. Pothos and A. J. Wills (New York, NY: Cambridge University Press), 65–87. doi: 10.1017/CBO9780511921322.004

Ashby, F. G., and Valentin, V. V. (2005). "Multiple systems of perceptual category learning: theory and cognitive tests," in *Handbook of Categorization in Cognitive Science* eds H. Cohen and C. Lefebvre (New York, NY: Elsevier), 547–572.

Ashby, F. G., and Waldron, E. M. (1999). On the nature of procedural categorization. *Psychon. Bull. Rev.* 6, 363–378. doi: 10.3758/BF03210826

Ashby, F. G., and Maddox, W. T. (2011). Human category learning 2.0. *Ann. N.Y. Acad. Sci.* 1224, 147–61. doi: 10.1111/j.1749-6632.2010.05874.x

Bauswein, E., Fromm, C., and Preuss, A. (1989). Corticostriatal cells in comparison with pyramidal tract neurons: contrasting properties in the behaving monkey. *Brain Res.* 493, 198–203. doi: 10.1016/0006-8993(89)91018-4

Bayer, H. M., and Glimcher, P. W. (2005). Midbrain dopamine neurons encode a quantitative reward prediction error signal. *Neuron* 47, 129–141. doi: 10.1016/j.neuron.2005.05.020

Bush, R. R., and Mosteller, F. (1955). *Stochastic Models for Learning.* New York, NY: Wiley.

Calabresi, P., Pisani, A., Mercuri, N. B., and Bernardi, G. (1996). The corticostriatal projection: from synaptic plasticity to dysfunctions of the basal ganglia. *Trends Neurosci.* 19, 19–24. doi: 10.1016/0166-2236(96)81862-5

Cools, R., Altamirano, L., and D'Esposito, M. (2006). Reversal learning in Parkinson's disease depends on medication status and outcome valence. *Neuropsychologia* 44, 1663–1673. doi: 10.1016/j.neuropsychologia.2006.03.030

Cunnington, R., Windischberger, C., Deecke, L., and Moser, E. (2002). The preparation and execution of self-initiated and externally-triggered movement: a study of event-related fMRI. *Neuroimage* 15, 373–85. doi: 10.1006/nimg.2001.0976

DeLong, M. R., and Wichmann, T. (2007). Circuits and circuit disorders of the basal ganglia. *Arch. Neurol.* 64, 20. doi: 10.1001/archneur.64.1.20

Draganski, B., Kherif, F., Kloppel, S., Cook, P. A., Alexander, D. C., Parker, G. J. M., et al. (2008). Evidence for segregated and integrative connectivity patterns in the human basal ganglia. *J. Neurosci.* 28, 7143–7152. doi: 10.1523/JNEUROSCI.1486-08.2008

Erickson, M. A. (2008). Executive attention and task switching in category learning: evidence for stimulus-dependent representation. *Mem. Cogn.* 36, 749–761. doi: 10.3758/MC.36.4.749

Erickson, M. A., and Kruschke, J. K. J. (1998). Rules and exemplars in category learning. *J. Exp. Psychol. Gen.* 127, 107–140. doi: 10.1037/0096-3445.127.2.107

Flaherty, A., and Graybiel, A. (1993). Two input systems for body representations in the primate striatal matrix: experimental evidence in the squirrel monkey. *J. Neurosci.* 13, 1120–1137.

Foerde, K., Knowlton, B. J., and Poldrack, R. A. (2006). Modulation of competing memory systems by distraction. *Proc. Natl. Acad. Sci. U.S.A.* 103, 11778–11783. doi: 10.1073/pnas.0602659103

Foerde, K., Poldrack, R. A., and Knowlton, B. J. (2007). Secondary-task effects on classification learning. *Mem. Cogn.* 35, 864–874. doi: 10.3758/BF03193461

Gerfen, C. (1992). The neostriatal mosaic: multiple levels of compartmental organization in the basal ganglia. *Annu. Rev. Neurosci.* 15, 285–320. doi: 10.1146/annurev.ne.15.030192.001441

Hélie, S., Paul, E. J., and Ashby, F. G. (2012a). Simulating the effects of dopamine imbalance on cognition: from positive affect to Parkinson's disease. *Neural Netw.* 32, 74–85. doi: 10.1016/j.neunet.2012.02.033

Hélie, S., Paul, E. J., and Ashby, F. G. (2012b). A neurocomputational account of cognitive deficits in Parkinson's disease. *Neuropsychologia* 50, 2290–2302. doi: 10.1016/j.neuropsychologia.2012.05.033

Hikosaka, O., and Isoda, M. (2010). Switching from automatic to controlled behavior: cortico- basal ganglia mechanisms. *Trends Cogn. Sci.* 14, 154–161. doi: 10.1016/j.tics.2010.01.006

Hintzman, D. L. (1984). MINERVA 2: a simulation model of human memory. *Behav. Res. Methods, Instrum. Comput.* 16, 96–101. doi: 10.3758/BF03202365

Homa, D., Rhoads, D., and Chambliss, D. (1979). Evolution of conceptual structure. *J. Exp. Psychol. Hum. Learn. Mem.* 5, 11–23. doi: 10.1037/0278-7393.5.1.11

Joel, D., and Weiner, I. (1997). The connections of the primate subthalamic nucleus: indirect pathways and the open-interconnected scheme of basal ganglia—thalamocortical circuitry. *Brain Res. Rev.* 23, 62–78. doi: 10.1016/S0165-0173(96)00018-5

Jones, E. G., Coulter, J. D., Burton, H., and Porter, R. (1977). Cells of origin and terminal distribution of corticostriatal fibers arising in the sensory-motor cortex of monkeys. *J. Comp. Neurol.* 173, 53–80. doi: 10.1002/cne.901730105

Jueptner, M., and Weiller, C. (1998). A review of differences between basal ganglia and cerebellar control of movements as revealed by functional imaging studies. *Brain* 121, 1437–49. doi: 10.1093/brain/121.8.1437

Kruschke, J. K. (1992). ALCOVE: an exemplar-based connectionist model of category learning. *Psychol. Rev.* 99, 22–44. doi: 10.1037/0033-295X.99.1.22

Lei, W., Jiao, Y., Del Mar, N., and Reiner, A. (2004). Evidence for differential cortical input to direct pathway versus indirect pathway striatal projection neurons in rats. *J. Neurosci.* 24, 8289–99. doi: 10.1523/JNEUROSCI.1990-04.2004

Lewandowsky, S., and Kirsner, K. (2000). Expert knowledge is not always integrated: a case of cognitive partition. *Mem. Cogn.* 28, 295–305. doi: 10.3758/BF03213807

Love, B. C., Medin, D. L., and Gureckis, T. M. (2004). SUSTAIN: a network model of category learning. *Psychol. Rev.* 111, 309–332. doi: 10.1037/0033-295X.111.2.309

Maddox, W. T., Ashby, F. G., and Bohil, C. J. (2003). Delayed feedback effects on rule-based and information-integration category learning. *J. Exp. Psychol. Learn. Mem. Cogn.* 29, 650–662. doi: 10.1037/0278-7393.29.4.650

Maddox, W. T., Love, B. C., Glass, B. D., and Filoteo, J. V. (2008). When more is less: feedback effects in perceptual category learning. *Cognition* 108, 578–89. doi: 10.1016/j.cognition.2008.03.010

Molnár, Z., and Cheung, A. F. P. (2006). Towards the classification of subpopulations of layer V pyramidal projection neurons. *Neurosci. Res.* 55, 105–15. doi: 10.1016/j.neures.2006.02.008

Mostofsky, S. H., and Simmonds, D. J. (2008). Response inhibition and response selection: two sides of the same coin. *J. Cogn. Neurosci.* 97, 751–761. doi: 10.1162/jocn.2008.20500

Nambu, A., Kaneda, K., Tokuno, H., and Takada, M. (2002). Organization of corticostriatal motor inputs in monkey putamen. *J. Neurophysiol.* 88, 1830–1842. doi: 10.1152/jn.00672.2001

Nosofsky, R. M. (1986). Attention, similarity, and the identification-categorization relationship. *J. Exp. Psychol. Gen.* 115, 39–57. doi: 10.1037/0096-3445.115.1.39

Packard, M. G., and McGaugh, J. L. (1996). Inactivation of hippocampus or caudate nucleus with lidocaine differentially affects expression of place and response learning. *Neurobiol. Learn. Mem.* 65, 65–72. doi: 10.1006/nlme.1996.0007

Parent, A., and Hazrati, L. N. (1995). Functional anatomy of the basal ganglia. I. The cortico-basal ganglia-thalamo-cortical loop. *Brain Res. Rev.* 20, 91–127. doi: 10.1016/0165-0173(94)00007-C

Parent, M., and Parent, A. (2006). Single-axon tracing study of corticostriatal projections arising from primary motor cortex in primates. *J. Comp. Neurol.* 496, 202–213. doi: 10.1002/cne.20925

Pitt, M. A., Kim, W., Navarro, D. J., and Myung, J. I. (2006). Global model analysis by parameter space partitioning. *Psychological Review, 113*(1), 57–83. doi: 10.1037/0033-295X.113.1.57

Pitt, M. A., Myung, J. I., Montenegro, M., and Pooley, J. (2008). Measuring model flexibility with parameter space partitioning: an introduction and application example. *Cogn. Sci.* 32, 1285–303. doi: 10.1080/03640210802477534

Poldrack, R. A. and Packard, M. G. (2003). Competition among multiple memory systems: converging evidence from animal and human brain studies. *Neuropsychologia* 41, 245–251. doi: 10.1016/S0028-3932(02)00157-4

Pollack, A. E. (2001). Anatomy, physiology, and pharmacology of the basal ganglia. *Neurol. Clin.* 19, 523–534. doi: 10.1016/S0733-8619(05)70032-3

Reiner, A., Hart, N. M., Lei, W., and Deng, Y. (2010). Corticostriatal projection neurons—dichotomous types and dichotomous functions. *Front. Neuroanat.* 4:142. doi: 10.3389/fnana.2010.00142

Reiner, A., Jiao, Y., Del Mar, N., Laverghetta, A. V., and Lei, W. L. (2003). Differential morphology of pyramidal tract-type and intratelencephalically projecting-type corticostriatal neurons and their intrastriatal terminals in rats. *J. Comp. Neurol.* 457, 420–40. doi: 10.1002/cne.10541

Riesenhuber, M., and Poggio, T. (1999). Hierarchical models of object recognition in cortex. *Nat. Neurosci.* 2, 1019–1025. doi: 10.1038/14819

Roland, P. E., Meyer, E., Shibasaki, T., Yamamoto, Y. L., and Thompson, C. J. (1982). Regional cerebral blood flow changes in cortex and basal ganglia during voluntary movements in normal human volunteers. *J. Neurophysiol.* 48, 467–480.

Romo, R., Scarnati, E., and Schultz, W. (1992). Role of primate basal ganglia and frontal cortex in the internal generation of movements. II. Movement-related activity in the anterior striatum. *Exp. Brain Res.* 91, 385–395. doi: 10.1007/BF00227835

Schultz, W., Dayan, P., and Montague, P. R. (1997). A neural substrate of prediction and reward. *Science* 275, 1593–1599. doi: 10.1126/science.275.5306.1593

Schultz, W., and Romo, R. (1992). Role of primate basal ganglia and frontal cortex in the internal generation of movements. I. Preparatory activity in the anterior striatum. *Exp. Brain Res.* 91, 363–84. doi: 10.1007/BF00227834

Schultz, W., Tremblay, L., and Hollerman, J. R. (2000). Reward processing in primate orbitofrontal cortex and basal ganglia. *Cereb. Cortex* 10, 272–283. doi: 10.1093/cercor/10.3.272

Smith, J. D., and Minda, J. P. (2000). Thirty categorization results in search of a model. *J. Exp. Psychol. Learn. Mem. Cogn.* 26, 3–27. doi: 10.1037/0278-7393.26.1.3

Takada, M., Tokuno, H., Nambu, A., and Inase, M. (1998). Corticostriatal projections from the somatic motor areas of the frontal cortex in the macaque monkey: segregation versus overlap of input zones from the primary motor cortex, the supplementary motor area, and the premotor cortex. *Exp. Brain Res.* 120, 114–128. doi: 10.1007/s002210050384

Tobler, P. N., Dickinson, A., and Schultz, W. (2003). Coding of predicted reward omission by dopamine neurons in a conditioned inhibition paradigm. *J. Neurosci.* 23, 10402–10410.

Tulving, E. (1972). "Episodic and semantic memory," in *Organisation of Memory*, eds E. Tuiving and W. Donaldson (New York, NY: Academic Press), 381–402.

Tulving, E. (1985). How many memory systems are there? *Am. Psychol.* 40, 385–398. doi: 10.1037/0003-066X.40.4.385

Turner, R. S., and DeLong, M. R. (2000). Corticostriatal activity in primary motor cortex of the macaque. *J. Neurosci.* 20, 7096–7108.

Waldron, E. M., and Ashby, F. G. (2001). The effects of concurrent task interference on category learning: evidence for multiple category learning systems. *Psychon. Bull. Rev.* 8, 168–176. doi: 10.3758/BF03196154

Waldschmidt, J. G., and Ashby, F. G. (2011). Cortical and striatal contributions to automaticity in information-integration categorization. *Neuroimage* 56, 1791–1802. doi: 10.1016/j.neuroimage.2011.02.011

Wallis, J. D., and Kennerley, S. W. (2010). Heterogeneous reward signals in prefrontal cortex. *Curr. Opin. Neurobiol.* 20, 191–198. doi: 10.1016/j.conb.2010.02.009

Yang, L.-X., and Lewandowsky, S. (2004). Knowledge partitioning in categorization: constraints on exemplar models. *J. Exp. Psychol. Learn. Mem. Cogn.* 30, 1045–1064. doi: 10.1037/0278-7393.30.5.1045

Zeithamova, D., and Maddox, W. T. (2006). Dual task interference in perceptual category learning. *Mem. Cogn.* 34, 387–398. doi: 10.3758/BF03193416

18

Procedural-Based Category Learning in Patients with Parkinson's Disease: Impact of Category Number and Category Continuity

J. Vincent Filoteo[1,2]* *and W. Todd Maddox*[3,4]

[1] Veterans Administration San Diego Healthcare System, San Diego, CA, USA
[2] Department of Psychiatry, University of California, San Diego, CA, USA
[3] Department of Psychology, University of Texas, Austin, TX, USA
[4] Institute for Neuroscience, University of Texas, Austin, TX, USA

Correspondence:
J. Vincent Filoteo, Veterans Administration San Diego, Healthcare System, Psychology Service 116B, VASDHS, 3350 La Jolla Village Dr., San Diego, CA 92161, USA
e-mail: vfiloteo@ucsd.edu

Previously we found that Parkinson's disease (PD) patients are impaired in procedural-based category learning when category membership is defined by a nonlinear relationship between stimulus dimensions, but these same patients are normal when the rule is defined by a linear relationship (Maddox and Filoteo, 2001; Filoteo et al., 2005a,b). We suggested that PD patients' impairment was due to a deficit in recruiting "striatal units" to represent complex nonlinear rules. In the present study, we further examined the nature of PD patients' procedural-based deficit in two experiments designed to examine the impact of (1) the number of categories, and (2) category discontinuity on learning. Results indicated that PD patients were impaired only under discontinuous category conditions but were normal when the number of categories was increased from two to four. The lack of impairment in the four-category condition suggests normal integrity of striatal medium spiny cells involved in procedural-based category learning. In contrast, and consistent with our previous observation of a nonlinear deficit, the finding that PD patients were impaired in the discontinuous condition suggests that these patients are impaired when they have to associate perceptually distinct exemplars with the same category. Theoretically, this deficit might be related to dysfunctional communication among medium spiny neurons within the striatum, particularly given that these are cholinergic neurons and a cholinergic deficiency could underlie some of PD patients' cognitive impairment.

Keywords: Parkinson's disease, category learning, implicit processes, procedural learning, striatum, basal ganglia

INTRODUCTION

It is now widely accepted that there are multiple category learning systems (Ashby et al., 1998, 2010; Smith et al., 1998, 2012; Ashby and Maddox, 2005, 2011) and that different neural systems play different roles in these systems (Knowlton et al., 1994, 1996; Poldrack et al., 1999; Ashby and Ell, 2001; Filoteo et al., 2001a,b, 2005a,b; Patalano et al., 2001; Keri, 2003; Reber et al., 2003; Shohamy et al., 2004a,b; Maddox et al., 2005a,b; Cincotta and Seger, 2007; Nomura et al., 2007; Price et al., 2009; Waldschmidt and Ashby, 2011). One of the more interesting, and potentially important lines of research in this area is the study of how some categories can be acquired without conscious awareness. This phenomenon, often referred to as procedural-based category learning, occurs when participants learn complex categorization rules, and despite highly accurate learning, they are unable to describe explicitly why any given exemplar belongs to a specific category.

The behavioral mechanisms of procedural-based category learning have received much attention in several recent studies with normal individuals (Gluck et al., 2002; Maddox and Ashby, 2004; Ashby and Maddox, 2005, 2011; Ashby and O'Brien, 2005). These studies have demonstrated that this form of category learning has distinct operating characteristics that differentiate it from other types of category learning processes, such as explicit category learning (Ashby et al., 2002, 2003a,b; Maddox et al., 2003, 2004a,b; Maddox and Ing, 2005; Worthy et al., 2013). For example, the perceptual similarity among exemplars has to occur along a continuum within each category for normal procedural-based learning to occur, whereas this is not the case for explicit category learning (Maddox et al., 2005a,b, 2007). Similarly, the number of categories to be learned does not differentially impact long-run accuracy in procedural-based category learning, but increasing the number of categories impedes the learning of explicit category rules (Maddox et al., 2004a,b).

Much has also been learned about the underlying neurobiology of implicit or procedural-based category learning by the functional imaging of normal individuals or by studying patients with neurological disorders. For example, fMRI studies with normal participants have identified the striatum as an important brain region for procedural-based category learning (Filoteo et al., 2006; Cincotta and Seger, 2007; Nomura et al., 2007; Waldschmidt and Ashby, 2011) and other studies have implicated midbrain dopamine regions in some implicit category learning tasks (Aron et al., 2004). Past work with patients with striatal dysfunction has also implicated this brain region in implicit forms of category learning. Knowlton et al. (1996), for example, demonstrated that patients with Parkinson's disease (PD) are impaired in learning probabilistically determined categories, a finding that has received considerable support in the literature (Shohamy et al., 2004a,b). Importantly, other patient studies have indicated that brain structure associated with explicit memory (hippocampus and diencephalon) do not contribute to the same extent to implicit forms of category learning (Knowlton et al., 1994) or the long-term retention of procedural-based categories (Filoteo et al., 2001b).

In our work we have conducted a series of studies designed to further understand the nature of procedural-based category learning deficits in patients with PD, and by extension, the role of the striatum in this process (Maddox and Filoteo, 2001; Ashby et al., 2003b; Filoteo et al., 2005a). We have primarily used the perceptual categorization task (Ashby and Gott, 1988) in which participants view simple two-dimensional stimuli often consisting of a single line that varies in length and orientation (or a Gabor patch that varies in spatial frequency and orientation; see **Figure 1**) and are asked to categorize stimuli into one of two categories (Category A or B), and then immediately following a response, feedback is given. The rule that dictates category membership depends on the nature of the relationship between the two stimulus dimensions. **Figures 2A,B** provide examples in which the optimal rule is linear or nonlinear, respectively. This figure provides scatter plots of Category A and B stimuli where the x-axis represents the length of the line (in arbitrary units) and the y-axis represents the orientation of the line (in arbitrary units). Closed squares represent stimuli from Category A and open circles represent stimuli from Category B. Each individual stimulus has the length value on the x-axis and the orientation value on the y-axis. The linear rule depicted in **Figure 2A** is represented as a linear function and provides an optimal separation of the Category A and B stimuli, whereas the nonlinear rule in **Figure 2B** is represented as a quadratic function that provides an optimal separation of the Category A and B stimuli. A participant who would adopt the linear rule in **Figure 2A** or the nonlinear rule in **Figure 2B** would maximize long-run accuracy. Note that both rules are procedural-based category learning rules because it is very difficult to verbalize either the linear or nonlinear relationship between the two stimulus dimensions when they are not in the same perceptual units (e.g., length and orientation).

The results of our first study using this paradigm (Maddox and Filoteo, 2001) found that PD patients were impaired in learning a categorization rule that was based on a nonlinear relationship between lines that varied in length and orientation, whereas they were normal in learning a linear rule. Similarly, in our next study (Ashby et al., 2003a,b) we used a somewhat different task but again found that PD patients were normal in learning linear procedural-based rules. Finally, in a third study (Filoteo et al., 2005a,b) we again examined linear and nonlinear category learning and found that the patients were impaired in the nonlinear condition but not in the linear condition. Importantly, task difficulty could not explain these findings since the more difficult task (based on the accuracy of the control participants) was the linear task, on which PD patients were normal. This series of studies suggest that PD patients are impaired in procedural-based category learning, but only when the rule that dictates category membership is nonlinear.

A surface-level explanation of our findings is that PD results in deficits in learning nonlinear procedural based rules, but it does not impact linear rule learning. Unfortunately this explanation

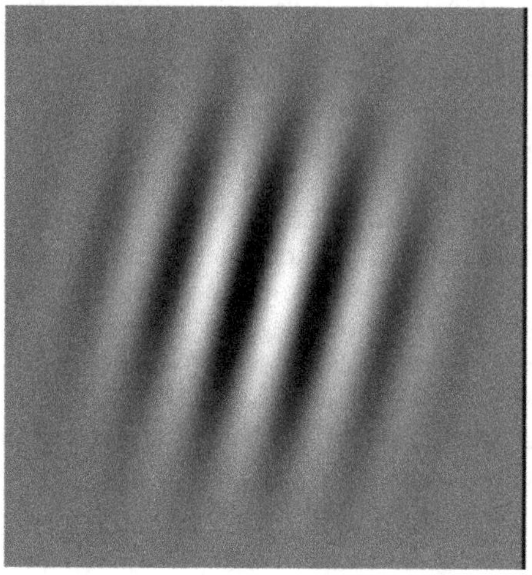

FIGURE 1 | **Example of a Gabor stimulus used in Experiments 1 and 2.**

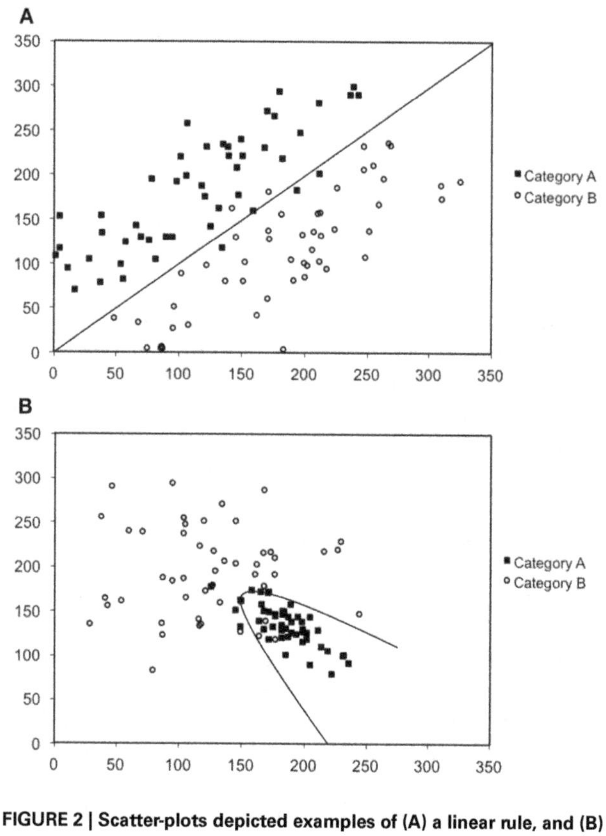

FIGURE 2 | **Scatter-plots depicted examples of (A) a linear rule, and (B) a nonlinear rule.** Note that the scales are in arbitrary units.

does not provide any insight into the possible mechanisms that might be driving these findings. To help interpret our past results we use the neurobiological and theoretical framework provided by the Striatal Pattern Classifier (SPC) model introduced by Ashby and colleagues (Ashby and Waldron, 1999). This model has been found to provide a good accounting of normal participants' response patterns in previous procedural-based category learning studies (e.g., Ashby and Waldron, 1999; Waldron and Ashby, 2001; Maddox et al., 2007; for applications to stimulus identification see Ashby et al., 2001; Maddox, 2001, 2002). The assumptions of this model are based on the neurobiology proposed to underlie the procedural-based category learning system in COVIS (Ashby et al., 2001). The SPC model, which is outlined in detail in Ashby and Waldron (1999), incorporates the knowledge of the many-to-one mapping of visual cortical cells onto cells in the striatum (Wilson, 1995). The model proposes hypothetical "striatal units" that are thought to represent the medium spiny cells in the striatum and provide a low-resolution map of the perceptual space. During procedural-based category learning the model assumes that these striatal units become associated with a category label and learn to associate a response with groups of cells in visual regions of cortex. It is important to be clear that the SPC is a computational model that is inspired by what is known about the neurobiology of the striatum. Because of this fact, the "striatal units" are hypothetical and could be interpreted within the language of some other computational model (e.g., as "prototypes" in a multiple prototype model).

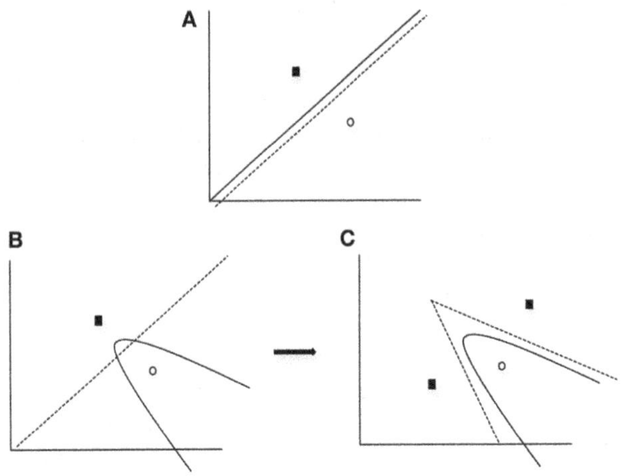

FIGURE 3 | Graphical example of the SPC modeling approach when (A) one unit per category is applied to a linear condition, (B) one unit per category is applied to a nonlinear condition, and (C) two units for one category and one unit for the other category is applied to a nonlinear condition. Solid line and curves represent the "optimal" rule, whereas the dashed line and curves represent the partition between categories provided by the units. Note with the use of additional units for the nonlinear condition (panel **C**), the optimal quadratic bound (represented as the solid curve) is approximated by piecewise linear bounds. In all cases, black squares represent Category A units and open circles represent Category B units.

One important finding from the application of the SPC to data obtained from normal individuals (Ashby and Waldron, 1999) is that a greater number of striatal units are typically needed to represent a nonlinear rule as compared to a linear rule. The SPC is a minimum distance classifier. This is depicted in **Figure 3A** in which a linear rule is approximated by one striatal unit representing Category A (closed square) and another striatal unit representing Category B (open circle). In this case a minimum distance "bound" is learned. Note in **Figure 3A** that only a single unit per category is needed to approximate a linear rule. In contrast, **Figure 3B** provides a graphic representation of how striatal units might approximate a nonlinear rule. As can be seen in the first panel of **Figure 3B**, a single unit per category does not provide a good approximation of the optimal nonlinear rule. However, in **Figure 3C** the addition of a second striatal unit allows for a better approximation of the nonlinear rule via the piece-wise combination of two linear bounds so that two minimum distance bounds are learned. Thus, the SPC model argues that additional striatal units are needed to represent nonlinear rules.

This observation raised the interesting possibility that dysfunction in PD within these model-based "striatal units" might also reflect the pathological manifestations of PD within actual medium spiny neurons that compose the majority of cells within the striatum. These cells are the primary input nuclei in the striatum from the cortex and are part of the direct and indirect pathways within the basal ganglia. Medium spiny neurons are thought to be impacted in PD through the dysfunction of their dendritic spines due to deafferentation effects following the loss of dopamine cells within the pars compacta of the substantia nigra (Deutch et al., 2007), although this change might only be reflected functionally in the later stages of the disease (Zaja-Milatovic et al., 2005). Given the involvement of the medium spiny neurons in PD, one manner in which this disease could impact the proposed units is that the actual number of functional medium spiny neurons has diminished in these patients, and because of this, nonlinear categories that require a greater number of units can no longer be adequately represented. Thus, procedural-based learning conditions in which a greater number of units are required would always place PD patients at a disadvantage. We refer to this as the "number of units" hypothesis.

An alternative, but somewhat related possibility, is that the number of functional medium spiny neurons is normal in PD (at least early in the disease), but somehow these neurons are unable to communicate in a manner that would enable learning to occur when a greater number of striatal units is needed to represent the categories, such as under nonlinear conditions. That is, the number of functional medium spiny neurons is sufficient to support nonlinear category learning, but impairment in the ability of these neurons to communicate results in impaired learning. We refer to this as the "communication among units" hypothesis. This hypothesis was initially based on the observation from our previous studies that the learning of nonlinear rules requires that certain stimuli that are less perceptually similar have to be grouped into the same category, whereas certain stimuli that are more perceptually similar have to be grouped into different categories. Such communication among medium spiny neurons would be needed for the striatum to output a consistent message regarding that category to which a particular stimulus belongs. That is, unless there were some sort of co-activation among medium spiny neurons that processed the percept of a stimuli belonging to the same category, the output of these neurons would theoretically send a unique message to other structures eventually responsible for generating a response (e.g., the globus pallidus), and these structures would have to somehow resolve the fact that different medium spiny cells are signaling that their representation belongs to the same category. Note that this would only be the case when multiple units are required to represent a category, because theoretically, no such resolution would be required when only single medium spiny neurons (or medium spiny neurons within close proximity of one another) are needed to learn, such as under linear conditions.

An important question that needs to be addressed, however, is what could allow the medium spiny neurons to communicate. One possibility is that cholinergic interneurons that connect medium spiny neurons within the striatum enable such communication, and under conditions in which it would be theoretically beneficial for such cells to communicate (i.e., nonlinear conditions), striatal interneurons are involved in the learning process. These neurons often referred to as tonically active neurons (or TANs, for their tonic firing rate at rest) comprise only a small percentage of neurons in the striatum but recently have been implicated in processes important to procedural-based category learning (Ashby et al., 2007; Ashby and Crossley, 2011; Crossley et al., 2013). Specifically, most studies suggest that these interneurons modulate the input of cortical cells onto striatal medium spiny neurons by decreasing (or pausing) their activity when a rewarding stimulus is processed within the striatum, which allows for increased reinforcement learning (Apicella, 2002; Joshua et al., 2008; Aosaki et al., 2010). However, another method by which these interneurons result in learning could be by controlling the number of potential responses that are selected by the striatum (Stocco, 2012) and would be more consistent with a broader view of these interneurons in various aspects of learning (e.g., Apicella, 2007). This proposed process could provide an appropriate mechanism by which the striatum is able to link perceptually distinct stimuli to the same category response. This process is also consistent with other models of basal ganglia function that suggest a role of the striatum in response selection (Mink, 1996; Stocco, 2012), with reinforcement learning being one aspect of selecting a response (Bar-Gad et al., 2003; Redgrave et al., 2011) or linking networks within the striatum that are important for learning (Graybiel et al., 1994). Although the exact effects of interneurons on medium spiny cell function is not completely known and likely very complex (see Oldenburg and Ding, 2011), these cells do appear to play an important role in normal striatal functioning. Importantly, animal models of PD suggest that the reduction of dopaminergic projections to the striatum result in abnormal interneuron activity (Raz et al., 2001; Pisani et al., 2003; Bonsi et al., 2011).

The purpose of the current study is to examine both the "number of units" hypothesis and the "communication among units" hypothesis described above. Experiment 1 examined the ability of PD patients and normal controls (NC) to learn a procedural-based task in which there were either four categories (Four-Category condition) or two categories (Two-Category condition). **Figure 4** displays the stimulus distributions for the Four- and Two-Category conditions. If PD results in a deficit in the number of hypothetical striatal units, then they should demonstrate greater impairment in the Four-Category condition as compared to the Two-Category condition. In contrast, Experiment 2 examined the "communication among units" hypothesis by determining the ability of PD patients and NC participants to learn categories that have either a discontinuous distribution of stimuli (Discontinuous condition) or a continuous distribution of stimuli (Continuous condition). **Figure 6** displays the stimulus distributions for the Discontinuous and Continuous conditions. A finding that PD patients are impaired in the Discontinuous condition relative to the Continuous condition would provide theoretical support for the "communication among units" hypothesis of procedural-based category learning deficits in PD.

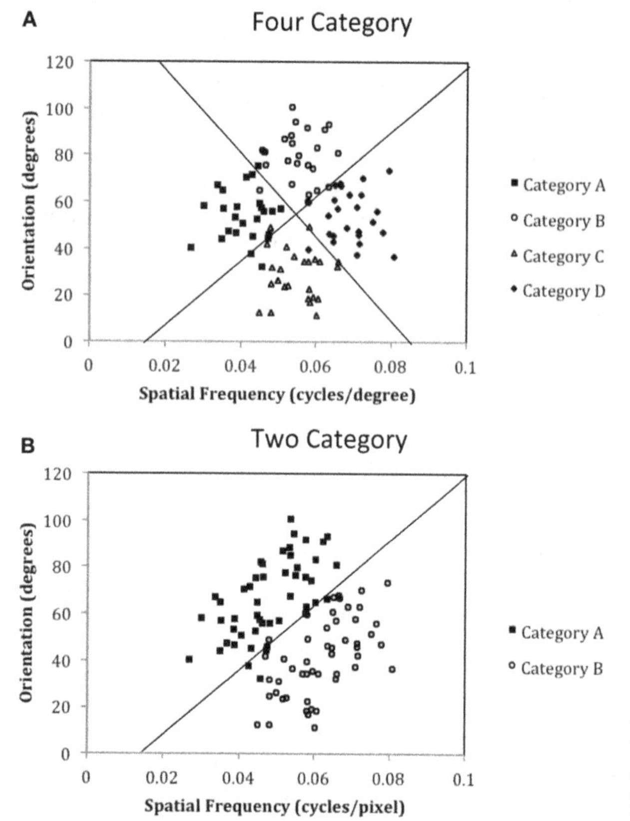

FIGURE 4 | Stimulus distributions for (A) the Four-Category and (B) Two-Category conditions in Experiment 1. The solid line(s) represent the optimal rule(s).

GENERAL METHODS

PARTICIPANTS

A total of 41 individuals participated in at least one of the two experiments: 20 PD patients and 21 NC participants. For the PD patients, 11 participated in at least one condition in both experiments and 9 participated in at least one condition in only one experiment. For the NC participants, 8 participated in at least one condition in both experiments and 12 participated in at least one condition in only one experiment. Participants were randomized to each experiment and in the case of those who participated in more than one experiment or in both conditions within an experiment, the order of administration of the experiments was randomized[1]. Participants were tested a minimum of 2 months apart between experiments or conditions. The specific numbers of individuals who participated in the two experiments are as follows. Experiment 1: Four-Category Condition, 12 PD patients (8 males and 4 females) and 12 NC participants (4 males and 8 females). Two-Category Condition, 11 PD patients (5 males and 6 females) and 11 NC participants (4 males and 7 females). Eight PD patients 8 NC participants were tested in both the Four-Category and Two-Category conditions. Experiment 2: Discontinuous Condition, 10 PD patients (6 males and 4 females) and 10 NC participants (4 males 6 females); Continuous Condition, 11 PD patients (8 males and 3 females) and 11 NC participants (5 males 6 females). Five PD patients and 7 NC participants were tested in both the Discontinuous and Continuous conditions.

The patients were recruited from Movement Disorder Clinics at UCSD and were diagnosed by a board-certified neurologist with subspecialty training in movement disorders. The diagnosis was based on UK Brain Bank Criteria (Hughes et al., 1992). PD patients were not included in the study if they scored above a cut-off of 11 on the Geriatric Depression Scale or if they scored below 130 on the Mattis Dementia Rating Scale (MDRS; Mattis, 1988). For Experiment 1, 14 patients were taking daily L-dopa medication, 8 were taking a dopamine receptor agonist, 5 were taking an MAO inhibitor, 5 were taking a COMT inhibitor as part of their L-dopa preparation, 5 were taking amantadine, and 1 was taking an anticholinergic. For Experiment 2, 14 patients were taking daily L-dopa medication, 8 were taking a dopamine receptor agonist, 3 were taking an MAO inhibitor, 6 were taking a COMT inhibitor as part of their L-dopa preparation, 5 were taking amantadine, and 1 was taking an anticholinergic.

Tables 1, 3 show the mean age, years of education, scores on the MDRS for the PD patients and NC participants who participated in Experiments 1 and 2, respectively, and the mean Hoehn and Yahr Rating Scale (HYRS; Hoehn and Yahr, 1967) score and the length of illness (LOI; years) for the PD patients. In both experiments, the PD and NC groups did not differ in age, education, scores on the MDRS, or gender distribution (all p's > 0.05).

STIMULI AND STIMULUS GENERATION

In both experiments, the stimuli consisted of a single Gabor patch (see **Figure 1**) that varied in orientation and spatial frequency. The stimuli were computer generated and displayed on a 21′ monitor with 1360 × 1024 resolution. Each Gabor patch was generated using MATLAB routines from Brainard's (1997) Psychophysics Toolbox, and each stimulus was 7 cm in diameter, which subtended a visual angle of about 8.8° from a viewing distance of 45 cm.

Both experiments used the randomization technique of Ashby and Gott (1988). For each experiment, an equal number of Category A and Category B stimuli were generated by sampling randomly from two bivariate normal distributions. Each random sample (x_f, x_o) was converted to a stimulus by deriving the frequency, $f = 0.0025 + (x_f/5000)$ cycles per pixel, and orientation, $o = 0.36x_o$ degrees. The scaling factors were chosen in an attempt to equate the salience of frequency and orientation based on our past experience with these stimuli. Each category distribution is specified by a mean and a variance on each dimension, and by a covariance between dimensions. For both category structures it was always the case that the covariance matrix for Category A was identical to the covariance matrix for Category B. The categories differed only in the location of their means.

The exact parameter values for the two experiments are listed in **Tables 2, 4**, and the category structures are displayed in **Figures 4, 6. Figure 4A** displays the category structures for the Four-Category condition in Experiment 1. Each filled square denotes the spatial frequency and spatial orientation of a Gabor pattern from Category A, each open circle denotes the spatial frequency and spatial orientation of a Gabor pattern from Category B, each closed diamond denotes the spatial frequency and spatial orientation of a Gabor pattern from Category C, and each closed triangle denotes the spatial frequency and spatial orientation of

Table 1 | Demographic characteristics and Mattis Dementia Rating Scale Scores of the PD patients and NC participants in the Four-Category and Two-Category Conditions of Experiment 1.

FOUR-CATEGORY CONDITION	Age		Education		MDRS		HYRS		LOI	
	M	*SD*	*M*	*SD*	*M*	*SD*	*M*	*SD*	*M*	*SD*
PD	67.1	7.6	16.5	1.9	139.7	3.1	2.0	0.5	7.3	4.6
NC	66.2	8.8	17.5	1.0	141.0	2.1	–	–	–	–
TWO-CATEGORY CONDITION	**Age**		**Education**		**DRS**		**HY**		**LOI**	
	M	*SD*	*M*	*SD*	*M*	*SD*	*M*	*SD*	*M*	*SD*
PD	64.2	7.9	16.3	2.0	140.5	2.5	2.1	0.5	6.3	3.6
NC	66.1	7.4	17.0	1.9	141.0	2.3	–	–	–	–

HY, Hoehn and Yahr Rating Scale score; LOI, Length of Illness.

Table 2 | Category distribution parameter values for Experiment 1.

FOUR-CATEGORY CONDITION					
Category	M_{sf}	M_o	SD_{sf}	SD_o	$cov_{sf,o}$
A	0.038	54.0	0.006	10.6	0
B	0.055	84.0	0.006	10.6	0
C	0.055	24.0	0.006	10.6	0
D	0.072	54.0	0.006	10.6	0
TWO-CATEGORY CONDITION					
Category	M_{st}	M_o	SD_{st}	SD_o	$cov_{st,o}$
A_1	0.041	54.0	0.006	10.6	0
A_2	0.055	79.5	0.006	10.6	0
B_2	0.055	28.6	0.006	10.6	0
B_2	0.069	54.0	0.006	10.6	0

[1] Additional analyses were conducted to determine if the order of administration of either the experiments or conditions could account for the pattern of results reported below and it was determined that this was not the case.

Table 3 | Demographic characteristics and Mattis Dementia Rating Scale Scores of the PD patients and NC participants in the Discontinuous and Continuous Conditions in Experiment 2.

DISCONTINUOUS CONDITION										
	Age		Education		MDRS		HYRS		LOI	
	M	*SD*	*M*	*SD*	*M*	*SD*	*M*	*SD*	*M*	*SD*
PD	65.4	6.9	16.0	1.8	138.5	3.3	2.0	0.2	6.8	2.9
NC	66.5	7.8	16.9	1.4	140.0	2.3	–	–	–	–
CONTINUOUS CONDITION										
	Age		Education		MDRS		HY		LOI	
	M	*SD*	*M*	*SD*	*M*	*SD*	*M*	*SD*	*M*	*SD*
PD	64.8	9.6	16.1	2.3	139.9	2.1	2.1	0.7	6.0	4.7
NC	66.6	7.2	16.3	2.5	141.0	2.5	–	–	–	–

HY, Hoehn and Yahr Rating Scale score; LOI, Length of Illness.

Table 4 | Category distribution parameter values for Experiment 2.

DISCONTINUOUS CONDITION					
Category	M_{sf}	M_o	SD_{sf}	SD_o	$cov_{sf,o}$
A_1	0.051	31.7	0.002	3.6	0
A_2	0.064	54.7	0.002	3.6	0
B_1	0.058	20.2	0.002	3.6	0
B_2	0.070	42.8	0.002	3.6	0
CONTINUOUS CONDITION					
Category	M_{st}	M_o	SD_{st}	SD_o	$cov_{st,o}$
A_1	0.051	31.7	0.002	3.6	0
A_2	0.055	39.2	0.002	3.6	0
B_1	0.058	20.2	0.002	3.6	0
B_2	0.062	27.7	0.002	3.6	0

a Gabor pattern from Category D. **Figure 4B** displays the category structures for the Two-Category condition in Experiment 1, and **Figures 6A,B** display the Discontinuous and Continuous conditions in Experiment 2, respectively. For these figures, each filled square denotes the spatial frequency and spatial orientation of a Gabor pattern from Category A, while each unfilled circle denotes the spatial frequency and spatial orientation of a Gabor pattern from Category B. The solid line(s) in **Figures 4, 6** denotes the location of the optimal decision bound(s). The use of the optimal bound in each of the four experiments maximizes long-run accuracy. Optimal accuracy in each condition was 95% given the categories overlapped to some extent, and thus were probabilistic.

EXPERIMENTAL PROCEDURE

For the Four-Category and Two-Category conditions in Experiment 1, 600 trials were presented in 6 blocks of 100 trials. For the Discontinuous and Continuous conditions in Experiment 1, 400 trials were presented and were broken down into 5 blocks of 80 trials. At the start of each condition, the participants were told that they were involved in a study that examined their ability to categorize simple stimuli, that a series of stimuli would be presented, and that they would be asked to categorize each as a member of Category A B, C, or D for the Four-Category condition of Experiment 1, or Category A or B in the Two-Category condition of Experiment 1, and both conditions in Experiment 2. They were also told that at the beginning of the experiment they may feel as though they were guessing, but as the experiment progressed, their accuracy would likely increase. Participants indicated their categorization responses by pressing designated keys on the computer keyboard. For each trial in both experiments, the stimulus was presented until the participant's categorization response was made and feedback was presented immediately after the response for 1 s that consisted of either the word "wrong" if their response was incorrect or "correct" if their response was correct. Once feedback was given, the next trial was initiated 1 s later.

EXPERIMENT 1: FOUR-CATEGORY vs. TWO-CATEGORY CONDITIONS

Experiment 1 was designed to examine the "number of units" hypothesis. In the Four-Category condition, the participant must learn to assign each stimulus to one of four categories. Theoretically, each category is represented by a single striatal unit that is linked to the corresponding response (A, B, C, or D). As can be seen in **Figure 4A**, these categories are derived from four clusters of stimuli with different means and standard deviations (see **Table 2**). In the Two-Category condition, these same four clusters of stimuli are again used, but now there are only two categories given that Category A and B stimuli from the Four-Category condition are collapsed into Category A for the Two-Category condition, and Category C and D from the Four-Category condition are collapsed into Category B for the Two-Category condition. Thus, the exact stimuli are held constant across the two conditions, as is the nature of the stimuli, the timing of the task trials, and the nature of feedback. The only thing that varied is the number of categories.

As noted above, it was anticipated that if PD patients' deficits in learning nonlinear rules was due to such rules requiring a greater number of units to represent nonlinearity (see **Figure 3**) and there was a deficiency in the number of units in PD patients, the "number of units" hypothesis would predict that PD patients would be differentially impaired in the Four-Category condition as compared to the Two-Category condition.

RESULTS

Accuracy rates for the Four-Category condition of Experiment 1 are displayed in **Figure 5A** and were analyzed using a 2 (group: PD vs. NC) × 6 (blocks 1–6) mixed-design ANOVA. Results revealed a main effect of block, $F_{(5,\ 110)} = 37.02, p < 0.001, \eta_p^2 = 0.63$, with both PD and NC participants' performance improving across the trials. However, there was no main effect of group, $F_{(1,\ 22)} = 0.08, p = 0.78, \eta_p^2 = 0.00$, and no group by block interaction, $F_{(5,\ 110)} = 0.35$, $p = 0.88$, $\eta_p^2 = 0.02$. Accuracy rates for the Two-Category condition are displayed in **Figure 5B** and were analyzed using the same ANOVA design. Results indicated a main effect of block, $F_{(5,\ 110)} = 11.88$, $p < 0.001$, $\eta_p^2 = 0.37$, but no main effect of group, $F_{(1,\ 22)} = 0.21, p = 0.65, \eta_p^2 = 0.00$, and no group by block interaction, $F_{(5,\ 110)} = 1.23, p = 0.30, \eta_p^2 = 0.06$.

DISCUSSION

The results of Experiment 1 suggest that PD patients are not impaired when learning either four or two categories. As can be seen in **Figures 4A,B**, participants initially demonstrate a disadvantage in learning four categories as compared to two categories, but this is due to the fact that participants are initially guessing early in learning and chance responding in the four category condition is 25%, whereas in the two category condition it is 50%. However, as learning progresses, performance improves in both the Four- and Two-Category conditions and asymptotes at approximately 80% during the last block of trials. These findings are consistent with our previous work with healthy younger adults that showed little impact of category number on procedural-based category learning (Maddox et al., 2004a,b). The most important finding, however, is that there was no difference between PD patients and NC participants in the pattern and extent of learning in either the Four- or Two-Category conditions. If we can assume that normal learning in the Four-Category condition required a greater number of functional striatal units, then these findings do not support the "number of units" hypothesis.

EXPERIMENT 2: DISCONTINUOUS CATEGORY vs. CONTINUOUS CATEGORY CONDITIONS

The purpose of Experiment 2 was to examine the impact of within-category discontinuity on procedural-based category learning in PD and NC participants. As noted above, we have found in three past studies that PD patients are not impaired in learning procedural-based category rules when the rule that dictates category membership is linear (Ashby et al., 2003a,b; Filoteo et al., 2005a,b) and our findings from Experiment 1 in this study provide further support for this observation. As we have argued above, one aspect of learning nonlinear rules is that participants must learn to categorize perceptual dissimilar stimuli into the same category so that they can activate the same response, and conversely, participants must learn not to categorize perceptually similar stimuli into the same category so that such stimuli can elicit a different response. This process is thought to occur through a response selection mechanism that is modulated by cholinergic interneurons within the striatum by inhibiting competing responses (e.g., Stocco, 2012). If there were a deficiency in communication among the medium spiny neurons within the striatum because of poor communication through the interneurons, then learning would be impaired. Again, we refer to this hypothesis as the "communication among units" hypothesis.

To test this hypothesis, we created a two-category condition in which a greater number of units would be needed to represent the stimuli within a single category but the rule was nevertheless linear. To do so, we created discontinuous categories by using two non-overlapping clusters within each category. As can be seen in **Figure 6A**, Category A stimuli (A_1 and A_2 clusters under

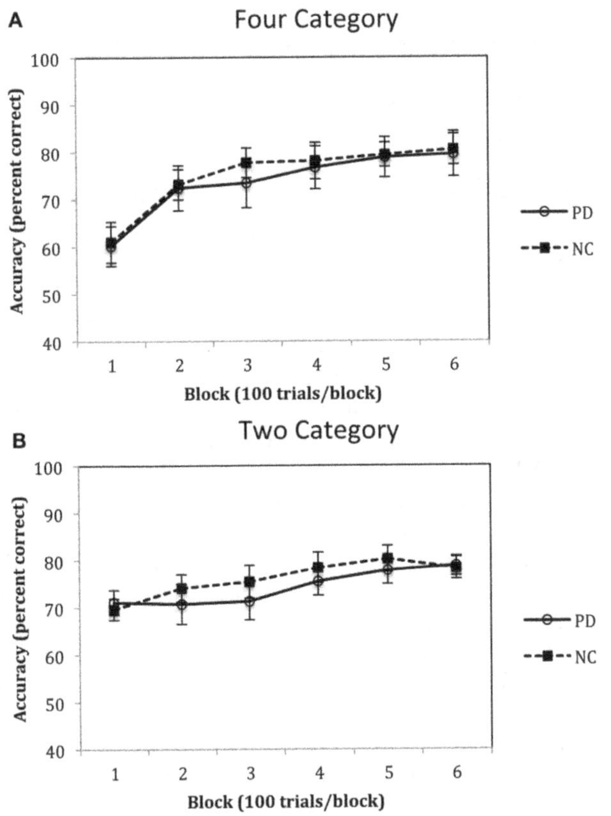

FIGURE 5 | Accuracy rates for PD patients and NC participants (A) Four Category and (B) Two Category conditions in Experiment 1. (Error bars are in standard error of the mean).

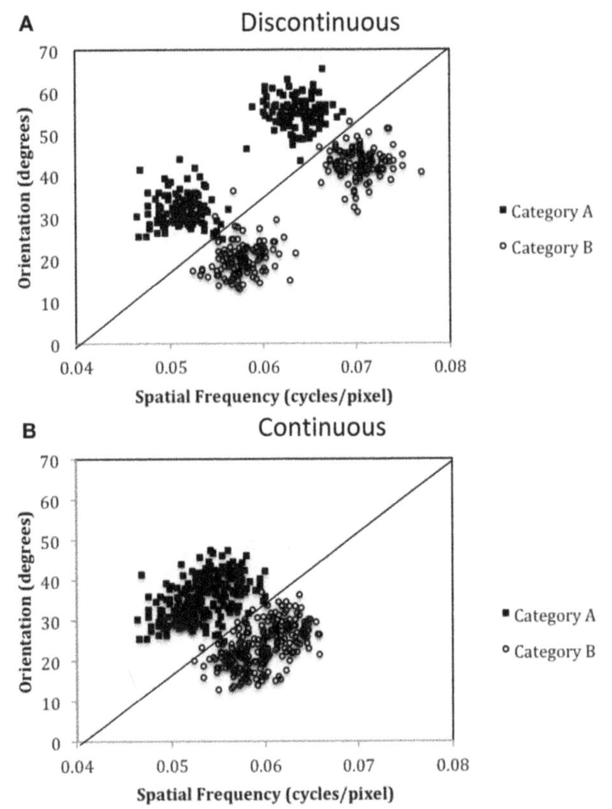

FIGURE 6 | Stimulus distributions for the (A) Discontinuous and (B) Continuous conditions in Experiment 2. The solid line represents the optimal rule.

Discontinuous condition in **Table 4**) compose two clusters as do Category B stimuli (B_1 and B_2 clusters under Discontinuous condition in **Table 4**). Importantly, stimuli from A_1 and B_1 are perceptually more similar than are A_1 and A_2 stimuli or B_1 and B_2. Thus, two important features of nonlinear rules are replicated: (1) perceptually dissimilar stimuli must be categorized together, and (2) more striatal units are needed to represent the categories; however, the rule is now linear. In contrast, in the Continuous condition, which served as the control condition, the categories were again composed of two clusters, but the clusters overlapped, which resulted in participants having to learn to categorize perceptually similar stimuli into the same category and a greater likelihood that only a single unit would be needed to represent the categories. If PD patients were differentially impaired in the Discontinuous relative to the Continuous condition, it would provide support for the "communication among units" hypothesis.

RESULTS

Accuracy rates for Experiment 2 are depicted in **Figure 7A** and were analyzed using a 2 (group: PD vs. NC) × 5 (blocks 1–5) mixed-design ANOVA. Results of this analysis identified a main effect of group, $F_{(1,\,18)} = 6.68$, $p < 0.05$, $\eta_p^2 = 0.27$, with PD patients performing worse than NC participants overall, and a main effect of block, $F_{(4,\,72)} = 11.06$, $p < 0.001$, $\eta_p^2 =$ 0.38, with both PD and NC participants' performances improving across the blocks. There was no group by block interaction, $F_{(4,\,72)} = 1.37$, $p = 0.25$, $\eta_p^2 = 0.07$. Performances in the Continuous Condition are shown in **Figure 7B** and were examined using the same mixed-design ANOVA as for the Discontinuous Condition. Results of this analysis indicated that there was there was a main effect of block, $F_{(4,\,80)} = 4.37$, $p <$ 0.01, $\eta_p^2 = 0.18$, but no effect of group, $F_{(1,\,20)} = 0.21$, $\eta_p^2 =$ 0.01, and no group × block interaction, $F_{(4,\,80)} = 0.85$, $p = 0.50$, $\eta_p^2 = 0.04$.

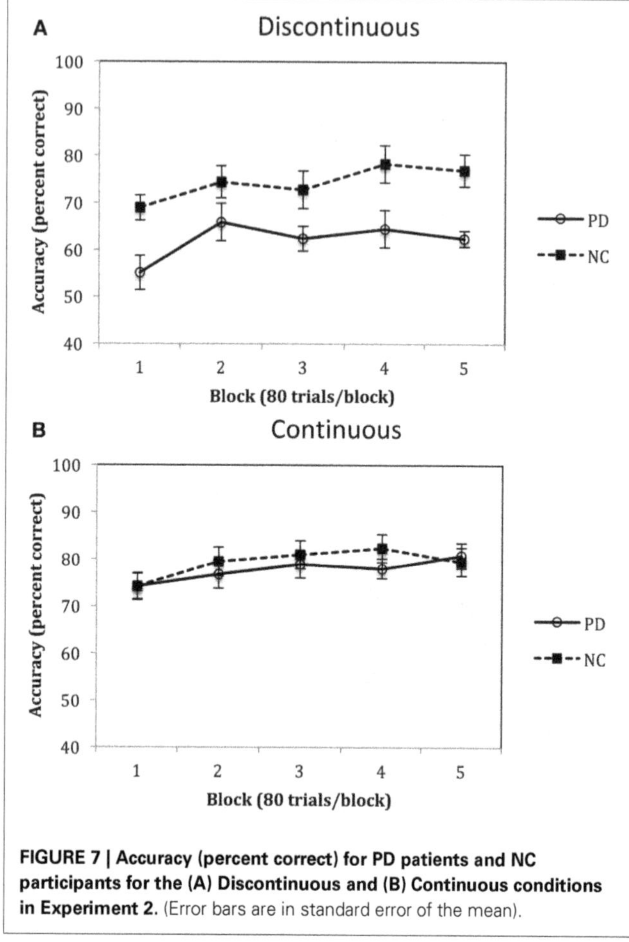

FIGURE 7 | Accuracy (percent correct) for PD patients and NC participants for the (A) Discontinuous and (B) Continuous conditions in Experiment 2. (Error bars are in standard error of the mean).

MODEL BASED ANALYSES

To further examine the results obtained in Experiment 2, we applied models to the final block of data separately from each participant (e.g., Estes, 1956; Maddox and Ashby, 1998; Smith and Minda, 1998; Maddox, 1999). The main class of model on which we focussed assumed that participants used an implicit procedural-based learning strategy—instantiated by applying the Ashby and Waldron's (1999) Striatal Pattern Classifier (SPC; see below for details). The model parameters were estimated using maximum likelihood (Ashby, 1992; Wickens, 1993) and the goodness-of-fit statistic was

$$AIC = 2r - 2lnL,$$

where r is the number of free parameters and L is the likelihood of the model given the data (Akaike, 1974; Takane and Shibayama, 1992). The AIC statistic penalizes a model for extra free parameters in such a way that the smaller the AIC, the closer a model is to the "true model," regardless of the number of free parameters. Thus, to find the best model among a given set of competitors, one simply computes an AIC value for each model, and chooses the model associated with the smallest AIC value (for a discussion of the complexities of model comparisons see (Myung, 2000; Pitt et al., 2002).

The SPC model has been found to provide a good computational model of participants' responding in previous information-integration category learning studies (e.g., Ashby and Waldron, 1999; Waldron and Ashby, 2001; for applications to stimulus identification see Ashby et al., 2001; Maddox, 2001, 2002). In addition, the assumptions of this model are based on the neurobiology proposed to underlie the procedural-based system (Ashby et al., 2001). The SPC-1 assumes that there is one striatal unit for each category, and the SPC-2 assumes that there are two striatal units for each category. Both models assume a single noise parameter that estimates the variability associated with the participant's responding, with large variability estimates being associated with less deterministic responding and small variability estimates being associated with more deterministic responding. These models were developed to examine the possibility that participants in the discontinuous condition might learn to associate the separate, and distinct, sub-clusters of perceptually similar stimuli with the appropriate category. We hypothesized that if there was a deficit in communication and recruitment among the medium spiny neurons via dysfunction of the interneurons, then the SPC-1 model should be more likely to account for the pattern of PD patients' responding in the discontinuous condition, whereas an SPC-2 model would be more likely to account for the NC participants' responding. In contrast, there should be no difference between the groups in the continuous condition.

The results of the model applications supported our prediction in that only 1 out of 10 of the PD patients' data sets in the discontinuous condition were better fit by the SPC-2 model, whereas 4 out of 10 of the NC participants' data sets were best fit by the SPC-2 model. Furthermore, for both groups, those participants whose data were best fit by the SPC-2 model demonstrated better accuracy than those whose data were best fit by the SPC-1 model (69.8 vs. 58.8% for the PD group; 87.2 vs. 70.0% for the NC participants). In contrast, in the continuous condition, 0 out of 11 PD patients' data sets were better fit by the SPC-2 model, and only 1 of the 11 data sets from the NC participants was best fit by the SPC-2 model. Thus, in the discontinuous condition, the SPC model with a greater number of units was more likely to account for NC data sets, and this model was also associated with greater accuracy rates[2].

DISCUSSION

The results from Experiment 2 indicated that, compared to NC participants, PD patients are impaired in procedural-based category learning when the categories are composed of discontinuous categories but are not impaired with continuous categories. **Figure 7** also demonstrates the slight advantage NC participants have when learning continuous vs. discontinuous categories, a finding that we observed in our previous studies with healthy younger participants (Maddox et al., 2007). Of note, if the category clusters from the discontinuous condition (see **Figure 6A**) were from four different continuous categories, as opposed to two discontinuous categories, we would predict that PD patients would be normal.

Note this is the first study in which we found PD patients to be impaired in learning a linear procedural-based rule, arguing against the surface-level explanation that PD patients' deficits in category learning are simply due to the linearity of the rule. Rather, the present results support the hypothesis that PD patients are impaired in procedural-based category learning when there is a need for communication among striatal units, thereby supporting the "communication among units" hypothesis. We now turn to a discussion of the theoretical implications of our findings.

THEORETICAL DISCUSSION

The main finding from the present set of experiments was that PD patients are impaired in learning discontinuous categories but are normal in learning continuous categories. In addition, these patients are not impaired when having to learn four categories. These findings provide initial support for our "communication among units" hypothesis. In contrast, the two groups did not differ in learning a procedural-based task with four categories, which does not support our "number of units" hypotheses.

The finding that PD patients are not impaired in learning either four- or two-category tasks suggests that the theoretical striatal units are functionally intact. This is consistent with the hypothesis that the medium spiny neurons were able to adequately represent multiple categories in our sample of PD patients. While it is known from PD animal models that the functional integrity of the medium spiny neurons can diminish in the absence of dopamine (Arbuthnott et al., 2000), post-mortem studies with actual PD patients suggest that structural changes to these neurons occurs only in later stages of the disease and may be the cause of motor complications secondary to dopaminergic treatment (i.e., dyskinesia). Specifically, Zaja-Milatovic et al. (2005) examined 9 PD patients post-mortem who had the disease a mean of 13 years and found that dendritic length of the medium spiny neurons was reduced in all striatal regions examined in PD patients relative to control post-mortem samples. The patients in our study tended to have the disease a mean of 6–7 years and were not displaying any complications of dopaminergic treatment (e.g., dyskinesia), so it is possible that the disease had not progressed in our patients to a point where the functioning of the medium spiny neurons had been impacted. This possibility raises the interesting question of whether PD patients with motor complications such as dyskinesia would be more likely to display deficits in the four-category condition given the possibility that their medium spiny neurons are less functional.

In contrast to the findings in Experiment 1, PD patients demonstrated a deficit in the Discontinuous condition in Experiment 2 but not in the Continuous condition. We have hypothesized that this is due to abnormal communication among the cholinergic interneurons in PD. We further hypothesized that normal interneuron communication is needed so that different medium spiny neurons that are processing perceptually dissimilar stimuli can resolve that they are representing stimuli that belong to the same category and are linked to the same response. This would only be required when there is a need for a greater number of the theoretical striatal units, such as when multiple units are needed to represent perceptually dissimilar exemplars from the same category (i.e., with discontinuous and nonlinear categories). Our assumption that striatal cholinergic interneurons are dysfunctional in PD is based on animal models that demonstrate increased activity of such neurons in the presence of reduced dopamine levels (Raz et al., 2001; Pisani et al., 2003; Bonsi et al., 2011). If this over activity of striatal interneurons is sufficient, improper signaling between medium spiny neurons would be likely to occur and the linking of perceptually dissimilar stimuli to the same response would be greatly compromised. This theoretical explanation is supported by other lines of research suggesting that the role of the basal ganglia, in general, and striatum, in particular, is to participate in response selection via the disinhibition of wanted responses and inhibition of unwanted responses (Mink, 1996; Stocco, 2012).

The possibility that cholinergic abnormality in PD underlies cognitive deficits in these patients is not new. However, the role of acetylcholine in PD cognition is not straightforward. On one hand there are previous studies indicating that medications

[2]It should also be noted that we applied a number of hypothesis-testing models that assumed the individual used an explicit approach to learning the categories. Although a few data sets were best fit by this class of models, the actual fits were close to those of the SPC models. Given specific questions we posed with the modeling and the small sample size we felt it was more important to focus on contrasting the SPC-1 and SPC-2 models.

that prevent the breakdown of acetylcholine (i.e., cholinesterase inhibitors) improve cognition in demented patients with PD (Emre et al., 2004; Bosboom et al., 2009; Possin et al., 2013). On the other hand we argue here that increased activity in cholinergic interneuron leads to a deficit in procedural-based category learning. Adding to this possible paradox are findings from a previous study where we demonstrated that impaired learning of a nonlinear procedural-based rule predicted future decline in global cognitive functioning in a group of nondemented PD patients (Filoteo et al., 2007). In addition, the fact that anticholinergic medications are often given to patients early in the course of the disease to improve motor symptoms by presumably reducing the over activity of the cholinergic interneurons also adds to the confusion as to how acetylcholine helps or hurts cognitive and motor functioning in PD. While we are unlikely to resolve these issues here, these possibilities raise the intriguing question of whether the administration of an anticholinergic would paradoxically improve nonlinear or discontinuous category learning in nondemented PD patients, or whether the use of a cholinesterase inhibitor would have any impact. These questions, and the general role of acetylcholine in PD cognition, certainly warrant further study.

It is important to note that the ideas tested in this paper are based on a hypothetical role of the function of cholinergic interneurons in the striatum and clearly represent an oversimplification of both the architecture and function of striatal medium spiny neurons and interneurons. At present, there is no neurobiological evidence to suggest that the specific role of these interneurons is to provide a conduit for which medium spiny neurons can link perceptually dissimilar stimuli to the same response. It may also be the case that the findings we report here are not due to such impairment but rather to some other mechanism, such as dysfunction in the output stage of response selection (e.g., Gurney et al., 2001). What is important is that we have further identified the experimental conditions under which PD patients demonstrate procedural-based category learning deficits, and that these data provide additional insights onto the mechanistic basis for some of our highly consistent previous results (Maddox and Filoteo, 2001; Ashby et al., 2003a,b; Filoteo et al., 2005a,b). In addition, the present work offers a potential computational understanding of the similarities between impaired nonlinear and discontinuous procedural-based category learning deficits in PD.

There are obviously several limitations to the present work. First, in regard to Experiment 1, it is possible that we did not tax the striatum sufficiently by the use of only four categories. It is possible that had we increased the number of categories we would have seen a deficit in the PD patients. As noted above, it is also possible that if we were to test patients in a more advanced stage of PD we would be more likely to see an impairment given the possibility that medium spiny neurons are only impacted in later stages of the disease (Zaja-Milatovic et al., 2005). Second, in regard to Experiment 2, there are several additional manipulations that could have been conducted to further examine the impact of discontinuity in PD patients' procedural-based category learning deficit. For example, in the present study we only examined one within category discontinuous separation and one between category separation. In other words, the within category cluster distance is fixed and so is the category (A vs. B) cluster separation. This issue could be examined parametrically to see what within and what between separations lead to a deficit. If, for example, we found that systematically increasing the between category separation decreases the magnitude of impairment in PD, this would further support the notion that perceptual similarity plays a key role in the observed deficit. Such manipulations are critical to further advance these theories. Third, in Experiment 2, the conditions did not only differ in terms of category continuity but also in terms of within-category range (i.e., how much of the stimulus space was occupied by category exemplars), which also could have explained the findings. However, in a previous study with healthy participants (Maddox and Filoteo, 2011) we found that category discontinuity had a greater impact on learning than did within-category range, suggesting that the results from the present study are less likely related to the degree of within-category range. Nonetheless, it will be important for future studies to directly examine this issue in PD.

In summary, the present study tested two theories of PD patients' deficits in procedural-based category learning. Our results and conclusions, while highly tentative and theoretical, suggest that PD patients are primarily impaired when learning requires perceptually dissimilar stimuli to be grouped in the same category, which may be due to dysfunctional communication among striatal units secondary to faulty communication.

ACKNOWLEDGMENTS

This research was supported in part by VA Merit Award and NINDS Grant (R01-41372) to J. Vincent Filoteo and NIMH Grant (R01-59196) to W. Todd Maddox.

REFERENCES

Akaike, H. (1974). A new look at the statistical model identification. *IEEE Trans. Automatic Control* 19, 716–723. doi: 10.1109/TAC.1974.1100705

Aosaki, T., Miura, M., Suzuki, T., Nishimura, K., and Masuda, M. (2010). Acetylcholine-dopamine balance hypothesis in the striatum: an update. *Geriatr. Gerontol. Int.* 10(Suppl. 1), S148–S157. doi: 10.1111/j.1447-0594.2010.00588.x

Apicella, P. (2002). Tonically active neurons in the primate striatum and their role in the processing of information about motivationaly relevant events. *Eur. J. Neurosci.* 16, 2017–2026. doi: 10.1046/j.1460-9568.2002.02262.x

Apicella, P. (2007). Leading tonically active neurons of the striatum from reward detection to contex recognition. *Trends Neurosci.* 30, 299–306. doi: 10.1016/j.tins.2007.03.011

Arbuthnott, G. W., Ingham, C. A., and Wickens, J. R. (2000). Dopamine and synaptic plasticity in the neuostriatum. *J. Anat.* 196, 587–596. doi: 10.1046/j.1469-7580.2000.19640587.x

Aron, A. R., Shohamy, D., Clark, J., Myers, C., Gluck, M. A., and Poldrack, R. A. (2004). Human midbrain sensitivity to cognitive feedback and uncertainty during classification learning. *J. Neurophysiol.* 92, 1144–1152. doi: 10.1152/jn.01209.2003

Ashby, F. G. (1992). "Multivariate probability distributions," in *Multidimensional Models of Perception and Cognition*, ed F. G. Ashby (Hillsdale, NJ: Lawrence Erlbaum Associates, Inc.), 1–34.

Ashby, F. G., Alfonso-Reese, L. A., Turken, A. U., and Waldron, E. M. (1998). A neuropsychological theory of multiple systems in category learning. *Psychol. Rev.* 105, 442–481. doi: 10.1037/0033-295X.105.3.442

Ashby, F. G., and Crossley, M. J. (2011). A computational model of how cholinergic interneurons protect striatal-dependent learning. *J. Cogn. Neurosci.* 23, 1549–1566. doi: 10.1162/jocn.2010.21523

Ashby, F. G., and Ell, S. W. (2001). The neurobiology of human category learning. *Trends Cogn. Sci.* 5, 204–210. doi: 10.1016/S1364-6613(00)01624-7

Ashby, F. G., Ell, S. W., and Waldron, E. M. (2003a). Procedural learning in perceptual categorization. *Mem. Cognit.* 31, 1114–1125. doi: 10.3758/BF03196132

Ashby, F. G., Ennis, J. M., and Spiering, B. J. (2007). A neurobiological theory of automaticity in perceptual categorization. *Psychol. Rev.* 114, 632–656. doi: 10.1037/0033-295X.114.3.632

Ashby, F. G., Noble, S., Filoteo, J. V., Waldron, E. M., and Ell, S. W. (2003b). Category learning deficits in Parkinson's disease. *Neuropsychology* 17, 115–124. doi: 10.1037/0894-4105.17.1.115

Ashby, F. G., and Gott, R. E. (1988). Decision rules in the perception and categorization of multidimensional stimuli. *J. Exp. Psychol. Learn. Mem. Cogn.* 14, 33–53. doi: 10.1037/0278-7393.14.1.33

Ashby, F. G., and Maddox, W. T. (2005). Human category learning. *Annu. Rev. Psychol.* 56, 149–178. doi: 10.1146/annurev.psych.56.091103.070217

Ashby, F. G., and Maddox, W. T. (2011). Human category learning 2.0. *Ann. N.Y. Acad. Sci.* 1224, 147–161. doi: 10.1111/j.1749-6632.2010.05874.x

Ashby, F. G., Maddox, W. T., and Bohil, C. J. (2002). Observational versus feedback training in rule-based and information-integration category learning. *Mem. Cognit.* 30, 666–677. doi: 10.3758/BF03196423

Ashby, F. G., and O'Brien, J. B. (2005). Category learning and multiple memory systems. *Trends Cogn. Sci.* 9, 83–89. doi: 10.1016/j.tics.2004.12.003

Ashby, F. G., Paul, E. J., and Maddox, W. T. (2010). *Formal Approaches in Categorization.* New York, NY: Cambridge University Press.

Ashby, F. G., and Waldron, E. M. (1999). The nature of implicit categorization. *Psychon. Bull. Rev.* 6, 363–378. doi: 10.3758/BF03210826

Ashby, F. G., Waldron, E. M., Lee, W. W., and Berkman, A. (2001). Suboptimality in human categorization and identification. *J. Exp. Psychol. Gen.* 130, 77–96. doi: 10.1037/0096-3445.130.1.77

Bar-Gad, I., Morris, G., and Bergman, H. (2003). Information processing, dimensionality reduction and reinforcement learning in the basal ganglia. *Prog. Neurobiol.* 71, 439–473. doi: 10.1016/j.pneurobio.2003.12.001

Bonsi, P., Cuomo, D., Martella, G., Madeo, G., Schirinzi, T., Francesca, P., et al. (2011). Centrality of striatal cholinergic transmission in basal ganglia function. *Front. Neuroanat.* 5:6. doi: 10.3389/fnana.2011.00006

Bosboom, J. L. W., Stoffers, D., Stam, C. J., Berendse, H. W., and Wolters, E.Ch. (2009). Cholinergic modulation of MEG resting-state oscillatory activity in Parkinson's disease related dementia. *Clin. Neurophysiol.* 120, 910–915. doi: 10.1016/j.clinph.2009.03.004

Brainard, D. H. (1997). The psychophysics toolbox. *Spat. Vis.* 10, 433–436. doi: 10.1163/156856897X00357

Cincotta, C. M., and Seger, C. A. (2007). Dissociation between striatal regions while learning to categorize via feedback and via observation. *J. Cogn. Neurosci.* 19, 249–265. doi: 10.1162/jocn.2007.19.2.249

Crossley, M. J., Ashby, F. G., and Maddox, W. T. (2013). Erasing the engram: the unlearning of procedural skills. *J. Exp. Psychol. Gen.* 142, 710–741. doi: 10.1037/a0030059

Deutch, A. Y., Colbran, R. J., and Winder, D. J. (2007). Striatal plasticity and medium spiny neuron dendritic remodeling in parkinsonism. *Parkinsonism Relat. Disord.* 13, S251–S258. doi: 10.1016/S1353-8020(08)70012-9

Emre, M., Aarsland, D., Albanese, A., Byrne, E. J., Deuschl, G., De Deyn, P. P., et al. (2004). Rivastigmine for dementia associated with Parkinson's disease. *N. Engl. J. Med.* 351, 2509–2518. doi: 10.1056/NEJMoa041470

Estes, W. K. (1956). The problem of inference from curves based on group data. *Psychol. Bull.* 53, 134–140. doi: 10.1037/h0045156

Filoteo, J. V., Maddox, W. T., and Davis, J. D. (2001a). A possible role of the striatum in linear and nonlinear category learning: evidence from patients with Huntington's disease. *Behav. Neurosci.* 115, 786–798. doi: 10.1037/0735-7044.115.4.786

Filoteo, J. V., Maddox, W. T., and Davis, J. D. (2001b). Quantitative modeling of category learning in amnesic patients. *J. Int. Neuropsychol. Soc.* 7, 1–19. doi: 10.1017/S1355617701711010

Filoteo, J. V., Maddox, W. T., Salmon, D. P., and Song, D. D. (2005a). Information-integration category learning in patients with striatal dysfunction. *Neuropsychology* 19, 212–222. doi: 10.1037/0894-4105.19.2.212

Filoteo, J. V., Maddox, W. T., Salmon, D. P., and Song, D. D. (2007). Implicit category learning performance predicts rate of cognitive decline in nondemented patients with Parkinson's diease. *Neuropsychology* 21, 183–192. doi: 10.1037/0894-4105.21.2.183

Filoteo, J. V., Maddox, W. T., Simmons, A. N., Ing, A. D., Cagigas, X. E., Matthews, S., et al. (2005b). Cortical and subcortical brain regions involved in rule-based category learning. *Neuroreport* 16, 111–115. doi: 10.1097/00001756-200502080-00007

Filoteo, J. V., Simmons, A. N., Zeithamova, D., Maddox, W. T., and Paulus, M. P. (2006). "Change in patterns of brain activity related to early and later learning of information-integration category structures," in *Paper presented at the Cognitive Neuroscience Society* (San Francisco).

Gluck, M. A., Shohamy, D., and Myers, C. (2002). How do people solve the "weather prediction" task? Individual variability in strategies for probabilistic category learning. *Learn. Mem.* 9, 408–418. doi: 10.1101/lm.45202

Graybiel, A., Aosaki, T., Flaherty, A., and Kimura, M. (1994). The basal ganglia and adaptive motor control. *Science* 265, 1826–1831. doi: 10.1126/science.8091209

Gurney, K., Prescott, T. J., and Redgrave, P. (2001). A computational model of action selection in the basal ganglia. I. A new functional anatomy. *Biol. Cybern.* 84, 401–410. doi: 10.1007/PL00007984

Hoehn, M. M., and Yahr, M. D. (1967). Parkinsonism: onset, progression and mortality. *Neurology* 17, 427–442. doi: 10.1212/WNL.17.5.427

Hughes, A. J., Daniel, S. E., Kilford, L., and Lees, A. J. (1992). Accuracy of clinical diagnosis of idiopathic Parkinson's disease: a clinico-pathological study of 100 cases. *J. Neurol. Neurosurg. Psychiatry* 55, 181–184. doi: 10.1136/jnnp.55.3.181

Joshua, M., Adler, A., Mitelman, R., Vaadia, E., and Bergman, H. (2008). Midbrain dopaminergic neurons and striatal cholinergic interneurons encode the difference between reward and aversive events at different epochs of probabilistic classical conditioning trials. *J. Neurosci.* 28, 11673–11684. doi: 10.1523/JNEUROSCI.3839-08.2008

Keri, S. (2003). The cognitive neuroscience of category learning. *Brain Res. Brain Res. Rev.* 43, 85–109. doi: 10.1016/S0165-0173(03)00204-2

Knowlton, B. J., Mangels, J. A., and Squire, L. R. (1996). A neostriatal habit learning system in humans. *Science* 273, 1399–1402. doi: 10.1126/science.273.5280.1399

Knowlton, B. J., Squire, L. R., and Gluck, M. A. (1994). Probabilistic classification learning in amnesia. *Learn. Mem.* 1, 106–120.

Maddox, W. T. (1999). On the dangers of averaging across observers when comparing decision bound and generalized context models of categorization. *Percept. Psychophys.* 61, 354–374. doi: 10.3758/BF03206893

Maddox, W. T. (2001). Separating perceptual processes from decisional processes in identification and categorization. *Percept. Psychophys.* 63, 1183–1200. doi: 10.3758/BF03194533

Maddox, W. T. (2002). Learning and attention in multidimensional identification, and categorization: separating low-level perceptual processes and high-level decisional processes. *J. Exp. Psychol. Learn. Mem. Cogn.* 28, 99–115. doi: 10.1037/0278-7393.28.1.99

Maddox, W. T., Aparicio, P., Marchant, N. L., and Ivry, R. B. (2005a). Rule-based category learning is impaired in patients with Parkinson's disease but not in patients with cerebellar disorders. *J. Cogn. Neurosci.* 17, 707–723. doi: 10.1162/0898929053747630

Maddox, W. T., and Ashby, F. G. (1998). Selective attention and the formation of linear decision bounds. Commentary on McKinley and Nosofsky (1996). *J. Exp. Psychol. Hum. Percept. Perform.* 24, 301–321. doi: 10.1037/0096-1523.24.1.301

Maddox, W. T., and Ashby, F. G. (2004). Dissociating explicit and procedural-learning based systems of perceptual category learning. *Behav. Processes* 66, 309–332. doi: 10.1016/j.beproc.2004.03.011

Maddox, W. T., Ashby, F. G., and Bohil, C. J. (2003). Delayed feedback effects on rule-based and information-integration category learning. *J. Exp. Psychol. Learn. Mem. Cogn.* 29, 650–662. doi: 10.1037/0278-7393.29.4.650

Maddox, W. T., Bohil, C. J., and Ing, A. D. (2004a). Evidence for a procedural-learning-based system in perceptual category learning. *Psychon. Bull. Rev.* 11, 945–952. doi: 10.3758/BF03196726

Maddox, W. T., and Filoteo, J. V. (2001). Striatal contributions to category learning: quantitative modeling of simple linear and complex nonlinear rule learning in patients with Parkinson's disease. *J. Int. Neuropsychol. Soc.* 7, 710–727. doi: 10.1017/S1355617701766076

Maddox, W. T., and Filoteo, J. V. (2011). Stimulus range and discontinuity effects on information-integration category learning and generalization. *Atten. Percept. Psychophys.* 73, 1279–1295. doi: 10.3758/s13414-011-0101-2

Maddox, W. T., Filoteo, J. V., and Lauritzen, J. S. (2007). Within-category discontinuity interacts with verbal rule complexity in perceptual category learning. *J. Exp. Psychol. Learn. Mem. Cogn.* 33, 197–218. doi: 10.1037/0278-7393.33.1.197

Maddox, W. T., Filoteo, J. V., Lauritzen, J. S., Connally, E., and Hejl, K. D. (2005b). Discontinuous categories affect information-integration but not rule-based category learning. *J. Exp. Psychol. Learn. Mem. Cogn.* 31, 654–669. doi: 10.1037/0278-7393.31.4.654

Maddox, W. T., Filoteo, J. V., Hejl, K. D., and Ing, A. D. (2004b). Category number impacts rule-based but not information-integration category learning: further evidence for dissociable category-learning systems. *J. Exp. Psychol. Learn. Mem. Cogn.* 30, 227–245. doi: 10.1037/0278-7393.30.1.227

Maddox, W. T., and Ing, A. D. (2005). Delayed feedback disrupts the procedural-learning system but not the hypothesis-testing system in perceptual category learning. *J. Exp. Psychol. Learn. Mem. Cogn.* 31, 100–107. doi: 10.1037/0278-7393.31.1.100

Mattis, S. (1988). *Dementia Rating Scale.* Odessa, FL: Psychological Assessment Resources.

Mink, J. W. (1996). The basal ganglia: focused selection and inhibition of competing motor programs. *Prog. Neurobiol.* 50, 381–425. doi: 10.1016/S0301-0082(96)00042-1

Myung, I. J. (2000). The importance of complexity in model selection. *J. Math. Psychol.* 44, 190–204. doi: 10.1006/jmps.1999.1283

Nomura, E. M., Maddox, W. T., Filoteo, J. V., Ing, A. D., Gitelman, D. R., Parrish, T. B., et al. (2007). Neural correlates of rule-based and information-integration visual category learning. *Cereb. Cortex* 17, 37–43. doi: 10.1093/cercor/bhj122

Oldenburg, I. A., and Ding, J. B. (2011). Cholinergic modulation of synaptic integration and dendritic excitability in the striatum. *Curr. Opin. Neurobiol.* 21, 425–432. doi: 10.1016/j.conb.2011.04.004

Patalano, A. L., Smith, E. E., Jonides, J., and Koeppe, R. A. (2001). PET evidence for multiple strategies of categorization. *Cogn. Affect. Behav. Neurosci.* 1, 360–370. doi: 10.3758/CABN.1.4.360

Pisani, A., Bonsi, P., Centonze, D., Gubellini, P., Bernardi, G., and Calabresi, P. (2003). Targeting striatal cholinergic interneurons in Parkinson's disease: focus on metabotropic glutamate receptors. *Neuropharmacology* 45, 45–56. doi: 10.1016/S0028-3908(03)00137-0

Pitt, M. A., Myung, I. J., and Zhang, S. (2002). Toward a method of selecting among computational models of cognition. *Psychol. Rev.* 109, 472–491. doi: 10.1037/0033-295X.109.3.472

Poldrack, R. A., Prabhakaran, V., Seger, C. A., and Gabrieli, J. D. (1999). Striatal activation during acquisition of a cognitive skill. *Neuropsychology* 13, 564–574. doi: 10.1037/0894-4105.13.4.564

Possin, K. L., Kang, G. A., Guo, C., Fine, E. M., Trujillo, A. J., Racine, C. A., et al. (2013). Rivastigmine is associated with restoration of left frontal brain activity in Parkinson's disease. *Mov. Disord.* 28, 1384–1390. doi: 10.1002/mds.25575

Price, A., Filoteo, J. V., and Maddox, W. T. (2009). Rule-based category learning in patients with Parkinson's disease. *Neuropsychologia* 47, 1213–1226. doi: 10.1016/j.neuropsychologia.2009.01.031

Raz, A., Frechter-Mazar, V., Feingold, A., Abeles, M., Vaadia, E., and Bergman, H. (2001). Activity of pallidal and striatal tonically active neurons is correlated in MPTP-treated monkeys but not in normal monkeys. *J. Neurosci.* 21, RCI129 (1–5).

Reber, P. J., Gitelman, D. R., Parrish, T. B., and Mesulam, M. M. (2003). Dissociating explicit and implicit category knowledge with fMRI. *J. Cogn. Neurosci.* 15, 574–583. doi: 10.1162/089892903321662958

Redgrave, P., Vautrelle, N., and Reynolds, J. N. J. (2011). Functional properties of the basal ganglia's re-entrant loop architecture: selection and reinforcement. *Neuroscience* 198, 138–151. doi: 10.1016/j.neuroscience.2011.07.060

Shohamy, D., Myers, C. E., Grossman, S., Sage, J., Gluck, M. A., and Poldrack, R. A. (2004a). Cortico-striatal contributions to feedback-based learning:converging data from neuroimaging and neuropsychology. *Brain* 127(Pt 4), 851–859. doi: 10.1093/brain/awh100

Shohamy, D., Myers, C. E., Onlaor, S., and Gluck, M. A. (2004b). Role of the basal ganglia in category learning: how do patients with Parkinson's disease learn? *Behav. Neurosci.* 118, 676–686. doi: 10.1037/0735-7044.118.4.676

Smith, E. E., Patalano, A. L., and Jonides, J. (1998). Alternative strategies of categorization. *Cognition* 65, 167–196. doi: 10.1016/S0010-0277(97)00043-7

Smith, J. D., Berg, M. E., Cook, R. G., Murphy, M. S., Crossley, M. J., Boomer, J., et al. (2012). Implicit and explicit categorization: a tale of four species. *Neurosci. Biobehav. Rev.* 36, 2355–2369. doi: 10.1016/j.neubiorev.2012.09.003

Smith, J. D., and Minda, J. P. (1998). Prototypes in the mist: the early epochs of category learning. *J. Exp. Psychol. Learn. Mem. Cogn.* 24, 1411–1436. doi: 10.1037/0278-7393.24.6.1411

Stocco, A. (2012). Acetylcholine-based entropy in response selection: a model of how striatal interneurons modulate exploration, exploitation, and response variability. *Fron. Neurosci.* 6:18. doi: 10.3389/fnins.2012.00018

Takane, Y., and Shibayama, T. (1992). "Structures in stimulus identification data," in *Multidimensional Models of Perception and Cognition*, ed F. G. Ashby (Hillsdale, NJ: Erlbaum), 335–362.

Waldron, E. M., and Ashby, F. G. (2001). The effects of concurrent task interference on category learning: evidence for multiple category learning systems. *Psychon. Bull. Rev.* 8, 168–176. doi: 10.3758/BF03196154

Waldschmidt, J. G., and Ashby, F. G. (2011). Cortical and striatal contributions to automaticity in information-integration categorization. *Neuroimage* 56, 1791–1802. doi: 10.1016/j.neuroimage.2011.02.011

Wickens, J. (1993). *A Theory of the Striatum.* New York, NY: Pergamon Press.

Wilson, C. J. (1995). *The Contribution of Cortical Neurons to the Firing Pattern of Striatal Spiny Neurons.*Cambridge: MIT Press.

Worthy, D. A., Markman, A. B., and Maddox, W. T. (2013). Feedback and stimulus-offset timing effects in perceptual category learning. *Brain Cogn.* 81, 283–293. doi: 10.1016/j.bandc.2012.11.006

Zaja-Milatovic, S., Milatovic, D., Schantz, A. M., Zhang, J., Montine, K. S., Samii, A., et al. (2005). Dendritic degeneration in neurostriatal medium spiny neurons in Parkinson disease. *Neurology* 64, 545–547. doi: 10.1212/01.WNL.0000150591.33787.A4

19

A Plastic Corticostriatal Circuit Model of Adaptation in Perceptual Decision Making

Pao-Yueh Hsiao*[1] *and Chung-Chuan Lo*[1,2]

[1] *Institute of Systems Neuroscience, National Tsing Hua University, Hsinchu, Taiwan*
[2] *Department of Life Science, National Tsing Hua University, Hsinchu, Taiwan*

Correspondence:
Chung-Chuan Lo, Institute of Systems Neuroscience, National Tsing Hua University, Life Science Building I, No. 101, Section 2, Kuang-Fu Road, Hsinchu 30013, Taiwan
e-mail: cclo@mx.nthu.edu.tw

The ability to optimize decisions and adapt them to changing environments is a crucial brain function that increase survivability. Although much has been learned about the neuronal activity in various brain regions that are associated with decision making, and about how the nervous systems may learn to achieve optimization, the underlying neuronal mechanisms of how the nervous systems optimize decision strategies with preference given to speed or accuracy, and how the systems adapt to changes in the environment, remain unclear. Based on extensive empirical observations, we addressed the question by extending a previously described cortico-basal ganglia circuit model of perceptual decisions with the inclusion of a dynamic dopamine (DA) system that modulates spike-timing dependent plasticity (STDP). We found that, once an optimal model setting that maximized the reward rate was selected, the same setting automatically optimized decisions across different task environments through dynamic balancing between the facilitating and depressing components of the DA dynamics. Interestingly, other model parameters were also optimal if we considered the reward rate that was weighted by the subject's preferences for speed or accuracy. Specifically, the circuit model favored speed if we increased the phasic DA response to the reward prediction error, whereas the model favored accuracy if we reduced the tonic DA activity or the phasic DA responses to the estimated reward probability. The proposed model provides insight into the roles of different components of DA responses in decision adaptation and optimization in a changing environment.

Keywords: perceptual decision, adaptation, speed-accuracy tradeoff, neural network model, corticostriatal circuit, spike-timing dependent plasticity

INTRODUCTION

To ensure survivability in complex environments, animals need to adapt to environments that may change with time. For example, when making decisions, animals have to choose a proper strategy that is optimal for the current situation, such as making quick but inaccurate decisions vs. making slow but accurate decisions. However, whether a decision strategy is proper or not may be subject- and environment-dependent. Indeed, at the behavioral level, speed-accuracy tradeoff (SAT) has been demonstrated in humans and animals in various decision experiments (Schouten and Bekker, 1967; Wickelgren, 1977; Palmer et al., 2005; Chittka et al., 2009; Balci et al., 2010). Although it has been suggested that a strategy can be optimized by maximizing the reward rate (Gold and Shadlen, 2002; Lo and Wang, 2006), several studies have demonstrated cases in which subjects adopt strategies that are faster (but less accurate) or slower (but more accurate) than the ideal one that maximizes the reward rate (Maddox and Bohil, 1998; Chittka et al., 2009; Bogacz et al., 2010).

At the neuronal level, numerous studies have shown correlations between the complex responses of dopamine (DA) neurons and reward-related information in decision making (Schultz, 2000, 2002; Arias-Carrión et al., 2010; de Lafuente and Romo, 2011). Furthermore, the responses of DA neurons do not simply depend on the presence of rewards, but also on various task-related factors such as the expected probability and magnitude of rewards and reward prediction errors (Hollerman and Schultz, 1998; Schultz, 1999; Kawagoe et al., 2004; Takikawa et al., 2004; Nomoto et al., 2010). However, how the DA system contributes to the mechanisms underlying the differential strategy chosen, and how the animals adapt their decision strategies to changes in the environment, remain unclear.

At the theoretical level, a number of mathematical models and neural network models have been proposed to account for decision behavior (Ratcliff, 1978; Bogacz et al., 2006; Lo and Wang, 2006; O'Reilly and Frank, 2006; Simen et al., 2006; Bogacz and Gurney, 2007; Roxin and Ledberg, 2008; Wang, 2008; Cohen and Frank, 2009; Deco et al., 2009; Hong and Hikosaka, 2011). In particular, a spiking neural network model consisting of an attractor cortical network for information accumulation (Wang, 2002, 2008; Wong et al., 2007; Wang et al., 2013) and a cortico-basal ganglia circuit mediating the decision threshold (Lo and Wang, 2006) have suggested that the threshold can be modulated by the strength of the corticostriatal pathway. Hence, this has provided insights into how SAT may be implemented in the neural circuits that perform perceptual decisions. This prediction has been subsequently supported by human functional magnetic resonance imaging (fMRI) experiments (Forstmann et al., 2010).

Despite this progress, we still lack an integrated model, with sufficient biological detail, that illustrates the neuronal mechanisms underlying how individual subjects choose their decision strategies differently, how their decision strategies adapt to changing environments, and how detailed DA neuron activity, including responses to expected reward probability or reward prediction errors, may play a role in behavioral flexibility. Although reward-dependent plasticity has been incorporated in a number of rate-based neural network models to account for various flexible behaviors (Simen et al., 2006; Cohen and Frank, 2009; Rao, 2010; Bogacz and Larsen, 2011; Wiecki and Frank, 2013), most of the models either do not address how the subjects adapt their decisions to changing environments, or were built based on relatively abstract learning rules that do not include complex real-time dopamine dynamics and spike-time based plasticity that has been observed empirically (Suaud-Chagny et al., 1995; Bi and Poo, 1998; Shen et al., 2008; Nomoto et al., 2010). Some of the models have been designed for simulating action-selection and executive control, which may involve very different mechanisms from the perceptual discrimination that we studied here.

We present a spiking neural circuit model that integrates a spiking cortico-basal ganglia model (Lo and Wang, 2006) and a DA system with complex dynamics that is consistent with empirical observations (Suaud-Chagny et al., 1995; Bi and Poo, 1998; Shen et al., 2008; Nomoto et al., 2010). We demonstrate that different decision strategies that are adopted by different animals can all be optimal in their own subjective sense which is weighted by their individual preferences for speed or accuracy. Furthermore, the interplay between the different temporal components of the DA dynamics supports the adaptation of the optimal strategies in response to changes in the environment.

MATERIALS AND METHODS

THE BASIC HYPOTHESIS AND LOGIC OF THE MODEL

In the present study, we did not investigate how a neural network can learn to achieve an optimal decision strategy, which has been addressed in various modeling studies, and we accepted that an optimal decision can be achieved by learning. Instead, we hypothesized that there is not just one, but many different optimal decision strategies that are weighted by individual's preferences for speed or accuracy. Our goal was to study how preferences were influenced by the detailed activity of the DA system and how dynamic balancing between different DA effects helped the subjects to adapt to changes in the environment when making perceptual decisions.

THE BEHAVIORAL TASK: RANDOM-DOT MOTION DISCRIMINATION

In order to investigate adaptive behavior in perceptual decision making and its optimization, we used the reaction-time version of the random-dot motion discrimination task (Newsome et al., 1989; Shadlen and Newsome, 1996; Roitman and Shadlen, 2002). In the task, a subject watches a display of randomly moving dots with a center fixation point and two saccade targets that are located on the two sides of the screen. A small fraction of the dots move coherently in one of two possible directions (right or left in our simulations), and the subject is required to determine the direction of the coherent movement while fixating on the center of the screen. The subject needs to make a saccade to the corresponding target (right target for right coherent movements and left target for the left coherent movements) as soon as a decision is reached.

The percentage of dots that move coherently is defined as the coherence level (c') or motion strength, and it represents the amount of evidence that is available to the subject during the decision process. Motion discrimination is easier in trials with a strong, compared to a weak, motion strength. We tested our model with two conditions: easy and difficult. The easy condition consisted only of trials with c' levels of 12.8, 25.6, and 51.2%, while the difficult condition consisted only of trials with c' levels of 3.2, 6.4, and 12.8%. The trials of the different coherence levels in each condition were pseudorandomly distributed with equal probability. The reaction time was defined as the interval between the start of the sensory input and the time when the subject made a saccade.

SINGLE NEURON MODEL

Neurons in the circuit model were simulated with the conductance-based leaky integrate-and-fire model that is described as follows.

The membrane potential $V(t)$ obeys the following equation:

$$C_m \frac{dV(t)}{dt} = -g_L\,(V(t) - V_L) - I_{\mathrm{syn}}(t),$$

where C_m is the membrane capacitance, g_L is the leak conductance, V_L is the resting potential, and I_{syn} is the total synaptic current. When the membrane potential $V(t)$ of each neuron reaches the threshold $V_{\mathrm{threshold}} = -50$ mV, a spike is emitted, and $V(t)$ is set to the reset potential $V_{\mathrm{reset}} = -55$ mV for a refractory period $T_r = 2$ ms. For inhibitory neurons, we used the following parameters: $C_m = 0.2$ nF, $g_L = 20$ nS, and $V_L = -70$ mV. For excitatory neurons, we used $C_m = 0.5$ nF, $g_L = 25$ nS, and $V_L = -70$ mV. I_{syn} is the total synaptic current and is given by:

$$\begin{aligned} I_{\mathrm{syn}}(t) &= g_{\mathrm{AMPA}} s_{\mathrm{AMPA}}(t)\,(V(t) - V_E) \\ &\quad + \frac{g_{\mathrm{NMDA}} s_{\mathrm{NMDA}}(t)\,(V(t) - V_E)}{1 + [Mg^{2+}]e^{-0.062V(t)/3.57}} \\ &\quad + g_{\mathrm{GABA}} s_{\mathrm{GABA}}(t)\,(V(t) - V_I) \end{aligned}$$

where (V_E (=0 mV) and V_I (= −70 mV) are the reversal potentials, $[\mathrm{Mg}^{2+}]$ (= 1.0 mM) is the extracellular magnesium concentration, g is the synaptic efficacy, and s is the gating variable. The subscripts in g and s denote the receptor type. The gating variables are described by

$$\frac{ds(t)}{dt} = \sum_k \delta\left(t - t^k\right) - \frac{s}{\tau}$$

for AMPA and GABA receptors and

$$\frac{ds(t)}{dt} = \alpha\,(1 - s(t)) \sum_k \delta\left(t - t^k\right) - \frac{s}{\tau}$$

for NMDA receptors, where $\tau = 2$ ms for AMPA, 100 ms for NMDA, and 5 ms for GABA. $\delta(t - t^k)$ is the delta function, and t^k is the time of the k-th pre-synaptic spike. The differential equations were solved numerically by the first-order Euler method with a time step of 0.1 ms.

THE CORTICO-BASAL GANGLIA NEURAL CIRCUIT OF DECISION MAKING

The model of the corticobasal ganglia neural circuit used in the present study was developed based on a previously described model (Lo and Wang, 2006), which consists of a cortical (Cx) circuit, a superior colliculus (SC) circuit, and a basal ganglia (BG) circuit (**Figure 1**). All parameters in the previous model (Lo and Wang, 2006) were preserved except for two changes made to CD neuron-related parameters due to the inclusion of the synaptic plasticity in the present model. First, we added NMDA receptors to the Cx-to-CD synapses and reduced the conductance for the AMPA-mediated current on the same synapse accordingly. Second, we increased the background noise for CD neurons in order to produce a baseline firing rate of several spikes per second. The small baseline activity is important for maintaining plasticity throughout the course of a trial. See **Table 1** for the parameters that were used in the circuit model. Three major neural processes described below are involved in the model:

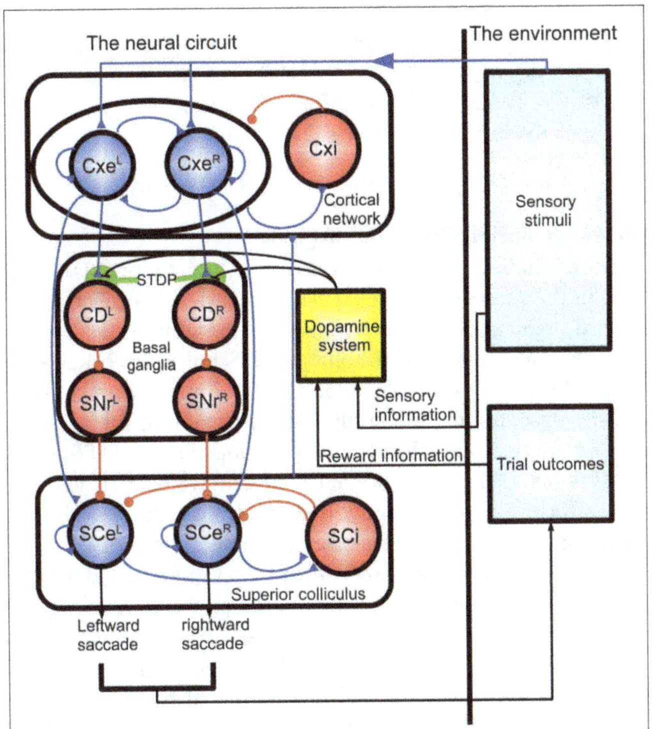

FIGURE 1 | Schematics of the computational model of decision optimization and adaptation for the random-dot direction discrimination task. The model is described by a close loop process that involves a neural circuit based on a dopamine system and a previously described cortico-basal ganglia circuit model (Lo and Wang, 2006). The neural circuit receives sensory input, accumulates sensory evidence (random dot movements), detects the threshold crossing, and then makes a decision (saccadic eye movements). The outcome of the decision determines the reward and thereby influences the dopamine system. The dopamine activity modulates the decision process by changing the Cx-CD synaptic strength through spike-timing dependent plasticity (STDP). Each circle represents a population of leaky integrate-and-fire neurons, and the dopamine system is a functional unit that is modeled by several equations. Cx, cortex; Cxe, excitatory cortical pyramidal neurons; Cxi, inhibitory cortical interneurons; CD, caudate nucleus; SNr, substantia nigra pars reticulata; SCe, superior colliculus excitatory neurons; SCi, superior colliculus inhibitory neurons. The L and R superscripts denote the neural populations responding to the left and right stimuli, respectively.

(1) Winner-take-all competition for sensory signals in the cortical network: After the stimulus onset, two signals representing the amount of leftward and rightward dot movements [presumably from the visual MT area (Britten et al., 1993)] project to the neural populations Cxe^L and Cxe^R in the Cx, respectively. The two decision populations, Cxe^L and Cxe^R, compete with each other through the inhibitory interneurons in Cxi. As a consequence, the decision population receiving the stronger sensory input has a higher chance to accumulate its activity (population firing rate) and suppress the other (Wang, 2002). The activity of the two decision populations are sent to the downstream regions (SC and BG) for further computation. There is a non-selective background population, CxeBg, that mimics neurons that are selective for directions other than the two forced-choice alternatives or to other stimuli that are irrelevant to the present study.

(2) All-or-nothing motor output in the SC: The neural circuit of the SC is similar to that of the Cx but with two important differences. First, the feedback excitation in SCe^L and SCe^R and the lateral inhibition between SCi and SCe^R/SCe^L are much stronger than those in Cx. Second, the lateral inhibition is endowed with short-term synaptic facilitation, as described in Lo and Wang (2006). These differences allow neurons in the SCe^R or SCe^L to develop a strong burst of spikes lasting for about 50 ms in response to input from the Cx. The activity resembles what has been observed in burst neurons in the SC of monkeys during various saccadic eye movement experiments (Munoz and Wurtz, 1995; Sparks, 2002). In the model, the saccadic eye movement was triggered, or a decision was made, when the population firing rate of SCe^R or SCe^L reached the threshold of 60 spikes/s. In addition to the excitatory input from the Cx, SCe^R, and SCe^L were constantly suppressed by feed-forward inhibition from the BG. Therefore, the Cx could only activate the SCe when it was disinhibited by the BG.

(3) Threshold-crossing detection and disinhibition: The $SNr^L$and SNr^R in the BG constantly exhibit inhibition over the SCe^L and SCe^R in the SC, respectively. This inhibition can be removed by GABAergic input from upstream caudate nuclei $(CD)^L$ and CD^R, which in turn receive inputs from the decision neurons in the Cx. Therefore, when the activity in the Cxe^L (or Cxe^R) is strong enough to activate CD^L (or CD^R), the activated CD^L (or CD^R) disinhibits the SC through the SNr^L (or SNr^R) and allows SCe^L (or SCe^R) to respond to input from the Cxe^L (or Cxe^R), thus producing a saccadic eye movement. The activation of the CD^L or CD^R indicates the detection of the crossing of the decision

Table 1 | Parameters of the circuit model.

Population name	Number of neurons	Membrane capacitance (nF)	Background input to AMPA receptors (frequency in Hz/conductance in nS)	Target population (receptor type/strength in nS)
SCe^{L}	250	0.5	1280/0.19	SCe^{L}(N/1.5), SCi (N/0.7), Cxi (N/0.11), Cxe^{L}(N/0.05), Cxe^{R}(N/0.05)
SCe^{R}	250	0.5	1280/0.19	SCe^{R}(N/1.5), SCi (N/0.7) Cxi (N/0.11), Cxe^{L}(N/0.05), Cxe^{R}(N/0.05),
SCi	250	0.2	1280/2.0	SCe^{L}(G/2.5), SCe^{R}(G/2.5)
SNr^{L}	250	0.5	3440/2.0	SCe^{L}(G/2.5)
CD^{L}	250	0.5	400/8.0	SNr^{L}(G/0.6)
SNr^{R}	250	0.5	3440/2.0	SCe^{R}(G/2.5)
CD^{R}	250	0.5	400/8.0	SNr^{R}(G/0.6)
CxeBG	1120	0.5	2400/2.1	CxeBG (A/0.05), CxeBG (N/0.165), Cxe^{L}(A/0.043825), Cxe^{L}(N/0.14462), Cxe^{R}(A/0.043825), Cxe^{R}(N/0.14462) Cxi (A/0.04), Cxi (N/0.13)
Cxe^{L}	240	0.5	2400/2.1	SCe^{L}(A/3.5), CD^{L}(N/0.2), CD^{L}(A/0.12), CxeBG (A/0.05), CxeBG (N/0.165), Cxe^{L}(A/0.085), Cxe^{L}(N/0.2805), Cxe^{R}(A/0.043825), Cxe^{R}(N/0.14462), Cxi (A/0.04), Cxi (N/0.13)
Cxe^{R}	240	0.5	2400/2.1	SCe^{R}(A_3.5), CD^{R}(N_0.2), CD^{R}(A_0.12), CxeBG (A_0.05), CxeBG (N_0.165), Cxe^{L}(A_0.043825), Cxe^{L}(N/0.14462), Cxe^{R}(A/0.085), Cxe^{R}(N/0.2805), Cxi (A/0.04), Cxi (N/0.13)
Cxi	400	0.2	2400/1.62	CxeBG (G/1.3), Cxe^{L}(G/1.3) Cxe^{R}(G/1.3), Cxi (G/1.0)

threshold. Hence, by varying the corticostriatal (Cx-CD) synaptic strength, we could change the level of the decision threshold. Specifically, a stronger Cx-CD strength resulted in a lower decision threshold, while a weaker strength resulted in a higher decision threshold.

In the model, the mean spike rate μ of each input to Cxe^{L}/Cxe^{R} depended on the motion strength of the stimulus linearly and followed the equations: $\mu = \mu_0 + \mu_A \times c'$ for the direction of the coherent motion and $\mu = \mu_0 - \mu_B \times c'$ for the opposite direction. The variable μ_0 (40 Hz) was the baseline input for the purely random motion, c' (between 0 and 100%) was the coherence level that characterized the stimulus motion strength, and μ_A (120 Hz) and μ_B (40 Hz) were the factors of proportionality, based on empirical observations (Britten et al., 1993).

In each trial, the reaction time was calculated by adding the decision time with a 250 ms non-decision time. The decision time was the time interval between the stimulus presentation to the model and the crossing of the response threshold in SCe neurons. The non-decision time represented the time that was needed for the sensory processing and the motor output that were not modeled in the present study.

In a previous study (Lo and Wang, 2006), we demonstrated that the major determining factor of the threshold is the Cx-CD synaptic strength and that there exists an optimal strength that results in the maximum reward rate (averaged number of rewards acquired per second). The optimal strength was different for the different task conditions. In the present study, the Cx-CD synapses were endowed with DA-dependent plasticity, and we investigated how the neural circuit adapted to the changing task conditions and remained optimized through the action of the DA system.

DOPAMINE-DEPENDENT SYNAPTIC PLASTICITY

Previous studies have demonstrated that the activity of DA neurons in the substantia nigra pars compacta (SNc) correlates with reward prediction error as well as with the stimuli that predict rewards (Hollerman and Schultz, 1998; Schultz, 1999; Kawagoe et al., 2004; Arias-Carrión et al., 2010; Nomoto et al., 2010). In the present study, we studied the behavior of fully trained subjects and assumed that they had developed a sense of the correlation between the performance (percentage correct) and the task difficulty (stimulus motion strength) Equation (1) below. Therefore, the subjects were able to estimate the probability of receiving a reward at the onset of the motion stimulus and thereby to evaluate the reward prediction error at the time of reward delivery/absence. Based on the hypothesis, the DA system in our model responded to the onset of the motion stimulus with a magnitude that correlated with the estimated reward probability as well as to the reward delivery/absence with a magnitude that correlated with the reward prediction error (**Figure 2A**). The hypothesized DA activity was consistent with a recent monkey experiment that used random-dot motion stimuli with a slightly different paradigm (Nomoto et al., 2010). In the present study, we did not model the activity of individual DA neurons. Instead, we directly modeled the DA levels at the Cx-CD synapses. Specifically, the DA system consisted of the following four processes:

(1) Estimated reward probability (reward prediction) as a function of motion coherence. After training, the subjects were able to estimate the probability of receiving a reward based on the motion stimuli. In order to simplify the computation of the model, instead of estimating the reward probability from the outcome of past trials, we used a preset function to estimate reward probability $p_{est}(c')$:

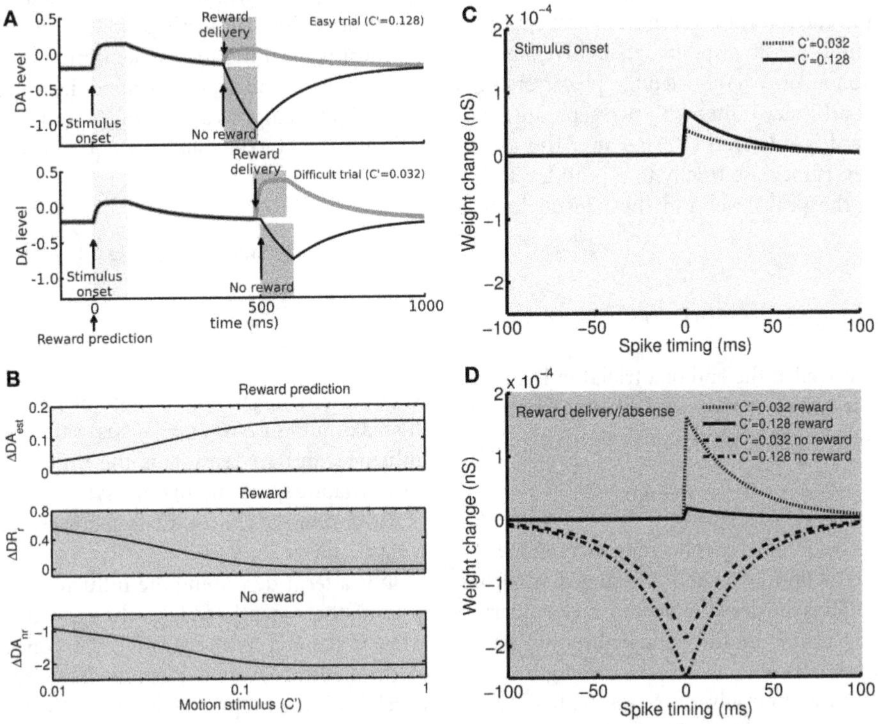

FIGURE 2 | The dopamine (DA) system and spike-timing dependent plasticity. (A) Example time courses showing that the DA levels (with respect to the neutral level, in arbitrary units) exhibit phasic activity in response to the stimulus presentation (light gray regions) and reward delivery/absence (dark gray regions). In an easy trial (top), the DA levels strongly respond to the stimulus presentation due to the large estimated reward probability but only result in a moderate increase in response to the reward delivery due to the small reward prediction error. In an erroneous trial, the absence of reward strongly suppresses the DA levels for the large and negative reward prediction error. In contrast, in a difficult trial (bottom), the DA levels increase moderately in response to the stimulus onset due to the small estimated reward probability, while the levels exhibit strong (or weak) responses for reward delivery (or absence). **(B)** The peak levels of the DA phasic responses to the stimulus presentation (top), reward delivery (middle), and reward absence (bottom) as functions of the difficulty of the task (stimulus motion strength). The responses to the stimulus presentation correlate with the estimate of reward probability, whereas the responses to the reward delivery and absence correlate with the reward prediction error. **(C)** Example STDP kernels (synaptic weight change Δw as a function of pre- and post-synaptic spike time difference) at the peak DA levels for the stimulus presentations. **(D)** Example STDP kernels at the peak/bottom DA levels for the reward delivery/absence.

$$p_{est}(c') = 1 - \frac{1}{2}e^{-(c'/\beta)^{\alpha}}, \tag{1}$$

where $\alpha = 1$ and $\beta = 0.047$. The function has been used to fit the simulated performance data that are produced by the same attractor network model (Lo and Wang, 2006). The parameter β was determined by fitting the equation to the overall performance of the model. We tested the model with different values of β and found that the behavioral outcome of the circuit model was not sensitive to the particular choice of the parameter. These results suggested that the model worked without the need to accurately estimate the reward probability.

(2) Phasic DA response to the motion stimulus. DA levels exhibit a phasic increase after the onset of the motion stimulus based on the estimated reward probability as we discussed above. The difference (in arbitrary units) between the peak DA level of the phasic responses and the neutral level, at which no synaptic weight change can be induced, correlates with the estimated reward probability $p_{est}(c')$ and is given by:

$$\Delta DA_{est} = c_{est} \times 0.15 \times r. \tag{2}$$

where

$$r = \frac{(p_{est}(c') - 0.5)}{0.5}, \tag{3}$$

and $c_{est} = 1$. c_{est} represents the sensitivity of the DA system to reward estimation and can be tuned to test how the sensitivity influences the decision behavior. Because the value of $p_{est}(c')$ falls between 0.5 and 1, the value of r falls between 0 and 1. Combining the equations for ΔDA_{est} and $p_{est}(c')$ described above, we determined that the peak level of the phasic DA response to the stimulus onset followed a monotonically increasing function of the motion strength c' (**Figure 2B**, top panel). Based on the observation of a quick increase in DA levels following DA neuron activity and slow reuptake (Suaud-Chagny et al., 1995), we further assumed that, after the onset of the motion stimulus, DA levels increase to their peak level exponentially (time constant = 10 ms) for 100 ms and then drop to the baseline level (−0.2) exponentially (time constant = 150 ms).

(3) Phasic DA response to reward delivery or absence. After the decision is made and the reward is received or not received, the DA neurons exhibit phasic responses that correlate with the reward prediction error. We modeled the phasic changes of the DA levels (in arbitrary units) with two separate functions. When a reward is delivered (100 ms after the choice is made), the DA levels increase briefly to a peak level. The difference between the peak level and the neutral level is given by

$$\Delta DA_r = c_{err} \times 0.71 \times (1 - r). \qquad (4)$$

When a reward is not received at the end of a trial, the DA levels decrease briefly to a lower boundary level. The difference between this lower boundary level and the neutral level is given by

$$\Delta DA_{nr} = c_{err} \times -1.5 \times r - 0.6. \qquad (5)$$

$c_{err} = 1$ in both equations. c_{err} represents the sensitivity of the DA system to the reward prediction error and is changed when we test how the sensitivity affects the decision behavior. Considering that r depends in a linear fashion on the estimated reward probability that positively correlates with the motion strength c', we determined that ΔDA_r monotonically decreases with c' while $|\Delta DA_{nr}|$monotonically increases with c' (**Figure 2B**, middle and bottom panels). Following our assumptions for DA release and reuptake, we here assumed that, after the reward is delivered, DA levels increase to their peak level ΔDA_r exponentially, with a time constant of 10 ms, for a period of 100 ms and then drop to baseline exponentially, with a time constant of 150 ms. In the absence of a reward, the DA levels reduce to their lower boundary level ΔDA_{nr} exponentially, with a time constant of 150 ms, for a period of 100 ms and then increase to the baseline level with the same time constant (150 ms). Combining Equations (1)–(5), we determined the temporal profiles of the DA levels (**Figure 2A**): at the stimulus onset, the DA levels increase intensely for easy trials but weakly for difficult trials. In contrast, when a reward is delivered in a correct trial, the DA levels increase weakly for the easy condition but intensely for the difficult condition. In erroneous trials, the DA levels exhibit a deep recession for the easy condition but a shallow recession for the difficult condition.

We note that the DA level changes (ΔDA_{est}, ΔDA_r, and ΔDA_{nr}) and the baseline level discussed above are defined with respect to the neutral level that represents the concentration of DA that does not induce synaptic plasticity (see below).

(4) DA modulated spike-timing dependent plasticity (STDP). Based on the extensive experimental evidence on the dopaminergic modulation of corticostriatal synapses (Fino et al., 2005; Calabresi et al., 2007; Pawlak and Kerr, 2008; Shen et al., 2008; Gerfen and Surmeier, 2011), we hypothesized that the stimuli and rewards modify the strength of Cx-CD synapses in the proposed model through DA-modulated STDP. A recent study has shown that, for D1 receptor-expressing striatal medium spiny neurons, high DA levels result in synaptic facilitation in the condition of positive spike timing (pre-synaptic spikes precede post-synaptic spikes), whereas low DA levels produce synaptic depression for both positive and negative spike timing (Shen et al., 2008). Based on these findings, we assumed that the STDP kernel (synaptic weight change as a function of spike timing) in our model is described by the following equations:

$$\Delta w = w_{max} \times \exp\left(\frac{-\Delta t}{\tau}\right) \times \Phi, \qquad (6)$$

$$\Phi = \frac{2}{1 + e^{-k\Delta DA}} - 1, \qquad (7)$$

where Δw is the weight change of Cx-CD synapses, w_{max} sets the maximum of Δw, ($\tau = 30$ ms) is the decay constant of STDP influence, and Δt represents the timing difference between the post-synaptic spike and the pre-synaptic spike, and is defined by:

$\Delta t =$ time of last post-synaptic spike—time of last pre-synaptic spike.

Φ is a term describing the influence of ΔDA over the amplitude of the synaptic weight change with a parameter ($k = 1$). ΔDA is defined as the relative DA concentration with respect to the neutral level. A positive ΔDA results in a positive Φ, which leads to synaptic facilitation ($\Delta w > 0$), whereas a negative ΔDA leads to synaptic depression ($\Delta w > 0$). At the neutral level ($\Delta DA = 0$), no synaptic weight change occurs. In addition, w_{max} takes different values for different spike-timing conditions and DA level conditions. Specifically, $w_{max} = 5.0 \times 10^{-4}, 2.0 \times 10^{-4}$, 0, or 2.0×10^{-4} (nS) for $\Delta t > 0$ and $\Phi > 0$, $\Delta t > 0$ and $\Phi < 0$, $\Delta t < 0$ and $\Phi > 0$, or $\Delta t < 0$ and $\Phi < 0$, respectively. The setting leads to a STDP kernel that produces synaptic facilitation for positive spike timing ($\Delta t > 0$) at high DA levels ($\Phi > 0$) but synaptic depression for both positive and negative timing at low DA levels ($\Phi < 0$).

After combining Equations (1)–(7), we obtained a reward- and stimulus-dependent STDP kernel (**Figures 2C,D**). After the stimulus onset, a strong motion stimulus results in a prediction of high reward probability that also results in strong synaptic facilitation for positive spike timing, while a weak motion stimulus results in a prediction of low reward probability that results in weak synaptic facilitation (**Figure 2C**). After the decision is made, if the motion stimulus was strong, the subject strongly expects a reward. Therefore, the delivery of the expected reward only results in weak facilitation. In contrast, if the reward is not delivered (due to a wrong choice), the unexpected reward absence leads to a strong depression (**Figure 2D**). However, if the motion stimulus is weak, the subject does not highly expect a reward, and, therefore, a reward delivery induces a strong facilitation while reward absence produces a weak depression (**Figure 2D**). Following the responses to the stimulus presentation and reward delivery/absence, the DA levels decay or increase to the baseline level, DA_b, which is set to be −0.2 with respect to the neutral level. The baseline DA levels result in a weak depression that slowly brings down the synaptic strength during the intertrial intervals (ITI).

Finally, we considered the empirical observations in which the relative change in the synaptic strength was smaller for a stronger synaptic strength when the synapse was facilitated, whereas the relative change remained constant when the synapse was depressed (Bi and Poo, 1998; van Rossum et al., 2000). In order to capture this property, for every pre/post-synaptic spike pair, if the resulting synaptic weight change was facilitation ($\Delta w > 0$), we used a simple additive rule, $\Delta g = g_{t+1} - g_t = \Delta w$, to update the efficacy g of the Cx-to-CD synapses, whereas if the resulting weight change was depression ($\Delta w < 0$), we used a multiplicative rule, $\Delta g = -g\,|\Delta w|$. The additive updating rule resulted in a percentage change that reduced with the synaptic strength ($\Delta g/g = \Delta w/g$), while the multiplicative rule resulted in a constant percentage change ($\Delta g/g = |\Delta w|$) (van Rossum et al., 2000). In the model, the efficacy g of the Cx-to-CD synapses is updated after each pre- or post-synaptic spike based on the STDP kernel Equations (6) and (7) with the multiplicative or additive rules stated above. The updates of the synaptic efficacy are long-term and do not change until the next pre- or post-synaptic spike.

We noted that, due to the noisy background input that each neuron receives, the weights of the Cx-CD synapses develop heterogeneity in the population under the effects of STDP (Kepecs et al., 2002). In order to avoid the complications that arise from the heterogeneity and that were outside of the scope of the present study, we implemented a "*mean-field*" approach in which each Cx-CD synapse followed a common synaptic strength that was updated based on the pre- and post-synaptic spikes that were pooled from every Cx neuron and every CD neuron.

REWARD RATE FUNCTION

We quantified the quality of the decision by calculating the conventional (objective) reward rate and a subjective reward rate, which was weighted by the subject's preference for speed or accuracy. The objective reward rate was defined as the average amount of reward received per unit time (in s) (Gold and Shadlen, 2002):

$$R_o = \frac{p_c}{T_{\mathrm{ITI}} + T_R + (1 - p_c)T_p} = \frac{1 - p_{\mathrm{err}}}{T_{\mathrm{ITI}} + T_R + p_{\mathrm{err}}T_p}, \quad (8)$$

where p_c represents the performance (percentage correct), $\mathrm{T_{ITI}}$ is the inter-trial interval (500 ms), T_R is the mean reaction time, T_p (2500 ms) is the penalty period that is appended to the end of every error trial, and p_{err} is the percentage error ($= 1 - p_c$). The objective reward rate R_o forms an inverted U-shaped curve as a function of the decision threshold (Gold and Shadlen, 2002) or the Cx-CD synaptic strength (Lo and Wang, 2006). Ideally, a subject should try to find the optimal threshold or synaptic strength that maximizes R_o (peak of the inverted U-shaped curve) in order to receive as much reward as possible in a given period of time. However, various studies have shown that individual subjects, including humans and animals, may favor speed over accuracy or vice versa (Kay et al., 2006; Rinberg et al., 2006). Therefore, the subjects may not seek to maximize R_o during the decision but rather to speed up or to increase their accuracy. In order to quantify such behavior, we need to measure the subjects' degree of preference for speed or accuracy. A number of studies have quantified the tendency for favoring accuracy over maximizing the reward rate for human subjects (Maddox and Bohil, 1998; Bogacz et al., 2006). We extended this idea by including the tendency for favoring speed and constructed a subjective reward rate function:

$$R_s = \frac{1 - k_a p_{\mathrm{err}}}{T_{\mathrm{ITI}} + k_s(T_R + p_{\mathrm{err}}T_p)} \quad (9)$$

where k_a and k_s are the weighting factors (with values between 0 and 1) representing the degrees of preference for accuracy and speed, respectively. R_s also forms an inverted U-shaped function of the Cx-CD synaptic strength with different peak locations for different values of (k_a, k_s) (**Figures 5A,B**). Therefore, if the Cx-CD synaptic strength of a subject converges to a specific value that corresponds to the peak location of R_s with a given (k_a, k_s), we can say that the subject's decisions were characterized by an optimization that was weighted by their specific preference represented by the factors k_a and k_s. A large $k_a (k_a > k_s)$ indicates that the subject is sensitive to the change in accuracy due to errors, whereas a large $k_s (k_s > k_a)$ indicates that the subject is sensitive to the change in the overall trial time due to slow decisions or additional penalty periods. We can recover the conventional (objective) reward rate Equation (8) by setting $k_a = k_s = 1$. In the present study, we showed that the optimal objective reward rate, R_o, for a given speed-accuracy preference (k_s, k_a) can be achieved in our model by tuning DA-related parameters.

RESULTS

DEPENDENCE OF THE SYNAPTIC WEIGHT ON THE TRIAL DIFFICULTY AND TRIAL OUTCOME

We tested the changes in synaptic weight in different trial conditions (**Figure 3**). In an easy trial (strong motion strength) in which the subject made a correct choice, the DA levels responded strongly to the stimulus onset due to the large estimated reward probability. However, the DA levels responded to the reward delivery only weakly because the reward was highly anticipated (**Figure 3A**). In contrast, in a difficult trial with a correct choice, the DA levels responded to the stimulus onset weakly, while the levels responded to the reward delivery strongly due to the less anticipated reward (**Figure 3C**). The overall effect of the synaptic weight changes for a correct choice in both easy and difficult conditions was facilitation. When the subject made an incorrect choice, even though the DA increase in response to the stimulus onset slightly facilitated the synapse, the absence of reward reduced the DA levels, which resulted in an overall synaptic depression (**Figures 3B,D**).

The plasticity rule that was used in our model was spike-time based, and, therefore, the synaptic weight change was sensitive to the variability of the spiking timing, which could be large in noisy neuronal environments. As a consequence, whether the synaptic strength was able to reach a stable level in a block of trials and whether the level of the stable synaptic strength depended on the task difficulty remained in question. To address the question, we tested the circuit model with blocks of trials with easy or difficult conditions. We set the initial Cx-CD synaptic strength to be 0.1 nS and found that, for the easy condition, the strength quickly reached a range of 0.3–0.6 nS, and the range remained stable afterwards (**Figure 4A**). In contrast, testing the model with the difficult condition also resulted in a stable but different range of Cx-CD synaptic strength (~0.1–0.3 nS) (**Figure 4B**). The results showed that the model was able to operate in stable

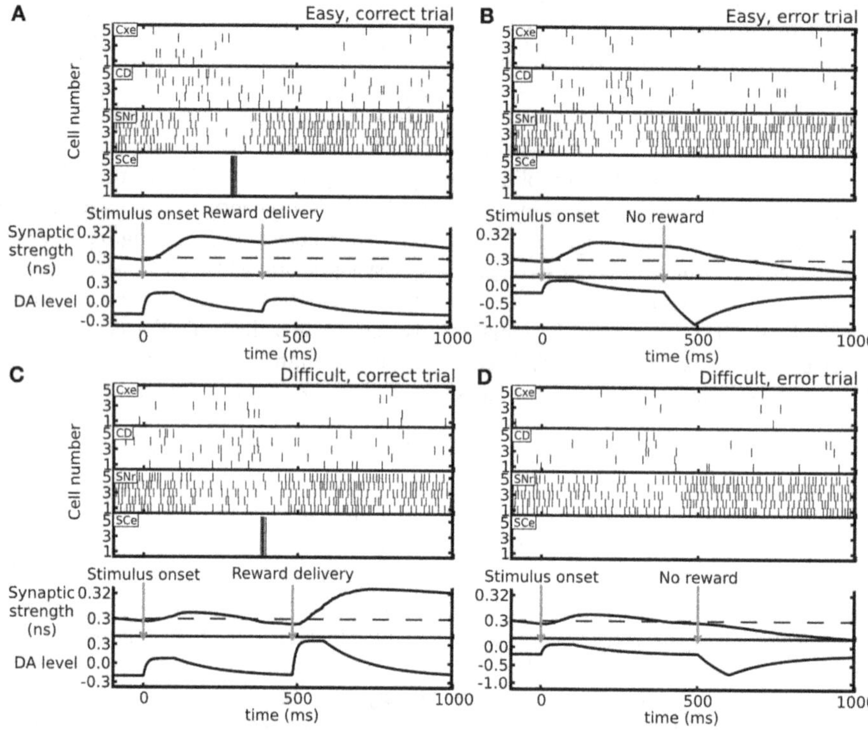

FIGURE 3 | Example trials showing distinct neuronal activity and resulting Cx-CD synaptic weights in the following four conditions. (A) An easy trial with a correct decision. **(B)** An easy trial with an incorrect decision. **(C)** A difficult trial with a correct decision. **(D)** A difficult trial with an incorrect decision. The top four spike rastergrams in each panel display the spike activity of neurons in the Cxe, CD, SNr, and SCe in the side that corresponds to the correct choice. The bottom two plots in each panel indicate the time courses of Cx-CD synaptic strength and DA levels (in arbitrary units). In general, correct trials result in synaptic facilitation, while error trials depress synapses.

but different ranges of Cx-CD strengths for different task conditions. Because the decision threshold is monotonically decreased with increased Cx-CD strength (Lo and Wang, 2006), the stronger Cx-CD strength in the easy compared to the difficult conditions indicated that the circuit model reduced the decision threshold for faster responses when the task was easy while it raised the decision threshold for a better performance when the task was difficult.

ADAPTATION TO THE CHANGE IN TASK DIFFICULTY

We showed that the circuit model tuned itself and operated at different levels of Cx-CD strengths when tested with trials involving either easy or difficult conditions. However, in natural environments, the task conditions may vary with time. Therefore, we asked whether the circuit model was able to adapt to environmental changes by testing the model with a sudden switch of the task condition from easy to difficult and vice versa (**Figures 4C,D**). We found that the circuit model was able to quickly change its Cx-CD strength after the task condition switched. Specifically, the Cx-CD strength decreased when the task condition changed from easy to difficult, while it increased when the change reversed. These results indicated that the circuit model was able to respond to the increased task difficulty by slowing down the decision speed, while it responded to decreased task difficulty by speeding up. Furthermore, we calculated how long the model took to complete the transition after the switch of the task condition. To this end, we counted the number of trials it took for the Cx-CD synaptic strength to reach the new average strength after the switch. We found that it took 30 ± 25 trials for the easy to difficult switch and 60 ± 28 trials for the difficult to easy switch.

DECISION OPTIMIZATION

The adaptive decision behavior shown in **Figures 4C,D** led to the fundamental question whether the adaptation was optimal. More specifically, does the decision strategy (the specific Cx-CD strength chosen by the circuit model) maximize the reward rate in both easy and difficult conditions? Our earlier study showed that the (objective) reward rate, as a function of Cx-CD strength, forms an inverted U-shaped curve. Therefore, there is an optimal Cx-CD strength that corresponds to the peak of the curve that gives rise to the maximum reward rate (Lo and Wang, 2006). We further found that the inverted U-shaped curve shifts or the optimal Cx-CD strength changes with different task conditions (Lo and Wang, 2006). Therefore, in the present study, we asked whether the model was able to automatically converge on the optimal Cx-CD strength when the task condition changed from easy to difficult. Indeed, we found that, when the task condition was easy, the model converged on the optimal Cx-CD strength (**Figure 5A**, thick black curve, $k_s = k_a = 1$). After we switched the task condition to difficult, the model quickly changed its

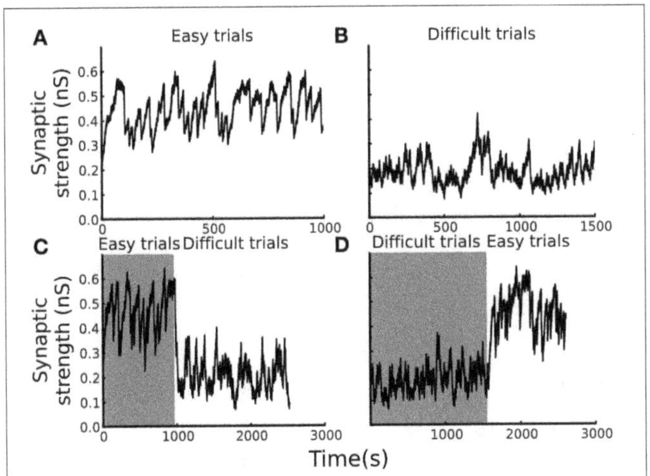

FIGURE 4 | Average Cx-CD synaptic strengths remain stable but exhibit different levels for different task conditions. (A) The time course of the synaptic strength in a block of trials with the easy condition. The synaptic strength converged to a range between 0.3 and 0.6 nS. **(B)** The time course of the synaptic strength in the difficult condition. The synaptic strength converged to a range (between 0.1 and 0.4 nS), which is lower than that in the easy condition. **(C)** When the trial condition switched from easy to difficult, or **(D)** from difficult to easy, the synaptic strength quickly converged to new range that is consistent with those shown in the **(A,B)**. The results show that the model exhibits stable and consistent adaptations to changes in task difficulty.

Cx-CD strength to a lower range that was optimal in the difficult condition (**Figure 5B**, thick black curve, $k_s = k_a = 1$).

One may argue that the optimization depends on the choice of the model parameters and ask what would happen if we chose different parameters. Below, we show that with different values of dopamine-related parameters our model still reached optimal decisions that were characterized by different weights for speed and accuracy.

SUBJECTIVE REWARD RATE

As discussed in the Introduction and Materials and Methods, human and animal subjects may not be ideal decision-makers that maximize their objective reward rate Equation (8). Rather, some individuals may favor more accurate decisions, while others may favor faster decisions. In other words, subjects may have their own *subjective* senses of optimization that are weighted by their preferences for speed or accuracy. We proposed a subjective reward-rate Equation (9) that can be used to quantify such preferences that are characterized by the values of the speed-weighting factor, k_s, and the accuracy-weighting factor, k_a.

We addressed the two following fundamental questions. First, what are the neuronal substrates that influence an individual's preference for speed or accuracy? This question is equivalent to finding the neuronal parameters that achieve maximum subjective reward rates for a given combination of k_s and k_a. Second, does the adaptive decision behavior remain optimal in terms of subjective reward rate when the task condition changes? This question is equivalent to asking, if a subject maximizes the subjective reward rate for given k_s and k_a in a task condition, does the subject still achieve the maximum subjective reward rate (for the same k_s and k_a) when the task condition changes? We addressed the questions with the following procedure:

(1) For each grid point on the (k_s, k_a) space (ranged from 0 to 1 with a grid space of 0.05), we calculated the subjective reward rate R_s Equation (9) for both easy and difficult conditions and then found the optimal Cx-CD synaptic strength that maximized R_s in each condition.
(2) We tuned the neuronal parameters, performed simulations, and then calculated the mean Cx-CD synaptic strengths for each task condition (easy or difficult). Here, we selected three DA-related parameters for tuning: (1) c_{est} in Equation (2), representing the magnitude of the DA responses to the stimulus onset (estimate of reward probability); (2) c_{err} in Equations (4) and (5), representing the magnitude of the DA responses to the reward delivery or absence (reward prediction error); and (3) The baseline DA level, DA_b. For each set of parameters (c_{est}, c_{err}, and DA_b) we found the mean and the standard deviation of the Cx-CD strengths for each task condition.
(3) Finally, by combining the results from 1 and 2, we looked for the (k_s, k_a) that gave rise to the optimal Cx-CD strengths that matched the simulated mean Cx-CD strengths for each parameter set (c_{est}, c_{err}, and DA_b) for both the easy and difficult conditions. We noted that the matched k_s and k_a may not fall exactly on a grid point in the (k_s, k_a) space. Therefore, we first located an area in the (k_s, k_a) space with the enclosed grid points that had optimal Cx-CD strengths very close to the simulated mean strengths (typically within 0.5 standard deviation). Then we had the center point of this area represent the matched (k_s, k_a).

We were able to identify the corresponding k_s and k_a for each model setting set that we tested (**Figures 5A,B**). We plotted the results for four representative settings. Setting **a** corresponded to the original setting (used in **Figures 3, 4**) in which $c_{est} = c_{err} = 1$ and $DA_b = -0.2$. Setting **b** represented enhanced responses to reward delivery and absence ($c_{err} = 1.8$). In setting **c**, we reduced the baseline DA level ($DA_b = -0.25$). Setting **d** represented the weakened responses to stimulus presentation ($c_{est} = 0.9$). The results showed that the different model settings represented the optimizations for different decision strategies (k_s and k_a combinations). Moreover, the circuit remained optimal for the same strategy when the task conditions changed.

Next, we examined how the neuronal parameters, c_{est}, c_{err}, and DA_b, affected a subject's preference toward either speed or accuracy. We found that the simulated subject favored accuracy ($k_a > k_s$) when we reduced the sensitivity, c_{est}, of the DA system to the estimate of reward probability as well as reduced the baseline DA level, DA_b. In contrast, the simulated subject favored speed ($k_s > k_a$) if we increased the sensitivity, c_{err}, to the reward prediction error (**Figure 5C**). We further analyzed the simulated result at the behavioral level and verified that, with a preference to accuracy ($k_a > k_s$), the percentage correct was larger but the decisions were slower than those in the ideal decision cases ($k_a = k_s = 1$). In contrast, with a preference to speed ($k_s > k_a$), the decisions

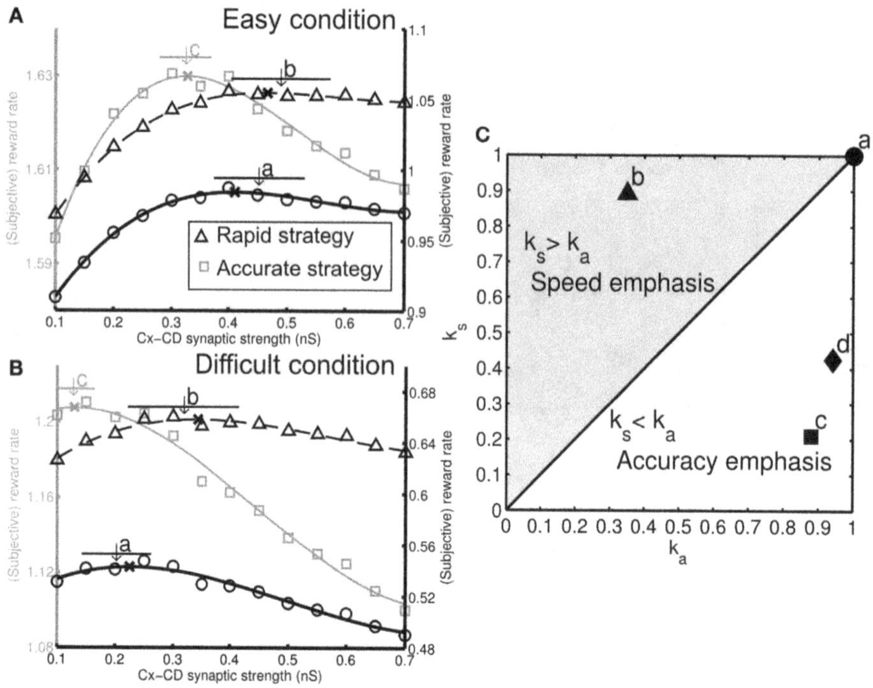

FIGURE 5 | Different decision strategies (characterized by favoring speed or accuracy) can be realized by tuning three dopamine-related parameters. (A) Each decision strategy can be represented by a subjective reward rate curve in the easy condition. We plotted curves for three different decision strategies (gray curve: left ordinate, solid and dashed black curves: right ordinate). **(B)** The same three decision strategies show shifted subjective reward rate curves in the difficult condition. We performed simulations for the model with three different model settings and found that each of the settings forms specific ranges of Cx-CD synaptic strengths in both task conditions (**a**, original as in **Figures 3**, **4**, **b**, enhanced responses to reward presentation/absence, and **c**, reduced baseline DA level. The arrows indicate the mean synaptic strength and horizontal bars represent the standard deviation). We found that each of the model settings corresponded to the optimization for a specific decision strategy (k_a, k_s). The x's indicate the peak locations of the curves. **(C)** Corresponding decision strategies for the three model settings [**a–c** in **(A,B)**] shown on a (k_a, k_s) plane. In addition, we tested the model by reducing the response of DA level to the stimulus presentation and found that the setting resulted in an accuracy-emphasis strategy (labeled by **d**), which is similar to that of the setting **c**.

were faster but the error rate was higher than those in the ideal decisions (**Figures 6A,B**).

DIFFERENTIAL RESPONSES TO THE SAME STIMULUS DUE TO ADAPTATION

In our task, the subjects were presented with stimuli with motion coherence levels of $c' = 3.2$, 6.4, or 12.8% in the difficult condition and $c' = 12.8$, 25.6, or 51.2% in the easy condition. The task design was unique in that the subjects encountered stimuli with $c' = 12.8\%$ in both conditions. Due to the adaptive behavior that brings the Cx-CD synaptic strength to different levels between the two conditions, we found that, for the same motion strength ($c' = 12.8\%$), the model circuit performed better in the difficult than in the easy conditions (**Figure 6C**). This observation provided a behavioral assessment that allowed us to easily assess whether a subject exhibited adaptive behavior when the task difficulty changed. We noted that this was a general result of adaptive behavior and was not specific to our model.

ROLES OF THE PHASIC RESPONSES OF DA LEVELS IN DECISION ADAPTATION

It is important to test individual contributions of the two phasic DA responses (to the stimulus presentation and to the reward delivery/absence) in the adaptive behavior of decision making. To this end, we performed two sets of simulations. In the first set, we tested the model by removing the DA responses to the stimulus presentation (estimate of reward probability), and, in the second set, we removed the DA responses to the reward delivery/absence (reward prediction error). We found that, without the phasic DA response to the stimulus presentation in the beginning of a trial, even though the Cx-CD strength was able to remain at stable levels in the difficult condition, the strength could not be maintained and quickly dropped to nearly zero in the easy condition (**Figure 7A**). This was because, in the difficult condition, the stability of the Cx-CD strength mainly relied on the balance between the facilitation that was due to the reward delivery (large positive reward prediction errors) and the depression that was due to the absence of the reward in the error trials and the baseline DA levels. Removing the DA responses to the stimulus presentation did not produce much impact on the circuit. However, in the easy condition, the reward delivery only weakly facilitated the Cx-CD synapses (due to small reward prediction errors), and the facilitation that was induced by the strong DA responses to the stimulus presentation (due to the large estimated reward probability) played a crucial role in maintaining the stability of the Cx-CD synapses. Removing the DA responses to the stimulus

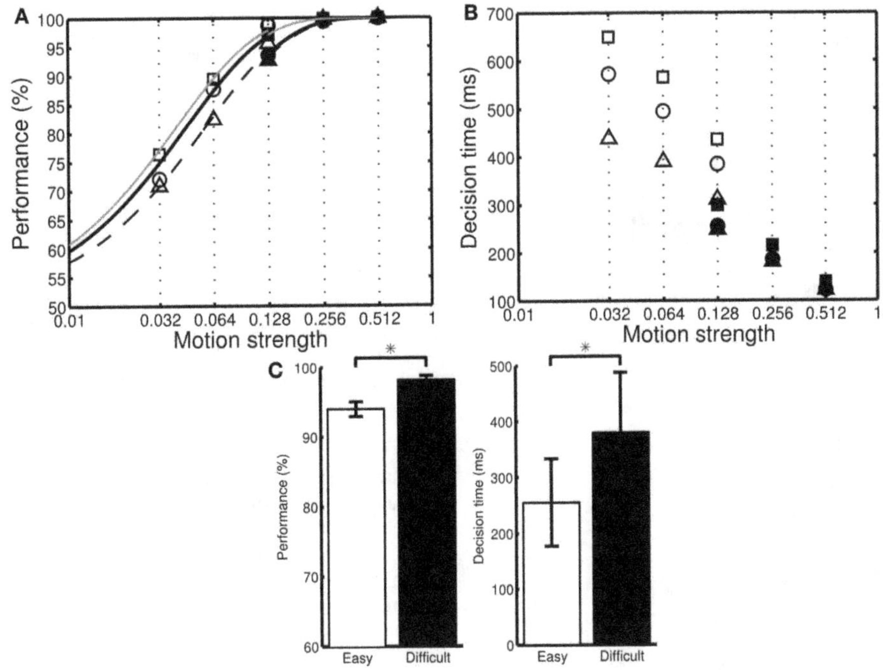

FIGURE 6 | The three different model settings (a–c in Figure 5) result in different behavioral performances. (A) The percentage correct is higher in the setting that emphasizes accuracy (squares: setting c, circles: setting a, triangles: setting b). Filled and open symbols indicate the data for the difficult and easy conditions, respectively. To help visualize the differences, the data were fitted separately in the two conditions using $p(c') = 1 - \frac{1}{2}e^{-((c')/\beta)}$ where β is a fitting parameter. **(B)** The mean decision times for the same model settings. The mean decision times are smaller in the setting that emphasizes speed. Both easy and difficult conditions include the stimulus motion strength of $c' = 12.8\%$. However, due to the decision adaptation, the neural circuit converges to different levels of Cx-CD synaptic strengths in the two task conditions. As a result, the behavioral performances for the same motion strength of $c' = 12.8\%$ in the two task conditions are different. **(C)** By analyzing the data from setting a, we found that the percentage correct (left panel) is higher, while the mean decision time (right panel) is larger in the difficult than in the easy conditions. $^*p < 0.05$.

presentation destroyed the balance between the facilitation and depression. As a consequence, the circuit was dominated by the depression that occurred when the DA level was at the baseline level and when the reward was not delivered in erroneous trials. In the second set of simulations, we removed the response of the DA levels to the reward delivery/absence and found that Cx-CD strength dropped to nearly zero in the difficult condition but was maintained at a reasonable level in the easy condition (**Figure 7B**). The imbalance between the facilitation and depression that occurred in the difficult condition was mainly due to the loss of the strong facilitation that was induced by reward delivery. The effect of the loss of depression that was induced by reward absence was relatively minor. These results suggested that both phasic DA responses were crucial for producing proper synaptic strength but that they contributed differently in the easy and difficult conditions. Thus, with only one phasic response, a subject may still be able to achieve optimal decisions in one condition but will fail when the task condition changes.

ADAPTATION ACROSS DIFFERENT INTER-TRIAL INTERVALS AND PENALTY TIMES

So far, we only tested the model by changing the task difficulty. We asked whether the same model also optimized decisions under other different task conditions involving, in particular, the temporal aspects of the task setting. The reason was that the subjects' perception to accuracy and time are two of the major factors that influence decision adaptation and optimization. Because we already tested the model by changing the task difficulty, the next objective was to test changing the speed or the pace at which the subjects performed the task. The easiest temporal parameters to manipulate are the ITIs and penalty times. Here, we used the difficult setting ($c' = 3.2$, 6.4, and 12.8%) and changed the task conditions by adding 300 ms to both ITIs and penalty times as well as by subtracting 300 ms from both of them. The model parameters followed those that were used in **Figures 3, 4** (or set **a** in **Figure 5**). We found that the subjective reward rate curve ($k_a = k_s = 1$) shifted toward the left as the ITI and the penalty time increased. Similarly, the model also exhibited the same trend by reducing the mean Cx-CD synaptic strength (**Figure 8**). We noted that a deviation between the simulated synaptic strength and the optimal strength was observed after adding 300 ms (ITI = 800 ms, penalty time = 1800 ms), which characterizes the limitation of the model. A possible solution to the deviation is discussed in the Discussion section.

DISCUSSION

In summary, we proposed a neural circuit model that was endowed with dopamine-modulated plasticity and that remained optimized (maximum subjective reward rates) in adaptation to changes in the task conditions. The ability is realized by the

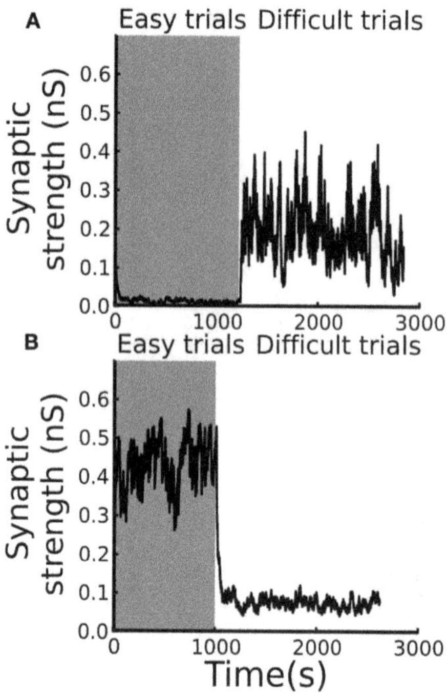

FIGURE 7 | Different contributions of the phasic responses to decision optimization. (A) By removing the response of the DA system to the stimulus presentation, the circuit model was not able to maintain a stable Cx-CD synaptic strength in the easy condition. **(B)** In contrast, when we removed the response of the DA system to the reward delivery/absence, the model failed when the task condition switched to difficult.

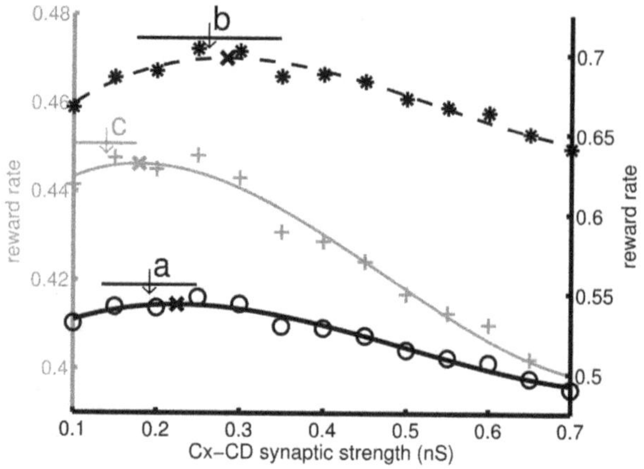

FIGURE 8 | Decision optimization under different speed settings by changing the intertrial interval (ITI) and the penalty time. a, The original setting (ITI = 500 ms, penalty time = 1,500 ms), **b**, the fast setting (ITI = 200 ms, penalty time = 1200 ms), and **c**, the slow setting (ITI = 800 ms, penalty time = 1800 ms). Circles, pluses, and asterisks indicate the corresponding subjective reward rates ($k_s = k_a = 1$) as functions of Cx-CD synaptic strength. As the ITI and the penalty times increase, the optimal Cx-CD synaptic strength that maximizes the reward rate reduces. Using the same parameters (set **a** in **Figure 5**) that optimize the objective reward rate ($k_s = k_a = 1$) under different difficulty settings, we found that the model also followed the same trend by lowering the average Cx-CD synaptic strength, as indicated by the shifted arrows. The horizontal bars represent the standard deviations of the synaptic strengths in the corresponding conditions.

effects of the following three DA components: (1) responses of DA to the stimulus presentation (estimate of reward probability), (2) responses of DA to the reward delivery/absence (reward prediction error), and (3) the baseline DA levels that causes slow synaptic depression. Balance between the facilitating and depression effects caused by these components is crucial for establishing a stable decision strategy (**Figure 9A**).

When a balance between the DA components is reached, the DA components that produce synaptic depression are compensated for by ones that facilitate synapses. Hence, changing the task condition results in changing the performance and tilting the balance between facilitation and depression. As a consequence, the adaptive behavior occurs when the Cx-CD synaptic strength shifts until a new balance is reached. We illustrate the process with an example. Assuming that the Cx-CD synaptic strength is in a stable state in the easy condition and if the task condition suddenly switches to difficult, the DA responses to the stimulus onset are weakened due to the lower estimated reward probability. The changes lead to less synaptic facilitation. In addition, the number of erroneous trials increases and the average trial time is prolonged (due to the punishment period). Both changes induce synaptic depression and effectively raise the decision threshold. As the threshold rises, the performance improves and the percentage of correct trials increases. The performance improvement leads to more positive reward prediction errors (more rewards than expectation) which facilitate the synapses. As a consequence, the depression and facilitation effects reach the balance and the Cx-CD strength is stabilized at a new and weaker level in the difficult condition. A similar argument can be made for the case in which the task condition switches from difficult to easy (**Figures 9B,C**).

By defining the speed and accuracy factors (k_s and k_a) for the decision behavior, we were able to identify DA-related parameters that accounted for the preference for speed or accuracy. Below, we discuss how the key DA components work to produce different optimal strategies during the decision process.

BASELINE DA LEVEL

In the model, the baseline DA level is slightly below the neutral level and results in a gradual decaying Cx-CD synaptic strength during the course of a trial and between the ITIs. Therefore, reducing the baseline DA level produces a faster decay in the Cx-CD synaptic strength, which leads to an increased decision threshold that improves the accuracy. A better accuracy produces more synaptic facilitation that balances with the strong synaptic depression caused by the lower baseline DA level. As a result, a lower DA level results in a better performance.

DA RESPONSES TO STIMULUS PRESENTATION

If we reduce the magnitude of the response, the synapses become more depressed, and, hence, the decision threshold increases. The change results in a higher percentage of correct decisions and reduces the synaptic depression that is caused by erroneous responses. As a consequence, the balance between facilitation and

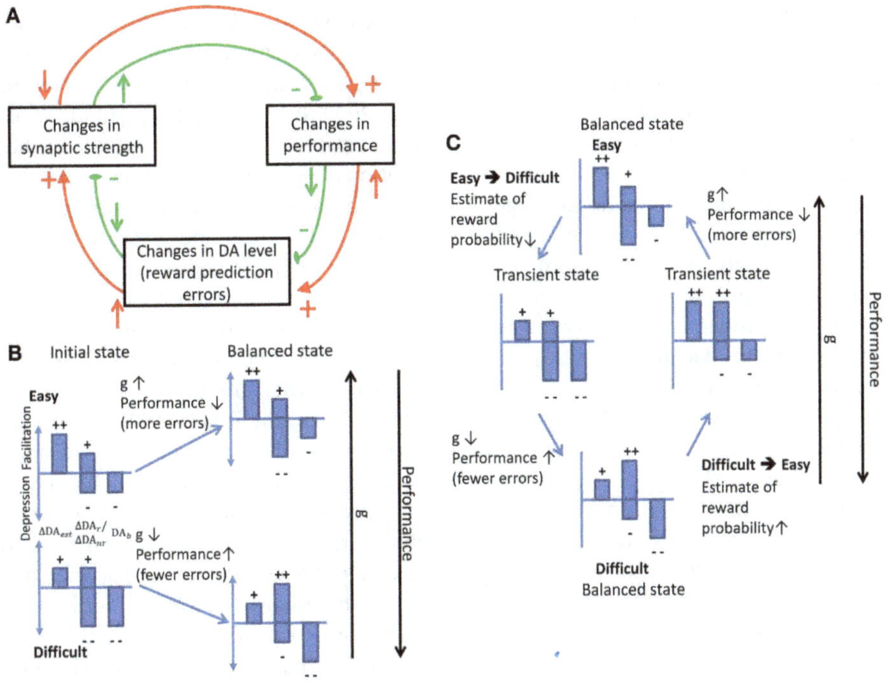

FIGURE 9 | Schematics showing how stability and adaptation are realized by the dynamic balance between different model components. (A) The stability of synaptic strength under a balanced condition. Any change in the synaptic strength (upper left rectangle) will alter the performance which will in turn change the DA level that leads to an opposite effect on the synaptic strength. The red and green circles indicate the flow of the processes induced by a decrease and an increase in the synaptic strength, respectively. The upward arrows represent an increase in the level of the source components while the downward arrows represent a decrease. Plus and minus signs indicate the facilitating and depressing effects on the target components, respectively. **(B)** The dynamic balance leads to a stronger synapse in the easy than in the difficult conditions. In each small bar chart, the left bar indicates the response of DA that represents the estimate of the reward probability (ΔDA_{est}). The two middle bars indicate the response of DA to the reward delivery (ΔDA_r) (the upper one) and to the reward absence (ΔDA_{nr}) (the lower one). The bar on the right represents the baseline DA level (ΔDA_b). The plus signs indicate the facilitating effect which is against the depressing effect indicated by the minus signs. The summation of the plus and the minus signs indicates the direction of change in the synaptic strength. When the task condition is easy, the high ΔDA_{est} level increases the synaptic strength which reduces the performance. As a consequence, ΔDA_{nr} becomes stronger and the synaptic facilitation stops. In contrast, the difficult task condition initially depresses the synapse. The depression leads to improved performance that induces more facilitating effect and, thus, the initial synaptic depression stops. **(C)** The balance shifts and re-established when there is a change in the task conditions. Such a dynamic balance underlies adaptive decision making.

depression is reestablished but with a better decision accuracy (an accuracy-emphasis strategy).

DA RESPONSES TO REWARD DELIVERY/ABSENCE

The responses of DA to reward delivery/absence induce synaptic facilitation in correct trials and depression in erroneous trials. However, the overall facilitating effect is stronger than the depressive one. Therefore, if we increase the magnitude of the DA responses, the net effect is to facilitate the synaptic strength. The change produces a lower decision threshold which leads to a faster decision or a higher error percentage. As a consequence, the balance between facilitation and depression is reestablished but with a faster decision (a speed-emphasis strategy).

The adaptive behavior results in a general prediction that can be tested experimentally. At the behavioral level, the model predicts that the performances (percentage correct) at the motion strength of $c' = 12.8\%$ are different between the easy block and the difficult block. The difference provides a quick and easy way to assess the existence of the adaptive behavior in decisions. Furthermore, the model suggests that the decision strategy (speed or accuracy emphasis) can be characterized by the accuracy factor k_a and the speed factor k_s. Although k_a and k_s are not directly measurable, it is possible to determine a subject's k_a and k_s indirectly by comparing the measured performance and reaction times with the proposed model.

In addition to the behavioral predictions discussed above, our model also makes specific predictions at the neuronal level. Specifically, the model suggests possible neural mechanisms that account for the intersubject and interspecies differences in decision strategies. For example, some animals make quick decisions rather than slower but more accurate decisions (Chittka et al., 2009). Apart from the issues in experimental design (Rinberg et al., 2006; Chittka et al., 2009) and in the differences between sensory modalities, one possible explanation is that the DA systems in animals respond strongly to the presentation of reward delivery/absence and, hence, shift the decision behavior to a speed-emphasis state. If a species, such as humans, tends to emphasize accuracy and make slow decisions, they may have relatively lower DA baselines that enhance the gradual Cx-CD depression and produce an overall weaker Cx-CD synaptic strength or a higher decision threshold. Alternatively, according to our model, the tendency can be accounted for if the subjects have weaker responses to the stimulus presentations.

Due to the lack of experimental data, we did not distinguish the relative contributions of the pre- and post-synaptic factors to the changes in the synaptic strength. According to Equations (6) and (7), the levels of the synaptic strength are affected by Δw, which is proportional to the multiplication between $w_{\max}$ and φ, which is a function of the dopamine levels (ΔDA). Physiologically, $w_{\max}$ characterizes the post-synaptic factors while φ corresponds to the pre-synaptic effect at the DA neuron side. Mathematically, the particular choice of the $w_{\max}$ values is not important as it can be compensated by changing φ. In the present study, we arbitrary set the values for $w_{\max}$ and then we tuned the magnitudes of DA responses, which effectively changed φ, to produce desired decision behavior. Detailed neurophysiological experiments are required to identify the relative contributions of the pre- and post-synaptic factors so that we can adopt more realistic values for $w_{\max}$ and φ.

For the sake of simplicity, we did not include in the proposed model the neural circuit that estimates the reward probability for each stimulus motion strength based on the past trial outcomes. Instead, we used a preset function Equation (1) of reward probability vs. stimulus motion strength. It will be interesting to construct such an estimator circuit in future studies as this circuit is useful in studying the learning process of decision adaptation. A possible solution is to implement a spiking and biologically realistic version of the value estimator as described in Rao (2010). Furthermore, the simulated average Cx-CD synaptic strength was slightly stronger in the easy condition and weaker in the difficult condition or the high ITI + penalty time conditions than the optimal values that were suggested by the objective reward rate curve (**Figures 5A,B, 8**). We expect that the small deviations could be corrected for if we implement an estimator circuit that can more accurately estimate the performance based on the trial history.

Several computational models for flexible decision behavior may relate to our work. In a firing-rate network model that exhibits rapid threshold tuning, researchers have demonstrated that their model is able to quickly converge to the optimal threshold that maximizes the objective reward rate under different task environments (Simen et al., 2006). However, the network needs prior knowledge about the reward rate-threshold relationships across different task environments, such as varying ITIs or varying difficulties. In contrast, our model does not need such information. Instead, the model requires a rough estimate of performance as a function of difficulty Equation (1), which is independent of the task environment. Compared to the reward rate-threshold relationships, performance as a function of difficulty seems to be the information that is more naturally and easily learned by subjects during training. This argument needs to be tested experimentally. Some other rate-based models have focused on action selection and executive control in BG circuits involving direct and indirect pathways (Cohen and Frank, 2009; Wiecki and Frank, 2013). The inclusion of the indirect pathway is a reasonable choice in their models as it is the pathway that has been associated with inhibitory control, the enhancement of action precision, or the avoidance of aversive stimuli (Hikosaka et al., 2000; Jiang et al., 2003; Hikida et al., 2010). Whether the indirect pathway plays a crucial role in the adaptation and optimization of perceptual discrimination tasks requires further tests. Furthermore, our model focuses on spiking neurons with detailed dopamine dynamics and STDP and is therefore able to provide experimental testable predictions on the correlation between cellular level factors and behavior performance.

We noted that a recent primate study has demonstrated that frontal-eye-field neurons change their ramping rates in a visual search task when the monkeys are cued for different decision speeds (Heitz and Schall, 2012). Their result suggested the possibility of another neuronal mechanism (other than changing the decision threshold) that might underlie the behavior of a SAT. Interestingly, we have recently shown that similar neuronal responses can be observed in the attractor decision model by applying a top–down control with balanced excitation and inhibition (Wang et al., 2013). We have suggested that the two mechanisms of SAT do not exclude each other. Rather, different SAT mechanisms may be implemented by the same subject under different task conditions. It is interesting to integrate the two mechanisms in a single model and to investigate whether the model is able to reproduce a wider range of empirical observations. Furthermore, a recent primate study has shown that neurons in the caudate nucleus encode complex information, including evidence accumulation, evaluation, and choice biases (Ding and Gold, 2010), during a random-dot task. With the combination of a top-down control mechanism (Wang et al., 2013), it is worth exploring how our model is able to reproduce these observations.

In conclusion, we proposed a neural circuit model for decision optimization and adaptation. The model is novel in several of the following aspects. First, the model optimizes (subjectively) the decision not just in a single environment but also in environments with changing task difficulties. Second, the model suggests neuronal substrates that correlate with the decision optimization in different task conditions. Third, the model provides an explanation at the neuronal level for why some subjects favor quick decisions while others favor accurate decisions.

ACKNOWLEDGMENTS

We thank the National Center for High Performance Computing (Taiwan) for providing computational resources. This work was supported by National Science Council grants 98-2311-B-007-005-MY3 and 101-2311-B-007-008-MY3.

REFERENCES

Arias-Carrión, O., Stamelou, M., Murillo-Rodríguez, E., Menéndez-González, M., and Pöppel, E. (2010). Dopaminergic reward system: a short integrative review. *Int. Arch. Med.* 3:24. doi: 10.1186/1755-7682-3-24

Balci, F., Simen, P., Niyogi, R., Saxe, A., Hughes, J. A., Holmes, P., et al. (2010). Acquisition of decision making criteria: reward rate ultimately beats accuracy. *Atten. Percept. Psychophys.* 73, 640–657. doi: 10.3758/s13414-010-0049-7

Bi, G., and Poo, M. (1998). Synaptic modifications in cultured hippocampal neurons: dependence on spike timing, synaptic strength, and postsynaptic cell type. *J. Neurosci.* 18, 10464–10472.

Bogacz, R., Brown, E., Moehlis, J., Holmes, P., and Cohen, J. D. (2006). The physics of optimal decision making: a formal analysis of models of performance in two-alternative forced-choice tasks. *Psychol. Rev.* 113, 700–765. doi: 10.1037/0033-295X.113.4.700

Bogacz, R., and Gurney, K. (2007). The basal ganglia and cortex implement optimal decision making between alternative actions. *Neural Comput.* 19, 442–477. doi: 10.1162/neco.2007.19.2.442

Bogacz, R., Hu, P. T., Holmes, P. J., and Cohen, J. D. (2010). Do humans produce the speed-accuracy trade-off that maximizes reward rate? *Q. J. Exp. Psychol. (Hove)* 63, 863–891. doi: 10.1080/17470210903091643

Bogacz, R., and Larsen, T. (2011). Integration of reinforcement learning and optimal decision-making theories of the basal ganglia. *Neural Comput.* 23, 817–851. doi: 10.1162/NECO_a_00103

Britten, K. H., Shadlen, M. N., Newsome, W. T., and Movshon, J. A. (1993). Responses of neurons in macaque MT to stochastic motion signals. *Vis. Neurosci.* 10, 1157–1169. doi: 10.1017/S0952523800010269

Calabresi, P., Picconi, B., Tozzi, A., and Di Filippo, M. (2007). Dopamine-mediated regulation of corticostriatal synaptic plasticity. *Trends Neurosci.* 30, 211–219. doi: 10.1016/j.tins.2007.03.001

Chittka, L., Skorupski, P., and Raine, N. E. (2009). Speed–accuracy trade-offs in animal decision making. *Trends Ecol. Evol.* 24, 400–407. doi: 10.1016/j.tree.2009.02.01

Cohen, M. X., and Frank, M. J. (2009). Neurocomputational models of basal ganglia function in learning, memory and choice. *Behav. Brain Res.* 199, 141–156. doi: 10.1016/j.bbr.2008.09.029

Deco, G., Rolls, E. T., and Romo, R. (2009). Stochastic dynamics as a principle of brain function. *Prog. Neurobiol.* 88, 1–16. doi: 10.1016/j.pneurobio.2009.01.006

de Lafuente, V., and Romo, R. (2011). Dopamine neurons code subjective sensory experience and uncertainty of perceptual decisions. *PNAS* 108, 19767–19771. doi: 10.1073/pnas.1117636108

Ding, L., and Gold, J. I. (2010). Caudate encodes multiple computations for perceptual decisions. *J. Neurosci.* 30, 15747–15759. doi: 10.1523/JNEUROSCI.2894-10.2010

Fino, E., Glowinski, J., and Venance, L. (2005). Bidirectional activity-dependent plasticity at corticostriatal synapses. *J. Neurosci.* 25, 11279–11287. doi: 10.1523/JNEUROSCI.4476-05.2005

Forstmann, B. U., Anwander, A., Schäfer, A., Neumann, J., Brown, S., Wagenmakers, E.-J., et al. (2010). Cortico-striatal connections predict control over speed and accuracy in perceptual decision making. *Proc. Natl. Acad. Sci. U.S.A.* 107, 15916–15920. doi: 10.1073/pnas.1004932107

Gerfen, C. R., and Surmeier, D. J. (2011). Modulation of striatal projection systems by dopamine. *Annu. Rev. Neurosci.* 34, 441–466. doi: 10.1146/annurev-neuro-061010-113641

Gold, J. I., and Shadlen, M. N. (2002). Banburismus and the brain. *Neorun* 36, 299–308. doi: 10.1016/S0896-6273(02)00971-6

Heitz, R. P., and Schall, J. D. (2012). Neural mechanisms of speed-accuracy tradeoff. *Neuron* 76, 616–628. doi: 10.1016/j.neuron.2012.08.030

Hikida, T., Kimura, K., Wada, N., Funabiki, K., and Nakanishi, S. (2010). Distinct roles of synaptic transmission in direct and indirect striatal pathways to reward and aversive behavior. *Neuron* 66, 896–907. doi: 10.1016/j.neuron.2010.05.011

Hikosaka, O., Takikawa, Y., and Kawagoe, R. (2000). Role of the basal ganglia in the control of purposive saccadic eye movements. *Physiol. Rev.* 80, 953–978.

Hollerman, J. R., and Schultz, W. (1998). Dopamine neurons report an error in the temporal prediction of reward during learning. *Nat. Neurosci.* 1, 304–309. doi: 10.1034/1124

Hong, S., and Hikosaka, O. (2011). Dopamine-mediated learning and switching in cortico-striatal circuit explain behavioral changes in reinforcement learning. *Front. Behav. Neurosci.* 5:15. doi: 10.3389/fnbeh.2011.00015

Jiang, H., Stein, B. E., and McHaffie, J. G. (2003). Opposing basal ganglia processes shape midbrain visuomotor activity bilaterally. *Nature* 423, 982–986. doi: 10.1038/nature01698

Kawagoe, R., Takikawa, Y., and Hikosaka, O. (2004). Reward-predicting activity of dopamine and caudate neurons—a possible mechanism of motivational control of saccadic eye movement. *J. Neurophysiol.* 91, 1013–1024. doi: 10.1152/jn.00721.2003

Kay, L. M., Beshel, J., and Martin, C. (2006). When good enough is best. *Neuron* 51, 277–278. doi: 10.1016/j.neuron.2006.07.015

Kepecs, A., van Rossum, M. C. W., Song, S., and Tegner, J. (2002). Spike-timing-dependent plasticity: common themes and divergent vistas. *Biol. Cybern.* 87, 446–458. doi: 10.1007/s00422-002-0358-6

Lo, C.-C., and Wang, X.-J. (2006). Cortico-basal ganglia circuit mechanism for a decision threshold in reaction time tasks. *Nat. Neurosci.* 9, 956–963. doi: 10.1038/nn1722

Maddox, W. T., and Bohil, C. J. (1998). Base-rate and payoff effects in multidimensional perceptual categorization. *J. Exp. Psychol. Learn. Mem. Cogn.* 24, 1459–1482. doi: 10.1037//0278-7393.24.6.1459

Munoz, D. P., and Wurtz, R. H. (1995). Saccade-related activity in monkey superior colliculus. I. Characteristics of burst and buildup cells. *J. Neurophysiol.* 73, 2313–2333.

Newsome, W. T., Britten, K. H., and Movshon, J. A. (1989). Neuronal correlates of a perceptual decision. *Nature* 341, 52–54. doi: 10.1038/341052a0

Nomoto, K., Schultz, W., Watanabe, T., and Sakagami, M. (2010). Temporally extended dopamine responses to perceptually demanding reward-predictive stimuli. *J. Neurosci.* 30, 10692–10702. doi: 10.1523/JNEUROSCI.4828-09.2010

O'Reilly, R. C., and Frank, M. J. (2006). Making working memory work: a computational model of learning in the prefrontal cortex and basal ganglia. *Neural Comput.* 18, 283–328. doi: 10.1162/089976606775093909

Palmer, J., Huk, A. C., and Shadlen, M. N. (2005). The effect of stimulus strength on the speed and accuracy of a perceptual decision. *J. Vis.* 5, 376–404. doi: 10.1167/5.5.1

Pawlak, V., and Kerr, J. N. D. (2008). Dopamine receptor activation is required for corticostriatal spike-timing-dependent plasticity. *J. Neurosci.* 28, 2435–2446. doi: 10.1523/JNEUROSCI.4402-07.2008

Rao, R. P. N. (2010). Decision making under uncertainty: a neural model based on partially observable Markov decision processes. *Front. Comput. Neurosci.* 4:146. doi: 10.3389/fncom.2010.00146

Ratcliff, R. (1978). A theory of memory retrieval. *Psychol. Rev.* 85, 59–108. doi: 10.1037/0033-295X.85.2.59

Rinberg, D., Koulakov, A., and Gelperin, A. (2006). Speed-accuracy tradeoff in olfaction. *Neuron* 51, 351–358. doi: 10.1016/j.neuron.2006.07.013

Roitman, J. D., and Shadlen, M. N. (2002). Response of neurons in the lateral intraparietal area during a combined visual discrimination reaction time task. *J. Neurosci.* 22, 9475 –9489.

Roxin, A., and Ledberg, A. (2008). Neurobiological models of two-choice decision making can be reduced to a one-dimensional nonlinear diffusion equation. *PLoS Comput. Biol.* 4:e1000046. doi: 10.1371/journal.pcbi.1000046

Schouten, J. F., and Bekker, J. A. M. (1967). Reaction time and accuracy. *Acta Psychol.* 27, 143–153. doi: 10.1016/0001-6918(67)90054-6

Schultz, W. (1999). The reward signal of midbrain dopamine neurons. *Physiology* 14, 249–255.

Schultz, W. (2000). Multiple reward signals in the brain. *Nat. Rev. Neurosci.* 1, 199–207. doi: 10.1038/35044563

Schultz, W. (2002). Getting formal with dopamine and reward. *Neuron* 36, 241–263. doi: 10.1016/S0896-6273(02)00967-4

Shadlen, M. N., and Newsome, W. T. (1996). Motion perception: seeing and deciding. *Proc. Natl. Acad. Sci. U.S.A.* 93, 628–633. doi: 10.1073/pnas.93.2.628

Shen, W., Flajolet, M., Greengard, P., and Surmeier, D. J. (2008). Dichotomous dopaminergic control of striatal synaptic plasticity. *Science* 321, 848–851. doi: 10.1126/science.1160575

Simen, P., Cohen, J. D., and Holmes, P. (2006). Rapid decision threshold modulation by reward rate in a neural network. *Neural Netw.* 19, 1013–1026. doi: 10.1016/j.neunet.2006.05.038

Sparks, D. L. (2002). The brainstem control of saccadic eye movements. *Nat. Rev. Neurosci.* 3, 952–964. doi: 10.1038/nrn986

Suaud-Chagny, M. F., Dugast, C., Chergui, K., and Msghina, M. (1995). Uptake of dopamine released by impulse flow in the rat mesolimbic and striatal systems *in vivo*. *J. Neurochem.* 65, 2603–2611. doi: 10.1046/j.1471-4159.1995.65062603.x

Takikawa, Y., Kawagoe, R., and Hikosaka, O. (2004). A possible role of midbrain dopamine neurons in short- and long-term adaptation of saccades to position-reward mapping. *J. Neurophysiol.* 92, 2520–2529. doi: 10.1152/jn.00238.2004

van Rossum, M. C. W., Bi, G. Q., and Turrigiano, G. G. (2000). Stable hebbian learning from spike timing-dependent plasticity. *J. Neurosci.* 20, 8812–8821.

Wang, C.-T., Lee, C.-T., Wang, X.-J., and Lo, C.-C. (2013). Top-down modulation on perceptual decision with balanced inhibition through feedforward and feedback inhibitory neurons. *PLoS ONE* 8:e62379. doi: 10.1371/journal.pone.0062379

Wang, X.-J. (2002). Probabilistic decision making by slow reverberation in cortical circuits. *Neuron* 36, 955–968. doi: 10.1016/S0896-6273(02)01092-9

Wang, X.-J. (2008). Decision making in recurrent neuronal circuits. *Neuron* 60, 215–234. doi: 10.1016/j.neuron.2008.09.034

Wickelgren, W. A. (1977). Speed-accuracy tradeoff and information processing dynamics. *Acta Psychol.* 41, 67–85. doi: 10.1016/0001-6918(77)90012-9

Wiecki, T. V., and Frank, M. J. (2013). A computational model of inhibitory control in frontal cortex and basal ganglia. *Psychol. Rev.* 120, 329–355. doi: 10.1037/a0031542

Wong, K.-F., Huk, A. C., Shadlen, M. N., and Wang, X.-J. (2007). Neural circuit dynamics underlying accumulation of time-varying evidence during perceptual decision making. *Front. Comput. Neurosci.* 1:6. doi: 10.3389/neuro.10.006.2007

Permissions

All chapters in this book were first published by Frontiers; hereby published with permission under the Creative Commons Attribution License or equivalent. Every chapter published in this book has been scrutinized by our experts. Their significance has been extensively debated. The topics covered herein carry significant findings which will fuel the growth of the discipline. They may even be implemented as practical applications or may be referred to as a beginning point for another development.

The contributors of this book come from diverse backgrounds, making this book a truly international effort. This book will bring forth new frontiers with its revolutionizing research information and detailed analysis of the nascent developments around the world.

We would like to thank all the contributing authors for lending their expertise to make the book truly unique. They have played a crucial role in the development of this book. Without their invaluable contributions this book wouldn't have been possible. They have made vital efforts to compile up to date information on the varied aspects of this subject to make this book a valuable addition to the collection of many professionals and students.

This book was conceptualized with the vision of imparting up-to-date information and advanced data in this field. To ensure the same, a matchless editorial board was set up. Every individual on the board went through rigorous rounds of assessment to prove their worth. After which they invested a large part of their time researching and compiling the most relevant data for our readers.

The editorial board has been involved in producing this book since its inception. They have spent rigorous hours researching and exploring the diverse topics which have resulted in the successful publishing of this book. They have passed on their knowledge of decades through this book. To expedite this challenging task, the publisher supported the team at every step. A small team of assistant editors was also appointed to further simplify the editing procedure and attain best results for the readers.

Apart from the editorial board, the designing team has also invested a significant amount of their time in understanding the subject and creating the most relevant covers. They scrutinized every image to scout for the most suitable representation of the subject and create an appropriate cover for the book.

The publishing team has been an ardent support to the editorial, designing and production team. Their endless efforts to recruit the best for this project, has resulted in the accomplishment of this book. They are a veteran in the field of academics and their pool of knowledge is as vast as their experience in printing. Their expertise and guidance has proved useful at every step. Their uncompromising quality standards have made this book an exceptional effort. Their encouragement from time to time has been an inspiration for everyone.

The publisher and the editorial board hope that this book will prove to be a valuable piece of knowledge for researchers, students, practitioners and scholars across the globe.

List of Contributors

Hagar Lavian and Alon Korngreen
The Leslie and Susan Gonda Interdisciplinary Brain Research Center, Bar-Ilan University, Ramat Gan, Israel
The Mina and Everard Goodman Faculty of Life Sciences, Bar-Ilan University, Ramat Gan, Israel

Hana Ben-Porat
The Leslie and Susan Gonda Interdisciplinary Brain Research Center, Bar-Ilan University, Ramat Gan, Israel

Shay Moshel
Department of Medical Neurobiology, IMRIC, The Hebrew University-Hadassah Medical School, Jerusalem, Israel
The Interdisciplinary Center for Neural Computation, The Hebrew University, Jerusalem, Israel
The Edmond and Lily Safra Center for Brain Sciences, The Hebrew University, Jerusalem, Israel
The Research Laboratory of Brain Imaging and Stimulation, The Jerusalem Mental Health Center, Kfar-Shaul Etanim, Hebrew University-Hadassah Medical School, Jerusalem, Israel

Reuben R. Shamir
Department of Medical Neurobiology, IMRIC, The Hebrew University-Hadassah Medical School, Jerusalem, Israel
The Edmond and Lily Safra Center for Brain Sciences, The Hebrew University, Jerusalem, Israel

Aeyal Raz
Department of Anesthesiology, University of Wisconsin School of Medicine and Public Health, Madison, WI, USA

Fernando R. de Noriega and Zvi Israel
Department of Neurosurgery, Center for Functional and Restorative Neurosurgery, Hadassah University Hospital, Jerusalem, Israel

Hagai Bergman
Department of Medical Neurobiology, IMRIC, The Hebrew University-Hadassah Medical School, Jerusalem, Israel
The Interdisciplinary Center for Neural Computation, The Hebrew University, Jerusalem, Israel
The Edmond and Lily Safra Center for Brain Sciences, The Hebrew University, Jerusalem, Israel

Renana Eitan
Department of Psychiatry, Hadassah University Hospital, Jerusalem, Israel

Sebastien Helie
Department of Psychological Sciences, Purdue University, West Lafayette, IN, USA

Srinivasa Chakravarthy
Department of Biotechnology, Indian Institute of Technology, Madras, India

Ahmed A. Moustafa
School of Social Sciences and Psychology, Marcs Institute for Brain and Behaviour, University of Western Sydney, Sydney, NSW, Australia

Liora Benhamou and Dana Cohen
The Leslie & Susan Goldschmied (Gonda) Multidisciplinary Brain Research Center, Bar-Ilan University, Ramat-Gan, Israel

Claire O'Callaghan
Neuroscience Research Australia, Sydney, NSW, Australia
Faculty of Medicine, School of Medical Sciences, University of New South Wales, Sydney, NSW, Australia

Sanne de Wit
Cognitive Science Center Amsterdam and Department of Clinical Psychology, University of Amsterdam, Amsterdam, Netherlands

James M. Shine and Simon J. G. Lewis
Parkinson's Disease Clinic, Brain and Mind Research Institute, University of Sydney, Sydney, NSW, Australia

Trevor W. Robbins
Department of Psychology, Behavioural and Clinical Neuroscience Institute, University of Cambridge, Cambridge, UK

Michael Hornberger
Neuroscience Research Australia, Sydney, NSW, Australia
Faculty of Medicine, School of Medical Sciences, University of New South Wales, Sydney, NSW, Australia
ARC Centre of Excellence in Cognition and its Disorders, Sydney, NSW, Australia
Department of Clinical Neurosciences, University of Cambridge, Cambridge, UK

Dorin Yael, Izhar Bar-Gad and Daniel Sand
The Leslie & Susan Goldschmied (Gonda) Multidisciplinary Brain Research Center, Bar-Ilan University, Ramat-Gan, Israel

Dagmar H. Zeef and Yasin Temel
Departments of Neuroscience and Neurosurgery, Maastricht University Medical Center, Maastricht, Netherlands

Anan Moran and Donald B. Katz
Department of Psychology, Volen National Center for Complex Systems, Brandeis University, Waltham, MA, USA

Yoshihisa Tachibana and Atsushi Nambu
Division of System Neurophysiology, National Institute for Physiological Sciences, Okazaki, Japan
Department of Physiological Sciences, Graduate University for Advanced Studies, Okazaki, Japan

Víctor Plata, Mariana Duhne, Jesús Pérez-Ortega, Ricardo Hernández-Martinez, Pavel Rueda-Orozco, Elvira Galarraga, René Drucker-Colín and José Bargas
Divisíón de Neurociencias, Instituto de Fisiología Celular, Universidad Nacional Autónoma de México, Mexico City, Mexico

Satomi Chiken
Division of System Neurophysiology, National Institute for Physiological Sciences, Okazaki, Japan
Department of Physiological Sciences, Graduate University for Advanced Studies, Okazaki, Japan

Samuel J. Gershman
Department of Brain and Cognitive Sciences, Massachusetts Institute of Technology, Cambridge, MA, USA

Elliot A. Ludvig
Princeton Neuroscience Institute and Department of Mechanical and Aerospace Engineering, Princeton University, Princeton, NJ, USA
Department of Psychology, University of Warwick, Coventry, UK

Ilana Molochnikov
The Leslie & Susan Goldschmied (Gonda) Multidisciplinary Brain Research Center, Bar-Ilan University, Ramat-Gan, Israel

Robert Merrison-Hort
Centre for Robotics and Neural Systems, School of Computing and Mathematics, The University of Plymouth, Plymouth, UK

Roman Borisyuk
Centre for Robotics and Neural Systems, School of Computing and Mathematics, The University of Plymouth, Plymouth, UK
Neural Networks Laboratory, Institute of Mathematical Problems in Biology, Russian Academy of Sciences, Pushchino, Russia

Benjamin Grieb
Department of Neurophysiology and Pathophysiology, University Medical Center Hamburg-Eppendorf, University of Hamburg, Hamburg, Germany
Department of General Psychiatry, Center for Psychosocial Medicine, University of Heidelberg, Heidelberg, Germany

Constantin von Nicolai
Department of Neurophysiology and Pathophysiology, University Medical Center Hamburg-Eppendorf, University of Hamburg, Hamburg, Germany
Centre for Integrative Neuroscience, University of Tübingen, Tübingen, Germany

Gerhard Engler, Andreas K. Engel and Christian K. Moll
Department of Neurophysiology and Pathophysiology, University Medical Center Hamburg-Eppendorf, University of Hamburg, Hamburg, Germany

Andrew Sharott
Department of Neurophysiology and Pathophysiology, University Medical Center Hamburg-Eppendorf, University of Hamburg, Hamburg, Germany
Medical Research Council, Anatomical Neuropharacology Unit, Department of Pharmacology, University of Oxford, Oxford, UK

Ismini Papageorgiou
Division of General Neurophysiology, Institute of Physiology and Pathophysiology, University of Heidelberg, Heidelberg, Germany

Wolfgang Hamel
Department of Neurosurgery, University Medical Center Hamburg-Eppendorf, University of Hamburg, Hamburg, Germany

Aude Retailleau
Sagol Department of Neurobiology, University of Haifa, Haifa, Israel

Thomas Boraud
Institut des Maladies Neurodegeneratives UMR 5293, University of Bordeaux, Bordeaux, France
Institut des Maladies Neurodegeneratives UMR 5293, CNRS, Bordeaux, France

Juan-Francisco Espinosa-Parrilla, Christelle Baunez and Paul Apicella
Institut de Neurosciences de la Timone, CNRS-Aix-Marseille Université, Marseille, France

Benjamin Pasquereau and Robert S. Turner
Department of Neurobiology, Center for Neuroscience and The Center for the Neural Basis of Cognition, University of Pittsburgh, Pittsburgh, PA, USA

Erick J. Paul
Beckman Institute for Advanced Science and Technology, University of Illinois at Urbana, Champaign, IL, USA

F. Gregory Ashby
Department of Psychological and Brain Sciences, University of California, Santa Barbara, Santa Barbara, CA, USA

J. Vincent Filoteo
Veterans Administration San Diego Healthcare System, San Diego, CA, USA
Department of Psychiatry, University of California, San Diego, CA, USA

W. Todd Maddox
Department of Psychology, University of Texas, Austin, TX, USA
Institute for Neuroscience, University of Texas, Austin, TX, USA

Pao-Yueh Hsiao
Institute of Systems Neuroscience, National Tsing Hua University, Hsinchu, Taiwan

Chung-Chuan Lo
Institute of Systems Neuroscience, National Tsing Hua University, Hsinchu, Taiwan
Department of Life Science, National Tsing Hua University, Hsinchu, Taiwan

Index

www.ingramcontent.com/pod-product-compliance
Lightning Source LLC
LaVergne TN
LVHW060546210926
848485LV00005B/1264